Uppity Women We Are!

100-YEAR HISTORY OF MEDICAL WOMEN
OF BRITISH COLUMBIA
(1893–1993)

To: Shauna Gold

from Eileen Nason Cambon, MD, CM

Eileen Cambon M.D.C.M.

For information contact:
Eileen Cambon
4346 Locarno Crescent
Vancouver, B.C. Canada
V6R 1G3
phone 604-224-3303

LIBRARY AND ARCHIVES CANADA CATALOGUING IN PUBLICATION

Cambon, Eileen Nason, 1926–

    Uppity women we are : 100-year history of medical women of British Columbia (1893–1993) / Eileen Nason Cambon.

ISBN 978-0-9694983-1-5

    1. Women physicians—British Columbia—History. 2. Women physicians—British Columbia—Biography. 3. Medicine—British Columbia—History. I. Title.

R464.A1C34 2008   610.82'09711   C2008-903414-7

Design and layout: Vancouver Desktop Publishing Centre Ltd.
Printed in Canada by Ray Hignell Services Inc.

This book is dedicated to all the women doctors of British Columbia,
past and present

and

to the loving memory of my husband, Dr. Kenneth Cambon,
who died on February 25, 2007 after six long years of illness.
He continually encouraged me in my career during the years
we practised together

and

to our daughters, Noreen and Marie,
who helped me to finally finish this book in 2008.

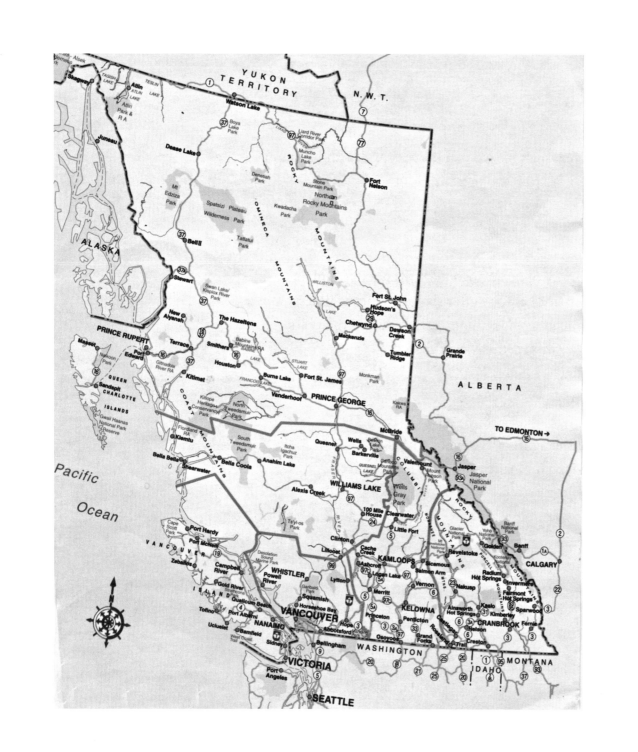

ACKNOWLEDGMENTS

First, I want to thank all the British Columbian women doctors who wrote their stories for this book. I had sent requests to over six hundred B.C. women doctors from 1999 to 2000, and over the years I received 160 stories from medical women who practised all over the province.

In 2000, I began research at the Library of the College of Physicians and Surgeons of British Columbia, which was then located at 8th Avenue and Hemlock. The Head Librarian, James Henderson, and his excellent staff are to be thanked for all their help in searching for every medical registry from the fragile 1880 papers to the 1990s, the early *Vancouver Medical Bulletins* from 1924 to 1958, and the *B.C. Medical Journals* from 1959. I had decided to have the book cover one hundred years from 1893 when the first woman doctor registered in B.C. to 1993, telling their own stories where possible.

The *VMA Bulletins* and *B.C. Medical Journals* provided stories of the doctors in the news, obituaries, and the occasional pictures. I thank both the *VMA* and *BCMA* for allowing me to include interesting facts and summaries for each decade.

I had great help from colleagues. Dr. Beverly Tamboline kindly edited the notes chosen from the early Bulletins and the Journals for each decade. I thank her for her help. I thank others who helped with stories and expertise: Richard Beck, Fred Bryans, Denys Ford, Joan Ford, Frances Forrest-Richards and husband Gerry Richards, Blair Fulton, Robert Hill, Patricia Rebbeck, Wally Thomas, and Adam Waldie (who died in 2001).

And special thanks to Dr. Stuart Kenny, archivist of the Victoria Medical Society, who helped with Dr. Eva Sutherland's story.

To Chunyee Li, who came to my rescue helping with computer work, preparing the disks for the editor and publisher, a special thanks.

Thanks to the editor, Linda Field, and page designer, Patty Osborne, who have been very patient through the several years it has taken me to finish the book.

Thanks to my late husband and our two daughters who all encouraged me to begin the project, and to the girls for assisting with editing and computer work over the years.

—*Eileen Cambon*

CONTENTS

INTRODUCTION

The definition for the word "uppity" in the Oxford dictionary is *self-assertive* and carries with it a long historical connotation of going against the grain of an established social order. Yes, uppity is what women had to be to think they could invade the domain of medical men. In English-speaking countries, the story of women attempting to break through the barrier of prejudice in medicine reflects all the determination and grit it takes for someone to go beyond their "station in life." In the late 1800s only a few women were accepted into medicine in Canada, and somewhat earlier in the United States. Still, Elizabeth Blackwell only succeeded in applying to Geneva Medical School in upstate New York by using her initials on her application. She turned up for classes, and graduated in 1849.

In an incident in America in the 17th century, a physician named Margaret Jones managed to set up in practice. She was so effective the Puritan fathers became suspicious. They sentenced her as a witch, and Margaret Jones was the first person to be executed in the New England colonies.

The prejudice against training women to become medical doctors was bitter, held not only by medical men of most countries, but by young male medical students. Hence, the shameful Surgeons' Hall riot of 1870 at the University of Edinburgh, and in our own Canadian Queen's University in 1880, when male students threatened to leave the university if the few women students remained. (Queen's University did not admit women again to study medicine until 1943.)

Dr. James Barry's story is fascinating as to what lengths a woman would go to practise her profession. Disguised as a man, she graduated from the University of Edinburgh in 1812, and entered the medical services of the British army as a male physician. After working in Jamaica, St. Helena, Trinidad, Malta, Corfu, and Crimea, Dr. Barry arrived in Canada in her sixties as a member of the Army Medical Department with the position of Inspector-General of Hospitals. Headquartered in Montreal, Dr. Barry made her rounds in the winter decked out in musk ox furs and travelling in a bright red sleigh.

This woman doctor, parading as a man, was the first female physician to practise medicine in Canada. (Her secret identity was not discovered until her illness and death in London, England.)

In Quebec, many of the French Canadian women who had the funds travelled to Paris or headed south for their medical training. Dr. Irma LeVasseur chose to attend Minnesota University College of Medicine in St. Paul, where many people of French descent had settled in the 1800s. Dr. LeVasseur graduated in 1900 and set up practice in New York, but later returned to Quebec where a bill was passed in the Quebec Legislative Assembly officially allowing her to practise in Montreal. She eventually took a course in pediatrics in Paris, France, returning to Montreal to establish a children's hospital, Hopital Ste-Justine.

Early on in the First World War, Dr. LeVasseur volunteered and embarked for Serbia, a country ravaged by a typhus epidemic. When the enemy advanced in 1915, she was part of the Serbian Great Retreat and returned to Quebec a First World War heroine. The experience of Dr. LeVasseur bolstered the reputation of all medical women active at the time, and the medical faculty of McGill University was so impressed by the record of Canadian medical women overseas in the First World War that from 1918 on, women were accepted into the Medical School.

Dr. James Barry's story is fascinating as to what lengths a woman would go to practise her profession. Disguised as a man, she graduated from the University of Edinburgh in 1812, and entered the medical services of the British army as a male physician.

Another early pioneer of medical women in Canada was Dr. Maude Abbott who became world-renowned for her work on congenital heart disease while curator of McGill's Medical Museum. An Arts graduate of McGill, she had hoped to enter medicine in 1889, but the faculty at McGill refused to admit women. The University of Bishop's Medical College in Montreal offered to take Maude Abbott as a medical student—their first woman student. She accepted, remained in Montreal, and had some of her disappointment assuaged by the fact that many of the courses were taught by McGill professors. Dr. Abbott was eventually hired by McGill University as Assistant Curator and worked closely with William Osler, who recognized her outstanding qualities. She became known internationally for her work on the clinical-pathological features of congenital heart disease and her career was another positive influence leading to the decision to have women admitted to McGill's Medical School.[1]

Although Queen's male students refused to allow women in the faculty, women students were taught by Queen's University professors in a separate building known as the Women's Medical College.

As the number of women medical graduates increased in Canada, the formation of the Federation of Medical Women of Canada (FMWC) came into being. The idea of a federation was first discussed in 1924 when the Canadian Medical Association had their annual meeting in Ottawa. Dr. Maude Abbott organized a group of founding members, which included herself, Dr. Janet Hall of Woodstock, Ontario, Dr. Jennie Smillie of Toronto, Dr. Elizabeth Bagshaw of Hamilton, Dr. Elizabeth Embury of Ottawa, Dr. Sarah McVean of Port Lambton, Ontario and Dr. Helen MacMurchy of Toronto. Dr. MacMurchy became the federation's first president.

The Medical Women's International Association (MWIA) was formed in 1920 and the FMWC joined as a member in 1924. At the 1947 conference of the MWIA in Amsterdam, the Medical Women of the Netherlands presented the FMWC with the Arnheim Medal, which subsequently became the presidential insignia of the federation. The medal was given in recognition of Canada's role in the liberation of Holland during the Second World War as well as a token of appreciation for the hospitality Canada gave to Queen Juliana and other members of Holland's Royal family during the war.

The FMWC continues to be active in the MWIA congresses, which are held every two to three years in various countries. Canadian members Dr. Beverley Tamboline was president of the MWIA from 1984 to 1987 and Dr. Shelley Ross was president from 2001 to 2004. In 1987, the MWIA met in Vancouver and was well-attended by women doctors from around the world. At the opening ceremony, B.C.'s own Dr. Mary Murphy piped the honoured guests to the stage.

The FMWC provides loans and academic awards to women medical students through the Maude Abbott Scholarship Loan Fund, established in 1939 to honour the memory of Dr. Maude Abbott. More recently, another prominent medical woman, Dr. Roberta Bondar, Canada's first woman astronaut, was made an honorary member of the FMWC when she attended the annual meeting in Calgary in 1993.

As the number of medical schools increased in Canada, so too did the opportunities for women to study medicine, albeit with limits. In eastern Canada during the 1880s and 1890s, the medical schools of Dalhousie, Bishop's, Queen's, University of Toronto, and Trinity each accepted small numbers of women every year. Although Queen's male students refused to allow women in the faculty, women students were taught by Queen's University professors in a separate building known as the Women's Medical College. The University of Toronto had the greatest number of women medical students in the early years. The Manitoba Medical College was established in 1893 and by 1928 there were sixteen female graduates in medicine. Manitoba's medical school was also the first institution in Canada to organize a special pre-medical studies program for Aboriginal students in 1979. By 1987, three of the graduates were women.

Elsewhere in the Prairies, Saskatchewan established a medical school in 1949, initially for the first two years of study with students transferring to other schools for the final two years. The University of Alberta Medical School graduated its first students in 1957, among them Dr. Leone McGregor. In 1978, she (as Dr. Leone McGregor Hellstedt) was instrumental in the publication of the book *Women Physicians of the World* for the MWIA.

---

1   Carlotta Hacker, the author of the *Indomitable Lady Doctors*, wrote an excellent history of pioneering women doctors in Canada as a project of the Federation of Medical Women of Canada to celebrate their Golden Jubilee in 1974.

British Columbia, with its rugged geography and isolation from the rest of Canada, took longer to establish its own medical school. Indeed, the area now known as British Columbia only came under formal British control in 1858 and expanded in population largely due to the discovery of gold. In 1871, the region became a province of Canada and construction for the western section of the Canadian Pacific Railway began in 1880. The first scheduled train from eastern Canada arrived in the new city of Vancouver on May 23rd, 1889.

By 1929, the Vancouver Medical Association, and later, the B.C. Medical Association, proposed the need for a medical school for British Columbia. But the discussion went nowhere and it was not until 1945, with returning veterans enlisting in pre-med programs, that the call for a provincial medical school was taken seriously. In 1950, fifty students were admitted, among them three women. In the following years, during the '50s and '60s, the presence of woman medical students in B.C. followed the general pattern of other medical schools in Canada, about ten percent of each class, reflecting an unwritten law among the medical establishment that limited the number of women allowed in. By the '70s and '80s the pattern began changing, and more women were admitted across Canada. By the 1990s women began outnumbering male students.

Even before B.C. had its own medical school, however, the province had its share of medical pioneers, and many of them included women. In 1893 when Dr. Mary McNeil registered with the B.C. College of Physicians and Surgeons, there was a total of 120 doctors practising in B.C. From 1916 to 1917, there were 643, with twelve women registered. Ten years later in 1927 there were 711 doctors and twenty-two of them were women. In 1940, forty-nine new registrants were women and by 1950 that number had more than doubled with 111 women registrants.

These included such women as Dr. Gladys Cunningham, who was a missionary obstetrician in China for many years before coming to Vancouver in 1952. Similarly, Dr. Mary Garner had a busy general practice in Vancouver with a special emphasis on obstetrics and covered extensively for her male colleagues' patients when many doctors joined up during the war years.

Dr. Isabel Day was another woman doctor in B.C. who was first a nurse with the Red Cross in the First World War and was decorated for gallantry. She also served in the Second World War as a commissioner in the St. John Ambulance Brigade. Dr. Josephine Mallek, a McGill graduate and endocrinologist, was the first woman doctor hired at St. Paul's hospital and a steadfast mentor for young women doctors throughout her career.

Dr. Ethlyn Trapp, born in New Westminster, was a pioneer in the treatment of cancer with radiation, the first woman to become president of the B.C. Medical Association from 1952 to 1953, and received the Order of Canada in 1968. Together with her colleagues, Dr. Olive Sadler (who trained in medicine after age of forty) and Dr. Margaret Hardie, Dr. Trapp was instrumental in researching treatment for breast cancer.

The first female neurologist in B.C., Dr. Ludmila Zeldowicz, arrived in Vancouver after the war from Poland, where she was a doctor in the Warsaw ghetto.

British Columbia also has its own famous military woman doctor, Dr. Wendy Clay, originally from northern B.C., who, after training as a flight surgeon (a doctor specializing in medical problems specific to fliers) became a Brigadier General in 1989 and commandant of the National Defense Medical Centre in Ottawa. In 1994, she was promoted to Major-General and Surgeon-General and became the only female General Officer in the forces at that time.

In the 1950s, following the upheaval of the Second World War, a large influx of doctors came into B.C. (and likewise the rest of Canada) from the British Isles and Europe, as well as other countries. Women doctors of all ages arrived with fascinating stories, like Dr. Laine Loo, a general practitioner from Estonia, who escaped to Sweden during the war, came to Vancouver, and had a busy practice for years. Dr. Julia van Norden, who arrived in Vancouver in 1951, was active in the underground resistance against the Nazis in Holland during the Second World War and went on to study medicine after the war ended. The first female neurologist in B.C., Dr. Ludmila Zeldowicz, arrived in Vancouver after the war from Poland, where she was a doctor in the Warsaw ghetto. Dr. Agnes Weston joined the British Army and later came to Vancouver and established the first public health geriatric clinic here. Other women doctors came to B.C. from China, South Africa, the Philippines, and Hungary.

By the late 1950s more women graduates began entering specialties, which became the pattern from the '60s onward. Women doctors are now represented in every specialty and also teach in medical faculties across the country. Most young women can follow their dream of studying medicine without facing the old prejudices of the past. Yet challenges still remain for immigrants, for First Nations People, and for others underrepresented in B.C.'s and indeed, Canada's medical establishment. It is my hope, in compiling this book, that the stories of these women doctors will be an inspiration to all, women and men, struggling to step beyond social boundaries to break new ground.

—*Eileen Cambon, MD, March 9, 2008*

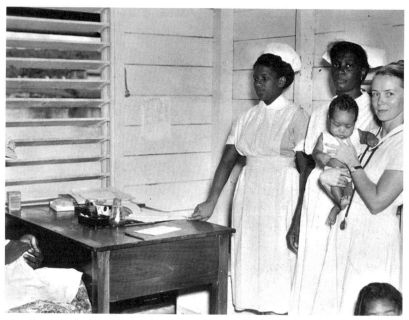

Dr. Eileen Cambon (1958) at the baby clinic, Mackenzie, British Guiana

Story from 1890 – 1899

Dr. Margaret McMillan (Mrs. Forster)

Year Registered & Name	Qualifications
1893: Dr. Mary McNeil, Victoria, B.C.	MD, Women's Hospital Medical College, Chicago, 1891
1896 Dr. Margaret McMillan (Mrs. Forster), Victoria, B.C. (later New Westminster) (see biographical note)	Trinity University, Toronto, 1895
1897 Dr. Isabel Arthur, Nelson, B.C.	MD, State University of Oregon, 1892
1897 Dr. Annie Verth Jones, Rossland, B.C.	MD, CM, Trinity University, Toronto, 1896; graduate of Woman's Medical College, Ontario, 1896; MCP&S, Manitoba, 1896

Dr. Annie Verth Jones practised in Rossland and Nelson, B.C. for 10 years. When her health failed, she returned to Ontario.

1898 Dr. Vera McPhee (Mrs. Green), Vancouver, B.C.	MD, CM, Manitoba, 1898; MC, PS, Manitoba, 1890; BA, Manitoba, 1886

In 1909, Dr. McPhee worked in Port Essington.

1899 Dr. Annie Chambers (Mrs. H. McKenzie Cleland), Victoria, B.C	MD, CM, Trinity University, Toronto, 1892; MCP&S, Ontario, 1892; Ontario Medical College for Women, 1892; LRCP &S, Edinburgh, Scotland, 1898; LFP&S, Glasgow, 1898

Dr. Chambers was a Christian Scientist; one of her duties was to sign all death certificates in Victoria, B.C.

c. 1899 Dr. Nancy Rodger Chenorweth, Michel, B.C. (left B.C. in 1911 for Chicago)	MD, CM, Trinity University, Toronto, 1894

DR. MARGARET McMILLAN (MRS. FORSTER)

Margaret McMillan graduated from Trinity, Toronto, in 1895. She was one of the earliest medical women in the west and practised in Victoria between 1896 and 1900. In 1900 she moved to New Westminster and then, in 1902, settled in Alberta. Of her three children, the two girls both entered medical fields; the elder (Dr. Sylling) studied medicine and the younger became a nurse.

Stories from 1900 – 1909

1906
Dr. Ruth Maude (McManus) Hall
1907
Dr. Helen Elizabeth Reynolds (Mrs. Thomas Ryan)
1908
Dr. Henrietta (Etta) Patterson Denovan
Dr. Katherine Joanne Mackay

REGISTRATIONS 1900 – 1909

Year Registered & Name	Qualifications
1903 Dr. Belle Holland Wilson, Port Essington, B.C.	MD, Keokuk College of Iowa, 1897; MD, Williamette, Salem, Oregon, 1903
1904 Dr. E.L. Anderson (Mrs. A.A. Wilson), Ladner, B.C. (later practised in Vancouver)	MB, Toronto University, Graduated in Women's Medical College, 1902; MCP&S, Ontario, 1903
1906 Dr. Georgina Urquhart, Vancouver, B.C.	MD, Toronto, 1905
c. 1906 Dr. Ruth McManus Hall, Vancouver, B.C. (see biographical notes)	Diploma in Nursing, Dr. Roger's Sanatorium of Chicago, Illinois, 1898; MD, National Medical University, Chicago, 1901; Bachelor of Clinical Surgery, National Medical University, Chicago, 1902; LMCC, 1902
c. 1907 Dr. Helen Elizabeth Reynolds Ryan, Victoria, B.C. (see biographical notes)	MD, CM, Queen's University, Kingston, 1885
1908 Dr. H.P. Denovan, Victoria, B.C. (see biographical notes)	MD, CM, Victoria College; MCP&S, N.W.T., 1892
c. 1908 Dr. Katherine Joanne MacKay, Port Coquitlam, B.C. (see biographical notes)	MD, CM, Dalhousie Medical College; A Pictou Academy graduate, 1895

1906

DR. RUTH MAUDE (McMANUS) HALL
(1867–1947)

Ruth Maude McManus was born in Iowa in 1867 and graduated from high school in 1886. In 1898, she was awarded a Diploma in Nursing by the Dr. Roger's sanatorium of Chicago, Illinois, and in 1900 spent some time in England at Queen Charlotte's Lying-In Hospital (founded in 1752), whose Patron was Her Majesty The Queen. In 1901, she received the Degree of Medicine from the National Medical University, Chicago, and in 1902 the same University conferred the Degree of Bachelor of Clinical Surgery. The Surgery Diploma was signed by the Professor of Clinical Surgery and Gynecology, the Professor of Orthopedic Surgery, and the Professor of Operational Surgery. In January 1902, Dr. McManus was licensed to practise in the State of Colorado, and in May 1902, at the age of thirty-three, she received her license to practise in the State of Illinois.

In September 1902, Dr. McManus married Thomas Proctor Hall (PhD & MD of Chicago, Illinois), a widower with three children. They came to Vancouver, British Columbia, shortly after their marriage. Dr. Thomas Hall registered in 1905 with the B.C. College of Physicians and Surgeons. Following the death of Dr. Ruth Hall's sister-in-law in Iowa in 1908, Ruth visited her brother and three nieces and was appalled at the physical condition of the three little girls. She promptly took matters into her own hands, and brought the girls to Vancouver.

The Halls resided at 1301 Davie Street, at the corner of Davie and Jervis Streets in Vancouver. They practised from their home and also operated a small private hospital. In time the five girls assisted when required, cleaning up after surgeries and helping nurse and care for patients (although none were nurses nor did they take up nursing as a career). Dr. Ruth Hall was very active in their practice, especially at a time when there were very few medical women (less than a dozen in Vancouver before the 1930s).

Dr. Ruth Hall died in Vancouver on September 8, 1942.

The information about Dr. Ruth McManus Hall and the dates of her training in the United States were provided by Joan Taylor Stace-Smith of Vancouver. Joan's mother was the niece of Dr. Hall, one of the three girls brought from Iowa in 1908 who lived with their aunt Ruth Hall and her husband until 1924. Joan also showed us the very ornate Diplomas and Certificates that had been awarded to Dr. Ruth Hall.

1907

DR. HELEN ELIZABETH REYNOLDS
(MRS. THOMAS RYAN)

Helen Elizabeth Reynolds graduated from Queen's with the degree of MD, CM in 1885. She made a success of her life in three different fields as a medical doctor, a suffragette, and a wife and mother. She was the first woman to be granted membership in the Canadian Medical Association, and she carried on a practice until 1907. Dr. Reynolds first worked with her brother in Mount Forest and then, after her marriage, ran an extensive practice in Sudbury, Ontario. She married Thomas Ryan and had five children. She and her family moved to Victoria, B.C. in 1907. In Victoria, she joined the local Council of Women and became very active in the franchise movement, travelling around British Columbia lecturing and drumming up support. Dr. Reynolds died in Victoria in 1947 at the age of eighty-seven.

1908

DR. HENRIETTA (ETTA) PATTERSON
DENOVAN

Henrietta Denovan graduated in 1892 with MD, CM from Victoria College which was later associated with the University of Toronto. She was one of the pioneer doctors in western Canada. She registered in the Northwest Territories in 1892 after she had sat a local exam as was normal policy, the exam being held in Calgary when Alberta was part of the Northwest Territories. She and her husband Rev. Dr. H. J. Denovan practised in various communities in Alberta, including Calgary, and in Red Deer from 1895 to 1903.

Dr. Denovan specialized in treating women and children patients in her general practice. She registered in British Columbia in 1908, practising in Vancouver until 1910, before moving to Victoria where she practised from 1910 to 1922.

Etta was a strong supporter of the extension of educational opportunities to all classes and to both sexes. Though firmly on the side of radical reform, she was much respected. She was a founding member of the University of British Columbia and became one of the pioneers of the early women's movement when she helped establish the Council of Women. She had a wide circle of friends, including such leaders as Sir Richard McBride, Dr. Henry Ession Young (both founding members of the University of British Columbia), and Mr. Carter Cotton, the first Chancellor of the University of British Columbia. She was honoured as a doctor, pioneer, feminist, and innovator.

Dr. Denovan's name is among the pioneer physicians of British Columbia on a plaque over the fireplace in the Memorial Room of the Woodward Library, the only woman listed.

Information about Dr. Henrietta Denovan was found with the help of Lee Perry, Librarian at the Woodward Library, UBC; and from the book *The Indomitable Lady Doctors* by Carlotta Hacker.

DR. KATHERINE JOANNE MACKAY
(D. 1925)

Katherine Joanne Mackay was the second woman to be granted an MD, CM from Dalhousie Medical College, and she was also a Pictou Academy graduate. Kate was one of ten children of whom one sister was a nurse, one brother was a doctor, and another an educator. Both brothers were anxious

for Kate to study medicine and offered to try to get her into McGill University, where no woman had ever been admitted to medical school.

Meanwhile, Kate went to Boston and graduated from the School of Nursing established by an associate of Dr. Elizabeth Blackwell.

Kate's certificate was signed by seven women doctors. Inspired again, Kate came back home and attended Dalhousie and obtained her MD, CM in 1895.

For a while, she practised medicine in New Glasgow with her physician brother, then she went to work in a government post in Honolulu, Hawaii, when the voyage was long and perilous around Cape Horn.

She sailed back to Canada and went home to Plainfield, Pictou County. In 1902, she married a former neighbour, John R. MacKenzie. Shortly thereafter, they moved to Edmonton where Kate practised medicine for a few years before they moved to B.C., finally settling in Port Coquitlam where her husband became the mayor, and she continued in general practice until she retired in 1918. She died in 1925 of septicemia. She was known as "one of the most highly respected public citizens in Port Coquitlam."

(Copied from the book Petticoat Doctors *by Enid Johnson MacLeod, with permission from the publisher, Pottersfield Press.)*

Stories from 1910 – 1919

1916
Dr. Eva Sutherland

1917
Dr. Margaret Gardner (Mrs. Hogg)

Year Registered & Name	Qualifications
1910 Dr. Mary B. Campbell	MD, Toronto, 1906; MCP&S, Toronto, 1908
1910 Dr. Maud McNaughton, Kelowna, B.C.	MB Ch, Glasgow University, 1899; MD, Glasgow, 1908
1910 Dr. M.L.M. Robertson (Mrs. T.F. Saunders), Baynes Lake, B.C.	MB, BS, Durham University, England, 1902
1912 Dr. Ella Scarlette-Synge, Vancouver, B.C.	LSA, London, 1901; DPH, Dublin, 1904; MD, Brussels, 1904

She saw active WWI war service; in 1915, she was Commander of the Vancouver Women's Volunteer Reserve at Batochina, Serbia.

1914 Dr. Gertrude Flumberfelt (Mrs. Jefferson), Victoria, B.C.	MRCP, London, 1912; MRCS, England, 1912
1916 Dr. E.M. Sutherland (Mrs. Alexander Sutherland), Ganges, B.C. (see biographical note)	MB, ChB, Edinburgh, 1903; MD, Edinburgh, 1908

She went to Bella Coola as a pioneer doctor, and died in 1944 (see story).

1917 Dr. Margaret Gardner Forrest (Mrs. M.Y. Hogg), Vancouver, B.C. (see biographical notes)	BM & S, Glasgow, 1904

She practised in Vancouver for many years and for a time worked for the city schools; in 1930, she died as a result of a motor accident.

In 1918, the LMCC (Licensure of the Medical Council of Canada) is required in B.C.

There were 758 doctors registered in B.C. in 1918, and 773 doctors in 1919.

DR. EVA SUTHERLAND
(1873–1964)

Dr. Eva Maud Sutherland was born in 1873 in Northumberland, England, the second of three daughters of William Snowball and Emma Davidson Snowball. She received her medical education at the Medical College for Women in Edinburgh. She was a brilliant student, having received the medals for Physics in 1898, Medical Jurisprudence in 1901, and Ophthalmology in 1902.

After graduation she and her first husband, T. Frances Cavanaugh, set up a joint practice in Liverpool. Shortly thereafter, he disappeared. Later, Eva, distraught and lonely, was told she had a brain tumour, and she decided to find her husband before she died. A private detective located her husband in Bella Coola, British Columbia, Canada. (In a recent book, *Healing in the Wilderness: A History of the United Church Mission Hospitals* by Bob Burrows, T. Francis Cavanaugh is mentioned as the second resident physician at Bella Coola.) Eva went to Bella Coola and nursed the ailing Frances until he died in November 1913, aged thirty-seven years. She stayed on in Bella Coola and was appointed physician in charge of the town hospital, registering with the College of Physicians and Surgeons in May 1916. She obviously was well enough to practise.

Dr. Sutherland met her second husband, Billie Sutherland, an Englishman, in Bella Coola. He enlisted in the navy in 1917 and was sent on the Atlantic Patrol, but was discharged two months later with tuberculosis.

It was about this time that Bella Coola was almost wiped out by a flood.

The Gulf Islands were urgently searching for a doctor for the Lady Minto Gulf Islands Hospital which had opened in 1914. A stipend of about $500 a year went with the position. The cottage hospital had been without a full-time physician since the fall of 1914, as both the doctor, Allan Beech, and the Matron (the only nurse), Miss Calhoun had gone on Active Service. Until Dr. Sutherland opened her practice in early 1918, the Gulf Islands had been serviced by Dr. Lionel Beech, the retired father of Dr. Allan Beech, and Dr. Fraser who came to Ganges a day or two a week from his home on Mayne Island. When Dr. Fraser was on Saltspring Island, he stayed at the boarding house of Mrs. Jane Mouat located near Ganges dock. He was known to always wear a kilt and dance the Highland Fling for guests.

When Dr. Sutherland arrived, she was expected to make routine trips to the Outer Islands. Her husband, Billie Sutherland, purchased a launch, reputed to be the largest in these waters, and he was able to transport her as needed.

Dr. Sutherland instituted a plan for training nurses at the Lady Minto Gulf Islands Hospital. Her plan was not considered a success by the hospital board, and was not repeated. A second physician arrived on Saltspring in the spring of 1923. The relationship between the two doctors was notably strained. Often the hospital was desperately short of funds, almost to the point of closure. During Dr. Sutherland's tenure of twelve years, the hospital had eleven matrons, few of whom met her standards.

Dr. Sutherland resigned as Health Officer in 1925, although she continued her private practice. Her increasing deafness and her husband's ill-health (Billie died in 1926) must have been difficult for her. Dr. Sutherland sold her practice, her house, and her 1928 Chevrolet to Dr. Raymond Rush for $4,000 in 1930. She went on an extended trip to England, and returned to Ganges where she rented a cottage. In 1932, she moved to Raeburn House on Rockland Avenue in Victoria. She died in 1964, aged ninety-one.

A private detective located her husband in Bella Coola, British Columbia, Canada. Eva went to Bella Coola and nursed the ailing Frances until he died in November 1913, aged thirty-seven years.

(Information regarding Dr. Sutherland came from Dr. Stuart Kenning, Chair of Victoria Medical Society. The story of Dr. Sutherland was written by Mrs. Susan Mouat for the Victoria Medical Society. Mrs. Mouat of Saltspring Island has given permission to use her information regarding Dr. Eva Sutherland.)

DR. MARGARET GARDNER (MRS. HOGG)

Margaret Gardner graduated from Glasgow University Medical School in 1904. She practised in Vancouver for many years and, for a time, worked for the city schools. Her death in 1930 was the result of a motor vehicle accident.

Stories from **1920 – 1929**

1920
Dr. Lillian Fowler
1925
Dr. Irene Mary Clearihue
1926
Dr. Isabel Day
Dr. Florence Evangeline Perry
1928
Dr. Ethlyn Trapp
1929
Dr. Irmla Kennedy-Jackson

Year Registered & Name	Qualifications
1921 Dr. Lillian Fowler, New Westminster, B.C. (see biographical notes)	MD, Rush Medical College, 1913; LMCC, 1921
1922 Dr. Margaret E.E. Bryant, Saltspring Island, B.C.	MB, BS, London, 1913; DTM & H Centab., 1915; LMCC, 1921
1922 Dr. Irene Baston Hudson, Luxton Po, Victoria	LRCP, London, 1914; MRCS, England; MB, BS, London, 1918; LMCC, 1922
1923 Dr. Dorothy Miller, Vancouver, B.C.	MB, ChBB, Glasgow, 1916; LMCC, 1923
1923 Dr. Dorothy M. Trapp, New Westminster, B.C.	MB, Toronto, 1922; LMCC, 1922
1925 Dr. Irene M. Clearihue, Victoria, B.C. (see biographical notes)	MRCS, London, 1922; LRCF, England, 1922; LMCC, 1925
1926 Dr. Isabel T. Day, Vancouver, B.C. (see biographical notes)	BA, Toronto, 1912; MB, Toronto, 1926; LMCC, 1926
1926 Dr. Emmal MacCrostie, Vancouver, B.C.	DO, Chicago College of Osteopathy, Illinois State, 1914; MDCM, McGill University, 1905

She died in the early 1960s.

Year Registered & Name	Qualifications
1926 Dr. Florence Perry, Vancouver, B.C. (see biographical notes)	MB, Toronto, 1925; LMCC, 1926

Year Registered & Name	Qualifications
1926 Dr. Tina Gardiner Head-Patrick, Vancouver, B.C.	MD, CM, Trinity Medical College, 1896; CP&S, N.W.T., 1903; CP&S, Alberta, 1906; LMCC, 1926

Dr. Head-Patrick died in 1932.

Year Registered & Name	Qualifications
1928 Dr. Ethlyn Trapp, New Westminster, B.C. (see biographical notes)	MD, CM, McGill University, 1927; LMCC, 1927
1928 Dr. Anna Henry, Vancouver, B.C.	MD, CM, Trinity, Toronto, 1898

After serving 30 years of missionary work in China and Japan, mostly in Chengtu in West China, Dr. Henry came to Vancouver where she worked among the Chinese and Japanese in Vancouver.

Year Registered & Name	Qualifications
c. **1929** Dr. Irmla Kennedy-Jackson, Vancouver, B.C. (see biographical notes)	MD, Toronto, 1919; LMCC, 1919; CP&S, Ontario, 1919

There were 651 doctors registered in British Columbia in 1922, 690 in 1926, and 711 in 1927. (See "Notes from *VMA Bulletins* 1924–1929" page 30)

1920

DR. LILLIAN FOWLER
(1881–?)

Dr. Lillian Fowler was born July 2, 1881 at Grenada, Kansas. She was the third of four children; the children in those days had to walk two miles to school. She graduated from Hiawatha Academy in 1899. For five years she taught sciences in high school. She received a BSc degree from Ottawa University, Ottawa, Kansas in 1904 and an MS degree from the University of Kansas in 1911, followed by an MD degree from Rush College which was associated with University of Chicago. The family moved to Oregon where she did general practice in Portland and gave anesthetics in the hospital of the Coffey Clinic. Dr. Fowler's brother became a widower and was left with two small children, so in October, 1919, Dr. Fowler moved to New Westminster, B.C. to help her brother raise the children

In late 1920 she was interviewed at the Vancouver General Hospital for a job in anesthesia. The doctor at VGH who interviewed her told her frankly that he did not approve of women in the medical profession and there was no place for her on staff. However, within a week Dr. Peter McLellan heard what had happened and asked her to come for another interview. She was accepted on the VGH staff and became the first female anesthetist there, beginning work on November 1, 1920. She received Certification in Anesthesia and worked with Dr. J.R. Neilson at the Haro Street Infants' Hospital as well as VGH until 1945, when she had problems with her health and resigned, after which she was made Honorary Member of the Consulting Staff. Dr. Fowler did some work with the Vancouver Medical Dental Hospital on Georgia Street and gave anesthesia for Dr. Ethlyn Trapp's radiotherapy patients. She received a Life Membership of the College of Physicians and Surgeons of British Columbia.

Dr. Fowler adopted a boy from the Children's Home and raised him along with her brother's children. She was a member of the University Women's Club of British Columbia and was active in the Soroptimist Club, which is the local unit of an International Service Club of Women whose objective is to provide homes for senior citizens of low income. She was a member of Ryerson United Church.

1925

DR. IRENE MARY CLEARIHUE
(1896 – 1978)

Curriculum Vitae

Born: June 17, 1896 in Rickmansworth, England; daughter of Minnie and George Henry Golding.

Education: attended Boarding School at St. Helens and St. Catherine; Finished school "Villa Erica," Lausanne, Switzerland, 1912–1913; A VAD, Red Cross nurse at Kempston, Eastbourne, 1914–1915. Admitted into London School of Medicine and the London Hospital when it first admitted women students; graduated as a physician followed by two years of General Practice with Dr. Basden, in Brook, Norfolk, 1919–1922; MRCP, LRCF, London, England, 1922.

Personal: July 30, 1924, married Joseph Badenoch Clearihue in London, England; daughter, Joyce Clearihue, born in 1927.

Certification: July 22, 1925 Member of the College of Physicians and Surgeons of British Columbia, and LMCC by examination.

Experience: Post-graduate training and worked in Anaesthesiology during and after World War II in Montreal, Chicago, and Victoria, B.C., at the Royal Jubilee Hospital, 1941–1953; a long-time member of the University Women's Club.

Died: June 7, 1978 in Victoria, B.C., aged eighty-one.

(Dr. Joyce Clearihue wrote the Curriculum Vitae of her mother, Dr. Irene Clearihue.)

1926

DR. ISABEL DAY
(c. 1892–1953)

Dr. Isabel Day was a brilliant student at college and a medalist in her final year at the University of Toronto. She graduated with a BA in 1912 and served with the British Army in France during the First World War as a VAD. She later went to medical school, earning an MB from the University of Toronto in 1926, and passed the LMCC exams in 1926. Dr. Day registered in British Columbia in 1926 and practised in Vancouver for many years. She had a large practice of people who thought highly of her, and as a public-spirited woman, consistently did her duty as she saw it in every department of life. In 1934 she was presented with a Jubilee Medal from His Majesty, George VI.

Dr. Day was on the staff of Grace Hospital and was associated with Children's Aid, the Greater Vancouver Health League, and the St. John Ambulance Society, of which she was Assistant Provincial Surgeon. She was an advisor for years with the Victorian Order of Nurses, elected President of the Federation of Medical Women of Canada in 1930 at the Annual Meeting in Winnipeg, and was liked and respected by all who knew her as well as being held in the highest esteem by her medical colleagues. In the Second World War she served as a Commissioner in the St. John Ambulance Brigade.

Dr. Day died in August, 1953.

DR. FLORENCE EVANGELINE PERRY
(1892–1966)

Dr. Florence Perry was born in Nova Scotia in 1892 but spent most of her life in British Columbia. She taught school for some years in B.C. and then went to the University of Toronto, where she graduated in Medicine in 1925. Coming back to Vancouver, she interned at the Vancouver General Hospital, one of the first medical women to do so in this hospital. She then went into private practice with Dr. Isabel Day, who was already a well-known family practioner in Vancouver. A competent and dedicated doctor, Dr. Perry was greatly interested in the Salvation Army Home, which later became Grace Hospital. She also worked with the St. John Ambulance Society and was a member of the Soroptomist Club.

Dr. Perry suffered for twenty years from rheumatoid arthritis. As one can imagine, her work as a doctor was doubly hard for this reason, but she faced the problem gallantly and and without complaint, working until 1962. She was greatly loved by her patients, to whom she gave great devotion and personal care. She was respected both as a hard-working doctor and as a person.

Dr. Perry died in April, 1966, at age 74.

1928

DR. ETHLYN TRAPP
(1891-1972)

The most famous woman doctor in British Columbia in the past hundred years was Dr. Ethlyn Trapp. Innovative and with the persistence to do what she believed in in her chosen field of radiotherapy for cancer treatment, she was highly respected in Canada and internationally.

Ethlyn Trapp was born in 1891, the daughter of Thomas John Trapp and Nellie Dockrill Trapp of New Westminster, a pioneer family whose foundations were built on service to the community. Monuments testify to her parents' generosity in the fields of education and recreation.

As a child of three years, before the days of X-rays, she had seriously damaged her hip in a sleighing accident on the hills of New Westminster. In spite of life-long lameness, she determinedly matched the activities of her four brothers and two sisters, and participated in the extracurricular life of skating and dancing at university. The only time she referred in public to her lameness was on the occasion of her delivery of the Osler Lecture in 1952. When the applause died down and the congratulations were flowing in, she said, "I am not sure of my lecturing ability, but I venture to say that I am the only Osler lecturer who has delivered the entire address standing on one foot." Dr. Trapp was the first woman doctor chosen by the Vancouver Medical Association to give the Osler Lecture since the annual memorial to Sir William Osler was established in 1921.

Ethlyn Trapp graduated from McGill University in 1913 with a B.A. During the war of 1914–1918, she did Occupational Therapy in Military Hospitals. She returned to McGill to study medicine and graduated in 1927 at the age of thirty-six years. She did post-graduate studies in Vienna and Berlin, then began the practice of pediatrics in New Westminster, B.C.

Early in her career, Dr. Trapp was convinced that one of the great deficiencies in medicine in B.C. was the treatment of cancer beyond surgery, namely X-ray and Radium Therapy. These treatments had been successfully applied for nearly two decades in European centres. She returned to Europe and spent three years at the Curie Institute in Paris, the Radium Hemmet in Stockholm, and the Holt Institute in Manchester. When she returned to Vancouver, as one of the first B.C. doctors to specialize in radiotherapy, she was well-equipped to bring these newer forms of cancer treatment into practice.

She would probably have preferred to have worked in the wider scope of an institution, but as with all pioneers of new concepts, she met with violent opposition from the existing medical establishment who regarded radium and X-ray therapy as dangerous and untried forms of treatment. In order to be able to treat her patients without the limits imposed by the existing bureaucracy, she used her private fortune to establish a modern and very well-equipped centre. In a short time she was able to demonstrate the great benefits of these new therapies. In her later years even her most severe critics sought her guidance in planning treatments.

During the struggle of these rather difficult years she bore no malice, but some of her close associates carried scars on her behalf, all of which were healed by the words of the late Dr. G.F. Strong, then President of the B.C. Cancer Foundation. In his address which marked the opening of the present Cancer Institute, he said: "This Institute is the fulfilment of a dream transposed into reality by many competent and willing people. All dreams start as a vision in one's mind and it takes energy, hard work, and great determination to keep this vision alive. Everyone here knows that this one person is Dr. Ethlyn Trapp."

Dr. Trapp had opened her new clinic in 1937. When the Second World War began in 1939, the director of the newly organized Cancer Institute, Dr. Max Evans, enlisted Dr. Trapp to take over his duties there in the mornings, and she worked in her private clinic in the afternoons as the only fully-trained radiotherapist in Vancouver. Her duties as Acting Director of the B.C. Cancer Institute ended with the war's end in 1945.

In 1945, in association with Dr. Olive Sadler, who later became her partner in her private clinic, along with Dr. Margaret Hardie, she began the first clinical research program on cancer of the breast to follow groups of women age eighteen to forty-five and to study various factors in their lives. The project was supported by the B.C. and Yukon Division of the Canadian Cancer Society. The Women's College Hospital in Toronto joined the project in 1946.

As with all pioneers of new concepts, she met with violent opposition from the existing medical establishment who regarded radium and X-ray therapy as dangerous and untried forms of treatment.

Dr. Trapp was National President of the Federation of Medical Women in 1945 and '46. The next year she became President of the British Columbia Medical Association, the first woman president of any of the provincial branches of the Canadian Medical Association. She was later a Senior Member of the C.M.A., and in 1952 became the sixth president and first woman President of the National Cancer Institute of Canada. As well, she was Director and Chairman of the Welfare Committee of the Canadian Cancer Society, B.C. Division, and a member of the Board of Directors of the B.C. Cancer Foundation. The Vancouver Medical Association awarded Dr. Trapp the honour of Prince of Good Fellows.

Among Dr. Trapp's many distinctions were Honorary Fellow of the Faculty of Radiologists of Great Britain and Honorary Degree of Doctor of Science of the University of British Columbia, conferred at the graduation ceremonies of the first graduating class of the Medical School on May 17,

1954. For service to her country, she received the Order of Canada medal from the Governor-General in 1968. The latter honour, conferred on her at the age of seventy-six, brought forth a typical comment: "There are lots of people who deserve a medal more than me."

Dr. Trapp, as President of the B.C. Medical Association, travelled and lectured all over British Columbia. A prominent radiotherapist and cancer specialist, she was invited to speak at medical meetings in many countries as well as lecturing to the local medical groups in Vancouver. Her official positions in the Canadian Medical Association enabled her to take part in policy-making for the national field of medicine, and her greatest sphere of influence was in the field of cancer treatment. She held official positions in the governing bodies of the treatment of cancer were held for her entire practising life.

When Dr. Trapp retired from active practice, she maintained an untiring interest in medicine as a whole, but now she was able to devote some of her time to other interests. She returned to university to take lectures in horticulture, anthropology, and sociology. "After all," she said, "you can get narrow-minded in the medical profession." She numbered among her friends Lawren Harris and Emily Carr; with Emily Carr's permission she had named her home in West Vancouver "Klee Wyck." She continued her interest in the United Nations Organization, in art, music, and literature.

Dr. Trapp travelled to the home of anthropology in South Africa. Her last trip with her friend since their McGill days, Ada McGeer, when both were touching eighty, was to the Galapagos Islands. A few months before her death she was taking Spanish lessons, hoping to explore the anthropological lore of Mexico.

Following in the family tradition and rounding out the circle of her life, Dr. Trapp left her valuable paintings to art galleries and her beautiful seven-acre gardens on the west bank of the Capilano River to her community of West Vancouver to be used as a park.

Dr. Ethlyn Trapp died in August, 1972 at age eighty-one years. Her friend, Ada McGeer, wrote: "On that last occasion when relatives and friends gathered to say their last goodbye to Ethlyn, my thoughts drifted back sixty years, to the time we shared as undergraduates at McGill University. In common with her fellow students, I was inevitably drawn to this gentle, quiet, yet magnetic person, who possessed such strength of purpose."

The British Columbia Branch of the Federation of Medical Women of Canada remembers her in the Ethlyn Trapp Scholarship Fund administered by the University of British Columbia. Two scholarships, the gift of the B.C. Branch FMWC, are offered annually in the Faculty of Medicine to women students entering the second, third, or fourth year of the program. They are awarded to students who have high standing and show promise of success in the medical profession. The winners are selected by the Faculty of Medicine in consultation with the Awards Office. (Initially the award was $500 each, but it has increased to $1000 each.)

*(The information of the life of Dr. Ethlyn Trapp was collected from articles by Dr. Olive Sadler [*B.C. Medical Journal, *Vol. 14, No. 8, August, 1972]; by Dr. Frances Forrest-Richards who included Dr. Ethlyn Trapp's story in the Pioneer Profiles for the FMWC Newsletters, and by Ada McGeer who wrote an article for* The Vancouver Sun *on Wed., Aug. 16, 1972 entitled "Many Thanks, Ethlyn" about her friend.)*

1929

DR. IRMLA KENNEDY-JACKSON
(c. 1897–1982)

Irmla Kennedy graduated in medicine from the University of Toronto in 1919. Her residency training was undertaken at the New York Hospital in White Plains. She quickly obtained her American Board certification in psychiatry and neurology, and later her Canadian certification. In 1927, she went to British Columbia where she was the only psychodynamic psychotherapy practitioner for years, and was on the staff at the Vancouver General Hospital. She was a role model for many women psychiatrists.

As Dr. Irmla Kennedy-Jackson, she returned to Ontario in 1951 to work at the Homewood Sanatorium in Guelph. She was involved in research, and was a regular participant in psychiatric meetings.

Although living in Hamilton, Dr. Kennedy-Jackson was one of the original members of the Toronto Psychoanalytic Study Circle formed in 1956. As a member of the Canadian Psychiatric Association, she petitioned successfully for the formation of a Section on Psychotherapy within the organization. A colleague, recounting her memories of Dr. Kennedy-Jackson, noted: "While she was unusual in many ways, she was both a wise and gifted psychotherapist."

Dr. Kennedy-Jackson practised privately in Hamilton until a few months before her death in 1982.

The information on Dr. Irmla Kennedy-Jackson was copied with permission from the book, *Pioneers All, Women Psychiatrists in Canada: A History*, by Dr. Judith H. Gold, Dr. Martine Michaud, and Dr. Odette Bernazzani.

(From the obituary in the BCMJ, *December, 1989, by Dr. Ardeth Hassel-Gran, Dr. George Elliot, and Dr. Mary K. Garner.)*

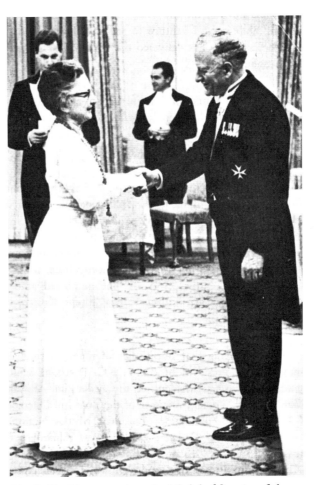

Dr. EthlynTrapp receives the Medal of Service of the Order of Canada from the Governor-General (1968).

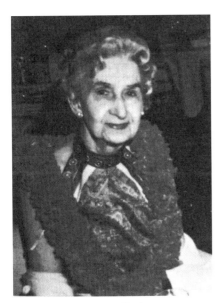

Dr. Irmla Kennedy-Jackson, 1927

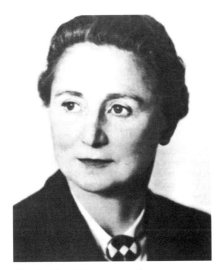

Dr. Ethlyn Trapp, 1928

Notes from VMA BULLETIN 1924 - 1929

The Vancouver Medical Association was founded in 1898 and incorporated in 1906. The *VMA Bulletin* began in October 1924 and represented the first attempt at a systematic medical publication in the Canadian west. The Editorial Board members were Dr. J.H. MacDermot, Dr. Stanley Paulin, and Dr. J.M. Pearson.

In 1921 in British Columbia there were 3,096 beds in public hospitals. The cost was $13.75 per day. The Workmen's Compensation Board had an industrial accident insurance plan for 150,000 workers. During the ten years ending December 31st, 1922, there were reported to the Health Department of the City of Vancouver 184 cases of smallpox, an average of eighteen per year. In the first ten months of 1924, 413 cases occurred among school children and vaccinations were begun in the schools. The *VMA Bulletin* began to report on the epidemics in the city.

The activities of the doctors and their comments were recorded in a column called *Bulletin*. There was a section on the B.C. Medical Association news, as well as several good articles in each *Bulletin* by the members of the medical profession.

October, 1924 The first note in the *VMA Bulletin* of a woman doctor concerned the marriage in September, 1924, of Dr. Dorothy Trapp of New Westminster to Dr. Roger S. Countryman, an intern at the Vancouver General Hospital during 1920, who later set up a medical practice in St. Paul, Minnesota.

January, 1925 The population of the City of Vancouver in November, 1924, was 123,000; Asiatics 9,875. Adding North Vancouver and New Westminster, the total was 237,000. Infant mortality was seven (rate 27.1). Diseases in the city: scarlet fever 127; diphtheria 20; mumps 24; TB 9 (new).

June, 1925 Vancouver General Hospital had the largest graduating class in Nursing in its history. (VGH was opened in 1906.)

July, 1925 The Vancouver Medical Association held its Summer School in July.

September, 1925 Savory Island is gradually becoming a very popular resort for medical men, who are building cottages there.

November, 1925 There is an increase in typhoid fever. Infant deaths under one year were 13 (rate 42.6), a high rate in 1925.

July, 1926 Dr. Maude Abbott of Montreal spoke to the Vancouver Medical Association members, on her way home after attending the CMA Annual Meeting in Victoria.

October, 1926 A measles epidemic occurred lasting for five months with 14 deaths.

June, 1927 Dr. Isabel Day, a popular general practitioner in the city of Vancouver, has left for a trip to her hometown, Toronto, and will do post-graduate studies in Obstetrics while there. Dr. C.H. Vrooman continues as President of the British Columbia Medical Association. (The BCMA was founded in 1900.)

December, 1927 There was a discussion of the long overdue establishment of a medical faculty at the University of British Columbia. Dr. George Seldon in his Osler Lecture urged that a medical school for Vancouver be considered.

January, 1928 There are 15 interns at the Vancouver General Hospital for 1928-29. The Maternity wing of the Vancouver General Hospital will be opened in January, 1929.

June, 1929 The new Medical-Dental building was opened in June. The VMA Library and the Vancouver Medical Association moved to the new building. Also, the B.C. Medical Association and College of Physicians and Surgeons have offices in the new building. At the VMA Annual Meeting (the thirty-second session of the VMA) there was a discussion about the pressing need for a medical faculty at the University of British Columbia.

Stories from 1930 – 1939

1930

Dr. Mary Kathleen (Woods) Langston

1931

Dr. Reba Willits (Mrs. Henryk Schoenfeld)

1932

Dr. Alice Evelyn Thorne

1935

Dr. Evelyn Gee

Dr. Alexa Eleanor Caroline Riggs-Wood

1936

Dr. Marian Noel Sherman

1938

Dr. Dorothy Saxton

1939

Dr. Christina (Fraser) Taylor

Fourteen new women registrants from 1930–1939 in B.C.

Year Registered & Name	Qualifications
1930 Dr. Mary K. Woods (later Langston), Vancouver & Port Coquitlam, B.C. (see biographical notes)	MD, Alberta, 1928; LMCC, 1929; re-registered as a specialist in 1949.
1931 Dr. Claire Madge R. Onhauser, Hollyburn, B.C.	MD, CM, Manitoba, 1925
1931 Dr. Reba E. Willits, Kelowna, B.C. (see biographical notes)	MD, Toronto, 1931; LMCC, 1931
1932 Dr. Alice Evelyn Thorne, Port Kells, B.C. (see biographical notes)	Dalhousie Medical School, 1924
1934 Dr. Ethel M. Robertson, Sooke, B.C.	MD, Toronto, 1923; LCP & S, Manitoba, 1923; LMCC, 1923
1935 Dr. Evelyn Stewart James, Vancouver, B.C.	MD, Toronto, 1931; Certified in Pediatrics
1935 Dr. Evelyn A. Gee, Tranquille, B.C. (see biographical notes)	MD, Toronto, 1930; LMCC, 1931
1935 Dr. Alexa Eleanor Caroline Riggs-Wood, Vancouver, B.C. (see biographical notes)	MD, Toronto, 1931; DPH, Toronto
1936 Dr. Marian Noel Sherman, Victoria, B.C. (see biographical notes)	London, 1917; MD, 1920; FRCS, England, 1922
1937 Dr. Alice McDonald, Vancouver, B.C.	BSc, Alberta, 1926; MD, Alberta, 1933; LMCC, 1933

Year Registered & Name	Qualifications
1937 Dr. Lois Stephens, Wells, B.C.	MD, Manitoba, 1936; LMCC, 1936
1938 Dr. Elaine B.M. Pugsley, Prince Ruport, B.C.	MD, Toronto, 1935; LMCC, 1936
1938 Dr. Dorothy E. Saxton, Ocean Falls & Victoria, B.C. (see biographical notes)	MD, Manitoba, 1936; LCP & S, Manitoba, 1936; MRCS, England, 1936; LRCP, London, 1936
1939 Dr. Christina A. Fraser, Vancouver, B.C. (see biographical notes)	MD, Toronto, 1932; LMCC, 1932

In 1930, there were 744 registered doctors, in 1932, 779.

DR. MARY KATHLEEN (WOODS) LANGSTON (1904–1991)

Dr. Kathleen Langston was born in 1904 in North Dakota. She moved to Canada where she graduated from the University of Alberta in 1928 with an M.D. After taking the LMCC exams in 1929, she registered with the B.C. College of Physicians and Surgeons in 1930 and practised general medicine in Port Coquitlam and New Westminster. With her husband Dr. Robert G. Langston, she left general practice to travel to England for post-graduate work: she in anesthesia and he in plastic surgery. The war began, and they joined the Emergency Medical Service of Great Britain in Scotland and served for five years. She obtained a Diploma in Anesthesia at Rooksdown Hospital where her husband was in a plastic surgery residency. Both returned to British Columbia and registered as specialists in 1949, joining the staff of Shaughnessy Hospital. Dr. Kathleen was one of the first certified anesthetists in British Columbia.

Dr. Kathleen Langston was a founding member of the B.C. Division of the Canadian Anesthetist Society and was granted an honorary lifetime membership. She was involved in a study of induced hypotension for surgery by IV drugs and was active in many women's organizations, especially the Voice of Women, sponsored by the United Nations.

In 1968, Dr. Kathleen and her husband were involved in a motor vehicle accident, which resulted in her losing a leg. Drs. Kathleen and Robert Langston have a son Leigh, a daughter Faith, and two grandchildren in Montreal. Dr. Kathleen Langston died on April 1991, twenty-six days prior to her husband's death.

(The above was written by Dr. H.B. Graves, for the BCMJ *of December, 1991.)*

DR. REBA WILLITS (MRS. HENRYK SCHOENFELD)

Dr. Reba Willets Schoenfeld was one of nine Canadian women chosen to write her story for the Medical Women's International book, *Women Physicians of the World*, a collection of autobiographies from ninety-one women doctors from around the world born before 1912. Her story is copied from this book which was published in 1978:

My parents are counted among the pioneers in Kelowna, British Columbia. My mother Ellen Carrie Bailey came to Kelowna with her family in 1893, when she was a little girl. My father Palmer Brooks Willits came in 1903 and went to work as a clerk in the village's only general store. He was a pharmacist and a year or so later he went into partnership to establish the drugstore that was named after him.

Father and Mother were married in 1905, and I was born the following year. We lived in an apartment over the drugstore until I was three, when we moved to a small farm on the edge of town. Mother and Father were farmers at heart, but Father continued his profession. It was a lonely life for me, as there were few neighbours and no children of my age nearby.

When I was six, my sister Mary was born. I have always felt a close bond with her and later developed an almost maternal attitude toward her. This interfered with a normal sisterly relationship, and it is only recently that I have overcome the tendency to "mother" her. This has resulted in an improvement in our feelings toward one another, and we are now very close.

When I was eight or nine, I became interested in medical things. We lived next door to the small cottage hospital that served Kelowna and the district. Father was on the board of directors and Mother on the women's auxiliary. I was frequently allowed to watch the babies being bathed, as even in those days women occasionally went to the hospital for delivery of their babies; but no one thought of the health hazard created by a child in the nursery. My interest was no doubt fanned by Father's attitude toward medicine. He would have studied for the profession had it been financially possible.

When I was ten or eleven, I met the girl who became one of my dearest friends—Audrey Knox. She was the eldest daughter of Dr. Benjamin Knox, whom I used to see around the hospital and who was a close friend of my father's. Audrey and I were inseparable until her marriage in 1930.

Kelowna's first physician, Dr. Boyce, had a marked influence on our family. He and my father were very close friends, and he was also our family doctor. All important decisions were discussed with him, and this included my education. When the time came for me to enter high school, there was serious talk about my future. Audrey's father and my father wanted us to go into medicine. My mother did not approve, and I cannot ever remember being asked what I wanted. It did not occur to me to go against my father's wishes, but I think that if I had been left to make my own decision, I would probably have studied nursing.

In June of 1922 Audrey and I passed our junior matriculation. We were both sixteen and too young to enter the University of Toronto, which had been picked as the most suitable of those accepting women in the medical course. As chemistry had not been taught in the Kelowna High School, we spent the year attending a private tutor to get a grounding, as we thought, in this subject, but even elementary chemistry without a laboratory is a poor introduction to a subject so vital to the study of medicine.

I shall never forget the thrill I felt the first time I was addressed as "Doctor." It was almost as though I had never believed I would become a qualified MD, and this convinced me.

Then came the great day when I left with my father for Toronto, over 2,000 miles away. Never will I forget my complete abandonment to tears as I said good-bye to my mother and sister. However, it didn't take me long to recover, and if ever there was a naïve and overprotected first-year student, it was I. We had to enroll in the first year arts course, as we had not been able to take the senior matriculation in Kelowna. This enabled us to live in Queen's Hall, the residence for girls in University College.

When we entered the medical course after obtaining our senior matriculation, we had to leave Queen's Hall and move to Argyll House, the residence for women medical students. Here the women were more serious-minded, and on the whole closer to our financial level. My family made a real sacrifice to send me to college, and most of the women at Argyll House were in the same position.

The course at Toronto that led to the degree of MD was six years in length. The first three years dealt primarily with the basic sciences and the last three with clinical subjects, to me the most interesting. In my class there were seven women and ninety men. I do not remember suffering any discrimination, but of course we did a certain amount of complaining. One incident in particular comes to mind. In our final year the women's names were put on the slate for Saturday evening emergency ward duty, and we grumbled about the men's unwillingness to give up their fun night. However, we were soon pleased with the arrangement, as the accident cases brought in on this night far outnumbered those on week nights, and the experience we gained was well worth the sacrifice of giving up our Saturday evenings.

I managed to involve myself in some of the social activities on the campus, taking an interest in the Medical Women's Undergraduate Association. I was vice-president in my fifth year and president in my final year.

During my college years I did not return home for Christmases, but spent them in the little village of Burford, Ontario, with my father's only sister and her family. I spent the summers at home. After I had started my clinical years, I made rounds with Dr. Boyce, who allowed me to assist with maternity cases and to observe at operations.

In May of 1931, I graduated without Audrey, as she had left college to be married. I shall never forget the thrill I felt the first time I was addressed as "Doctor." It was almost as though I had never believed I would become a qualified MD, and this convinced me. The highly charged atmosphere of bidding farewell to so many dear friends and college associates, of being the centre of attention as the envied graduate, and most of all of starting out on my career at last made graduation an occasion I don't think I will ever forget. I had an appointment at the Vancouver General Hospital for a rotating internship, and the thrill of being in the west again equalled that of starting to work, even in the lowly position of an intern. It was my first taste of having a job with a paycheque.

Although the Vancouver General Hospital was not a teaching hospital, the staff and many visiting doctors were most generous in sharing their knowledge and experience with us. There were about thirty interns, and only two of us were women. I enjoyed my two years at the hospital both for the experience and knowledge that I gained and for the social life I enjoyed as part of the large hospital.

I had planned to continue working at the Vancouver General Hospital for a third year, but Dr. Boyce was anxious for me to come into practice with him, and this was in the middle of the hungry thirties. These things combined to launch me into practice in Kelowna in the spring of 1934. Father built an office at the back of his drugstore. Half the space accommodated Dr. Boyce's office and ophthalmic chair. I had an examining room and a consulting room, and we shared a small laboratory and waiting room. It was with mixed feelings that I undertook practice in my native town and working with the doctor who had delivered me. As it turned out, my practice was a mixture of men and women, children and adults, old friends and new acquaintances. I was the first medical woman most of them had encountered and so was a bit of a novelty; in fact, some of my patients came out of curiosity. However, many of them came because they preferred to attend a woman doctor. Dr. Boyce was endeavoring to confine his practice to ophthalmology, and he referred the other patients to me, but there were some who would have none of that. This was particularly true of people in the older age group and of the Indians. Well do I remember having to deliver an Indian woman of a retained placenta in a dirty home, without any assistance from the disgruntled husband because the "old man" hadn't come.

Dr. Knox and Dr. Boyce would still on occasion take home deliveries. However, I didn't like maternity work at the best of times, so I began to try to educate the women on the advantages of going to the hospital for delivery. Eventually I won out, and Dr. Boyce was converted.

The night work I found very trying. It was the interference with my sleep that troubled me rather than the unpleasantness of being out alone at night. At first it was a real challenge to get out of the house and away on the call before my mother could get dressed to come with me. Eventually I persuaded her to let me out on my own. I think she always imagined that the call came from a dope addict who was waiting to "do me in." Even in Kelowna, which at that time had a population of about 3,000 to 4,000, we had transient dope addicts.

Twice in the five years I practised there, my medical kit was stolen from my car. Each time the bag was recovered minus the morphine and heroin. Some of the very early morning calls in the summer provided me with beautiful experiences, reminding me of the horseback rides that Audrey and I used to take when we were at school.

Another aspect of general practice that bothered me was the irregular hours at work and the resultant interference with my private life. In a small town with a central telephone operator it was almost impossible to get away from the telephone. Central, as we called her, knew who my friends were, in many cases knew my patients, and seemed to be able to ferret me out if I had purposely neglected to leave word at home as to where I might be found. General practice was so demanding and so discouraging because few people could afford medical care, and thus I looked about for a change.

During this time I had been conducting a "well-baby clinic," which was sponsored by the Women's Institute. Here babies were weighed and measured, health habits were discussed, and mothers were advised about general health. I found this very satisfying and more meaningful than patching up sick children. I had also been appointed to be visiting physician at the small local preventorium. The patients were young children who

General practice was so demanding and so discouraging because few people could afford medical care, and thus I looked about for a change.

were malnourished and therefore, in those days, considered to be susceptible to tuberculosis. This work I also found rewarding, and so my interest in preventive medicine began.

At the beginning of World War II, I gave up my practice and went back to Toronto to study public health. I was the only woman in the class of about thirty men and had the advantage of having done general practice. I think this gave me a greater appreciation of the value of the preventive side of health care, and I thoroughly enjoyed the courses. In May of 1940, I obtained my diploma in public health; I was the first woman in British Columbia to do so.

Most of the men had been granted fellowships through their city or provincial health departments. I had applied for one to the provincial officer of health in British Columbia, but he did not bother to answer my letter. Two young men were granted fellowships, however. With my mother's financial help and all my savings, which at the end of the thirties didn't amount to much, I had scraped through, but again a job was essential. There were two prospects: the first was a National Research Fellowship to work with Dr. Ronald Hare on the War Wound Commission, to study streptococcal infections in war wounds; the other opening was with the Provincial Department of Health in British Columbia. The new provincial health officer told me he would never employ a woman as a health officer, so that left the War Wound Commission.

The research project under Dr. Hare's guidance proved fascinating and was a year well spent, but I missed working with people and longed for the west, so at the conclusion of the grant I returned to Vancouver.

Dr. Stewart Murray, senior medical health officer of the Metropolitan Health Committee of Vancouver, did not share Dr. Amyot's views on employing women and took me on his staff without hesitation. Nevertheless, the newspapers reported my appointment with the headline "Woman Takes Man's Job." In September of 1941, I started to work in Vancouver as a health-unit director, and so began twenty-three years of satisfying and exciting work. The city and the surrounding districts were divided into units, and each had a director who supervised public health nurses, nursing staff, and clerical workers. The area that I directed was a large working-class district with many health problems. I was responsible for the examination of school children, acted as consultant for well-baby clinics, and advised the public health nurses on their work.

In 1942, the director of School Health Services retired, and Dr. Charles Gundry, who was director of mental hygiene, was appointed; in his absence overseas I was made acting director. This meant I had two positions, for as staff was difficult to obtain, no one was available to take over the health unit. The broader scope of the new position added greatly to its interest, even though it meant much extra work. Everyone was working hard during the war years, and the excitement of being on the planning level of so many projects made up for the inconvenience.

When, at the end of the war, Dr. Gundry returned from overseas, he retained his title, but did not take any responsibility for its direction. He continued to direct the Division of Mental Health. In recognition of my direction of the service my title was changed to associate director.

After the war years the doctors returned, and I was able to turn over the health unit to its previous director and confine myself entirely to the School of Health Service. This afforded the opportunity of co-ordinating the various aspects of health care with the outpatient department staffs of the Children's Hospital and the Health Centre for Children at the Vancouver General Hospital. I also took part in the medical examination of students at the University of British Columbia, where the Metropolitan Health Committee conducted the Student Health Service. The university was booming, as men and women recently returned from the war were taking their re-establishment credits, and we were faced with examining hundreds of new students.

Another very interesting part of my work was the medical supervision of the students of the Provincial School for the Deaf and Blind. There had been very little communication between the medical and education professions in the field of diagnosing and educating these children, particularly the deaf. When the university established its medical school around 1950, there was an influx of top-flight doctors and an upswing in new plans for health care of children.

One of the most exciting medical discoveries was the development of the Salk vaccine for protection against acute anterior poliomyelitis. Only someone who had practised medicine before the day of Salk vaccine could fully appreciate the relief from anxiety that it afforded. In 1955, as soon as the vaccine became available, we held clinics throughout the metropolitan area. The vaccine was in short supply, so we could not immunize all school children the first year, but in a matter of two or three years the vaccine was available at no charge to all infants, children, and young adults.

About this time, there was a reorganization of the health department; I was transferred from the school-board staff back to the Metropolitan Health Committee, and my title was changed to director of medical services. I was then in charge of child-health conferences, preschool children, school health services, and the pre-employment examination of teachers.

With the establishment of the medical school at the University of British Columbia came the involvement with the medical students who attended school health examinations. During these we stressed, as always, the preventive aspects of health care.

Although Dr. Murray did not appear to have any prejudice against employing women on his medical staff, he had certain reservations about giving them much authority. This was brought home to me very forcibly when his assistant was about to retire. My position was next in line, but I did not want the job, as I preferred the work I was doing in the schools. I told Dr. Murray that I was not going to apply. Nevertheless, he advised the Metropolitan Health Committee against employing me on the basis that a woman was not suitable for the position.

In 1964, I retired. I was only fifty-eight, but I felt the pressure of change and was eager to plan my retirement. In 1947, I had bought a lakeshore property in Kelowna for my dream home and was impatient to get on with it and the garden. A most suitable young man with certification in pediatrics, as well as in public health, was found for my replacement.

The staff gave me a big farewell party, at which I shed copious tears—tears of sentiment, not sorrow—through which I was able to laugh. It was one of the highlights of my life.

It was again with mixed feelings that I took the next step, that of selling my West Vancouver house, where I had been so happy, and moving away from all the wonderful friends I had made. Mother was living in Kelowna, crippled by a car accident, and there was my beautiful property, so this seemed the wise thing to do. When I finally moved in, there was plenty to be done, especially in the garden.

A retired person in a town like Kelowna need never want for something to do, as there are many agencies that need volunteers. I had worked in Vancouver for the United Way and was soon at it again here. There were other groups that I worked with, and soon I volunteered for the Elizabeth Fry Society and to drive for Meals on Wheels.

While I was in Vancouver the women in the normal school would ask me how to meet young men who were single. I always advised them to join a church group. One would almost imagine that I was taking my own advice, as it was at the Unitarian Fellowship that I met Henryk Schoenfeld, who was a Polish chemical engineer. It wasn't "love at first sight," but we were certainly attracted to each other from the beginning. Six months later we were married at the Unitarian Church in Vancouver. Henryk had been a widower for three years and was lonely, and so was I. We marveled at our good fortune in finding each other and settled happily into the house built for my retirement. We enjoyed our common interests, going to concerts and travelling to Vancouver to hear visiting artists. We enjoyed our friends and took trips back to London, Ontario, to visit Henryk's elderly mother and his old friends there. My mother was still alive and was delighted over our marriage.

It was too good to last. In March of 1970, Henryk was stricken with symptoms of a brain tumor, from which he died in March of 1971. I was shattered. I had waited so long to enjoy the love and close companionship of a respected and highly intelligent man—and to have him snatched away so soon seemed most tragic to me.

However, the passage of time has modified my grief, and my friends have rallied around, so that I once again find life worthwhile as I sit here alone in my lakeside home, writing about the things I have done.

1932

DR. ALICE EVELYN THORNE

Alice Evelyn Thorne was born on October 23, 1890, in Karsdale in the Annapolis Basin, Digby County, Nova Scotia, one of thirteen children of Joseph and Lydia Wooster Thorne, a Loyalist family who farmed and operated weirs. The Thorne farm is still in operation today.

After attending a one-room school, Alice went to Acadia University and obtained a teacher's licence before she was accepted into Dalhousie Medical School. In the year she graduated, 1924, she was found to be suffering from pulmonary tuberculosis, for which the only treatment in those days was bed rest.

Alice returned home to Karsdale and stayed there until she recovered. Once she was well again, she went as an intern to the Tuberculosis Sanatorium in Qu'Appelle, Saskatchewan, but found the Prairie winters so harsh that she moved to the milder climate of British Columbia and made her home with her sister, Mrs. Herberts.

Alice took an internship in the Vancouver General Hospital, but in the male-dominated hospital there was no accommodation for women doctors, so she boarded in the nurses' residence. When her nephews went to visit her, although only little boys, they had to sit with her on the porch outside because males were not allowed to set foot inside the nurses' residence.

Meanwhile, two young men from Digby County had settled in Port Kells, fourteen miles form Vancouver, up the Fraser River in British Columbia. They had set up a lumber mill where they cut ties and tie sets for the Canadian National Railway. The men shipped timber to the overseas market and dressed lumber for local buyers, running a profitable business even during the Great Depression years.

One of the men, Norman Wade, was from Karsdale. He had been a friend of the Thorne family when Alice was a girl. When he learned that two of the Thorne girls were in Vancouver, he called at the Herberts' home and met Alice again. They were married in 1932; Alice went to live in Port Kells, where she cared for the medical needs of the mill hands who were in a hazardous occupation. She was a pioneer occupational medicine specialist.

The marriage was short-lived. Norman Wade died of a coronary thrombosis in 1937 and Alice was left to carry on the business as manager and as a spare hand in the mill when needed. She helped on the green chains—one of the less strenuous jobs.

David Herberts, one of her nephews who, as a boy, had visited her at the nurses' residence, recalled in later life: "She was the only lady mill operator: she was popular but strict, always acting and dressing as a lady. She maintained community respect, and she supplied lumber gratis to churches, community halls, and charities."

Alice's nephews visited her every summer vacation and lived in the bunkhouse with the mill hands while they worked at the mill. They were expected to do as much or more than the other employees. They remember that she kept a barrel of dulse from Karsdale, Nova Scotia, on hand as a treat for them.

Impressed and inspired by their Aunt Alice who "helped put us through medical school," the boys eventually became doctors. Both Dr. Edward

David Herberts and Dr. Lewis Herberts specialized in urology and are now retired, living in B.C.

Alice remarried and her second husband, Harold Morrison, was a sawyer in the mill.

At the age of sixty-one, on April 8, 1952, Alice died of cancer of the pancreas and was buried in the Church of England graveyard at Cloverdale. She had no children.

(From Petticoat Doctors *by Enid Johnson Macleod, revised, with permission from the publisher, Pottersfield Press, pps. 98-100.)*

DR. EVELYN GEE
(1905-1988)

Dr. Evelyn Gee graduated from the University of Toronto Medical School in 1930. She interned at Vancouver General Hospital and did a residency in Pathology. She worked as an assistant pathologist under Dr. H.H. Pitts, and was certified by the Royal College as a Specialist in Pathology. In 1940, she contracted tuberculosis and spent two years as a patient in Tranquille Sanatorium. After dischage she joined Tranquille as a pathologist and clinician. When Tranquille Sanatorium closed in 1958, Dr. Gee came to Vancouver and worked with the Travelling Tuberculosis Clinic, travelling to central and northern B.C. and the south Okanagan area.

A life member of the Alpine Club of Canada, Dr. Gee loved the mountains and made eight treks to Nepal. She was also an artist. Her friends fondly described her as "having the energy of a herd of mules." She died in 1998 at the age of eighty-three.

(From the obituary in the BCMJ, *Dec. 1989, by Dr. Ardeth Hassel-Gran, Dr. George Elliot, and Dr. Mary K. Garner.)*

DR. ALEXA ELEANOR CAROLINE RIGGS-WOOD
(1908 – 1982)

Dr. Riggs-Wood was born in Vancouver in 1908. She received an MD from Toronto in 1931, and qualified in Public Health and Medical Microbiology. Registered with the College of Physicians and Surgeons of British Columbia in 1935, she worked in many cities across Canada, including Vancouver, Toronto, Halifax, and Montreal. She returned to Vancouver when she retired in 1974.

Dr. Riggs-Wood died on May 22ND, 1982. She is survived by her husband, one daughter, and one son.

1936

DR. MARIAN NOEL SHERMAN

Dr. Marian Sherman was born Marian Noel Bostock in England, and came to Canada when she as a very young child. She was the eldest of eight children of the late Hewitt Bostock, pioneer of Monte Creek, British Columbia. Bostock ran in the election of 1896 and won the federal seat of Yale-Cariboo in the government of Wilfred Laurier. After getting into financial difficulties, the energetic, progressive Bostock resigned his seat, and went to Monte Creek (near Kamloops), where he and his wife ran a cattle ranch. His family grew up on the ranch. In 1904, Hewitt Bostock was made a Senator and was Speaker of the House for the last seven years of his life.

At the age of fifteen, Marian went back to England for school, and later to become a medical student at St. George's Hospital in London, qualifying as a doctor in 1917. Later, she received her M.D. degree in London, became a Fellow of the Royal College of Surgeons in 1922, and was appointed house surgeon at St. George's—a distinction for a woman at that time. She worked in India as a medical missionary from 1922 until 1927, where she met her future husband, Victor Sherman, then a bank manager. The couple married in 1928 and returned to India to live in Agra and Lucknow until she retired in 1934. She and her husband then lived in England for two years and came to Victoria, British Columbia in 1936. During the Second World War, Dr. Sherman worked with Dr. G.F. Kincaid at the TB Pavilion in Victoria for three years. Dr. Dorothy Saxton worked with her at the same institution during the war years.

Dr. Sherman became a Humanist in the 1940s, and a pioneer in that movement in Western Canada. During her forty years in the Victoria area, she devoted herself freely to many humanitarian and progressive causes. She was named Canadian Humanist of the Year a short time before she died at the age of eighty-three years.

1938

DR. DOROTHY SAXTON

I graduated in 1934 from the University of Manitoba Medical School. There were three women in our class of eighty-eight students. When the required internship year was completed at the Winnipeg General Hospital, I did a brief locum in Winnipeg. My first patient was a young man miserable with poison ivy following a Sunday picnic with his girlfriend. I was reminded of the wise words of our lecturer in skin diseases: "Hang on to your skin patients: they will always be with you." As the weeks passed I realized how inadequate my skills were, so I returned to the Winnipeg General to do a senior residency in Obstetrics, Gynecology, and Pediatrics. Then I was on the staff of the Manitoba Sanatorium at Ninette, Manitoba for a year. During this period I also had the opportunity to do a few obstetric cases in the surrounding countryside.

For one case I had to set out with a pony and sleigh in a snowstorm. The snow was so deep it was impossible to follow the road. The anxious first-time father gave instructions about the general direction and advised that he would hang a lantern out to guide me across the snow-covered landscape. Eventually a flicker of light appeared on the darkening horizon, and I arrived in time to make minimal preparation for the impending delivery. The husband was the only person available to help. He was becoming very anxious, as the labour had gone on for hours and it was getting late and dark, the only available light being two kerosene lamps. I decided a few whiffs of chloroform would help. We carefully set the lamps as far away as possible, administered a few drops, and in short order a healthy baby girl arrived. Everything worked out beautifully.

Another interesting case had occurred in the heat of summer with horses neighing and the buzz of horseflies coming through the open windows of the farmhouse. Again the only help available was a tired husband. Fortunately, everything went smoothly and a healthy baby arrived, and the father was finally relieved.

There were very isolated prairie farms with very limited facilities. Follow-up visits were made and supplies taken in regularly.

Life at the San on the other hand was interesting, as new treatment methods were being introduced. I believe we did some of the first thoracoplasties there as well as using the Iron Lung.

During this time, room, board, and laundry facilities were provided, so I was able to save enough funds to purchase a third-class passage on the Empress of Britain to England. It was an exciting trip as it was 1936, the year of both the Olympics in Munich and the memorial celebrations at Vimy Ridge for the Canadians who lost their lives during the First World War. Many notable characters and several Olympics teams were on board. The Queen's Own Cameron Highlanders Band provided many evenings of Scottish dancing and funny escapades, and they also later played at the Vimy Ridge memorial. There was a great sense of revelry by night and day, which went on for ten days as we crossed the Atlantic Ocean from Montreal to Southampton. It was a busy port, and the skyline presenting endless rows of chimney pots was a unique sight to a Canadian.

We boarded the boat train to London and found our way to Garing's Private Hotel on Russell Square where we had reservations for bed and breakfast at 10/6—about $2.50 in Canadian funds at that time. The breakfasts were enormous and gave us enough to last all day. We learned about interesting eating places in Soho Square and how to get inexpensive tickets to the theatres and musicals. We registered at Canada House where we hoped to pick up mail and get information on events. Of course, I also registered at the British Medical Association and made inquiries about residencies. Within two weeks I was on my way to the new Sussex Women's Hospital in Brighton. I spent nine months there having a great variety of medical experiences while working under some wonderful women surgeons, physicians, and a pathologist.

Occasional days off were spent exploring Brighton and cycling through the neighbouring villages. Although I had been advised that fraternizing with the nurses was not allowed, we managed to have some happy adventures. The chief surgeon—a woman to whom I was responsible—had given me her full approval. She lived in London and drove out twice a week in her chauffeur-driven Rolls Royce to do her surgical cases. At least sixty-five years old, she was still very active. She seemed very old to me.

Following this residency I was married to George D. Saxton in Gloucester where he was on a surgical program. After two weeks in Switzerland and Italy, we returned to Gloucester where George continued his surgical training. I went on to Birmingham where I had been appointed as an obstetrical resident in the maternity hospital, which was part of the University of Birmingham Medical School. As the second largest city in England, Birmingham offered a great range of obstetrical experiences—in hospital where only complicated cases were admitted, as well as in the vast slum areas where we travelled day and night by bicycle, with loaded saddle bags. We usually had five or six medical students who came out to see the deliveries. During my time there, one of the medical students who had a vintage Rolls Royce arrived in great style in the slum areas with the other students. He parked his car near my bicycle and joined me in the small birthing chamber. For many of these students it was a very humbling experience. On returning the next day to follow up on mother and child, we would often find the mother on her hands and knees scrubbing the floor, or if she had been forewarned of our arrival, she would be in bed with her boots on. Mothers and babies usually thrived under the tender care of the midwives and nurses in spite of their sordid surroundings.

In early 1938, we decided to return to Canada and settled in British

Columbia. We arrived in Vancouver in April. Fortunately, we were offered the opportunity to practise in Ocean Falls, a paper mill town of 2,500 people on the west coast of B.C. at the end of Dean Channel. At this time access was only possible by boat. There was a well-equipped seven-bed cottage hospital with an operating room, X-ray department, two doctors' offices, and a very capable nursing staff to serve the local community and patients who came in by boat from the isolated villages in the area. It was a diverse and interesting multi-national population and provided a rich experience not only medically, but in human relationships too.

We left Ocean Falls in 1942 for Victoria, B.C. George joined the Canadian Army Medical Corps and I worked in the Royal Jubilee Hospital in the Tuberculosis Unit. In 1943, George was posted overseas. We moved to Vancouver as we had decided to make our home there. On the ferry en route from Victoria to Vancouver we met Dr. Don Williams, Director of the Division of Venereal Disease Control for B.C. He had just been commandeered by the Canadian Armed Services in Ottawa to organize and direct a V.D. control program and needed someone to take over his duties in Vancouver immediately. The V.D. control program was co-ordinated with the Army, Navy, and Air Force V.D. control offices. A very important part of the program was the epidemiological procedures—the reporting and treatment of all cases of V.D. and the follow-up and treatment of all contacts. It was a mammoth job, interesting, heartbreaking, and exhausting, but the co-operation of the wonderful staff of doctors, nurses, medical social workers, and office staff never failed. They were all willing to work overtime when necessary to control the sexually transmitted diseases that caused more loss of manpower in the armed forces than the actual warfare. The advent of the spectacular effect of new drugs—the sulfa drugs, Prontasil and Penicillin—which rendered the patients non-infectious so quickly and reduced the tedious long-term treatment regimes was a great breakthrough. Unfortunately, there was always the possibility of these patients becoming re-infected, and it did happen.

There are many interesting tales and horror stories to tell of this period, but finally the war was over and we returned to civilian life. I took time out to have three daughters, eventually doing some part-time work with the Metropolitan Health Services of Vancouver until the girls were in school.

Then I increased my working hours, but remained on a sessional basis.

I became involved in community activities, the United Church, the YWCA and the Children's Aid Society where I became a member of the Board, the Volunteer Bureau, the Early Childhood Education Program, and covered short-term volunteer commitments in the health field. George was busy with his surgical practice doing thoracic surgery and teaching programs. We had many interesting years because of his involvement with the B.C. and Canadian Cancer Societies, and the B.C. and Canadian Lung Association. When he became ill with cancer in 1976, I resigned and we had a peaceful time until his death in March 1977.

I continued to do volunteer jobs and seminars and took courses at UBC in literature, music, art, and history. Family activities, reading, and travel have kept me well-occupied.

1939

DR. CHRISTINA FRASER TAYLOR
(1908-1982)

Born in Edinburgh, Christina Fraser emigrated to Canada at the age of three. She received her MD from the University of Toronto in 1932 and took post-graduate training in Radiology. She was chief and often the sole Radiologist for the Seymour Clinic and the Children's Hospital for approximately thirty years and worked at Vancouver General Hospital as well.

Chris's primary intention to become a medical missionary was sacrificed to caring for her widowed mother until the latter's death.

She devoted time and energy to the less fortunate: she financed an X-ray machine and training of technicians for a hospital in Nigeria, she was active in setting up homes for seniors in Vancouver through the Soroptomist Club, and was a member of the Presbyterian Church—"A real lady in the finest sense of the word."

Reverend W. Taylor and Chris were married in 1976. Chris developed renal failure and died on June 6, 1982.

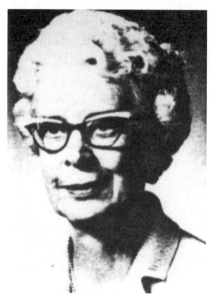

Dr. Reba Willits, 1931

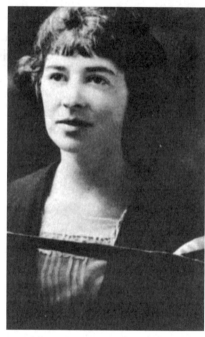

Dr. Alice Thorne, 1932

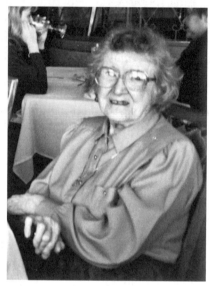

Dr. Dorothy Saxton, 1938

Notes from VMA BULLETIN 1930–1939

July, 1930 Statistics: Vancouver population 240,421, Asiatics 9,335. Infant mortality February 46.30, March 65.28, and by June reduced to 33.94.

September, 1930 Dr. Isabel Day was elected President of the Federation of Medical Women of Canada at the Annual Meeting in Winnipeg.

January, 1931 Dr. Irmla Kennedy discussed the paper of Dr. J.G. McKay, "Treatment of Psychoses" at the meeting of the Vancouver Medical Association held in November, 1930. Dr. Kennedy will address the B.C. Academy of Science on January 21st, 1931, on "Personality Study." The Outpatient Department of the Vancouver General Hospital had 7,000 patients in 1929, and 15,000 in 1930. There are 35 interns, including six senior interns at Vancouver General Hospital. Dr. Thomas Alexander Wilson died on January 16, 1931. He was associated with Indian Affairs for over 30 years in British Columbia. He spent six years in Fort Simpson. In 1888 he married Dr. Belle Holland. They had two sons, Dr. Ray Wilson, a dentist, and Dr. P.M. Wilson, a physician at Britannia Beach, B.C.

November, 1931 Dr. Isabel Day is on a six-month appointment in Obstetrics and Gynecology at the Lying-In Hospital in Chicago. Dr. Day expects to resume practice in Vancouver in the spring.

February, 1932 There were 1,059 cases of measles in the Vancouver area.

May, 1932 Dr. Isabel Day has been appointed to the Advisory Board of the Victorian Order of Nurses, a standing committee of VMA.

1933 Statistics: Population of Vancouver 247,251. Asiatics listing now is separated into Japanese 8,429, Chinese 7,759, Hindu 251.

January, 1934 Dr. Ethlyn Trapp has just returned from an intensive post-graduate study in radiation therapy, notably with radium. She informs us that all she needs now is for the Provincial Government to provide the radium.

November, 1934 The VMA meeting had as speaker Dame Janet Campbell, DBE, MDMS of England, an authority on Maternal and Child Welfare.

June, 1935 Dr. Isabel Day was presented with a Jubilee Medal by His Majesty George VI; Drs. R.E. McKechnie and George Seldon also received Jubilee Medals.

August, 1935 The Government of British Columbia Council is to study a Draft Act of Health Insurance now being considered by the Government. Dr. Isabel Day, at the 1935 Annual meeting reported for the Victorian Order of Nurses. Dr. J.H. MacDermot of the *VMA Bulletin* Editorial Board has written an "Early Medical History of the B.C. Coast."

1936 February and March each had one death from smallpox. In April there were three deaths from diphtheria.

April, 1936 It was noted that a Bill has been presented in March on an Act to provide for the establishment of a Provincial Health Insurance System.

August, 1936 Dr. Elinor Riggs has moved to the Medical Dental Building to practise with her father. She was previously with the Vancouver General Hospital Laboratory Staff.

January, 1937 There was a measles epidemic with 1,593 cases and five deaths in 1936.

May, 1937 Drs. Dorothy Miller and Claire Onhauser are members of the North Vancouver Medical Society.

June, 1937 There were 16 medical graduates from B.C. at eastern universities: four at Queens University, four at University of Toronto, and eight at McGill University.

July, 1937 Dr. J.C. Poole and Mrs. Poole (Dr. Lois Stephens) are going to Fraser Lake to take over the practice vacated by Dr. W.C. Pitt's departure. Both were interns at the Vancouver General Hospital. Dr. Reba Willits is in practice with Dr. Boyce in Kelowna. Dr. Ethlyn Trapp, at a

VMA meeting gave an account of her post-graduate studies in cancer therapy during the two years she spent in Europe. She stated, "The absolute necessity of centralization as *sine que non* of efficient cancer work has been established. Here in British Columbia we are tragically behind the times, but we have the tremendous advantage of beginning from nothing, with nearly 30 years of the trial and error of other places by which to profit."

November, 1937 Dr. Alice McDonald has returned from Toronto where she did post-graduate work in the Physiotherapy Department of the University of Toronto. She is now with the Physiotherapy Department of the Vancouver General Hospital.

January, 1938 Dr. Ethlyn Trapp has opened offices in the Medical Dental Building and will confine her practice to X-ray and radium treatment of cancer. Dr. Trapp is installing high-voltage deep therapy equipment. The BCMA Committee on the Study of Cancer for 1937–1938 has as Chairman, Dr. A.Y. McNair, Vancouver and as Secretary, Dr. Ethlyn Trapp.

February, 1938 Dr. Lois Stephens (Mrs. J.C. Poole) is conducting the practice single-handed at Fraser Lake during her husband's absence, while he is covering Dr. Brummet's practice in Smithers. Dr. Brummet is ill in Vancouver.

March, 1938 Dr. Bliss McQuarry was married to Dr. L.J. Pugsley of the Fisheries Experimental Station, Prince Rupert, where they will reside. She will commence medical practice in Prince Rupert. Dr. Ethlyn Trapp spoke on "Trends of Radiation Therapy in Europe" at a meeting in Victoria of Radiologists of B.C. and Alberta.

April, 1938 At the VMA monthly meeting Dr. Evelyn Gee spoke on "Physiology of the Liver and Gall Bladder."

June, 1938 Dr. Dorothy Saxton, wife of Dr. George Saxton, has registered recently with the College of Physicians and Surgeons of B.C. She did post-graduate work in Obstetrics and Gynecology in England. Sulfanilamide therapy has been introduced to treat infections.

November, 1938 BCMA Lecture Tours visited the Okanagan, and East and West Kootenays. Dr. Reba Willits is the Honorary Secretary-Treasurer of the Kelowna Medical Association. Dr. A. Maxwell Evans is to take charge of the Cancer Clinic which will open in Vancouver on November 5th.

February, 1939 The population of Vancouver is 263,974; Japanese 8,891, Chinese 7,728, and Hindu 389. The BCMA membership has shown an increase of 45% in new members.

April, 1939 Dr. Kathleen (Woods) Langston and her husband have left New Westminster for extended post-graduate study, first to the University of Alberta, and then to Europe. At the VMA meeting of April, 1939, Dr. Ethlyn Trapp gave the report of the Department of Cancer Control.

June, 1939 Dr. Evelyn Gee and Dr. D.S. Munroe presented a "Report on Clinical Pathological Cases" at the VMA meeting.

July, 1939 St. Vincent's Hospital is opened.

August, 1939 Dr. Lois Stephens of Wells, B.C., attended the Annual Meeting of the Central Medical Society, Prince George, B.C.

September, 1939 WAR IS DECLARED.
  Dr. Eleanor Riggs who was on her way to England and had reached Montreal, has postponed her sailing. At the BCMA Annual Meeting in September, Dr. Evelyn Gee gave a lecture on "The Friedman Modification of the Aschiem-Zondek Test." Again, there was discussion on the need for a medical school in British Columbia. Dr. Ethlyn Trapp will attend the International Cancer Congress to be held at Atlantic City, and will visit hospitals in the Boston area and New York.

October, 1939 The British Medical Association asks for information regarding the acceptance into homes of Canadian doctors of the children of British doctors. The B.C. Commission for Evacuation of Overseas Children received a splendid response. At this date it is providing for the care of 200 children of British doctors.

Stories from **1940 - 1949**

1941

Dr. Josephine (Schacher) Mallek

1942

Dr. Mary Kay Garner

Dr. Olive E.M. Sadler

1943

Dr. Elda Lindenfeld

Dr. Marguerite B. Shea (Carroll)

Dr. Agnes Black Weston (Mrs. Kenneth Campbell)

Dr. Margaret Buchanan Forster Sylling

1944

Dr. Florence Nichols (Haines)

Dr. Margaret Florence Burridge Hardie

Dr. Evelyn May (Woodman) Fox

1945

Dr. Lucille G. Ellison

1946

Dr. Margaret Adele Mullinger

Dr. Mary Viola Rae

1947

Dr. Ardeth E. Robertson Hasselgren

Dr. A. Pauline Hughes

Dr. Jean Templeton Hugill

Dr. Mary A. Murphy

1948

Dr. Anna Farewell

Dr. Anne Steele

Dr. Ludmila (Lola) Fishaut Zeldowicz

1949

Dr. Kathleen Belton

Dr. Honor (Molly) Kidd

Dr. Valentina (Vaya) Marken

Forty-seven new women registrants from 1940–1949 in B.C.

Year Registered & Name	Qualifications
1940 Dr. Ella Cristall (later Evans), Vancouver, B.C.	BS, Alberta, 1930; MD, Alberta, 1937; LMCC, 1937
1941 Dr. Mary C. Luff, Vancouver, B.C.	MRCS, England; LRCP, 1925; MB, BS, London, 1926; MD, London, 1930; LMCC, 1941

She had been an evacuee from England during the war.

Year Registered & Name	Qualifications
1941 Dr. Josephine Mallek, Vancouver, B.C. (see biographical notes)	BA, McGill University, 1932; MD, CM, McGill University, 1936; MSc, McGill University, 1937; LCP & S, Quebec, 1938; GMC, Great Britain, 1939
1941 Dr. Flora Barr, Penticton, B.C.	DO, College of Osteopathy, Los Angeles, U.S.A.
1942 Dr. Olive Edmonson MacLean Sadler, New Westminster, B.C. (see biographical notes)	MD, McGill University, 1940
1942 Dr. Mary K. Garner, Deep Cove, B.C. (later Vancouver, B.C.) (see biographical notes)	BA, Saskatchewan, 1934; MD, Manitoba, 1942; LMCC, 1942
1943 Dr. Agnes Black (later Weston), Vancouver, B.C. (see biographical notes)	MB, ChB, Glasgow, 1933; MD, Glasgow, 1935; DPH, Royal College P & S, England, 1940; LMCC, 1943; FRCP, 1956
1943 Dr. Kathleen S. Graham, Vancouver, B.C.	BSc, Alberta; MD, Alberta, 1943; LMCC, 1943
1943 Dr. Elda Lindenfeld, Vancouver, B.C. (see biographical notes)	MD, Vienna, 1923; LMCC, 1943

Year Registered & Name	Qualifications
1943 Dr. M.B.F. Sylling, Tranquille, B.C. (see biographical notes)	MB, Toronto, 1925; LCP & S, Ontario, 1925; MD, Toronto, 1930; LMCC, 1942
1943 Dr. Marguerite Shea, Vancouver, B.C. (see biographical notes)	MD, Toronto, 1935; LMCC, 1942
1944 Dr. Hazel Krause, Vancouver, B.C.	MD, Manitoba, 1930; LMCC, 1930

She was a medical officer in the armed forces; married to Dr. J.R. Farish.

Year Registered & Name	Qualifications
1944 Dr. Eve Susan May McMaster, Vancouver, B.C.	MCCN, Berlin, 1934; LMCC, 1930
1944 Dr. Agnes O'Neill, Vancouver, B.C.	University of Toronto, 1943; LMCC, 1943
1944 Dr. Margaret F.B. Hardie, Vancouver, B.C. (see biographical notes)	MB, University of Toronto, 1924; LMCC, 1944
1944 Dr. Florence Nichols (see biograghical notes)	MD, c. 1944
1944 Dr. Evelyn Woodman (later Fox), Harrison Hot Springs, B.C. (see biographical notes)	MD, Manitoba, 1944; LMCC, 1944; Canadian Army Corps
1945 Dr. Lucille Ellison, Victoria, B.C. (see biographical notes)	MD, Manitoba, 1944; LMCC, 1945
1945 Dr. Marion Gertrude Irwin, Kaslo, B.C.	MD, Alberta, 1934
1945 Dr. C. Elizabeth Mahaffy, Vancouver, B.C.	MD, Alberta, 1930; LMCC, 1930; Flight Officer, #8RMB, Jericho Beach, Vancouver, B.C.

Year Registered & Name	Qualifications
1945 Dr. Elizabeth Sprung, Vancouver, B.C.	MD, Alberta, 1939; LMCC, 1939; LCP & S, Alberta, 1942
1945 Dr. Winnifred Van Kleek, Vancouver, B.C.	BSc, Alberta, 1941; MD, Alberta, 1945; LMCC, 1945

Lieut. Winnifred Van Kleek and Lieut. G.B. Wilson were married in 1946.

Year Registered & Name	Qualifications
1946 Dr. Elizabeth Fleck, Vancouver, B.C.	BA, UBC, 1940; MD, Western, 1946; LMCC, 1946
1946 Dr. (Vi) Mary Viola Rae, Vancouver, B.C. (see biographical notes)	MD, Alberta, 1929; LMCC, 1929; BSc, Toronto, 1933; FRCP&S (Canada) in Pathology, 1946
1946 Dr. Gertrude Lillian Hutton, Vancouver, B.C.	MD, Toronto, 1945
1946 Dr. Margaret A. Mullinger, Vancouver, B.C. (see biographical notes)	MD, Toronto, 1946; LMCC, 1946
1946 Dr. Jean Singleton, Vancouver, B.C. (later Nairobi, Kenya)	BA, UBC, 1941; MD, McGill, 1945; DPH, Toronto, 1946; LMCC, 1946
1946 Dr. Agatha Wilford, Chilliwack, B.C.	MD, Toronto, 1945
1946 Dr. Kathleen Cecilia Lewis, Minneapolis, U.S.A.	MD, Manitoba, 1942
1946 Dr. Marion Elizabeth Griffiths, Vancouver, B.C.	MD, Alberta, 1944
1947 Dr. Ardeth E. Robertson (later Hasselgren), Tranquille, B.C. (see biographical notes)	MD, McGill, 1945

Year Registered & Name	Qualifications
1947 Dr. Mary Frances Callaghan, Long Beach, California	MD, Kansas, 1947
1947 Dr. Helen Elizabeth Hughes Johnston, Vancouver, B.C.	MD, Toronto, 1946
1947 Dr. Annie Pauline Hughes, Essondale B.C. (later New Westminster, B.C.) (see biographical notes)	MD, Toronto, 1947
1947 Dr. Jean T. Hugill (see biographical notes) Vancouver, B.C.	BSc. Alberta, 1943; MD, Alberta, 1946; LMCC, 1946; Certified in Anesthesia
1947 Dr. Mary A. Murphy, Hedley, B.C. (see biographical notes)	BA, UBC, 1940; MD, UBC, 1943; MD, U of Western Ontario, 1947; LMCC, 1947
1947 Dr. Helen B.L. Zeman, New York, U.S.A.	MD, Toronto, 1944
1948 Dr. Elizabeth Nora McKay, Toronto, Ontario	MD, McGill, 1940
1948 Dr. Alice Murray	BSc, Saskatchewan, 1927; MD, Manitoba, 1931; LMCC, 1931; MRCOG, London, 1938
1948 Dr. Ludmila Zeldowicz, Vancouver, B.C. (see biographical notes)	MD, Warsaw, 1930; LMCC, 1948
1948 Dr. Laura Muir Coleman, Toronto, Ontario	MD, McGill, 1947
1948 Dr. Anne Steele, Victoria, B.C. (see biographical notes)	MD, Edinburgh, 1944

REGISTRATIONS 1940–1949

Year Registered & Name	Qualifications
1948 Dr. Doreen May Davidson	MD, Sydney, Australia, 1947
1948 Dr. Anna E. Farewell, Chilliwack, B.C. (see biographical notes)	MD, Manitoba, 1944
1949 Dr. Honor Kidd, Vancouver, B.C. (see biographical notes)	BA, UBC, 1926; MD, CM, McGill, 1947; LMCC, 1949
1949 Dr. Jean MacLennan, Vancouver, B.C.	MB, ChB, Edinburgh, Glasgow, 1934; MD, Edinburgh, 1937; LMCC, 1948
1949 Dr. Kathleen Belton (see biographical notes)	MD, McGill, 1941; certified in Anesthesia in 1946: Royal College
1949 Dr. Valentina (Vaya) Marken (see biographical notes)	MD, Petrograd, 1917; joined Pacific Region Indian Health Service of Canada in 1949
1949 Dr. Mary Woods Langston, Vancouver, B.C. (see biographical notes)	MD, 1930; DA, England, 1940; re-registered as specialist in Anesthesia, Canada, 1949

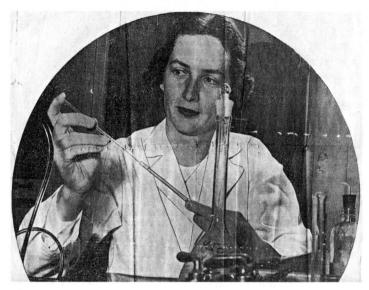

Dr. Margaret Mullinger, 1946

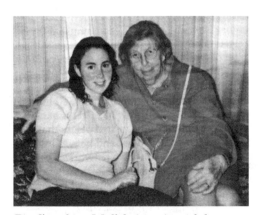

Dr. Josephine Mallek (1941), with her granddaughter

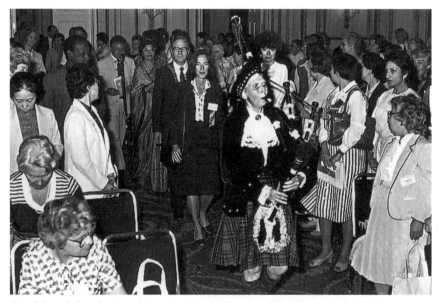

Dr. Mary Murphy (1947) piping in the honoured guests at the MWIA Congress, August 1984

DR. JOSEPHINE (SCHACHER) MALLEK

Dr. Josephine Mallek was a Vancouver doctor who practised for over fifty years and experienced more changes in medicine and more so-called new diseases than most doctors ever will.

Dr. Mallek was born in Montreal in 1912 to Russian immigrant parents who were both doctors. They practised medicine from their home so that Josephine and her sister were literally brought up in a doctor's office. Her experience in medicine began in infancy, and she did not consider any other option than to become a doctor.

Josephine's mother, trained as a teacher in Russia, had more than her share of struggles to become a doctor. Like her brother, she wanted to go to medical school. They both had disadvantages: they were Jewish and she was a woman—no Russian medical school wanted her. Only five feet tall, Josephine's mother worked her way to France and eventually was admitted to Montpelier Medical School. She supported herself by teaching Russian to the diplomats who hoped to serve in the French embassy in Leningrad (Petrogad). Meanwhile, she was learning French, because when she became a doctor she wished to practise in France. But at this time the Dreyfus affair smothered France in a storm of anti-Semitism, preventing her from obtaining French citizenship, a requisite to practise medicine in France. She decided to emigrate to a French-speaking country and chose Quebec as her next destination. Josephine's mother made a living through teaching French to immigrants, which is how she met her future husband, a young doctor who had moved with his parents from New York. To obtain a licence to practise medicine in Quebec, a doctor had to pass an examination in French.

Josephine's father had been born in Austria, and his family emigrated first to America, then to Canada. The couple eventually married. They borrowed twenty-five dollars as a down-payment for a four-storey house in the east end of Montreal, set up their offices in their home, and were busy from then on. With many immigrants arriving from central Europe, the Montreal Jewish community was very active in helping newcomers, and the Schacher's household was always filled with immigrants as well as family members. Hospitalization was not easy or affordable for many pregnant women. Josephine's mother went from house to house doing deliveries, sometimes five a day. Both doctors had busy practices as they could communicate with the new Canadians from central Europe.

Josephine was a bright student and went on to McGill University, graduating with a BA in 1932. She was accepted into medical school at McGill despite the unwritten restriction of admitting only five percent women students and five percent Jews. She had been presented with the medal for Biochemistry as an undergraduate and graduated in the top five of her class of over one hundred students.

Josephine had decided that since she had never travelled beyond New York, she was going to spread her wings and intern outside of Montreal. She was accepted by the Dr. Reese Hospital in Chicago. However, the Dean of Medicine at McGill wanted her to stay and urged her to contact Dr. J.S.L. Browne, a famous research doctor at the Medical Research Laboratory at Royal Victoria Hospital in Montreal. He promptly gave her a research job. Dr. Browne had developed a technique of extracting estrogen from urine. The product was marketed by a then unknown local laboratory, Ayerst McKenna, and eventually the refined product was sold worldwide to millions of menopausal women. Josephine also had the opportunity to work with Hans Selye who was developing his theory about "non-specific stress" and the body's adaptation to stress. He demonstrated that the adrenal gland produced a hormone which was essential to fight stress. Josephine worked for two years with the research team which included Dr. Collip and earned a Master of Science degree in 1938. Among her teachers at McGill were Dr. Eleanor Percival and Dr. Jessie Boyd Scriver, and Josephine also remembered Dr. Maude Abbott who had just retired as the Curator of the McGill Medical Museum.

Josephine met medical student Howard Mallek from Victoria, British Columbia, in her final year. Howard had contracted tuberculosis and was admitted to the Ste. Agathe Sanatorium. A long-distance courtship followed. Despite the opposition of the Superintendent at the sanatorium, they were married when Josephine completed her Master's research.

Doctors Josephine and Howard Mallek decided to go to England to finish their specialty training, he in Ophthalmology at Moorfields Hospital, and she in Internal Medicine at St. Bartholomews Hospital in London. St. Bartholomews was very much a male bastion since its beginning in 1100 AD; women doctors were not allowed on the wards or to do clinical work there. Josephine's research was on the excretion of corpus luteum hormone in females following ovulation and its absence in anovulatory cycles. She caused great consternation by appearing on the wards and at one time she thought she might have been instrumental in starting the Second World War! After a year the laboratory research was stopped due to lack of funds at the beginning of the war. Josephine was refused commissions in both the British and Canadian armies and was assured that women doctors would never be needed. Instead, she got a rotation internship position at the Post-graduate Medical School for the next year.

The Malleks had two children. In order to look after the children, they opened one of the first private nursery schools in the basement of their home.

After their two years in England, Josephine and Howard returned to Montreal. Howard was given a commission in the Canadian Army Medical Corp, but was turned down for wartime service because of a tubercular lesion. He was offered a job at St. Paul's Hospital in Vancouver to work with Dr. Anthony. Howard later became the first Jewish Chief of Staff of a hospital in British Columbia.

Josephine had difficulties getting work at the Vancouver General Hospital, which did not encourage women doctors, until she met Dr. West who was a specialist in diabetes. He gave her a job in the Diabetic Clinic, which she enjoyed. When Dr. West joined the armed services she was left in charge until another male doctor announced he was taking over the clinic. Josephine left VGH and was immediately taken on staff at St. Paul's as its first medical woman. The one condition was that she must not attend the all-male annual dinners or the Christmas party. As time passed, Josephine was joined by Dr. Doris Kavanagh on staff, and since neither were invited to the Christmas party, they gathered the female interns and made a night of celebration. First they had an expensive dinner at the Swiss Chalet, then went to the Opera, and then returned to the restaurant to eat and drink some more. They sent the bill to St. Paul's Hospital medical staff. From then on the meetings and dinners became co-ed!

The Malleks shared adjoining offices for over fifty years in Vancouver, first in the Birk's Building, and later in the Vancouver Block. Josephine practised medicine with a special interest at Endocrinology, while Howard practised his specialty of Ophthalmology.

The Malleks had two children. In order to look after the children, they opened one of the first private nursery schools in the basement of their home. They employed professional teachers and enrolled most of the infants in their neighbourhood. It was a successful co-operative effort and operated for four years.

Josephine was the President of the B.C. Branch of the Federation of Medical Women of Canada before the '60s and was most gracious in loaning her home for dinner meetings and parties for the women doctors in the '60s and '70s. She was the Osler lecturer at the Vancouver Medical Association's 65th Osler Dinner, the third woman to be so honoured. As the "Lady Osler," she delivered a delightful, witty presentation. President of the Vancouver Medical Association from 1989–1991, for years she also was the Medical Administrator of the Louis Brier Home for the aged, an accredited chronic facility with 216 beds. (The Louis Brier Home serves as a model for other such facilities in western Canada.) Josephine served on the Seniors' Advisory Council at City Hall and on subcommittees on Housing Needs and for the elderly. She was an Honorary Senior Member of the Canadian Medical Association, and honoured member of the College of Physicians and Surgeons of British Columbia, and also of the Federation of Medical Women of Canada.

The Doctors Mallek travelled extensively. They were proud of their two children, a son who is an Ophthalmologist like his father, and a daughter who has a special interest in drama and fine arts and teaches mentally handicapped children. There are four grandchildren; one granddaughter studied medicine in Calgary and is pursuing the specialty of Ophthalmology in Vancouver. The Malleks had fifty-seven happy years of marriage, and as Josephine said, they "practised medicine during the Golden Age when it was an honoured profession." Howard died in August 1995, and shortly after that Josephine retired from medical practice. She kept busy with committee work, the McGill Alumni Associations, and the Vancouver Medical Association, as well as enjoying her annual winter vacation in Hawaii.

(Dr. Mallek was interviewed during the year 2000 for this story. She died July 24, 2004.)

1942

DR. MARY KAY GARNER
(1913–2005)

Dr. Kay Garner was one of the very busy doctors in Vancouver during the war years. She took over the practices of Dr. Sid Hobbs and Dr. Fred Saunders—both busy Obstetrical practices—in 1942 when they joined the armed services. She delivered about 250 babies a year during that time.

Kay was born in Toronto in 1913, grew up in Saskatoon, and graduated from the University of Saskatchewan in 1934 with a Bachelor of Science degree. She married a businessman in 1935, and had two children, a son and a daughter. She later decided to study medicine, and attended the two pre-clinical years at the University of Saskatchewan with two other women in a class of twenty-four. Since the University of Saskatchewan did not have a full medical course in those days, she transferred to the University of Manitoba, where she was one of four women in a class of sixty. Kay graduated in medicine in 1941 and interned at the Vancouver General Hospital in June 1942. She was the only female intern that year until she was joined by Dr. Elizabeth (Monty) Akhurst. The accommodation for women interns was located on the first floor of the Maternity Building. When Maternity became busy, Kay and Monty were transferred to a room in the nurses' infirmary where the nurses in the private ward pavilion took all calls for them. When Margaret Alexander and Olive Sadler came as interns in the following year, the "girls" moved to the interns' quarters. Kay did additional training in Obstetrics and Pediatrics, and began her practice in the Medical Dental Building at 925 West Georgia.

During the war, Kay made house calls all over Vancouver and its vicinity, despite the rationing of gas. She delivered a few babies in the homes of mothers who could not afford to stay in the hospital for ten days at the rate of $3.00 a day and fifty cents for the babies. Maternity beds were also scarce; patients in labour were not always admitted to the hospital of their choice. Besides making house calls, Kay worked at the Grace Hospital Outpatient Clinic with Dr. Isabel Day, a highly respected general practitioner, and at the Salvation Army Maywood Home for unwed mothers. Doctors worked seven days a week in those days, and most had visiting privileges in all the city hospitals.

On her off days, Kay and her husband liked to escape to Texada Island; while they were away, she generously lent her home to the B.C. Branch of the Federation of Medical Women of Canada for some of their social get-togethers and dinners.

In 1969 Kay retired for the first time to Texada with her husband where they had built a retirement home by the sea. But their retirement plan was postponed when Kay was persuaded to organize the opening of a large medical clinic, built at Gillies Bay by the Kaiser Company that owned the Iron Mine on Texada. The clinic had remained empty because of the difficulty in recruiting a doctor. Kay accepted the offer, as the clinic was well-equipped and less demanding on her hours of work. She retired from the clinic in 1971 after another doctor came to take over, but continued to do locums for the Island's doctors until she retired permanently in 1980.

Kay remained on Texada after her husband died in 1979. She enjoyed taking part in community activities, and frequently drove to Vancouver to visit her daughter and friends, and to attend the opera, "Thanks to two hearing aids, two lens implants, and a pacemaker," said Kay.

(Dr. Garner died in November 2005.)

DR. OLIVE E.M. SADLER

Dr. Olive Sadler was born in Ottawa in 1898 (a year made famous by Marie Curie's discovery of radium and polonium), the same night that Eddie's Match Factory across the river in Hull exploded.

After moving from Ottawa to Victoria, British Columbia as a child,

Olive went on to gain an MSc in bacteriology and chemistry from the University of British Columbia. She met her future husband, Professor Wilfred Sadler, an agricultural scientist studying pasteurization of milk, while she was working in the laboratory of the Vancouver General Hospital. They were married happily for ten years before his tragic death in 1933.

Olive graduated from McGill University Medical School in 1940. She interned in Montreal, at the Children's Hospital in San Francisco, and at the Vancouver General Hospital. For four-and-a-half years, she had a private practice in Vancouver and worked part-time at the B.C. Cancer Institute.

A new chapter of Dr. Sadler's life began when, while studying radiation therapy, she met Dr. Ethlyn Trapp, a radiotherapist, and joined her research project on breast cancer. Olive went on to residency programs in therapeutic radiology at the Mount Sinai and Sloan Kettering Institute in New York and the State Cancer Hospital in Columbia, Missouri. In 1949, she joined Dr. Trapp as a partner in her private practice of radiotherapy. Dr. Sadler opened the Radiotherapy Department at the Royal Columbian Hospital in New Westminster in 1954 and worked there part-time, becoming full time in 1957, when Dr. Trapp retired and the private clinic closed.

Dr. Sadler's kindness to patients was legendary. She set up the Olive Sadler Fund to help cancer patients in the days when they had to pay for their chemotherapy. In some cases, patients from remote regions stayed at Dr. Sadler's home as guests while they underwent treatment. Her cheerful calm and unaffected generosity comforted the sick, and many of these patients became her friends for life.

Dr. Sadler's philosophy was to help her patients live and be useful while they still could. According to one story, to forestall the departure of a patient whose birthday fell within the course of treatment, Dr. Sadler arranged a candlelight dinner complete with champagne for the woman, her husband, and their dog.

Anecdotes about this marvellous lady abound. As an intern in San Francisco, she and her fellow interns often worked for seven days around the clock. Because they were not allowed to leave the grounds while on duty, Olive organized rooftop barbecues. On one occasion, seeing smoke coming from the roof, the administrator called the fire department. All the guilty interns were threatened with dismissal until Olive managed to persuade the Board to be lenient.

Olive's spirit was not dampened by this encounter. During her internship at Vancouver General Hospital, she was known to sneak her dog into her room, and once, in keeping with the spirit of the season, she managed to steam a Christmas pudding in an old sterilizer at the Royal Columbian Hospital!

Olive's retirement as a radiotherapist in 1969 did not mean the end of her medical career. After discovering that her island paradise, Thetis, did not have a physician, Dr. Sadler returned to her hospital emergency ward for a refresher course in emergency medicine and surgery. With the help of a nurse and later a retired fireman, she established first-aid stations at various points on the island. The summer flood of visitors brought with them no lack of work and, although she was now in her seventies, Dr. Sadler placed herself on twenty-four-hour call. Many times her own guests had to wait while she stitched a laceration in the utility-cum-emergency room in her home.

In 1975, at the age of seventy-seven, Olive died from leukemia in Vancouver after a full and rich life. Highlights of her professional career included being physician to the nursing school at Vancouver General Hospital, an appointment to the B.C. Cancer Institute, Certification in Therapeutic Radiology by the Royal College of Physicians and Surgeons of Canada, and active involvement in the Federation of Medical Women of Canada, the Red Cross Society, St. John's Ambulance, and the British Columbia Medical Association. She was also paid the unusual tribute of a testimonial banquet by the medical staff of the Royal Columbian Hospital and was made a Senior Member of the Canadian Medical Association.

(The story of Dr. Olive Sadler was written by Dr. Frances Forrest-Richards for the Pioneer Profile section of the FMWC Newsletter *issue of Spring 1993. Dr. Forrest-Richards gave her permission to include her most informative and delightful profile of Dr. Sadler in this book.)*

1943

DR. ELDA LINDENFELD

Elda Lindenfeld was born in Trieste in 1898 and received her medical degree in Vienna in 1922. In 1939, she escaped from Germany to Canada with her young son Peter, leaving her husband behind in a concentration camp. Barely able to speak English, Dr. Lindenfeld ran a small electrolysis practice in Vancouver, British Columbia, until the B.C. Medical Association agreed to allow her to sit the examinations of the Medical Council of Canada. The association insisted, however, that Dr. Lindenfeld would have to attend a Canadian medical school for one year before taking the exam. This condition was not applied to immigrant men doctors. Even her husband, a dermatologist, was able to establish a practice shortly after emigrating to Canada at a later date. Although Dr. Lindenfeld had been offered an "enabling certificate" to sit the examinations by the Premier of Alberta, Bill Aberhart, she chose not to circumvent the decision of the British Columbian Medical Association in this way, fearing that she might face hostility upon her return.

Thanks to a loan from the Vancouver Jewish community, Dr. Lindenfeld was able to pay for one year's tuition at the University of Manitoba Medical School. After completing her supplementary studies in 1942, she worked briefly at provincial mental hospitals in Portage La Prairie and Brandon, Manitoba. Upon her return to Vancouver, she sat and passed the Medical Council and board examinations, and began instructing nursing and social work students at the University of British Columbia. Later she was hired as a clinical instructor by the university when the medical school opened in 1950.

According to her son Peter Lindenfeld, his mother always felt like an outsider in the medical profession, not only because she was a woman, but also because she was an immigrant espousing foreign methods and theories. She had worked with Alfred Adler in Vienna, and was later sympathetic to the views of Freud. For these reasons, she often found it difficult to deal with the medical establishment in Vancouver. Despite such obstacles, she enjoyed her work and was admired by many.

Dr. Elda Lindenfeld died in 1967. Her son Peter prepared an evocatively-written memorial address, designed as a letter to his children about their grandmother.

Dear Tommy and Naomi,

This letter is for you because you are her grandchildren.

You know Elda as a grandmother whom you saw only for a few days at a time. I want you to know a little more about her, about the kind of person she was, and about the kind of life that she lived.

I am flying over Canada, passing over the country which I first crossed with her, nearly thirty years ago. I was about as old as you are now, Tommy, but I was a thin tuberculous child. I was all she had—my father was in a concentration camp in Germany that few survived—and she fought and worked like an animal protecting her young to get me and herself away from the horror that was descending on the Jews in Europe.

We were in the train from Montreal to Vancouver for four days—I still remember the black seats and the stuffiness of the air. Another boy gave me some comic books. I had never seen any and didn't understand them. We were in a country that had only been a page in a geography book for us, where people spoke a language Elda knew only slightly, and I not at all.

She had to start a completely new life. There were many people who helped, but it was her courage, her drive and determination which I want to tell you about today.

Her eyes had always been bad, but now she worked for years, squinting and straining, removing hair from women's faces. She hated the work, but it was a start, and in the meantime I could go to school.

She believed that what the world needed most was more sanity. She worked all her life to bring people closer to sanity, to an understanding of themselves and an understanding of others. She believed that on the largest scale peace between people and between peoples would come when more individuals had this understanding, this sanity themselves.

She brought her whole warmth and humanity to this work and it was here that she came closest to fulfillment. She helped many people, and she was loved and admired by many people for it.

It is a rare kind of person who has the wisdom and insight that this work requires. She had this gift to a very high degree. Sometimes it failed her; sometimes she was not able to use it with herself or some of those closest to her.

Elda only rarely came close to inner peace and serenity. She always wanted more—more physical activity, more mental activity—to see more, to do more, to help more, to give more, and to understand more. She might have been happier had she been able to be more passively accepting, but that was not her way.

I believe, as she believed, that our lives have meaning only through our contact with others.

(The biography was copied with permission from the book: Pioneers All, Women Psychiatrists in Canada: A History, *by Judith H. Gold, CM, MD, FRCPC; Martine Lalinec-Michaud, MD, FRCPC; and Odette Bernazzani, MD, CSPQ, FRCPC, PhD., published by the Canadian Psychiatric Association, 1995. The Memorial Address by Peter Lindenfeld to his children was quoted with his permission. Peter Lindenfeld has retired from Rutgers University after forty-six years of teaching in the Physics Department.)*

DR. MARGUERITE B. SHEA (CARROLL) (1905–1987)

Dr. Marguerite B. Shea was born in 1905 and graduated in medicine from the University of Toronto in 1933. She married Russell Shea, a school teacher, and was widowed with two small children. In 1943, she came to Vancouver to live with her parents, Colonel and Mrs. Brown, in Shaughnessy. Working as a general practitioner, she assisted Dr. David Freeze as a part-time anesthetist at Vancouver General Hospital, completing her anesthesia training under Dr. M.D. Leigh at VGH in 1949. Dr. Shea married Dr. John Carroll who later became Head of Anesthesia at Grace Hospital and Burnaby Hospital. She gave up full-time practice in 1950 and retired in 1959 after assisting her husband for a few years.

Staff members and residents remembered the kindness exhibited by Marguerite and her parents in the late 1940s and early 1950s; she received

the Emily Award for her Thespian activities. She had two sons, four grandchildren, and two great-granddaughters at the time of her death in 1987.

DR. MARGARET BUCHANAN FORSTER SYLLING (1899–1978)

Dr. Margaret Sylling was born in Victoria, B.C. in 1899. Her mother was Dr. Margaret MacMillan Forster who graduated from Trinity in Ontario in 1895 and practised in Victoria between 1896 and 1900. Dr. Sylling graduated from the University of Toronto with an MB in 1925, LCP&S, Ontario in 1925, and an MD from Toronto in 1930. After graduation she practised as a medical missionary in Hunan, China, for several years, and served during the years of the China-Japanese war in north China.

She returned to Canada and in British Columbia passed the LMCC exams and registered with the B.C. College of Physicians and Surgeons in 1943. Dr. Sylling worked in Tranquille, B.C. for a short time prior to establishing a very busy general practice in Vancouver. She married Captain Kaare. Dr. Sylling practised medicine in B.C. for a total of twenty-five years and died on May 5, 1978 at the age of seventy-nine.

DR. AGNES BLACK WESTON (MRS. KENNETH CAMPBELL) (1910–2003)

Agnes was born on May 1, 1910, the fifth child of a Scottish couple, Henry and Margaret Black, in New Jersey, U.S.A. Her father was a naval architect, much in demand in the British Isles and in North America. During her pregnancy with Agnes, her mother travelled with her father twice across the Atlantic to England. At the age of seven, Agnes remembered meeting Thomas Edison, a friend of her parents, in New Jersey.

The family moved to Dunblane, Scotland, in August 1920. The children were sent to boarding schools—the girls to Bridge of Alan and the boys to

Perth. It was a sad time for everyone. Jim, aged eight, developed diphtheria in his first term, followed by a palatal paralysis. In 1925, Agnes and her sister Margaret went to school in Lausanne-Suisse. At the age of sixteen, she returned to Glasgow, Scotland, to start the study of medicine. In the pre-clinical years she studied zoology, biology, physics, and chemistry.

An honour in her early teens was an invitation to christen the CSL ship SS Kamloops. The life and tragedy of this ship is well documented in the book *Passage to the Sea* by Edgar Collend.

In 1927 and 1929, Agnes journeyed to Vancouver, British Columbia. The first visit was to attend the wedding of her brother, William Black, who later became head of the accounting firm of KPMG. The second visit was to see her niece Maureen, born in 1928, who was later to become a senator in the state of New Jersey, marry Robert Ogden, and have three wonderful boys.

Agnes graduated in medicine in 1933 with a MB, ChB. She did a post-graduate year as a Senior Resident at the Hospital for Sick Children in Glasgow which she enjoyed, and researched into the causes of hypertension in elderly people for a year. She remembered Prontosil being a great saver of lives in 1936/37; puerperal fever was prevalent at that time. She was especially interested in Bacteriology, and after a vacation spent with her parents at Ste. Agathe in Quebec and Nassau, in 1936 she returned to England and was offered a job as a bacteriologist for the London City Council.

In the summer of 1939, Agnes crossed the Atlantic again to visit her parents in Toronto where she saw her father for the last time, as he died in 1940. Three days after leaving New York while returning to England, war broke out, and the ship *Aquatania*, zigzagged across the Atlantic Ocean to avoid detection. She was recruited into the army RAMC as one of the first women doctors and was posted to Folkstone as Lieutenant, and later to Brighton, Bournemouth, Tidworth, Bath, and Bristol where she was promoted to Captain. Her mother was ill in Vancouver, B.C. and Agnes was released from the army on compassionate grounds in January, 1943, to assist her mother. At that time four of her brothers and a nephew were in the services. Dr. Agnes Black lived with her mother on 6th Avenue in Vancouver, and in the same year was appointed by Dr. Stewart Murray, head of the Metropolitan Health Service, as the first woman Medical Health Officer in Burnaby, B.C., which was then a small town.

In June 1946, Agnes was married to G.H. Weston. A son, Bruce, was born in 1947 and a daughter, Margo, was born in 1948. Agnes and her family moved to Duncan and then to Courtenay, where she continued in Public Health as Dr. Agnes Weston. A Mrs. Sorenson became a great family friend and stayed with the family for eight-and-a-half years, caring for the children while Agnes worked. Agnes covered a wide territory from Campbell River to Courtenay, and had to fly by seaplane to more isolated villages.

Divorced in 1952, Agnes went to eastern Canada to look for work, but decided to return to B.C. Dr. Reba Willits and Dr. Stewart Murray were very good to her, and along with providing employment also encouraged her to take the Fellowship exam. She became a Fellow of the Royal College of Physicians of Canada in 1956. This was a tremendous feat for a single mother of two children: to work and study and successfully obtain a Specialist degree. Agnes continued her career in Public Health and did a great deal of preventative work in Psychiatry and Geriatric Medicine, stressing the need for greater health for the aged. The Metropolitan Health Service of Greater Vancouver, in an effort to meet this need, established a "60 and up" Health Centre in November 1966. The response to this augmentation of the health services was so great that it was extended to include the five health units within the City of Vancouver at that time. Agnes enjoyed her work with Dr. Murray, and at the Outpatient Department at Vancouver General Hospital.

Agnes was recruited into the army RAMC as one of the first women doctors and was posted to Folkstone as Lieutenant, and later to Brighton, Bournemouth, Tidworth, Bath, and Bristol where she was promoted to Captain.

Agnes and her family lived on Laburnum Street in Vancouver for fifteen years. By then Bruce and Margo had graduated from their respective schools. In 1970, Bruce married and subsequently had three children; Margo became a Psychologist. Both still live and work in Vancouver.

The rule at the Metropolitan Health Service was that women had to retire at sixty years of age while men could continue until the age of sixty-five. The B.C. Branch, Federation of Medical Women of Canada presented a brief to the government by President Dr. Patricia Rebbeck to appeal this rule, without success. Agnes was now sixty years of age and was compelled to retire. She was then offered a job with the Workmen's Compensation Board in 1970. The same year she married Kenneth Campbell, who had three grown sons who all had worked for CUSO at one time or another. Agnes had bought a cottage on Bowen Island in 1965. She and Kenneth lived in their condo in West Vancouver, and shared many enjoyable times both there and on Bowen Island. Ken loved to fish; Agnes was an enthusiastic golfer from the age of ten until age seventy-five when a back injury forced her to retire from the game. The Marine Drive Golf Club had been her course for many years.

On a flight home from a winter vacation in 1983, Agnes developed a thrombosis in the left leg along with an embolus to the lung and was very ill. Some years later Kenneth became ill with cancer of the liver; he died in 1992. Agnes gave the cottage and property on Bowen Island to Bruce and Margo and moved to Arbutus Manor where she lived for five years. In 1994 Agnes developed asthma and this required her to move to the Windermere Care Centre where she resided for ten years. Even in her nineties she managed her arthritis, asthma, and a hearing problem, and was mentally alert and still very engaged in life and learning.

Travels during her life were always interesting. They included a 500-mile cycling trip with her sister in 1932 to the magnificent Highlands of Scotland, Canada from ocean to ocean, and almost all of the U.S.A. In 1973, she also journeyed to the Far East with Ken Campbell, who had two sons in Thailand and friends in Japan and Hong Kong. In 1978, she enjoyed a cruise through the Panama Canal, ending at Christmas with her brother Jim and his wife Hope at "Little Orchard" in Tyron, North Carolina.

On May 1, 2000, Margo and Bruce hosted a Black family reunion to celebrate Agnes' ninetieth birthday. About fifty relatives and friends from as far away as the Yukon, New Zealand, Switzerland, Scotland, and several locations in the U.S. came to Vancouver. It was a wonderful tribute to Agnes and a great event for the Black clan.

During most of her medical career she was Dr. Agnes B. Weston, MB, ChB, MD, DPH, LMCC, FRCP—a very special person who stressed that she had a wonderful life and great support from her children.

(The story of Dr. Agnes Weston was written from interviews with her in 2000, and with help from her daughter, Margo. Dr. Weston died in January, 2003, in her 93rd year.)

DR. FLORENCE NICHOLS (HAINES)
(1913-1987)

Florence Nichols was a medical missionary. In 1944 she was the first female psychiatrist missionary in the small coastal towns of British Columbia. Later she developed a magnificent department of psychiatry in a Christian medical college in Vellore, India. She was a prolific writer and an astute clinician, who never allowed religious dogma to obscure her clinical judgements.

A realist with a vision, in Canada Dr. Nichols persuaded her colleagues to start family therapy in the prison setting long before the Canadian Penitentiary Service officially adopted the policy of conjugal visits. She laid the foundation that would subsequently form the basis of the Ethical Principles of Prison Health Care Officials (enshrined in the Oath of Athens).

With her husband, Douglas Haines, she again came to British Columbia to work with Dr. C. Roy at a maximum prison psychiatric hospital in Abbotsford, B.C. From 1974 until her retirement in 1979 she pioneered the treatment of sex offenders in federal prisons. Her book *Understanding Sexual Attacks* was a Canadian first.

(The above information was copied from the In Memoriam column of the BCMJ of July, 1988, written by Dr. C. Roy.)

DR. MARGARET FLORENCE BURRIDGE
HARDIE
(1898–1984)

Margaret (Mardi) Burridge was born November, 1898, in Saint John, New Brunswick. She grew up in Victoria where she received her early education. She obtained a Teacher's Certificate and taught school in Victoria for several years, then went off to Toronto to study medicine where she graduated in 1924 with an MB. Mardi likely saw insulin being given for the first time as well as earning her big "T" as the champion women's tennis player.

Mardi married Roderick Campbell Hardie in 1924. Rod was an electrical engineer who had also graduated from the University of Toronto. They returned to British Columbia to live in Vancouver where they had three children: Jean (1927), Nan (1928), and Rod (1937).

Due to health reasons and raising a young family, Dr. Hardie did not return to medicine until 1942 during the Second World War. She was asked by Dr. Ethlyn Trapp to come and help out at the B.C. Cancer Institute. She did some interning at the Vancouver General Hospital while working at the BCCI and passed her Licensure of the Medical Council of Canada in 1944. This was quite an accomplishment considering the years since her graduation, working, and running a busy household with two teenage daughters and a seven-year-old boy.

Mardi soon took a special interest in gynecological cancer. In the early 1950s she studied in Manchester, England, and in Uppsala, Sweden. Successfully writing her specialist examination in therapeutic radiology in 1953 at age fifty-five, she became one of three female therapeutic radiologists in the province at the time. Mardi ran the gynecological service at the BCCI until her retirement in 1962. Her other main interest was dermatological malignancies. She was also a Clinical Instructor, Department of Surgery, in the Faculty of Medicine at the University of British Columbia.

Mardi helped get the cytology program started at the BCCI, along with Dr. Maxwell Evans, Dr. Herb Fidler, and Dr. Alex Agnew. This program has gone on to have an international reputation.

In the late 1940s consultative clinics were started in the province. Dr. Hardie drove to the Okanagan Clinics in all kinds of weather for many years. This was a great service to the local doctors and their patients, allowing them to be followed in their own community and preventing needless travel.

Mardi, as she was known to all, was a long time supporter of the B.C. and Yukon Division of the Canadian Cancer Society. Early on she became aware of the emotional and family needs of women, especially young women with ovarian cancer. To this end she was instrumental in starting the first Patient Services Program of the Cancer Society, and was chairperson of the Patient Services Committee for many years.

Mardi was a very gracious and friendly person, dedicated to her patients as they were to her. There was a quiet dignity about her, a great attribute in a clinical setting. One of her daughters said that she had "healing hands." Those who knew her would agree.

On retirement Mardi and her husband went around the world on a freighter. At the Club Med in Agadir, Morocco, where the language was French of which they knew little, they became the bridge champions of North Africa. On their return they moved to their home—"Yellow Cedars" at Yellow Point on Vancouver Island. They had a huge garden and sold produce to the local stores, and both regularly and successfully fished for salmon. They enjoyed duplicate bridge and would travel up and down the island many miles for a game. "Yellow Cedars" was a fun place to visit for their children and grandchildren, and Rod and Mardi spent many happy years there. Only latterly did they return to Vancouver, where Mardi died at the age of eighty-five in 1984 and Rod a few years later at ninety-two.

(The above was written by Mardi's son-in-law, Dr. Richard Beck.)

DR. EVELYN MAY (WOODMAN) FOX
(1920–1986)

During her years in General Practice and as Alcan Medical Officer, Evelyn visited Kemano, the village where the power station for the Kitimat smelter works was located, to attend medical clinics for the Alcan employees in Kemano. This necessitated many trips by boat and/or helicopter in all kinds of weather, at times very nerve-wracking. She served the medical needs of the people of the First Nations in Kitimat Village—some of whom became her long-term friends. As Kitimat had a population of young people in the early days, Evelyn's medical practice was largely maternity, and she delivered many babies into the world.

When Evelyn was in the Army and posted at Harrison Hot Springs, she lectured in many places in B.C., one of which was Prince Rupert. As Charles R. approached graduation from UBC in 1949 and went job hunting, Evelyn told him that she would go anywhere in Canada with him except northwestern B.C. Little did she realize that in 1953 she would move with her family to Kitimat and reside there (in northwestern B.C.) for the next twenty-four years!

In addition to her medical practice, Evelyn was Cub Leader for the 2nd Kitimat Cub Pack, Commissioner for the Kitimat Girl Guides, Chair Person of the Conquer Cancer campaign, Vice-President of the Kitimat Red Cross, President of the Canadian Citizenship Committee, President of the Kitimat Business and Professional Women Club, and in 1974 was nominated as Kitimat Citizen of the Year.

Charles Fox writes an amusing story about his wife Evelyn:

"When Evelyn first arrived in Kitimat in December 1953, she decided to take a rest from General Practice for awhile. At that time there was only one doctor in Kitimat (Dr. Phil Margetts) who looked after the populace composed of construction workers and a few of their families. Within the first two weeks the resident doctor had to leave Kitimat for an extended period (his wife had died suddenly). Evelyn was required to enter practice again. One incident that she was called upon to attend was an attack (actually a rape) on one of the female residents of the community.

Even though she never really condoned working mothers, she admitted she enjoyed her medical work. Her father believed that all girls should be educated for making a living, she said, and she believed that this is still good advice.

"Some time later the court case was convened in Prince Rupert and Evelyn was summoned to act as a witness for the prosecution. As Evelyn didn' know how long the case would go on, she packed her suitcase to prepare for a lengthy stay. At that time medical expenses were entered on IBM cards which were submitted for payment, so she included a load of IBM cards to be filled out from her records, to work on during idle time.

"In those days there was a passenger train running from Kitimat to Terrace, and passengers were separated, the men in the back cars and the females in the front.

"So off Evelyn went with her loaded suitcase heading for Terrace and on to Prince Rupert. The conductor started to collect tickets at the back of the train and then forward to the front car, asking if there was a Dr. Fox on the train. Evelyn identified herself and the conductor advised her that he had just received a message that the accused had pled guilty and that she was not required to go to Prince Rupert. Evelyn had no desire to go to Terrace or Prince Rupert to wait for the next train back to Kitimat, so she asked the conductor to stop the train and let her out, as she thought they had just left the Kitimat Station. She assured the conductor that that was what she wanted, so the train was stopped and she got out with her suitcase. Only as the train disappeared out of sight did she realise that she was miles from the station in the middle of nowhere, with dusk falling, rain falling, and bears all around. So off she set to walk back to the station and only then did she notice the weight of her suitcase, and how ill-equipped she was for walking.

"For this trip she had worn a new light raincoat, high-heels, and a suit, none of which was the proper gear for walking miles down the track in pouring rain. At one point she met some workers heading in the direction of Terrace and heard one say to the other, 'Wonder if she walked all the way from Terrace.' After walking several miles worrying about bears, she arrived back at the Kitimat Station and asked the Station Master to phone her husband to come and get her. She overheard the Station Master saying 'there is someone here who says she is your wife and wants you to come and get her.' I went to the station and found my wife soaking wet, with very sore feet and ready to throw her suitcase at anyone who laughed. Later she vowed never again to get off a train in the middle of nowhere or to walk on a railroad track in high-heels or take a load of IBM cards with her on a trip."

In 1960, in an interview for the *Sentinel*, the Kitimat newspaper, Dr. Evelyn Fox described her arrival in Kitimat in 1953. The Smeltersite Hospital at Kitimat could accommodate about ten patients, with an operating room, dentist office, and offices for herself and Dr. Margetts. Now (1960) there was a big, new hospital, a wonderful thing for Kitimat. Even though she never really condoned working mothers, she admitted she enjoyed her medical work. Her father believed that all girls should be educated for making a living, she said, and she believed that this was still good advice.

In 1976, the B.C. Legionnaires made a donation to the Kidney Foundation of Canada (Vancouver) of a $35,000 mobile home and dialysis machine, to be used on a first come, first serve basis for one's holidays. There was no charge, other than gasoline and operating expenses, for its use. In September 1976, for the first time since 1970 when Evelyn began dialysis, she and Charles were able to travel free of the inconvenience of booking into hospitals for the four-and-a-half hours of treatment three times a week, Monday, Wednesday, and Friday. Thanks to the Pacific Command of the Royal Canadian Legion, Evelyn was able to accompany her husband to the annual meeting of the Association of Professional Engineers of B.C. at Fairmont Hot Springs and continue on their two-week holiday through the southern part of B.C. In the early 1960s, Evelyn came under the care of Dr. J.D. Price in Vancouver, and she and her husband made annual visits to Vancouver for her medical check-ups. We were told that when Evelyn's creatinine level reached a certain point that she would have to go on hemodialysis. In the fall of 1969 we were told that Evelyn's kidneys were failing, her creatinine level was up, and we should prepare for hemodialysis. That was a long and sad trip back to Kitimat, as we faced an uncertain future and Evelyn was far from well. Her husband continues with her story:

"In November 1969 Evelyn went to Vancouver and on the 24th had her first peritoneal dialysis. She commenced a two-month period of getting her blood chemistry back to normal and learning how to handle a hemodialysis machine. I went to Vancouver in January, 1970, to take a two-week course on machine maintenance and how to be the care-giver, machine operator, helper, or whatever it took to administer a home dialysis program. Possibly it was because Evelyn was a doctor and I was an engineer that we were the first couple, other than those in the Vancouver and Victoria areas, allowed to go home and carry out a Home Dialysis Program.

'During seventeen years there were many changes to the equipment used, the systems of blood stream entry, and the medications. The physician problems and operations with many trips to Vancouver General or the Royal Jubilee Hospitals had to be endured, and the one aspect of dialysis that cannot be under-rated is the mental strain and the fact that three times a week, come hell or high water, you have to be connected to a machine for a length of time, and all other activities have to make way for that. At times Evelyn would just pray that she could have a week free from the machine, but then we would have to get back on schedule, Monday, Wednesday, and Friday. The same today, tomorrow, and forever!"

Evelyn's husband describes so well the ordeals of such a severe kidney condition and has nothing but praise for the medical and other staff in the Central and Home Dialysis Units at the Vancouver General and Royal Jubilee Hospitals. Evelyn had dialysis number 2,612 on August 8th, 1986, and she died on August 9th, 1986.

(Charles R. Fox, husband of Dr. Evelyn Fox for thirty-nine years, provided the above story of his wife in July 2000, along with copies of clippings and pictures of this amazing woman who defied ill-health for so long. I am sure their son Charles and daughter Jean gave Charles great support during his writing and collecting material in response to my request. I know the project must have been difficult for him.—E.C.)

Personal: Born in Pinawa, Manitoba, 1920; married Charles R. Fox in Fort Frances, Ontario, 1947; son Charles W. born in Arvida, 1950; daughter F. Jean born in Arvida, 1953.

Early education: Fort Frances, Ontario, 1926.

Medical studies: Premedical studies for two years, 1939; Medical School, University of Manitoba, 1941; Joined Royal Canadian Army Medical Corps, Camp Borden, Ontario, 1943; graduated from Medical School, University of Manitoba, posted to Canadian Women Army Corps, Harrison Hot Springs, B.C., and lectured to WACs throughout B.C. on the perils of VD, 1944; discharged from the Canadian Army and began a Residency in Shaughnessy Hospital, Vancouver, B.C., 1946.

Professional: Entered General Practice in Arvida, 1949; moved to Isle Maligne, PQ, with Charles and continued in General Practice in both Arvida and Isle Maligne, 1951: began a General Practice in Kitimat, BC., 1954; diagnosed as having polycystic kidneys, retired from General Practice and was appointed as Medical Officer for Alcan, Kitimat, 1960; renal failure, she and Charles trained in Home Dialysis at Vancouver General Hospital and were the first dialysis team allowed out of the Vancouver-Victoria area to practise Home Dialysis, 1969.

Retirement: She and Charles moved to Victoria, B.C. and Evelyn retired from all medical work, 1977; after seventeen years on hemodialysis (home program), Evelyn died in 1986. At that time, she had been on Home Dialysis longer than any patient in B.C.

DR. LUCILLE G. ELLISON
(1922–2005)

Lucille Ellison (nee Sheps) was the fourth of five children and the only girl. Three of her brothers went into medicine—the other went to law school. When Lucy applied to medical school at the University of Manitoba she had to contend with a form of double discrimination in the selection process, that against Jews and other ethnic groups as well as that against female applicants, since quotas were applied to both, leading to fierce competition for places. During WW II as a medical student, she was a private in the Army, in an accelerated course, and graduated in 1945.

She and Dr. Earl Ellison, a dentist, were married in December 1943. Their coming together required special permission as marriage between officers and other ranks was not commonly allowed. Earl was then posted to England for the rest of the war.

After medical school she interned in Victoria, reasonably close to where Earl was then stationed and was promoted to Lieutenant. Her brother recalls that she asked her mother to come to Vancouver to stay with her in a hotel while she studied the materials for the licensing exam—out loud! Victor Mature, a movie idol of their mother's, was in the next room and, from their mother's viewpoint, saved the day as she had no clue about what Lucy was memorising and was totally bored. She was then posted to Camp Borden near Toronto, an advanced training centre for the Canadian Armoured Corps and the Army Service Corps.

After they were both demobilised, Lucy and Earl came to Vancouver. Lucy said that having left Winnipeg at forty degrees below and arriving in Vancouver only to be invited to play tennis the next day, she had no doubts about where she wanted to stay!

A stroke of good fortune occurred in February 1947 when she was appointed to the medical staff at the B.C. Cancer Institute (BCCI) where she remained for forty years! During this time she left an indelible mark on many aspects of the BCCI (later to become the B.C. Cancer Agency).

Lucy's main clinical interest was the hormonal management of patients with breast cancer, but perhaps her most enduring contribution was to medical records. She established the first comprehensive database of patient information in the form of punch cards and took upon herself the arduous and unpopular job of reviewing all new patient charts for completeness. Her personality was such that she managed to obtain compliance. There were many jokes about the "greenslips" on the front of the charts, but when any of us or our residents wanted to review charts for outcome or complications of treatment, we recognised the importance of her supervision and the discipline of record keeping.

When she retired, Lucy asked that her leaving present be in the form of a prize for the best suggestion to enhance patient comfort. Many relatively small changes due to these suggestions have been made with disproportionate effect, for example a bench by the entrance to the parking lot. A group of her old patients clubbed together to endow a Book Prize for the resident delivering the best presentation at the Annual Resident's Day of the Division of Radiation Oncology. It is listed among the awards offered by the University of British Columbia. Her contribution to the people of British Columbia was recognised by the College of Physicians and Surgeons in 1988 when she was made an Honorary Life Member—the highest award offered by the College.

Despite Lucy's very busy professional life she raised two children—Russell (who also became a physician) and Roslyn, who lives in Vancouver, and was a major support to her mother during her final illness.

The above comments would not be compete without mentioning her dedication to the cancer patients of B.C., and her loyalty to her colleagues and friends, among whom I have the honour to count myself and my family.

(Written by Vivien Basco, who also acknowledges the contributions of Sheldon G. Sheps, MD; Stewart Jackson, MD, in his book Radiation as a Cure for Cancer; *and Sarah H. Tobe from a conversation with Dr. Ellison for the Jewish Historical Society.)*

1946

DR. MARGARET ADELE MULLINGER

I graduated from the University of Toronto in February, 1946. We were the last war-time class in medicine. There were few places for women to intern because of returning servicemen, so I came to the Vancouver General Hospital along with six others from Toronto.

We were all housed in the interns residence on Heather Street, opposite the hospital's drive-in gate. There were an interesting group of residents and interns at that time. The rotating internship was very good in its wide variety. At that time the children's wards were divided; B was the boys' ward, C was for toddlers, and D was for older girls. The infants were housed in the Infants' Hospital on Haro Street (now long gone). In pediatric rotation the teaching was done by the practising pediatricians, so the quality was a reflection of their training, experience, and interest. I remember Dr. John Davies, Dr. Ted Curtiss, Dr. Gordon Mathews, Dr. Joe Grant, and Dr. Reg Kinsman. Dr. Reg Wilson and Dr. Archie Hardyment joined this flotilla, followed eventually by Dr. Harold Krivel and Dr. Ben Shuman when they returned from the armed services. I cannot remember any women pediatricians, but I have vivid memories of Dr. Ethlynn Trapp and Dr. Margaret Hardie who worked at the Cancer Agency. The women doctors were always very kind to the women interns and residents, and invited them to meetings and social get-togethers, which sometimes were held at the home of Dr. Josephine Mallek.

When I finished my intern year, Dr. Kinsman asked me to work with him until a young doctor in pediatric training would join him. This I did, and he kindly taught me the art of actually practising pediatrics. However, I finally got an appointment to work in the Department of Pediatrics of the Massachusetts General Hospital in September 1947, to work under Dr. Samuel Butler and Dr. Gertrude Riesbach. That was a stimulating experience because I could also attend all the Grand Rounds in adult medicine and mingle with people from all over the world who were doing their specialty training. In July 1948, I trained at the Hospital for Sick Children in Toronto under Dr. William Donohue and Dr. Ted Roy for a year. I continued at the same hospital as resident in pediatrics under Dr. Allan Brown for two years. I then became a Research Fellow at the Sick Children's Hospital in Toronto and at St. Christopher's Hospital, Temple University, Philadelphia for 1952-1953, under Dr. Waldo Nelson, working with Dr. Helen Reardon.

I joined the Faculty of Medicine in the Department of Pediatrics, University of British Columbia in July 1953. I was a Research Fellow under Dr. Jack McCreary, doing research in neonatology. I obtained Certification in Pediatrics by the Royal College of Physicians and Surgeons of Canada and later FRCP(C).

During the subsequent years until retirement from the University I rose in the academic ranks to Associate Professor in 1966. I worked with the Cystic Fibrosis Clinic at the Health Centre for Children at the Vancouver General Hospital, developed the division of Pediatric Gastroenterology, and continued with research in gastroenterology. During the last fifteen years before retirement I was in charge of the teaching program for pediatrics in the third-year student program. I continued to do consultations and teaching until retirement in 1986.

I married Dr. Abraham Bogoch and we have three children, Sarah, David, and Ruth. A life member of Vancouver Hadassah, I served as president of Shalom chapter for two years each on two different occasions, campaigned for Youth Alijah, and served on the board of education for Vancouver Talmud Torah School for several years. I have been a member of the Beth Israel sisterhood for over thirty years, and have worked on the board for the Canadian Friends of the Hebrew University.

I was made a Prince of Good Fellows in 1987 by the Vancouver Medical Association and, with my husband Dr. A. Bogoch, I was awarded the University of Judaism Community Service Award in 1987. On my retirement, the Department of Pediatrics and colleagues established an annual award in my name to the student in third year who showed excellence in pediatrics.

Curriculum Vitae

Present Rank: Associate Professor, Faculty of Medicine, Department of
Pediatrics.

Birth place and date: October 22, 1921, Toronto, Ontario.

Undergraduate Education: University of Toronto, 1940-1946, MD.

Special Professional Education: Harvard Medical School; Massachusetts
General Hospital, Post-graduate course, 1946-47; Hospital for Sick
Children, Pathology-Intern, 1947-48; Junior Intern, 1948-49; Senior
Intern, 1949-50; Senior Intern, 1950-51.

Graduate Education: CRCP, 1953; FRCP(C), 1972.

Professional Employment: Research Fellow, Hospital for Sick Children,
Toronto, 1951-52; Research Fellow, St. Christopher's Hospital,
Temple University, 1952-53; Research Fellow, Department of
Pediatrics, University of British Colombia, 1953-55; Teaching
Fellow, Dept. Paediatrics, UBC, 1955-56; Demonstrator, Dept.
Paediatrics, UBC, 1956-57; Clinical Instructor, Dept. Paeds., UBC,
1957-59; Instructor II, Dept. Paeds., UBC, 1959-62; Assistant
Professor, Dept. Paeds., UBC, 1962-66; Associate Professor, Dept.
Paeds., UBC, 19___.

Memberships: Western Society for Paediatric Research, Northwest
Society for Clinical Research, North Pacific Paediatric Society,
Canadian Paediatric Society, B.C. Branch Federation of Medical
Women, Canadian Medical Society, B.C. Division and Paediatric
Division, Nutrition Committee—B.C. Division, CMA (1958:
Member; 1959-65: Chair; Nutrition Committee, CMA, corresponding
member, 1962; Canadian Gastroenterology Association; B.C.
Paediatric Society.

Awards and distinctions: Certification in Paediatrics by the Royal College
of Physicians and Surgeons of Canada, 1952; American Paediatric
Boards, 1953.

Other: Co-ordinated 3-year teaching program in Paediatrics since 1971.

List of Publications:

Cold Hypersensitivity, *CMAJ* May 1948.

Adrenal Insufficiency in Childhood, *CMAJ* 65: 353; 1951.

Cretinism, *CMAJ* 66: 560; 1962

A Survey of the Rh Problem in Toronto 1947-52, *Am. J. Obs. & Gynae*
67: 233; 1954.

Regional Enteritis Involving the Duodenum with Clubbing of the
Fingers and Steatorrhoea, *Gastroenterology* 32: 917; 1959.

Contributor to *Pediatrics*, J. B. Lippincott Co, Philadelphia, pps. 85-96,
121-123; 1957.

Comparison of Arterial & Arterialized Blood in Normal Newborn
Infants and Children with Congenital Heart Lesions, *J. Ped.* 56: 630,
1960.

Gastrectomy in Early Childhood, D.L. Collins, J.H. Black, M.A.
Mullinger, *AMAJ Dis. Child.* 109, 149; 1965.

The Effects of Exogenous Pancreatic Enzymes on Fat Absorption, *Ped.*
42: 523; 1968.

DR. MARY VIOLA RAE
(c. 1905–1984)

Dr. Mary Viola Rae, (Vi, as she was known), graduated from the University of Toronto with a BSc and from the University of Alberta with her MD in 1929. She specialized in pathology and bacteriology, receiving Certification as a specialist from the Royal College of Physicians and Surgeons of Canada in 1946. Vi was the associate director of pathology at Shaughnessy Hospital, Vancouver from 1944 until retirement. She died at age seventy-nine.

1947

DR. ARDETH E. ROBERTSON HASSELGREN

I had no idea when I applied to Medical School at McGill how many applicants they receive annually and how few females were admitted. I had been in Montreal on an NRC scholarship in Botany at McGill, thanks to the efforts of Dr. Bill Argue, head of Botany at the University of New Brunswick. Dr. McIntosh, whose acquaintance I had made while working in the biochemistry laboratory at Royal Victoria Hospital, told me about the loans the government was making available at that time, and blissfully unaware of how slim my chances were, I applied. Guess who the man I had for my interview was: this same Dr. McIntosh! He was a fellow Maritimer, bless him.

My time at McGill was short, due to the war. I started my career in the anatomy lab by being assigned a locker in the men's section, much to the consternation of the delightful old Irishman who made the mistake many people do when your hair was as short as mine was and they don't look below the neck. That mistake was quickly remedied. There were ten girls in my class of 120 (twenty delegated as dental students-to-be), half of them American. I joined the army as soon as possible and thanks to their great cold weather uniforms, I had the coziest winter yet in that city. In the summer we looked like unmade beds.

I received my MD in 1945 and became an intern at the Royal Victoria Hospital. I was handed a very reasonable rotation, but after two months at the prestigious Allan Memorial in Psychiatry, I managed to trade all but two months in Medicine and had ten happy and most enjoyable months working under Dr. D. Ewen Cameron. And no matter what they have accused him of since his death, he was an inspiration to work for. I decided to make my career in Psychiatry, moving west to be the first woman ever hired on the staff at Essondale, under Dr. Crease, another notable man in his day.

After being told by the Specialty Board that I needed all kinds of other training to specialize in the one field in which I had most experience so far, and less further training to specialize in Medicine, I got so annoyed I decided to go for more training in Medicine. I applied to the Vancouver General Hospital and became assistant resident under Dr. G. F. Strong. At the end of the year I was wondering "what next" when Dr. Stuart Stalker from the TB Sanatorium out of Kamloops was looking for staff. I registered with the B.C. College of Physicians and Surgeons in 1947. I liked the idea of working for him and said "why not." There was another female doctor on staff already, Evelyn Gee, a pathologist and surgeon, as well as Dr. Bill

Trapp (Dr. Ethlyn Trapp's nephew) and Dr. Alec Marshall. I had five-and-a-half wonderful years there and made friends for life. It was a great time.

I left that position to get married. My husband had a hotel in Quesnel, most noted for the size of its beer parlour. I only spent a few days at a time in Quesnel and did not have a medical practice there.

My last stint in the medical field was in Victoria. I was offered part-time work in Administration at the Jubilee Hospital, which was most interesting. The head nurses, most Vancouver General Hospital graduates, were a great help to me in that job. When the regular administrator came back, it wasn't long until I was able again to work part-time for Dr. Norman Lockyer, a wonderful man, as an assistant at the Cancer Clinic. That turned out to be a full-time job for fifteen years. All the staff were great to work with, especially the head nurse, Dorothy Sullivan, "Sully" to one and all.

I seem to have wandered from one field to another, but I have no regrets about that. I enjoyed every bit of it and made lifelong friendships along the way.

I seem to have wandered from one field to another, but I have no regrets about that. I enjoyed every bit of it and made lifelong friendships along the way. One of the memorable highlights of my time at the Cancer Clinic was when my teen-aged son came in to call with his hair dyed blue and in cut-offs, he and his friend looking like street kids. They got the bum's rush out the back door so the patients in the waiting room didn't have to gaze on their splendor!

DR. A. PAULINE HUGHES

Dr. Hughes saw many changes in attitudes towards the mentally challenged over the years since she first worked at Woodlands in 1949. With society's attitude of dumping mentally handicapped babies in institutions, by 1968 Woodlands had a waiting list of 500. With 100 babies in a ward, it was hard to give them all the cuddling they needed, recalled Dr. Hughes in an interview for the *Royal City Record/Now* of April 2, 1995. At its height, Woodlands had

1,400 residents. Attitudes began to shift and by the late 1970s Woodlands no longer accepted babies or children. Its new policy stated that no one should be admitted or remain in Woodlands if their needs could be met elsewhere. When Dr. Hughes started at Woodlands, the prevailing belief was that the mentally challenged were incapable of growth and would always remain children mentally. She said in the interview: "By the time I retired in 1984, philosophies had shifted to recognize that each person had the power within them to grow and mature. The objective was to find ways to help them achieve that growth. For some, growth meant learning enough life skills to be able to live on their own and earn their own living. For the severely mentally challenged, growth could mean just learning to swallow. Sometimes, with the proper approach and encouragement, even the profoundly retarded can grow. And that can be a major challenge when the person cannot feed themselves, cannot walk, and has no control over their bowel or bladder."

Today, when a child is born mentally challenged, the parents are encouraged to keep the child at home. And as Dr. Hughes said, with services available to them through the Infant Development Program, these youngsters are likely better off than those placed in a ward with 100 other babies. In regards to deinstitutionalization, Dr. Hughes agreed that smaller units are preferable to massive institutions.

When Dr. Hughes looks back on her years at Woodlands, she fondly remembers the many good times and the great love and appreciation shown by the residents. She claims that if a worker remained for a couple of months, they would be hooked. It was a great place to work and a hard place to leave.

Curriculum Vitae

Education: Bachelor of Science, University of Alberta, Edmonton, Alberta, 1945; Medical Degree, University of Alberta, Edmonton, Alberta, 1948; Specialist Certificate in Psychiatry by the Royal College of Physicians And Surgeons of Canada, 1955.

Career History: Ward Physician, Ponoka Mental Hospital, Alberta (six months), 1948; Physician, Provincial Mental Hospital, New Westminster, B.C. (later called Woodlands), 1949; Physician, Provincial Mental Hospital, Essondale, B.C., 1952; Psychiatric Residency, University of Toronto (year spent in out-patient clinic of the Toronto Psychiatric Hospital) 1953; Travelling Clinic from the Child Guidance Clinic, Vancouver, B.C. (six months), 1954; appointed Deputy Medical Superintendent, Woodlands School, 1955. Retired 1959; part-time Physician, Cancer Clinic, Vancouver, B.C. (approximately six months), 1960; Psychiatrist at Mental Health Clinic, Burnaby, B.C., 1961; Psychiatrist at Woodlands School, New Westminster, B.C., 1962; Director of Psychiatric Services, Woodlands School, New Westminster, B.C., 1965; appointed Medical Superintendent, Woodlands School, New Westminster, B.C., 1968. Retired 1984.

Professional Affiliations & Memberships: College of Physicians and Surgeons of B.C., licensed 1949. Retired 1984; Life Member B.C. and Canadian Medical Associations; previous member of B.C. Psychiatric Association. Director at Large for two years, American Association on Mental Deficiency (AAMD). Joined 1955 and now a Life Member: Region 1 AAMD (WA, OR, ID, AK, B.C.). Chairman 1957–1958 and 1968–1969, Federation of Medical Women of Canada; B.C. Branch President 1966-1967.

Community Involvement & Memberships: Board of Directors, Douglas College, New Westminster, B.C. 1984–1991;. Chairman 1988–1990. Director of CKNW Orphans Fund 1974 to present; University Women's Club of New Westminster; Canadian Club of New Westminster and Fraser Valley; President 1987.

Hobbies & Interests: Grandchildren, family history, gardening, travelling.

DR. JEAN TEMPLETON HUGILL

Jean Hugill was born in 1922 in Calgary, Alberta. Her father was a lawyer who practised in Alberta from 1900 to 1949, and was Attorney-General from 1935 to 1937. Her mother, born in Ontario, worked in Montreal, Chicago, and Calgary worked as a nurse. Jean attended public schools in

Calgary, and the University of Alberta in a combined course BSc-MD from 1940 to 1945 (because of the war the medical course was speeded up). She was the winner of the Paul McLeod prize in organic chemistry in 1942, and joined the Canadian Women's Army Corp in 1943. Dr. Hugill interned in the Edmonton University Hospital and Edmonton General Hospital, and obtained an MD degree in January, 1946. She held the position of Captain RCAMC in 1946, stationed in Currie Barracks, Calgary.

Post-graduate work included the McGill Diploma course in Anesthesia 1946-1949, and resident training at the Montreal General Hospital, Vancouver General Hospital, Shaughnessy Hospital, and the Children's Memorial Hospital in Montreal. She received the Specialist Certification in 1950 and FRCP in 1972 and became a Diplomate of the American Board of Anesthesiology in 1951.

Dr. Hugill practised in Port Alberni at the West Coast Hospital July, 1949 to December, 1950 where, as the first trained anesthetist in the community, she founded the Department of Anesthesia. She then became a Clinical Instructor at the Vancouver General Hospital, and later an assistant Professor at the University of British Columbia and VGH. Dr. Hugill was Head of Obstetrical Anesthesia at VGH from 1951 to 1974, and she continued in all areas of anesthesia and teaching until August, 1985 when she retired.

Her special interests included pioneering the use of spinal and peridural anesthesia in Obstetrics; resuscitation of the newborn and pediatric anesthesia; anesthesia for surgery of adrenal tumours (thirty cases), especially Pheochromocytoma. In research she investigated the problems of water retention during TUPR resection when water was used for irrigation (1958-1962); administered the first intra-arterial transfusion at VGH in 1952; and investigated the hepatitis toxicity of Halothane (1960-1966).

Her publications: Hugill, J.T. and Gillespie, C., "Nupercaine Spinal Anesthesia in Obstetrics," published in the *Canadian Medical Association Journal* in 1948; "Liver Function in Anesthesia," (Thesis for the McGill Diploma Course 1950), published in the *American Journal of Anesthesiology*; Englebrecht, E.R., Hugill, J.T., and Graves, H.B., (1966), "Anesthetic Management of Pheochromocytoma," published in the *Canadian Anesthesia Society Journal*.

Dr. Hugill presented many papers at UBC and VGH refresher courses in Obstetrical Anesthesia, Resuscitation of the Newborn, and other topics related to anesthesia. At the First European Congress of Anesthesiology in Wiens (Vienna) in 1962, she gave a paper on "Reactions to Irrigating Fluid in Prostatic Resection—Anesthetic Considerations." At Banff in 1966 at the Annual Meeting of the Canadian Anesthesia Society she presented a paper on "Anesthetic Managenment of Pheochromocytoma." She attended many national as well as international meetings in Britain, U.S.A., Austria, Germany, and Japan.

Dr. Hugill was awarded a Senior Membership of the Canadian Anesthesia Society in 1990. She established the Jean Templeton Hugill Chair in Anesthesia at UBC in 1991. More recently, in 2002 Dr. Hugill returned to the campus of the University of Alberta and unveiled a plaque recognizing her outstanding financial contributions in making the Multidisciplinary Pain Centre in the Department of Anesthesiology and Pain Medicine a reality.

Dr. Hugill's extracurricular activities are varied: she was a judge of figure skating and dance to the gold medal level for twenty years; she skated and curled at the Arbutus Club from 1968 to 1984; was owner and breeder of English Cocker Spaniels, siring and breeding over thirty champions and top English Cockers in obedience for three years; and was an honorary member of the English Cocker Spaniel Club of Canada as well as a member of the British Columbia Club. (Her kennel name is Beaverlodge; she and her dogs have visited many Extended Care facilities.) Dr. Hugill is a gardener who specializes in fruit tress, and has been active in St. Anselm's Church for over forty years.

DR. MARY A. MURPHY

I was born in Calgary, Alberta on October 16, 1918. My Scottish father worked on farms during the First World War and later became a warehouseman in the wholesale grocery business. My mother and her sister had come to Canada from Belfast during the war to work as domestic help. The family, including a sister a year younger than myself, moved to Vancouver when I was about two.

I grew up near Kitsilano beach and spent a lot of time close to and in the ocean. Summer days were spent at the beach and playgrounds. Our fifteen cents bought us a box of chips and one piece of fish. No one had to worry about what might happen to us—how times have changed.

Childhood was uneventful, or at least I don't remember much of it. My primary school was Henry Hudson a few blocks from where we lived, and from Grades 7 to 12 were spent at Kitsilano High School. I wasn't a particularly outstanding student; one of my math teachers told me I would never get through high school because I was such a disaster in his subject, but I did pass it.

I took dancing lessons and competed in the Highland Games. After learning to play the bagpipes, I became a member of the Vancouver Ladies Pipe Band and later the Glengarry Girls Pipe Band.

I will never forget the first day in anatomy class. The professor was a tall, imposing, stern-looking man with white hair. He stared down at the three female students huddling in the front row and said pointedly, "Don't expect any favours—nobody asked you here." We didn't; two of us topped the class.

After my mother died when I was fifteen, I took over running our household. I remember scrubbing clothes on an old-fashioned scrubbing board and using a hand wringer.

When I graduated from high school in 1936 my father asked me if I was going to go to Normal School (teacher training) or to UBC. Since Normal School had already started, I applied to UBC and was accepted. Along with the required basics, I took mainly biological sciences, and graduated in 1940 with a BA degree. I continued on to obtain a Master of Arts degree in 1943.

During this time I instructed in the biology labs and taught first year University biology at a private night school in Vancouver as well as making most of the slides for the UBC biology classes. My MA thesis was about plant chromosome abnormalities—how much more we know now. There was a war on and I was given the job of sectioning and mounting tissue for a 'hush-hush project.' It was lung tissue that had been exposed to poisonous gas.

When I completed the Masters degree, my professor asked me if I was going to take a PhD and teach, or go to medical school. I had applied for a Government Research position and was told that my name was second on the list, but that I would never get the job because I was a woman. Since I couldn't imagine being a teacher, I applied to the University of Western Ontario in London, Ontario and was accepted as a medical student. My future was determined.

It was quite an experience arriving by train on a dark evening with nothing more than a list of possible boarding homes that took in students. Railway stations are seldom in the most desirable part of town and London was no exception. I phoned a few places, but since the medical school classes started before the rest of the university, the landladies were not prepared to accept students at that time. I finally found a woman who seemed dubious, but since I must have sounded desperate, she told me to come over. I took a taxi to her place, which wasn't far from the station. The house was elderly, as was the proprietor. I was ushered into a gloomy, musty parlour with dark red drapes and carpet, old furniture, and one small lamp on a table in the far corner. One of the first questions the landlady asked was what church I went to. I can't remember how I got out of that one, and I was ready to hop back on the train. But that wasn't possible, and besides, there was nothing to go back for.

The next day I contacted the university and got the addresses of a few boarding houses near the medical school, which was at the other end of town. I ended up staying with two sisters in a small apartment within walking distance of the school. One of the girls had just graduated from the University business school, and the other was a secretary at Kelloggs (the cornflakes one). For two years I slept on a trundle bed and burned the midnight oil there.

Classes started a few days after I moved in. I will never forget the first day in anatomy class. The professor was a tall, imposing, stern-looking man with white hair. He stared down at the three female students huddling in the front row and said pointedly, "Don't expect any favours—nobody asked you here." We didn't; two of us topped the class.

I was called back to Vancouver in late September of 1943, my first year in London, because my father was ill. He had myelogenous leukaemia with the white cell count so high that it interfered with the oxygen supply to his brain, causing severe dementia. His room was in the basement at Vancouver General Hospital—they called it Ward R. It was a very dark small room, with a little barred window in the door; overhead were large pipes. It was very oppressive. My father opened his eyes once and said, "Mary, you're a bonny lassie"—the only communication that occurred. He died on Dec 23rd; I didn't have the money to return for his funeral.

Back at Western, I carried on. We did the four academic years in three; classes were accelerated because of the war. Even then, the number of women in the classes was restricted to ten percent. We worked away quite diligently, liking some subjects and definitely not others. Public health was a joke, but it gave some of us a chance to catch up on our sleep.

The summers were quite short. The first one I spent at Port Stanley, a resort on Lake Erie, dispensing pop and hot dogs. The next summer I was a waitress at the Bigwin Inn in the Muskoka Lake area. The waitresses were under the charge of a large German woman who ruled with military precision. The chefs ran the kitchen. I remember an American woman who ordered well-done roast beef, and when I asked for that, the chef slapped a beautiful piece of rare roast beef on the plate, emphatically stating, "My roast beef is always well done." How can you argue with that?

In my last year at the medical school I lived as an undergraduate intern at the Mental Hospital just outside London. Another of my classmates was there as well. We assisted at any surgery that was done, we immunized the entire hospital against typhoid because of an outbreak there a few years previously, and sutured cuts if a patient had shoved his hand through a window, or if a chair had been broken over someone's head. I became an expert at giving intravenous glucose in the middle of the night to vastly overweight patients convulsing as a result of their insulin shock therapy.

In our final year we lived in at the University Hospital during surgical and obstetrical services. I was put in a small room at a turn in the stairs; the nurses called it the "biscuit box." It obviously had been intended for a broom closet—it was awful. But I was stuck there because I was a female student. There were, however, two pleasant rooms for students in another part of the hospital, one of which was occupied by a male student. Without asking anyone I moved myself into the empty room. I heard by the grapevine that this caused quite a stir, with the Dean of Medicine saying he was not responsible for the morals of the female students. I never did hear anything directly.

I was still on the obstetrical service at the end of the school year when I got quite sick with right lower quadrant pain typical of appendicitis. I was transferred to the surgical ward. The professor of surgery removed my appendix under spinal anaesthesia. There were a couple of surgical interns from the year ahead of me making snide remarks about what they were finding, but it wasn't anything more interesting than an acute appendix. I moved back to my room downstairs a couple of days later and was told that I didn't have to write the final exams. But I couldn't see sitting around while everyone else was busy doing exams, so I wrote them anyway. Only ten days after the operation, I went to the graduation dance and bumped into a surprised professor of surgery in the middle of the dance floor.

I applied for an internship at Vancouver General Hospital. The Catholic hospitals didn't accept female interns at that time. Happy to be back in familiar surroundings, I had really missed the ocean and mountains.

At the interns' residence across the street from the hospital, I was given a basement room. We were paid the magnificent sum of $25 a month plus room and board. One of my chief memories of the year was the food. Every Thursday we were served a heavy brown bread and baked beans; I haven't eaten either since. The kitchen also had some secret method of vulcanizing the fried eggs they served at breakfast.

That was a busy year. We struggled through the polio epidemic of 1948 and became experts at doing lumbar punctures. One poor paralyzed woman came in and when I did a physical exam I found a large breast lump. She didn't have polio, she had metastatic breast cancer. A chiropractor had told her not to worry, the lump was only gristle.

During the year another intern from Montreal and I started going downtown to get a decent meal when we could afford it. This friendship led to a decision to get married. We married at the end of February at the courthouse in Vancouver, gathering up a couple of secretaries to act as witnesses. Since married interns were not allowed to live in residence, we didn't tell anyone. He lived on the third floor and I still lived in the basement, and we got together once in a while when we weren't too exhausted. We finally got away for a weekend on the 24th of May.

On the Emergency rotation I was called one evening to look after a logger who had been in a bar-room brawl. He was well-anaesthetized and docile and didn't need a local anaesthetic, so I sutured the extensive knife wounds on his arms. After I finished he was considerably sobered, and he hauled a roll of bills out of his pocket, peeled off several, and handed them to me. I assured him I was not allowed to accept money and returned it. His retort was, "If you don't take them, Doc, some other babe will just roll me for them."

The intern year was long and arduous, but we all survived it. The friends I had known four years before had all gone their separate ways. We had no money to set up a practice in the city. Our only wedding present was from a woman resident in anaesthesiology who gave us a couple of aluminum pots and a few pieces of cutlery stamped VGH. (I still have one spoon.) We went to Victoria to see if there was an opportunity there. We were definitely discouraged by the local physicians who didn't seem to want any competition.

We eventually settled in Hedley, a gold mining town in the Similkameen Valley, half-way between Princeton and Keremeos, B.C. It had been a boom town at one time. The doctor in Hedley was leaving his practice and my husband Ed took it over. There were two mines operating at that time, the Kelowna Exploration and the Hedley Mascot. Because this was before there was any medical insurance, there was a private contract between the doctors and the companies. The single miners paid $1.50 a month and the married men with families paid $2.50. For this the doctor was expected to supply basic medications. Fortunately the drugs were relatively simple at the time and the patients on the whole were healthy. Needless to say I carefully saved any drug samples that came along. I practised in Princeton twenty-five miles away, with two doctors located there. There was a hospital in Princeton which served the Similkameen Valley. The nearest hospital in the other direction was in Penticton fifty miles away. We also looked after the Aboriginal people in the Similkameen Valley, for which we were paid fifty percent of the 1929 schedule of fees—this was about $25 for complete maternity care, including delivery and post-partum care.

The farmers and residents in the valley not connected with the mines sometimes paid the few bills I sent out, but frequently we didn't bother. Mostly it was subsistence living for them. One winter we were given a hind quarter of a moose which hung in the shed frozen solid. I hacked off bits of this gamey beast and tried assorted ways to make it edible, but eventually gave up. Even our two cocker spaniels wouldn't eat it. I don't recall how we eventually disposed of it.

When we first arrived in Hedley in 1948, there had been a flood and a lot of property damage. We lived for a short time in an upstairs suite in a mine company building opposite the ore crusher. The machinery went night and day, so there was no escaping the din. The local pharmacist had a small empty house that had been in the path of the flood at the bend of the river. It was still standing, but the floor was covered with three inches of sand and the small basement with its sawdust burner furnace was full of river rocks. We worked hard, cleaned out the sand and debris, and painted all the floors. We acquired a bed, a kitchen table, two chairs, a two-burner hot plate, a record player, and that was it for furniture. We then stared to cart the rocks out of the basement by the bucketful. It was still early in the year, so we didn't need a heat supply. Just about the time we got the furnace cleaned out, the Department of Highways came along and decided that was where the highway should run, and the house was demolished.

An old house that had been a mine manager's residence was empty, so we moved there. It was two storeys with an attic, and no insulation whatsoever. The whole place had been painted an ugly beige shade, so we decided to remedy that. Ed didn't mind painting walls, but refused to do any ceilings, so the ceilings were my job. Perhaps because of cheap paint and poor preparation, the whole place had a poorly-stippled surface, rough and uneven—I have never painted a ceiling since. It was getting colder, so at the same time we gathered all the newspapers we could find and lugged them up to the attic to put between the beams. I suppose that helped a bit, but it was still a cold place in the winter.

We didn't have a car for a short while, so the same kindly pharmacist who rented us the first house lent us a little old Ford truck. There was only a gravel road between Hedley and Princeton and it was very rough in spots. The truck's battery terminal was loose and a good bump in the road would dislodge the little piece of wood we wedged in to keep the contact. The truck of course stalled, so someone had to get out and find another little stick, position it, then restart the truck.

I had a wonderful little Austin A40 which served nobly for the six years we were in Hedley. It was a great car and would go over icy roads even when the buses got stuck. The chief problem was the heater, which was next to useless. At forty below outside, the temperature in the car was probably thirty below, with drafts coming though the floor boards and swirling about your legs. But when nothing else could get up the slippery mountain roads to the camp at Copper Mountain, that little car could do it.

Ed bought a Pontiac in Vancouver. He had never driven a car before and had one driving lesson before we started up the recently flooded Fraser Valley to Princeton. There was no Hope-Princeton road then; the route was through the Fraser Canyon. With many scary detours because of road wash-outs in the lower valley, it was a trip we weren't likely to forget, but we made it without any major problems.

The communications systems have certainly changed since that time long ago. We had three telephones in the house: one was for the Nickel Plate Mine, one for the Hedley Mascot, and the third was the outside line. These were the models with two large bells at the top and a mouth piece below, a receiver on a hook on the left side, and a handle to crank on the right side. Each of the telephones had a slightly different sound and each had its own ring. If you heard the mine manager's ring in the middle of the night, it usually meant trouble. The next ring would probably be ours—one long and two shorts—that called the doctor. That didn't happen very often, luckily. Other than at the mines, the only other outside lines were at the gas station and the drug store. Occasionally the townsfolk came to the house if they needed to make a long distance call.

The office in Hedley was upstairs above the gas station. It was a large open room with a very old examining table, a few cabinets stocked with some very basic tools, and some simple medications. It also had an ancient unshielded glass X-ray tube which we used very occasionally, since the nearest other machine was in Princeton twenty-five miles away. The office heating system depended on a furnace at the gas station, but when it was fired up in very cold weather, the pipes leaked and soot drifted over everything in the place. There was no janitor service, so that too became part of my job.

My routine at the Princeton office was three days a week for formal office hours in town. One day a week was spent at the mining camp at Copper Mountain up a narrow switchback road that could be very hazardous, particularly in the winter. Many of the miners and their families lived at the camp. I went up to the camp with one of the doctors I worked with. We did any necessary house calls, then stopped at the mine offices at Granby part-way down the mountain. Sometimes my little Austin was the only car that could safely get up there, so I did the driving. There was a little Scottish nurse living at the camp with her accountant husband. She was a gem who had been a field nurse in the First World War. She kept us informed of any serious problems at the camp.

I looked after a fair percentage of the maternity patients in Princeton, and since we had no rotation arrangement, if a patient was in labour or even expected to go into labour soon, it meant staying close to the telephone. When the roads were treacherous I spent many nights in the hospital. It didn't make sense to drive twenty-five miles home then have to turn around and go back again. The women appreciated having someone standing by and someone to talk to. Whenever possible I had the husbands come into the case room as well. This was not the accepted thing to do at that time and it did raise some eyebrows, but I just ignored that. There weren't many high risk pregnancies, and I only recall a couple of real disasters, but not with my patients.

When one of the two doctors I worked with was away on holiday, I stayed at his house and didn't get back to Hedley for the duration. It was usually in the winter time, so the conditions could be difficult. One New Year's Day I was on call and started out on a house call. It was forty below and everything was frozen solid. We used block heaters so the car started, but before I got to my destination, I skidded and wound up in a snow bank. There were no such things as cell phones in those days, so it took me three hours to shovel my way out of the icy mess. No one came by, as it was at the edge of town, and it really wasn't any emergency when I did get there.

There was a similar sort of private contract with company employees in Princeton as we had in Hedley. The senior doctor I worked with was called out on an emergency one night. When he got to the house outside of town, the woman just wanted him to drive her to Princeton. She figured that

It was a great car and would go over icy roads even when the buses got stuck. The chief problem was the heater, which was next to useless. At forty below outside, the temperature in the car was probably thirty below, with drafts coming though the floor boards and swirling about your legs.

doctors had to come out when they were called, and that would be cheaper than calling a taxi. I have no idea what the doctor's response was, but the woman didn't get her ride.

Only two doctors were in practice in Princeton when my husband and I arrived in the area. The senior one had been a surgeon in an advanced field hospital overseas during the war and had lots of experience in traumatic surgery. The other one had been a classmate in my early days at UBC in a biology class. He had gone to medical school after finishing his BA, whereas I had completed a Masters degree in Botany and Zoology in 1943, so he graduated in Medicine three years before I did. He had had some instruction in giving anaesthetics which was very useful in a small rural hospital. When I joined the others I did mostly assists, but gave the occasional anaesthetic by dripping ether onto a mask. That was the extent of the sophistication in that field except for the occasional use of intravenous pentothal for short procedures. I once had to give an anaesthetic to a very old man with a strangulated inguinal hernia. During the procedure he quit breathing when his tongue slipped backwards. I got a clamp on his tongue to pull it forward and he woke up to the point of being able to swear at me with every invective he could think of. I was never so happy to hear anything in my life. We all survived the experience.

While we were living in Hedley, the Hope-Princeton road opened. Before that the way from the coast was through Merritt. There were many accidents on the new road, as there were some steep hills with curves at the bottom. When the road signs said "Slow to 30," that's what it meant. That was thirty miles per hour, but it was frequently ignored. One night a loaded gasoline tanker truck went off the road and caught fire. The driver was pulled out, but didn't make it. My senior partner said it was as bad as anything he had seen during the war. We did our best and that was all anyone could do. Some of the car accidents were dreadful, and the young RCMP officers seemed to take great delight in calling me out to them if they needed a doctor.

I will say this for the police officers, when I was doing a lot of travelling between Hedley and Princeton at all hours of the night and day they seemed to keep a watch out. They usually knew when I had taken the old Hedley road, which was still a gravel surface, instead of the 'new' one which

was shadier and more likely to be slick with black ice. I appreciated that. On one very icy day I was travelling the new road and a small deer was having difficulty getting across it, and since stepping on the brake would have been disastrous, I skidded into the poor creature and broke its leg. When I got to Princeton I notified the game warden and the animal was picked up. (A few days later we had a wonderful venison roast at the hospital—they had an excellent cook there.) The police suggested they should charge me with hunting with a dangerous weapon—to wit—one Austin!

The people associated with the mines in Hedley and Princeton had often lived in other mining towns in B.C. Their history of mining was often of small mines that had shut down; there were tales of Sandon and Blakeburn and other areas. We met some old prospectors who went out every year to try their luck, hoping to strike it rich, but I never met anyone who succeeded. There was one old fellow who used to come into Princeton every fall and turn up at the hospital. He was never in very good shape so he would be taken in. His clothes had to be cut off him because he had worn them continuously since he'd put them on in the springtime. It took about a week of daily baths administered by the nurses to get him cleaned up. Then he usually stayed in the hospital until spring when he was issued new clothes and off he went again. Nobody seemed to know what he did in the summer, but he was a seasonal patient for a number of years.

The country around Princeton and Hedley was a pleasant place to be most of the year. There were creeks with small trout in them and interesting old roads to explore. The six years there were a good experience: my husband and I came out of there with two old cars and $2,000 in my savings.

Ed had gone to Seattle to take post-graduate training in surgery. The mines were shutting down and I had stayed on while they closed operations, still working at Princeton and also looking after the miners and families in Hedley. I had one son a year old, and the lady who had been baby-sitting moved into my house with her two children aged about eight and ten. I was a boarder in my own home.

After the mines closed I moved to Seattle for about a year, while Ed continued his studies. We lived in a rickety mouldy little house on the border of the Italian and Black sections of town. My second son, born in Seattle, was registered as a Canadian citizen born abroad. The other residents' wives couldn't understand why I was determined to return to Canada. I had to subscribe to a Vancouver paper to make sure that Vancouver and Canada were still up there—there was no sign of them in the U.S. papers.

I didn't practise in Seattle for that year, just looking after my children. We returned to Canada in 1957 to a practice in Cloverdale in Surrey, about thirty miles from Vancouver. Cloverdale was mainly an agricultural centre. The three doctors practising there all left to specialize in anaesthesiology at the same time; we took over one of the practices. I did a locum for another physician in North Surrey for a couple of weeks who was well-known for his colourful use of the English language. I was seven months pregnant at the time when a rough-looking patient was ushered in to see Dr. Murphy (me). He let out a couple of expletives, saying, "Are you the doctor? I was expecting to see a big strapping Irishman!" He simmered down and we got along fine.

I now had three children and practised part-time. My husband hadn't completed his certification in surgery because he decided he preferred general practice. There was no hospital in Surrey, so we travelled to the Royal Columbian and St. Mary's hospitals in New Westminster when the patients needed hospital care. I delivered a few patients in Langley and White Rock and we did house calls all over Surrey, driving for many miles.

Finding household help was difficult. We had a sweet little old Dutch lady as Oma for a couple of years, but it got to be too much for her. Later a sixteen-year-old German girl came to live in with us to look after the children, but she had no idea how to cook. I must have been a reasonably good instructor as she became quite good at it.

We both practised as family physicians from the same office which we had set up to do minor surgery. It was more convenient for both the patients and ourselves since there was no emergency department within miles. I once sutured an ear back to where it was supposed to be after it was nearly ripped off. Another impatient patient came to the office after trying to pull something from under his lawnmower while it was still running. The bone was cut through and the thumb dangled from a bit of dorsal flesh and skin. I cleaned it, put it back in place, sutured and splinted it, and it healed beautifully. Another time a young sailor was brought to the office one night by friends, following a desperate phone call. He didn't want to go to a hospital or have anyone else know of the occurrence. He had been in a pub fight and had numerous deep knife slashes on his back. I used up nearly all the suture material and a lot of local anaesthetic to suture the wounds. I asked him to come back in a few days, but never saw him again, nor did I get paid anything for my efforts. That was my good deed for the day.

When we first started in Cloverdale the government paid fifty percent of the schedule of fees for seniors and people on social assistance. It wasn't long before seniors from one of the other offices were coming to our office, having been told that they should see someone new for a fresh opinion on their many problems. Soon after, the fees became the same for everyone; someone must have complained.

My daughter was born in January 1958 in New Westminster, and Surrey Memorial Hospital was opened later that year. My husband and I were among the original members of the medical staff. Ed did a considerable amount of surgery at first, but as general surgeons and specialists joined the staff, that became less frequent. We were twenty miles from the hospital and still did a lot of minor emergency surgery at the office. If an emergency patient did turn up at the hospital it meant travelling there and back, sometimes for nothing much more than a scratch. It was years before emergency physicians arrived on the scene. We both did obstetrics, but as time went by I handled a greater portion of it. Before I gave up delivering babies, I was onto the third generation. A few years ago a Chinese lady came to the office with two fancy t-shirts, wanting me to choose one of them. After I had picked one, she explained that I had stayed with her all night twenty-five years before when she had her first son.

I looked after some of my patients for forty years and we grew old together. They trusted me and my advice so it was a happy association. In later years I found I was doing more counselling as well as trying to cope with my aging patients' increasing problems. When the 'walk in' clinics

I looked after some of my patients for forty years and we grew old together. They trusted me and my advice so it was a happy association. In later years I found I was doing more counselling as well as trying to cope with my aging patients' increasing problems.

became popular I was asked to verify that the pills from the clinic were the right ones. More than once I had to explain that ulcer pills wouldn't do anything for a sick gallbladder. But it was all in the day's work.

The years went by, the children grew up and went their way. The municipality grew tremendously and now calls itself the City of Surrey. My husband retired in 1992 and died two years later. I carried on with a smaller practice until 1998 when the Medical Services Plan retired older physicians by taking away their billing numbers. Medicine has changed a great deal, but it was a wonderful and fascinating fifty years, and I never got tired of it.

1948

DR. ANNA FAREWELL
(1910-1980)

Born in 1910, Anna Farewell had her preliminary education in Saskatchewan. In 1920, she and her family moved to Texas, where she graduated Phi Beta Kappa in 1930 at the University of Texas. She then went to Minneapolis where she was trained and worked as a medical technologist until 1939. In that year she entered Medicine at the University of Manitoba and received her MD in 1944. Dr. Farewell worked with Bruce Chown in his Rh laboratory, and at Toronto Sick Children's Hospital. She was certified in Pediatrics by the Royal College of Physicians and Surgeons of Canada, and registered with the B.C. College of Physicians and Surgeons in 1948.

Since then, Anna worked in British Columbia at the Coqualeetza Hospital, in Pediatric practice in Chilliwack, and at Woodlands School until her retirement in 1976. An active member of B.C. Medical Association, she was made a Life Member of the BCMA. Anna was much liked and admired by her fellow workers and patients throughout her career.

She died on December 28, 1980, survived by her husband, Mr. Fleet Farewell, in Surrey, B.C.

(Written by Dr. Archie Hardyment for the BCMJ *of March, 1982.)*

DR. ANNE STEELE
(C. 1920-1959)

Dr. Anne Steele graduated in medicine from Edinburgh Medical School in 1944. After graduation she joined the Red Cross and was sent to Malaya to be in charge of a hospital in Johore State. She then came to British Columbia, interned at St. Josph's Hospital in Victoria, and registered with the College of Physicians and Surgeons of B.C. in 1948. She entered into private practice in Victoria.

In 1959 Dr. Steele had a horrible accident: a fall from her horse resulted in a coma, from which she never recovered. She died September 6, 1959, leaving her family, friends, and patients.

DR. LUDMILA (LOLA) FISHAUT ZELDOWICZ
(1905–1992)

Ludmila (Lola) Fishaut was born into a family of doctors and dentists in Warsaw in 1905; her older brother became a neurologist. Lola studied medicine at the University of Warsaw—unusual for a Jewish girl between the years of 1924 and 1930. She specialized in neurology and became an assistant to a professor in a hospital in Warsaw. In 1935, she was married to Dr. Henry Zeldowicz who had received his medical training in Rome, Italy. When the Germans invaded Poland in 1939, Henry was called up by the Polish army. The ghetto where the Jewish people lived was divided into several areas, the largest housing the Judenrat, a group in charge of running the ghetto and advocating order and organization as a way of easing life for the Jews. A smaller area was taken up by the Schultz Company, with the workers now working for the Germans. Between the areas was a no-man's land patrolled by the German armed guards.

Lola lived in the smaller area, and as a doctor she was able to move between the ghettos. The mass deportation of the Jews had begun, and the ghetto population was decimated. In the large area bunkers were built underground as hiding places to avoid forced evacuation. In January 1943, Lola survived in one of these bunkers for four days. As a doctor she had had to stay overnight in the big ghetto on a special permit to attend a very sick child. A German blockade was established and the first armed resistance in the streets took place. Lola and a friend escaped in a hearse drawn by horses; the driver whipped through the gate guarded by a German into the territory of the Schultz Company. Friends of the underground hid her, moving her from town to town in hair-raising escapes.

Finally, the war was over for Poland. Lola was mobilized to the Polish army in Lublin where the provisional government was being formed. She was appointed Inspector Neurologist of the Polish base hospitals and spent many months moving westward with the army. It was not until the autumn of 1945 that she returned to her position with the Neurology Department of Warsaw University.

In the meantime, Henry worked with the Polish forces as a doctor, and later with the British military hospitals in Egypt, North Africa, and Italy. Through their mutual friends, Lola found out that Henry was safe in Italy, and was on his way to England to be demobilized. Lola's decision to emigrate was firm. She considered that there was now no room for Jews in Poland. She left Warsaw for Prague on May 4, 1946, and eventually reached England where she joined Henry to move to Canada.

Since Henry had been with the allied forces in Italy and later British hospitals, his command of the English language was very good. When they arrived in Vancouver where Lola's brother was already established, Henry began training in psychiatry at Shaughnessy Hospital and attained certification in his specialty. Lola, however, had to learn English in order to obtain her specialist certification in neurology. She was the first woman neurologist in British Columbia, and over the course of her career, wrote thirty-eight medical publications on research and clinical work. Lola was on the staff of Vancouver General Hospital and taught at the University of British Columbia as well as running a busy private practice and becoming an authority on Multiple Sclerosis.

Lola and Henry enjoyed winter trips to Hawaii. After their retirement, Henry became ill with cancer and Lola nursed him at home until his last days in March 1986. She stayed in her condo until she had a fall. After hospitalization at the UBC Hospital, she was transferred to the Extended Care where she lived for two years. She died on April 18, 1992.

(The information of Lola's years during the Second World War is from the book In the Warsaw Ghetto: The Memoirs of Stanislaw Adler. *This manuscript was given to Lola before she left Poland and she arranged for its translation and publication. She presented this book to the library of the College of Physicians and Surgeons of British Columbia in 1982. Mr. Paul Heller of Vancouver, a friend of Henry and Lola, kindly gave me further information.)*

1949

DR. KATHLEEN BELTON
(1916-1980)

Dr. Kathleen Belton was born in Grand Coulee, Saskatchewan. She was trained in medicine for two years at the University of Saskatchewan, and completed her MD at McGill University in 1941. She studied anesthesia at Toronto General Hospital, continued her post-graduate work in pathology at Montreal General Hospital, and was certified in anesthesia in 1946. She became Assistant Director of Anesthesia at Children's Memorial Hospital in Montreal and a member of McGill teaching staff. Moving to Vancouver when Dr. M.D. Leigh of McGill became Head of the Anesthesia Department at Vancouver General Hospital, she soon became anesthetist-in-charge of pediatric anesthesia at Vancouver's Children's Hospital. In collaboration with Dr. Leigh, Dr. Belton published the first textbook on pediatric anesthesia in 1948.

In 1954, Dr. Belton resigned from Vancouver Children's Hospital to work at Los Angeles Children's Hospital and was Assistant Professor of Anesthesia at the University of Southern California Medical School until 1960. She then began her private practice in Oxnard, California, until her retirement in 1978. Despite illness, she continued to promote pediatric anesthesia in Vietnam and Tunisia. In 1979, she was honoured with a Woman of the Year award in Oxnard.

Dr. Belton died of carcinomatosis on August 19, 1980, at age sixty-four.

DR. HONOR (MOLLY) KIDD
(1907–1977)

Dr. Honor Kidd graduated with a BA from the University of British Columbia in 1926. Much later, she studied medicine at McGill University Medical School and graduated with an MD, CM in 1947. Her main interests centered on pathology and research investigations which she carried on for many years at the Vancouver General Hospital and Cancer Institute Laboratory. Dr. Kidd was also a business woman.

The B.C. Medical Association extended congratulations to her on winning the Osler Medal from the American Association of Historical Medicine in 1946. Dr. Kidd was the first woman and the first Canadian to win this award.

Dr. Wally Thomas, who worked with her at Vancouver General Hospital, very kindly wrote about her as follows: "My old friend Molly Kidd was really a delightful person. Indeed as I sit here writing I have a smile on my face and a warm feeling inside. She had a great zest for life and loved to travel. I first met Molly when we were both doing a year of Pathology at Vancouver General Hospital. Perhaps my first impression of her was one of vigour—and a cigarette—she was busy every moment. At that time, we had journal club meetings that were excellent, but which were also a bit of a social event. Having one at her home was rather special as she always served us delicious dinners.

"As we sat around the room doing our journal review, we could be sure that at some point we would have a visit from the racoon family—indeed, many families, as they awaited their evening treat of marshmallows—bags of them!

"It turned out that Molly's interest was in the lymphomas and she became part of the Lymphoma Clinic with Mac Whitelaw as Chair, Bob Moffat, Harry Perry, Dick Beck, Vivien Basco, Ian Plenderlieth, and others. Her special interest was the plasma cell. Morphology and special stains were of great importance at that time. She had a laboratory on the third floor of the Cancer Institute, and here she pursued this interest with a grant from the Canadian Cancer Foundation. One of the problems in finding some clumps of plasma cells was to distinguish between a reactive process

and the disease myeloma. Molly found that much could be done with special stains, but she also found that there was a peculiarity to the shape of the clumps in myeloma, and she named this formation 'Kidd's Squiggle.' She presented her findings at the annual Cancer Foundation meeting at Honey Harbour—a mosquito-ridden resort in northern Ontario. All this time she was running the OverWaitea [later called Overwaitea] business—the name came from her mother's habit of always putting in an extra amount of tea when weighing out this item in the store. In later years, I think that Molly found herself more involved in the business."

Molly Kidd died in April, 1977, at age 70.

DR. VALENTINA (VAYA) MARKEN
(1891–1986)

For the last three years of her life Dr. Valentina Markin was lost in the company of strangers at the old folks' home. When she died at age ninety-five in December of 1986, her brilliant and colourful career as a pioneering ophthalmologist among the Native peoples of this province was some ten years behind her. Without family or known relatives, she had buried two husbands, and counted on only God and "Kaya," her beloved dog, as the final repositories for her affection.

Afflicted with a failing memory and unable to see clearly because of macular degeneration, it must have been especially lonely for her at the end—the present obscured by a white milky haze, her past rolling up like a frayed carpet behind her.

Still, "Vaya," as she was known to her friends, would not want to be remembered as a tragic figure. It was how she lived her life, not how it ended, that commands our respect. The great events of history can make losers and then victims of some, but it also goads others to develop great strength of character—to be outstanding against all odds. By all accounts Dr. Valentina Markin was such a person.

Born on March 1, 1891 at Kasan, Troezk, a Russian settlement at the foot of the Ural mountains, Valentina was the daughter of Nicholai Wnukow, a medical doctor, and Katherina Tupicina, a lady of Tartar extract. She obtained her own medical degree with honours at Leningrad (Petrograd) on April 29, 1917, just as Russian participation in the First World War was ending and the Bolshevik Revolution was beginning. Her first residency was spent in military field hospitals, caring for wounded soldiers who were dying under deplorable conditions. During that tour of duty she met and married a doctor named Pietzenko, who took her with him to Cracow, Poland, where she continued to practise medicine and obtained her ophthalmic training. The move, unfortunately, did not signal the start of a new life for Valentina and her husband, but rather the end of one, for he became ill shortly after they had established their medical practice and died suddenly.

More hardship was to come. By the closing months of the 1939–45 war, Valentina had again married, this time to Dr. Alexander Markin. Left penniless amid the general ruination of Poland under the Third Reich—soon to be engulfed by the now advancing Soviets—Valentina and her husband decided to flee to Germany with the retreating Nazis, where they existed as refugees and continued to work as physicians until 1948. In April of that year, the couple applied for refugee status, hoping to start a new life together in Canada or the United States. Unfortunately, by October Valentina was alone again. Alexander Markin had followed her first husband to the grave after a sudden illness.

Now widowed twice and still without a country, Valentina made preparations to cross the ocean alone that year. Having been sponsored by Canada, she travelled to British Columbia, where she finally received her landed immigrant certificate in December, 1948. She celebrated by taking a position as ophthalmologist for the Pacific Region with the Vancouver based Indian Health Service.

At the time she took the job, trachoma was endemic among the Native peoples of British Columbia, a situation the federal government had been trying to rectify by building regional hospitals at Coqualeetza, Nanaimo, and Millar Bay, and by establishing health centres on the reserves. The government's smartest move, however, at least to her colleagues and friends, took place the day it hired Dr. Valentina Markin.

From 1949 to 1959, when she retired, Valentina was revered as the "workhorse" of Indian ophthalmology in the Pacific region. To those who knew and worked with her—the doctors, nurses, and countless Indian folk—she was the one who made a difference: the "prime mover" who all but eliminated most of the acute trachoma among the Native peoples of British Columbia.

Still there is more to her accomplishments than simply what she did. She was well-equipped for the job by her training and what she had already experienced—the horrible conditions on the reservations could not have been much worse than the maggot-infested field hospitals she had worked in during the Russian Revolution.

Speaking little English, Valentina travelled to the remote Indian settlements with dictionaries and grammar texts as part of her medical kit bag. She did not simply want to treat her patients. She passionately studied the language of her new country so she could meet and know them as people.

A religious woman fond of the fine arts and music, she thought nothing of climbing into a canoe or a fisherman's gill netter or flying by the seat of her pants with a bush pilot through rugged mountain passes in any kind of weather. For Valentina, the cause she embraced in the service of others was always more important than the effect it might have on her own health.

Call it spirit or life force or whatever you like, but that, in the end, is what Valentina had and probably would be most pleased to be remembered by—not as a faltering old lady doddering toward death, blinded by eye disease she had worked so selflessly to prevent in others. The end demeaned Dr. Valentina Markin and one would have thought she deserved better, for it was in the life she led that we find her true testament. She upheld the human values of simple courage, unflagging compassion, and that all-too scarce currency of life called plain old-fashioned spunk.

(Permissions were given by Mr. Rick Campbell, editor of the Medical Post, *and Dr. John R. Kellet, an ophthalmologist who worked for the Pacific Region of the Indian Health Service from 1959 to 1978, to print his story, "Her Brilliant Career: 'Vaya' gave strength, vision to Canada's native Indians," written for the* Medical Post, *May 17, 1988.)*

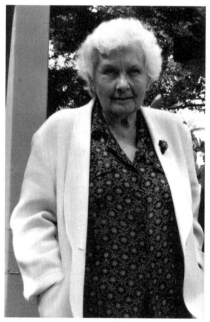

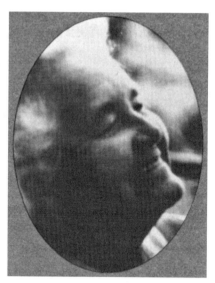

Dr. Olive Sadler, 1942

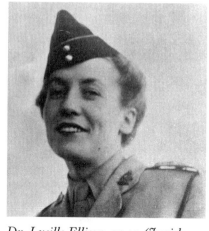

Dr. Lucille Ellison, 1945 (Jewish Historical Society)

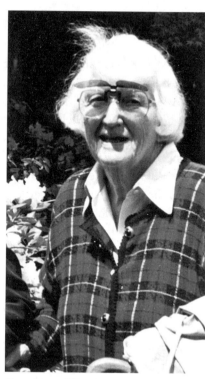

Dr. Mary K. Garner, 1942

Dr. Agnes Weston, 1945

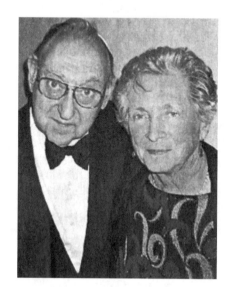

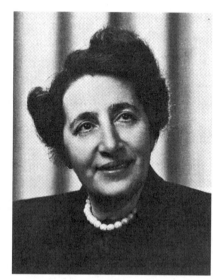

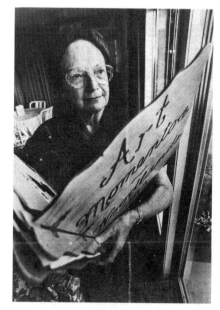

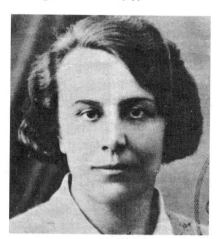

Dr. Margaret Mullinger Bogoch (1946) with her husband

Dr. Elda Lindenfeld, 1948

Dr. Pauline Hughes, 1949

Dr. Valentina Markin, 1949

Notes from VMA JOURNAL 1940–1949

April, 1940 Statistics: Population of Vancouver is 269,454; Japanese 9,094, Chinese 8,467, Hindu 339. The Drs. Poole (Dr. Lois Stephens) have moved from Wells to Revelstoke, B.C. Dr. Reba Willits has completed her course in Public Health at the University of Toronto and is now doing research in War Wound Infections at the same University. There was praise for Dr. Evelyn Gee's work for the past 8 years on the Aschiem-Zondek Test. The report was given by her at the BCMA Annual Meeting.

September, 1940 The Annual Meeting of the BCMA will be held in Nelson, B.C., September 9–11.

October, 1940 Medical Services Association has opened their office.

June, 1941 Dr. Ethlyn Trapp will present a paper to the Victoria Medical Society on "The Radiation Treatment of Carcinoma of the Uterus." Dr. Trapp is the chairman of the BCMA Standing Committee on Cancer. Dr. Claire Onhauser of West Vancouver is now the Vice-President of the North Vancouver Medical Society. Attending the 1941 Annual Meeting of the British Columbia Medical Association were Dr. Josephine Mallek, Dr. Claire Onhauser, Dr. Florence Perry, Dr. Olive Sadler, Dr. Dorothy Saxton, Dr. Lois Stephens, and Dr. Ethlyn Trapp.

November, 1941 Dr. H.G. Farrish, Surgeon Lieutenant, of Vancouver, and Dr. Hazel Krause of Montreal were married in October, 1941. There is a rapid increase in insurance organizations. The following have made contracts with the medical profession of B.C. through its organization, B.C. Medical Association: B.C. Telephone, the B.C. Electric, the Vancouver School Teachers, and the Medical Services Association. All other insurance companies that are advertising have not made contracts with BCMA, and doctors must realize this.

There are 12,000 doctors in Canada. About 12%, or 1,400, have enlisted and are engaged full time in one of the armed services. There are 750 doctors in British Columbia, of these there are 130 enlistments among medical men in the province, or some 17% of our total enrolment.

December, 1941 At the Annual Dinner of the Vancouver Medical Association on November 20, 1941, 150 men enjoyed the dinner and entertainment. The Board of Directors of BCMA met on November 19, 1941. Dr. Ethlyn Trapp gave a report on "The Study of Cancer," outlining the programme which is being carried out. Dr. Ethlyn Trapp and Dr. Christina Fraser attended the meeting of the Committee on The Study of Cancer in B.C. A new, short form for reporting cases of cancer in B.C. was approved and will be distributed by the Provincial Board of Health to all doctors in B.C.

Japan bombs Pearl Harbor. WAR IS DECLARED AGAINST JAPAN.

January, 1942 A committee of the VMA has been formed regarding the organization of local medical men for action in the event of an air raid on the city or neighbouring municipalities. The city is divided into twenty-three air raid districts, each with an ARP post. A medical officer-in- charge whose home is in his ARP district has been chosen. The hospitals in Victoria are organized and ready for any emergencies that might arise from enemy attack.

February, 1942 Dr. Reba Willits is now associated with the Metropolitan Health Board in Vancouver.

March, 1942: At the Annual Meeting of the Honorary and Attending Staff of the B.C. Cancer Institute, Dr. Ethlyn Trapp, medical superintendent, gave the report of the Institute. During February and March there were epidemics of mumps.

April, 1942 Gas Rationing has begun. At the Annual Meeting of the BCMA, in June at Jasper, Dr. Isabel Day gave the report of the VON Advisory Board. Dr. Ethlyn Trapp gave a report of the Committee on the Study of Cancer at the BCMA Meeting. Dr. Lois Stephens Poole of Revelstoke also attended the BCMA meeting.

July, 1942 There were epidemics of mumps in April, May, and June. Dr. Eleanor Riggs, formerly of Vancouver, contributed an excellent paper on "Methods for the Diagnosis of Nutritional Deficiencies." Dr. Riggs is now clinical assistant in the Department of Nutrition, School of Hygeine, University of Toronto.

August, 1942 Dr. Belle Holland Wilson, widow of the late Dr. T.A. Wilson and mother of Dr. P.M. Wilson, died on June 22, 1942. Dr. Dorothy Miller is now a Medical Officer with the RCAMC. She was formerly of North Vancouver, and more recently had an office in Vancouver. The meeting of the Board of Directors of BCMA took place in August, 1942. Dr. Ethlyn Trapp is a member of the Board, and is Chairman of the Cancer Committee. Dr. Isabel Day is Chairman of the St. John's Ambulance Association.

September, 1942 The new president of the North Shore Medical Society is Dr. Claire Onhauser. Honorary Secretary is Dr. Christina Fraser. Attending the Annual Summer School medical lectures in September were Dr. Dorothy Saxton of Victoria, Dr. Isabel Day, Dr. Claire Onhauser, and Dr. Ethlyn Trapp. There were 239 registered.

October, 1942 "Attention! All Doctors under 60 years of age: Department of National Defence has instructed Divisional Advisory Committee in this province (British Columbia) to notify the profession that all doctors (under 60) should be boarded and categorized. These doctors are strongly urged to present themselves for examination by the Army Medical Board. Please communicate with the Army Medical Board at the earliest possible date and secure appointment."

November, 1942 Dr. Ella Cristall, wife of Captain S.E. Evans, will act as part-time Director of the Health Unit in North Vancouver.

April, 1943 Female physicians are now being accepted into the Royal Canadian Army Medical Corp, both as specialists and general practitioners. Female medical students are now permitted to enlist in RCAMC under the government's accelerated plan of medical education as members of the Canadian Women's Army.

May, 1943 Dr. Ethlyn Trapp is acting medical superintendent of the B.C. Cancer Institute during Dr. Maxwell Evans' absence overseas. Dr. Margaret Hardie presented a review of cases of "Cancer of the body of the Uterus" at the Annual meeting of the Honorary Attending Staff of the B.C. Cancer Institute. Four hundred have registered for the VMA Summer School June 22–25, 1943.

June, 1943 The population of Vancouver is 288,542; Chinese 5,541, Hindu 301. (All Japanese had been evacuated by the end of December, 1942. Dr. M. Frizell of Blue River is caring for the Japanese in that area). Dr. Ethlyn Trapp attended the Canadian Medical Association General Council Meeting in Montreal in June.

July, 1943 Civilian doctors have increasing patient load. There are 3,100 doctors in Canada and 30% are in the armed forces.

September, 1943 BCMA Annual Meeting had 500 attending. Dr. Isabel Day continues on the VON Advisory Board.

October, 1943 Vancouver accepted the ruling of the Dominion Public Health Authorities that the water supply of the City and its neighbours North Vancouver and New Westminster be chlorinated as a war measure. The ruling stirred up a hornet's nest as the public is gradually developing an ever-increasing degree of a genuine fear of chlorinated water, a marked hostility to this measure, and a marked hostility to those who are responsible for it. We deplore the attitude of certain members of the City Council towards the Health Officer, Dr. Stewart Murray.

Pre-medical work at University of British Columbia is not yet satisfactory for eastern medical schools. Hospital teaching is down because there aren't the usual number of internes. Dr. K.D. Panton says the obvious solution is to form a medical faculty at UBC. He states that 150 men a year leave B.C. to study medicine. Several associations have developed their own non-profit Health Insurance Plans.

December, 1943 The December *Bulletin* is called by the editors the "Military Bulletin," as several articles are written by men in the medical units of the Canadian Forces. The Ottawa authorities gave their consent to the publications of the articles, and we have been greatly helped by Col. Wallace Wilson, CMO, Pacific Command.

In the *Bulletin* Dr. Agnes W. Black, MHO Burnaby, Metropolitan Health Commission, described "A Localized Outbreak of Diphtheria." Dr. Ethlyn Trapp stresses that the Cancer Institute is in its fifth year and still has no bed accommodation, so it is urgent that arrangements must be made.

January, 1944 Congratulations to Major Edna E. Rossiter, RCAMC, Principal Matron in the Pacific Command, who has received a Royal Red Cross in the New Year's Honours in recognition of her services. (Doctors who have worked with her at Shaughnessy Hospital remember her with fondness and respect.)

February, 1944 The public has been told that for $12 per year per person Health Insurance can be given to everyone.

At the Annual Meeting of the Honorary Attending Staff of the B.C. Cancer Institute, Dr. Ethlyn Trapp, acting Medical Director, presented the report. There were 415 patients admitted for cancer treatment in 1943 compared with 348 in 1942. There are plans for long-term research investigation on cancer of the breast under Dr. Olive Sadler's direction. There are American reports on the use of diethyl-stilbesterol treatment for cancer of the prostate, and the practical application of chemotherapy in the treatment of cancer. It was reported there is a rising incidence of cervical cancer during menopause and the post-menopausal period.

Dr. F.R.G. Langston is now working with Sir Harold Gillies at the Plastic Unit at Basingstoke, England. Dr. Kathleen (Woods) Langston is at the same hospital working in anesthesia.

March, 1944 Streptococcal meningitis is being treated with penicillin. Epidemics of chickenpox occurred in January, February, and March, 1944. Dr. A.A. O'Neil and Dr. Agnes J. Eagles, internes at Vancouver General Hospital, were married recently.

May, 1944 The fee at the Annual Summer School for doctors was $7.50. There are 321 members of the Vancouver Medical Association. Dr. Ethlyn Trapp, a member of the CMA General Council, and Dr. Josephine Mallek attended the Canadian Medical Association Annual Meeting in Toronto.

July, 1944 The population of Vancouver is 299,460; Chinese 5,728, Hindu 227. There is an increase in venereal disease in B.C., especially gonorrhea.

September, 1944 Dr. Ethlyn Trapp attended the BCMA meeting and gave a report of the Committee on the Study of Cancer. Also attending the meeting were Dr. Irene Clearihue of Victoria, Dr. Ella Cristall Evans, and Dr. Claire Onhauser.

BCMA officers for 1944-45 include Dr. Ethlyn Trapp as second Vice President. Dr. Trapp served actively for a number of years as a member of the Board of Directors of the BCMA and during recent years was Chairman of the Committee on Cancer and Honorary Treasurer 1934–35. She was also a member of the General Council of the Canadian Medical Association.

October, 1944 Dr. Christina Fraser was appointed secretary-treasurer of the North Shore Medical Society. Many doctors are returning from the war and going back into medical practice. MSA (Medical Services Association) has had a 65% increase in enrolment during the past year with many companies in Vancouver joining MSA.

November, 1944 Dr. F.R.G. Langston, and his wife, Dr. Kathleen (Woods) Langston have returned to B.C. after several years spent in England doing specialty training during the war years.

December, 1944 The people of Bella Bella and surrounding district recently honoured Dr. George E. Darby upon completion of thirty years' service as a missionary doctor in that area.

January, 1945 A Medical School for British Columbia is again under discussion. Canada has nine Medical Schools graduating 530 to 550 annually. There are 201 students at the University of British Columbia who wish to study medicine. Thirty-eight will be accepted in eastern schools. The University of Toronto Medical School has closed its door to any but Ontario Students. To study medicine costs $1,500 a year. The B.C. Government has allotted $1,500,000 for the construction of permanent medical buildings to be erected as soon as building materials are available. Dr. K.D. Panton is head of the committee for a UBC Medical School.

February, 1945 At the VMA forty-seventh Annual Meeting Dr. Ethlyn Trapp spoke on "Carcinoma of the Cervix." Dr. Ernest Boxall, interne at Vancouver General Hospital, gave a report to the meeting of the Clinical

Section of VGH on the results of the "Use of Penicillin at the Vancouver General Hospital." The third Western Canada Conference on VD Control informed those attending that Sweden has 14 cases per 100,000 of syphilis, whereas Canada has 175 cases per 100,000.

March, 1945   Vancouver's population is now 311,799.

April, 1945   The new Vancouver Military Hospital, adjacent to Shaughnessy Hospital, opened with 400 beds, and 200 beds at the Annex at the University. Lt. Col. F.E. Cox is Head, Lt. Col. Rocke Robertson is Head of Surgery, Major C.B. Rich is Head of Medicine, and Major Andrew Turnbull is Head of Radiology.

May 5th, 1945, 8 a.m. European time: WAR IS OVER IN EUROPE.

May, 1945   Measles epidemic continued since March with one death in 415 cases. Parents were advised to keep children home for 6 weeks. Dr. Ethlyn Trapp was elected President of the Federation of Medical Women of Canada. Summer School (for Doctors) Registrants included Drs. Mary Callaghan, Lillian Hutton, Violet Myers, Margaret Nelson, Olive Sadler, Ethlyn Trapp, Angela Waselek, and Helen Winsor, all of Vancouver.

July, 1945   The Law School at UBC has opened.

August, 1945   WAR IS OVER IN THE EAST, as the Japanese surrender. Chlorination debate—City Council wants to discontinue the protective measure. Drs. Amyot and Claude Dolman urge continuing chlorination.

September, 1945   Dr. Ethlyn Trapp becomes First Vice President of the Canadian Medical Association. Medical Office space is scarce. There is a need for medical staff to share space with returning veteran medical doctors. Cancer is now a reportable disease. The Health Department notes a very high rate of syphilis and gonorrhea in Canada. In British Columbia there are 21,976 cases of gonorrhea and 15,911 cases of syphilis. The Canadian Prisoners of War of the Japanese have been repatriated back to Canada.

November, 1945   Dr. Margaret Hardie was the speaker at the Annual Meeting of the Vancouver Medical Association. Her subject was "Research on Breast Cancer." Dr. G.E. Kidd's "History of The Vancouver Medical Association" is excerpted in the *VMA Bulletin*.

December, 1945   First advertisement of Premarin noted in this *Bulletin*.

January, 1946   Canadian Anesthesia Society, B.C. Division recently organized. Dr. Isabel Day continues on the Board of the Victorian Order of Nurses.

February, 1946   VMA presents a symposium on "Cancer of the Breast." Dr. Margaret Hardie spoke on "Research on Breast Cancer."

March, 1946   Another epidemic of chickenpox occurred in January, February, and March. An outbreak of smallpox of the hemorrhagic type which has recently occurred in Seattle with eight fatalities to date, has produced a very notable demand for vaccination in this province. Population of Vancouver is now 323,850.

April, 1946   Dr. Ella Cristall Evans and Dr. Sydney Evans of Vancouver have left for England for a year of post-graduate studies. The Committee on Medical Education consists of chairman Dr. K.D. Panton and members Dr. C.G. Dolman, Dr. A.B. Schinbein, Dr. G.F. Strong, and Dr. Frank Turnbull. In 1946 only 20 of the 70 UBC pre-med students were accepted by medical schools in eastern Canada.

May, 1946   The Vancouver Medical Association now has 366 members.

June, 1946   During the debate about the Medical School hospital a comment was made: "The University area is the last place that should be chosen for such a hospital." BCMA Annual Meeting was held at Banff. Dr. Ethlyn Trapp was elected President of the B.C. Medical Association, the first woman to be elected to such a high office in organized medicine in Canada. Also attending the Banff meeting were Drs. Christina Fraser, Margaret Hardie, Claire Onhauser, Florence Perry, and Olive Sadler.

September, 1946   The VMA Summer School registration included Drs. Christina Fraser, Mary K. Garner, Margaret Hardie, Irmla Kennedy-

Jackson, Josephine Mallek, Margaret Mullinger, Agnes O'Neil, Olive Sadler, Margaret Sylling, and Ethlyn Trapp. Many Medical Officers from the Armed Forces received their discharge and returned to British Columbia.

October, 1946 Dr. Trapp spoke on "Cancer of the Skin" at the West Kootenay Medical Association Annual Meeting, the East Kootenay Annual Meeting, the Southern Interior Medical Association, and the Victoria Medical Society.

November, 1946 Dr. Trapp is off to Havana as speaker at the Inter-American Congress of Radiologists. Lt. Winifred Van Kleek and Lt. G.B. Wilson were married, and after discharge from the Medical Corp, commenced practice at Harrison Lake and Agassiz. Dr. Elizabeth Johnson recently joined staff of the Tranquille Sanatorium. Dr. Elizabeth Sprung has been elected to VMA membership.

April, 1947 Dr. Ethlyn Trapp, President of BCMA, spoke at meetings in Prince George and Prince Rupert.

June, 1947 Dr. Honor M. Kidd is to be congratulated on winning the Osler Medal from the American Association of Historical Medicine. She is the first woman and first Canadian to win this award.

June, 1947 The Summer School registrants included Drs. Elizabeth Fleck, Honor M. Kidd, Josephine Mallek, Susan May, Margaret Mullinger, Agnes O'Neil, Elaine Peacock, Marguerite B. Shea, and Ethlyn Trapp.

July, 1947 Dr. Marion G. Irwin has come from Moose Jaw, Saskatchewan to practise in Kaslo, B.C. A survey of physicians in Canada reported there are 1,012 physicians in British Columbia. Population per physician in B.C. is 938.

September, 1947 The first Travelling Clinic of the Children's Hospital went to the Okanagan Valley. It was composed of an Orthopedic specialist and a Pediatrician. Kamloops, Vernon, Kelowna, and Penticton were visited, and a total of 76 patients were examined. There are 1,417 Medical Officers returning to Canada from the services, 130 from B.C. The Health Centre for Children was formed in 1947 under the Societies Act of British Columbia.

October, 1947 The retiring President of BCMA, Dr. Ethlyn Trapp, in addressing the members, stated, "There are 8,482 members in the Canadian Medical Association. In B.C. there are 715 members. In Canada there is one physician to 1,017 residents." Dr. G.A. Kidd continues his "History of The Vancouver Medical Association."

November, 1947 The Children's Hospital Travelling Clinic visited the Kootenay and the Cariboo districts.

February, 1948 Epidemic of rubella with 331 cases was reported. Members elected to Vancouver Medical Association include Dr. Agnes O'Neil and Dr. Marguerite Shea.

March, 1948 Vancouver population is now 354,045. An epidemic of measles has begun, and rubella cases continue as well. In March a two-week post-graduate course for General Practitioners was held at Shaughnessy Hospital. Forty-six doctors registered.

April, 1948 The Academy of Medicine building was approved. Dr. Kathleen C. Lewis has left Vancouver to take up residence in Los Angeles. Dr. Dorothy Miller, formerly of Parksville, B.C., has begun a practice at Sooke, on Vancouver Island, B.C.

May, 1948 Dr. Helen Zeman was appointed Medical Health Director of the Okanagan Health Unit at Kelowna. The BCMA Board of Directors meeting was held on May 3rd. Past President Dr. Ethlyn Trapp attended.

June, 1948 Summer School registrants included Drs. Mary K. Garner, Irmla Kennedy-Jackson, Elda Lindenfeld, Susan May, Mary Murphy (VGH interne), Claire Onhauser, Elaine Peacock, Lois Pearce, Margaret Sylling, and Ethlyn Trapp. Registration fee was $10. Dr. Isabel Day continues as representative for VON. B.C. Flood Emergency Fund Committee advises chlorination of wells.

August, 1948 Dr. M. Viola Rae will speak on "Aspiration Techniques in the Diagnosis of Cancer" at a course of lectures being held at Shaughnessy Hospital in October, 1948 and will do so again in May, 1949. The World

Medical Association has 37 member countries, as mentioned in the Annual Report of the Canadian Medical Association Executive by BCMA Past President and now the BCMA representative on the Executive, Dr. Ethlyn Trapp. There are 8,502 members of the CMA, and British Columbia has 850 members in the CMA.

September, 1948 Establishment and Recognition of Sections is requested, with application to the BCMA Board of Directors. There are 1,544 doctors in B.C., 690 in Vancouver.

October, 1948 Dr. Marion Irwin of Kaslo is the Vice-President of the West Kootenay Medical Association, the first woman to hold office in this district.

January, 1949 Dr. Elizabeth Mahaffy has been appointed assistant Medical Health Officer of the Union Board of Health in Victoria. There was a chickenpox epidemic in October, November, and December 1948.

February, 1949 Beginning March 1st, 1949, a new venture is taken for the medical care of all those who come under Social Assistance plans. It is entirely under the control of the medical profession whose representative body, the B.C. College of Physicians and Surgeons, is handling it through its Council. The Minister of National Health and Welfare, Hon. Paul Martin, said that the Federal Government will contribute $122,000 toward the cost of equipping the new Crease Clinic of Psychological Medicine and of providing additional equipment for the Provincial Mental Hospital at Essondale.

March, 1949 The Dean of the Medical Faculty of the University of British Columbia has been chosen. He is Dr. Myron K. Weaver from Minnesota. The first class of the UBC Medical School is to be admitted in the fall of 1950. Dr. J.A. Singleton married Dr. Jean Agnes Morrison and they are off to work in Nairobi, Kenya. Dr. Mary Callaghan left British Columbia to do post-graduate work at the Mayo Clinic in Rochester, Minnesota. Dr. Jean Hugill is doing post-graduate work in anesthesia at the Childrens' Memorial Hospital in Montreal. Population of Vancouver is now 376,000. Chickenpox and measles epidemics occurred in January and February.

April, 1949 Drs. James and Libuse (Jublicek) Tyhurst are doing post-graduate work in Psychiatry in Montreal.

June, 1949 At the Canadian Medical Association meeting in Saskatchewan it was reported by the Federation of Medical Women of Canada that there are 700 women doctors in Canada. At the FMWC Annual Meeting, Dr. Elda Lindenfeld of Vancouver was elected as one of the Vice-Presidents.

July, 1949 The medical profession of Vancouver will be greatly interested to hear that Dr. Olive Sadler, who was formerly associated with Dr. Ethlyn Trapp in Radiology, has recently returned to Vancouver after a two and a half years' absence and will again be associated with Dr. Trapp on Georgia St. Dr. Sadler did post-graduate study in various large U.S. centres on a Fellowship. She has been studying the latest work in X-ray and radium therapy, including the new work on radioactive isotopes. Vancouver welcomes her back. Dr. Leila Goulden of Miller Bay, B.C. was certified as a Specialist in Diagnostic Radiology by the Royal College of Physicians and Surgeons of Canada.

July, 1949 Dr. Jean Hugill who has recently completed a post-graduate course at Children's Memorial Hospital in Montreal is now on staff at the West Coast General Hospital in Port Alberni, B.C., as an anesthetist. In 1949 fewer than 30 of every 1,000 children died before reaching the age of one year, whereas in 1922, 68 of every 1,000 children born failed to survive. Infant mortality has been reduced by over 50% in British Columbia.

August, 1949 Dr. Marion Irwin, President of the West Kootenay Medical Association, has been appointed as representative to the BCMA Board of Directors. She is the second woman in B.C. to hold a position of this nature.

Stories from **1950 – 1959**

There were 130 new registered women doctors from 1950 to 1959.

1950
Dr. Eve Forrest Gulliford
Dr. Elaine J. (McLean) Stefanelli
1951
Dr. Lois Davies
Dr. Barbara Pead Kraft
Dr. Estelle M. Stevens
1952
Dr. Margaret Jean Hardie Beck
Dr. Gladys Story Cunningham
Dr. Tonka (Toni) Kamburoff
Dr. Shirley Baker Thomas
1953
Dr. Jacoba (Julia) van Norden
1954
Dr. Joyce Golding Clearihue
Dr. Joan Ford
Dr. Anne Lees
Dr. Laine Loo
Dr. Patricia A. Radcliffe
1955
Dr. Margot Boothroyd
Dr. Madeline (Huang) Chung

Dr. Helena Bozena Hale
Dr. Sarah Louise (Sally) Hemming
Dr. Margaret Maier Hoehn
Dr. Marjorie E. Dupont Jansch
Dr. Ruth Roffmann
Dr. Bluma Tischler
1956
Dr. Frances Forrest-Richards
Dr. Joyce Mavis Teasdale
1957
Dr. Margaret (Dobson) Cox
Dr. Ailsa Thurgar
1958
Dr. Eileen Nason Cambon
Dr. Dorothy M. (Simpson) Goresky
Dr. Margaret (Peggy) Manson (Mouat) Johnston
1959
Dr. Judy Hornung (Mrs. Frank Kalla)
Dr. Doris Kavanagh-Gray
Dr. Lois MacKenzie-Sawers
Dr. Margaret Trembath
Dr. Bernice Wylie

DR. EVE FORREST GULLIFORD
(1917–1997)

Born in January 16, 1917, Dr. Eve Forrest Gulliford is a legend in the Pitt River area, Port Coquitlam, Oliver, and Salmon Arm towns of British Columbia. After running tugs on the river for four years, Eve wrote her Master's papers and became Captain Eve Forrest. She decided to go into medicine after struggling through her high school education by correspondence, and finished her medical training at the University of British Columbia in 1944 (MD, CM) and Queen's University in 1950. Dr. Eve Forrest Gulliford says in the book *Saltwater Woman at Work*, by Vickie Jensen:

"My parents were Samuel and Hilda Forrest. Father was tough and efficient. He came to New Westminster in 1910, which was then full of muddy streets and potholes. He had come from Ontario and used to tow the ore barges from Port Arthur to Duluth on Lake Superior. During the war, he worked for Dawe's and Mercer's, just below New Westminster on Lulu Island. He also logged part-time with horses on Annacis Island. Apparently we lived in a tent for a while. My sister Mildred and I were born in New Westminster. She married and had two children, and died at age thirty-eight. Father had built a little boat. It wasn't a tugboat, but it had a little towing bit that he could use for towing. I don't think it even had a name, just a number. He built another boat at Pitt River. By this time we were living in a float-house and we ended up going ashore right there at the mouth of the Pitt River. My brother Harvie was born there and Father named the tug *Harvie W* after him. The *Harvie W* had a 40-horsepower Vivian gasoline motor. Unfortunately, my father

That was the way we got our work. There was nothing written—no contract, nothing. I started to run the smaller Harvie W *because I had to be home sometimes with Mother, who was now also quite ill with cancer.*

went into this at the time when diesels were just coming out. Gasoline was forty cents a gallon, and fuel oil that people used in diesels was five cents. (He always had small jobs, but never got in on the big ones.) Years later, Dad also had the hull of *Old Faithful* built and launched at the Pitt. But he just left her sit there when he got sick with cancer. He died when my brother was sixteen and I, eighteen. We inherited a pile of debts and a second tugboat without an engine. Harvie was the greatest teacher, but I never dreamed of being on a boat and making a career of it. We had to find a diesel motor for the *Old Faithful*. A family friend offered to get a loan for us if Mother would sign for it. I worried about owing $3,000, which was quite a burden in those days. But that was what we did. We found one at J.B. Hoffer's on Georgia Street—this great hunk of iron sitting right on the floor. It was a Fairbanks Morse and taller than we were. We had no choice but to take it. Neither of us knew how to run it, so Hoffer's let us have an engineer to start us out. We both had to learn. There was no manual, no nothing. $1,500 gave us the motor, the shaft, the propeller, and everything we would need to put it in working condition. It started with compressed air, which was the bane of my existence. In 1937, the *Old Faithful* was taken to Benson's shipyard to get the motor installed and be finished off, which was why people thought it was built in Vancouver.

"Bill Rennie, the head boom man at Fraser Mills, said, 'Get that boat up there and start towing these logs to the Pitt. You can't pay for a boat if you don't have work.' That was the way we got our work. There was nothing written—no contract, nothing. I started to run the smaller *Harvie W* because I had to be home sometimes with Mother, who was now also quite ill with cancer. But I could still take the log-scalers out and assist with whatever they needed on the booms. Later in that summer, both of our boats were gone on a day when I was home looking after Mother. I saw this other boat across the way between Pitt Meadows and Douglas Island. It was getting late and the tide was just starting to flood. Floodtide on the Pitt was always very powerful, so I was a little worried about that boat. It looked like a pleasure yacht, and I thought if the fellow on board couldn't get it started, the boat was going to go up on the Pitt Bridge. So I went over to a fellow who lived on the shore, and asked him if he would go and row the boat somewhere safe or tie it up. He protested that maybe the man wouldn't have any money, and I told him, 'Well we can't let him go up on the bridge. I'll pay you if he doesn't have any money.' Not that I had that much, but I did have the two dollars I could pay. When the fellow came home from towing the boat, he told me, 'The guy said thanks very much; his name is Brown and he paid me already.' Well, that didn't mean a thing to me. Then about 11 o'clock that night, the phone rang, and a voice said, 'This is Brown speaking. Send your boat up to Hammond Cedar to pick up some boom sticks and take them up to the head of Pitt Lake.' I was thinking, Good Lord, was he the same man? So we did that—for years. There never was a contract. In the following fall, we realized we needed another boat. Stanley Park Shipyards gave us a price of $2,800 for the *Wayfarer*. We got a 75-horsepower direct-reversing Fairbanks engine, a twin motor to our other one, so we could have interchangeable parts.

"One day, I took *Wayfarer* to Vancouver to clear customs, and Angus Fadden, a fine man at the customs, said, 'By the way, I think you and your brother should get your Master's papers because you've been reported running tugboats that are over tonnage. You've got two boats, so both of you will have to go to the school of navigation in Vancouver.' We'd heard terrible stories about how tough Captain Lindsay, the examiner of Masters and Mates, was. My brother had been injured at school and was blind in one eye, so all the guys on the tugs had always told him he would never be able to get his Master's papers. But we had to find out, so I went over to see Captain Lindsay. I was just terrified, but there was the nicest girl at the desk and I thought, 'Well, he can't be *that* bad.' So I talked to him about my brother's blind eye and told him that my brother needed his ticket. 'Well, that's no problem, but I understand there are two of you working on the tugboats, so you will both have to get your sea time and your tickets.' We had to get two people on the river to certify that we had indeed been running tugs on the river for four years. Once we got our sea time certified, he told me to talk to Captain Norman Young, who was the principal of the school of navigation in Vancouver. When I went there, the place was row upon row of men at their desks. I suppose there were thirty of them in one big room, but it looked like a thousand to me. I said to Captain Young, 'I just *can't* come here!' So he let my brother and me work in his office. This was in 1941, and I was twenty-four years old. We worked out of his office for two days. After that we got friendly with all these people. Every afternoon, they'd say, 'OK, it's our break time; let's go to the Ivanhoe.' But Harvie and I didn't drink, so we'd go to the ice-cream parlour! They laughed about it, but they accepted it quite well. We wrote the Master's examination. Captain Young and Captain Patrick were the examiners. We passed and that was it. For the most part, people sort of took us under their wing. We were known as the Pitt River Towing Company.

"I knew I wasn't going to be working on the river for my whole life. My father didn't believe in education for women higher than Grade 8, but I wanted to get my Grade 12 and go on to university, so I was doing courses by correspondence. When I got my Master's papers Captain Young told the newspapers, and Jack Nilan came to interview me. He told me about his friend D.B. Turner at Connaught High School, who would help me to enroll there. I thought I'd die a thousand times, being twenty-four in Grade 12. In the end I was ten credits short to graduate because I didn't have any electives. Mr. Calder was the principal, and he said, 'If they give credits for music and art I can't see why you couldn't get credit for your navigation papers.' He wrote Victoria and they agreed. So I was off to the University of British Columbia and then Queen's. I missed the river terribly; I can remember every year feeling this fierce restlessness around the end of May and finally realized, 'I know, the freshet's on!' Eventually I married, became a doctor, and had five children. My husband, who was also a doctor, was not enthusiastic about my work on the river. He was born in Newfoundland, and I guess they thought that was a terrible thing for a woman to be doing. Today, nobody would worry about it. He became an alcoholic and later died of

When I went there, the place was row upon row of men at their desks. I suppose there were thirty of them in one big room, but it looked like a thousand to me. I said to Captain Young, 'I just CAN'T come here!'

cancer. I raised my five children mostly by myself when they were four, five, six, seven, and eight years old. I don't think I was remarkable, just single-minded and determined. I think I had the best of all worlds, and I still love the river."

Eve Forrest married fellow medical student, Campbell Gulliford, in 1948, during their fourth year of medical school. They received their medical diplomas in 1950, and had their first child. Their second daughter was born when they did their internships at Hotel Dieu, Kingston, and Kingston General Hospital. Finally licensed to practise medicine, they moved to Oliver, B.C, to set up a general practice. Meanwhile, three more children were born, the last two were boys. The Gulliford family then moved to Salmon Arm in 1957, where Eve worked part-time as much as her young family allowed. She described the old Salmon Arm Hospital as "a very cozy place where everyone did everything." The laundry was all hand-washed by the nurses and hung to dry in the back yard, and a large garden provided fresh vegetables in season.

Mom never turned any of these people away for lack of money. She would provide them with some of the sample medications she had in the office, left by the pharmaceutical salesmen.

After her divorce in 1962, Dr. Eve Gulliford tackled the job of running a full-time medical practice and raising five young children. She set her office in her home so that she could remain close to her children. She hired Mabel Laws to help her. Mabel ran the house and looked after the kids even though she was about sixty-five years old. Mabel lived to see all the children graduate and married.

Dr. Gulliford was active in the Salmon Arm community. She served a term as Chief of Staff at the hospital and on the school board, and was also an environmentalist who encouraged the development of McGuire Park. She was instrumental in the acquisition of the Herald Park property by the provincial government during the early 1970's, and fought for the construction of the Salmon Arm Senior High School. A religious woman from the days when she taught Sunday School at Trinity United Church, Port Coquitlam, she applied one fast rule to her towing business—no work is performed on Sundays. At the time of her decision to become a doctor, her dream was to operate a mission boat to give medical aid to remote B.C. coast settlements.

Dr. Gulliford continued to practise part-time after the age of seventy from her country home, Happy Acres. She had many elderly patients who required house calls. She claimed, "House calls are a tremendous learning experience for doctors; you learn so much about people and the conditions they live in, the stresses which we don't even know about"; and, "Medicine was just something I wanted to do and general practice is the best of all worlds."

Dr. Gulliford retired in 1996. Four of her children live in Salmon Arm and one daughter lives in Quesnel. Dr. Gulliford loved her extended family of animals, especially her donkey, Molly. She lived her final years at Happy Acres with her tugboat *Memorabilia* and prints of her grandchildren proudly displayed. Eve Forrest Gulliford died in 1997 at home with her children and grandchildren. Her ashes rest in Pitt River. Her eldest daughter Anne Lloyd writes, "Our Mom would rise from her ashes in the Pitt River if we tried to sensationalize her life in any way. She was a private person but fought many 'political' battles over the years, very publicly! She was a member of the local School Board and the Medical Staff of Shuswap Lake General Hospital, and provided anaesthetic services there for many years. Her greatest satisfaction and happiness was in her children and grandchildren."

Anne continues: "Mom practised medicine in the 1950s and early 1960s before Medicare came into being. We as children remember many of Mom's patients coming to the house with a sick child, an ill spouse, even just seeking information as to what to do because they could not afford to pay the doctor. Mom never turned any of these people away for lack of money. She would provide them with some of the sample medications she had in the office, left by the pharmaceutical salesmen. Within days or weeks, she would receive a sack of carrots or potatoes or some chickens for the freezer. Eggs were another prized commodity, as was homemade bread. People would leave these items for Mom and her five children in exchange for the drugs that helped these families.

"House calls are mainly a thing of the past now, but Mom firmly believed in seeing people in their own setting, their own milieu. She said you could learn far more about what was really bothering a person if you saw them with their spouse, children, siblings, etc. Today we call this holistic, family care. Again, there was no charge for the house call, but she would have some fresh baking or produce pushed into her hands on her way out the door.

"Families loved having a woman doctor, she often said, especially a woman who had five children of her own and understood what they were going through. Because few could afford a Vet for their pets, Mom often helped with the pets of our friends. Children would bring a cat or a rabbit to her to figure out what was wrong with it. Often she would tell me that the animal was pregnant and wondered how she could explain this to these little seven- to ten-year-old children. In those days, you didn't discuss those subjects with someone else's children!

"Mom had her office in a couple of different buildings in downtown Salmon Arm, but eventually decided to have her office in her home. That way, she was available when we came home from school. If there were any emergencies in our daily lives, she could start supper in the afternoon and continue seeing patients until the end of the afternoon. For years, she had people stop by for a chat and a cup of tea. She helped more families, men, women, and young people with a cup of tea and her willingness to listen to them than many prescriptions would have done. Having her office in her home made it seem less like a formal office where you had an appointment and only so many minutes with the doctor. Sometimes she would take the individual into the office, but if it appeared they needed more of the family touch, she sat them at the kitchen table near the wood stove and talked as she made the tea and produced cookies or bread and jam cut in small, dainty pieces. All of us children grew up running around the house, just yelling 'hi' to anyone we saw having tea with Mom.

"Dr. Eve, as she was known, or Doc to some of the younger generation, was an incredible woman, a physician beyond her time in many ways who had a firm belief that 'the Lord will provide if we say our prayers.' Between her and her Lord, several generations of her patients and their families were extremely well cared for over the years. Eve Gulliford practised in Salmon Arm for nearly fifty years."

(Permission was given by publisher Douglas and McIntyre Ltd., and author Vickie Jensen to print information about Dr. Eve Gulliford from Saltwater Women at Work. *Anne Lloyd kindly provided clippings from local newspapers that she had saved.)*

ELAINE J. (MCLEAN) STEFANELLI (1923–1992)

Elaine McLean was born July 8, 1923 in Pincher Creek, Alberta. She attended Mount Royal College in Calgary, then graduated in medicine from the University of Alberta in Edmonton in 1948, after which she interned at the University Hospital in Edmonton for two years. On July 1, 1950, she married her classmate, Dr. John Stefanelli from Trail, British Columbia.

They worked together for a time in the C.S. Williams Clinic in Trail, where she was the first lady doctor to practise in the Kootenays. She had done extra training in anaesthesia in Edmonton, so her professional work was largely limited to that area. When John left to continue graduate work in surgery, she accompanied him on his residences in Philadelphia and Salt Lake City.

Elaine took a number of years away from practice as she undertook to raise her five boys. Eventually she renewed her licence in order to pursue an interest in the practice of acupuncture when it first came into British Columbia, but she readily admitted she could never understand it. "The cases I think are going to work don't, and the cases I think are going to fail get better. I don't understand it."

Perhaps the most remarkable accomplishment of her life was to have raised her five sons to professional careers—three doctors, a lawyer, and a mathematician. David is a pathologist in Kamloops, Michael is a psychiatrist in Burnaby, and Mark is an internist and neurologist in Newfoundland. Andy graduated in honours mathematics and computer science and Tom is a lawyer in medico-legal work.

Elaine was a well-read person, and had collected a considerable library covering a wide range of subjects. She had a hip replacement at a comparatively young age because of a congenital disorder. She died September 15, 1991 of a breast malignancy.

(The late Dr. Adam Waldie, a long-time friend of Elaine and her husband, kindly wrote this information about Elaine, confirmed by her husband.)

DR. LOIS DAVIES

Curriculum Vitae

Born: Toronto, March 6, 1923.

Early education: Elementary and High School in Toronto; Grade 13 at Bloor Collegiate Institute.

University: MD University of Toronto Medical School 1946.

Post-Graduate: Rotating Internship, St. Joseph's Hospital, Victoria, B.C. 1946–1947; Junior Residency in Anaesthesia, Royal Victoria Hospital, Montreal; Montreal Neurological Institute 1947–1948; Residency in Anaesthesia, Vancouver General Hospital; Shaughnessy Hospital Vancouver, 1948–1949; Senior Resident in Anaesthesia, Children's Hospital, Montreal; Herbert Reddy Hospital, Montreal, 1949–1950; Middle Registrar in Anaesthesia, Westminster Hospital, London, England 1950–1951.

Graduate degrees: MD University of Toronto, 1946; Diploma in Anaesthesia, McGill University, Montreal, 1950; Certification in Anaesthesia, Royal College of Physicians and Surgeons of Canada, 1952; Diplomate, American Board of Anesthesiology, 1956.

Professional Work: Clinical Instructor in Anaesthesia, Department of Anaesthesia, Faculty of Medicine, University of British Columbia, at Vancouver General Hospital, appointed May 1951.

Professional Memberships: Royal College of Physicians and Surgeons of Canada; Canadian Medical Association; Canadian Anaesthetists' Society (member of Sub-committee on Accreditation of Hospitals); Federation of Medical Women of Canada (active on committees); Medical Protection Society.

Awards: Golden Jubilee Membership Medical Women's International Association 1998; Senior Honorary Member Federation of Medical women of Canada.

Personal: Married Dr. F.W. (Bill) Arber in 1957; two daughters, Karen and Catherine; divorced in 1976; widowed 1986.

DR. BARBARA PEAD KRAFT

I practised medicine in Kitimat for almost twenty years, while my husband, Bob, was Technical Director at the Aluminum Plant. In 1949, following our marriage, Bob was sent by his employer to Vancouver as part of a team studying the feasibility of establishing an Aluminum smelter in the province. Technically it was a challenge, boring a hole through the Coast Range to serve as a penstock for the powerhouse, and building a power transmission line across a glacier. The excitement of the day was augmented by the hope of job creation. There were many returned servicemen looking for an opportunity to put down roots. The depression was still freshly in mind, and hope for permanent jobs prevailed.

In 1951 a pile driver went to the head of Douglas Channel, a dock was created, and enough trees cut for a camp site. More land was cleared, temporary housing was built, and a temporary hospital. Clearing was done for the smelter, then, at a slight distance, for a town. The plant was constructed, permanent homes built. The smelter commenced producing aluminum ingots in August 1954. The people who came to work, along with their families, arrived from everywhere, and numerous ethnic-Canadian social clubs came to exist. The general optimism of the times seemed to have a bonding influence.

That was the setting in which health services were established. There was a temporary hospital from 1951 to 1960, well-equipped and staffed. The health problems were about what one would expect for the age group—generally young adults with increasing numbers of children. I recall the efforts of the doctors who were there to maintain a high standard of health care. We worked at gaining hospital accreditation from the then joint Canadian and U.S. accrediting body. In 1958 we gained temporary accreditation, limited by the physical plant, which was the temporary structure, and received full accreditation in 1960 when the permanent hospital was opened. Kitimat was the second hospital outside the Metropolitan areas of Victoria and Vancouver-Burnaby-New Westminster to gain this standard. Powell River was the first. These bigger hospitals tended to be teaching and referral institutions in Metropolitan areas. In such locations there tend to be tens of doctors to share the service load associated with the accreditation program. When this is translated to a smaller community institution, the incessant demands on a few of doctors creates the living reality of the threat of acute fatigue and its possible effect on judgement. We are proud today of our "prepaid" medical system, but paying the bills of hospitals, laboratories, X-ray facilities, and professional fees does not solve the problem of the fatigue involved.

When it came time for us to leave Kitimat after nearly twenty years in the 'sticks,' I elected to see what the academic world was teaching in prevention. My search took me to the University of Toronto School of Hygiene in the second to last year of existence of that historic body. This led to an interesting diversity of work in Montreal and later, Vancouver, until I retired in 1989.

Curriculum Vitae

Education: BA McGill University 1943; MD, CM McGill University 1947.
Post Graduate Training: Rotating Internship Queen Elizabeth Hospital, Montreal 1947–1948; Anaethesia Residency Royal Victoria Hospital, Montreal July 1948–Dec. 1948; Montreal General Hospital, Montreal Jan. 1949–June 1949; Vancouver General Hospital, Vancouver Sept. 1949–Jan. 1950; Vancouver General Hospital, Vancouver Jan. 1951–June 1951; Public Health School of Hygiene, University of Toronto 1973–1974.
Qualifications: Certification Royal College of Physicians and Surgeons, Canada 1952 Anaesthesia; Fellowship American College of Anaesthesiology 1954; Diploma Public Health, University of Toronto; Diploma Public Health, University of Toronto 1974.
Practice: Anaesthesia Staff: Shaughnessy Hospital, Vancouver, B.C. 1951–1953; Staff: Kitimat General Hospital, Kitimat, B.C. 1954–1964; Staff: Kitimat General Hospital, Kitimat, B.C. 1968–1973; Family Practice Staff: Kitimat General Hospital, Kitimat, B.C. 1969–1973;

Community Health: Ville de Montreal Mar.–Oct.1975, Division de la Medecine Preventive, Service des Affaires Sociales; Departement de Sante Communautaire: Oct. 1975–May 1976, Hopital Ste. Justine, Montreal; Occupational Health Physician in Charge: June 1976–Sept. 1978, McGill Staff Health Service, McGill University, Montreal; Chief Physician: Oct. 1979–Oct. 1980, Employee Health Service, Douglas Hospital, Montreal; Geriatrics: Douglas Hospital June 1976–Oct. 1980, Montreal (psychiatric), Geriatric and Medical Services; Administative Pension Medical Examiner: July 1981–1989, Medicine Veterans Affairs, Canada, Vancouver District Office.
Date & Place of Birth: March 29, 1921, Lowell, Massachusetts, U.S.A.
Citizenship: Canadian.
Marital status: Widowed (Husband: Robert W. Kraft, Professional Engineer, deceased 1999).
Children: Three.

DR. ESTELLE M. STEVENS

Curriculum Vitae

Born: Toronto, Ontario, September 1926.
Education: Davisville Public School, Toronto, ON; Humber Heights Consolidated School, Weston, ON; Weston Collegiate and Vocational School, Weston, ON; Oakville High School, Toronto, ON.
Degrees: University of Toronto, MD 1949; University of Toronto LMCC 1949; University of British Columbia, Royal College of Physicians and Surgeons–FRCP(C), March 1978.
Internships: Hamilton General Hospital: Junior Rotation 1949-50; Regina General Hospital: Senior Resident, Anaesthesia and Internal Medicine
Post-Graduate Training: Ottawa University: Senior Resident Child Psychiatry 1959–60 (half-time); Senior Resident Adult OPD Psychiatry 1960–61 (half-time); Psychiatry under Prof. R. Chalke. Dalhousie University: Senior Resident Child Psychiatry, Atlantic

Child Guidance Centre 1966–67 (half-time); Psychiatry under Prof. R.O. Jones, London University, Medical School, England; Post-graduate course in Neurology at Maida Vale and Queen's Square Hospital (1975). University of British Columbia: Fourth Year Resident (full-time); Health Sciences Centre Hospital 1977; Shaughnessy Hospital, 1977; Psychiatry under Prof. M. Miller.

Experience: General Practice, St. Catherines, ON, 1953–58; Child Psychiatrist, Winnipeg Guidance Clinic, Winnipeg, MB, 1968–70; Child Psychiatrist, B.C. Youth Developmental Centre (The Maples), Burnaby, B.C. under Dr. Allan Cashmore, Director 1970-73; Consultant Psychiatrist: Bonn, West Germany 1973-76. This period involved frequent consultations with German psychiatrists and American doctors working with the American overseas community. There was also extensive group work with women (consciousness raising), and Parent Effectiveness Training Groups; Sessional Psychiatrist, Shaughnessy Hospital, B.C., 1977; Sessional Psychiatrist–Children and Adolescents: Surrey Mental Health Centre and Langley Mental Health Centre, B.C., April 1978 to May 1980; Consultant Psychiatrist in Adolescent Residential Treatment Centre: B.C. Youth Development Centre (The Maples) 1980–81; Sessional Psychiatrist Consultating in Schools, Vancouver Department of Health 1981–1992; Private Practice in Child and Adolescent Psychiatry: Delta, B.C. 1978–1981; Private Practice in Child and Adolescent Psychiatry: Vancouver 1981–1993.

Retired: June 1993.

Hospital Appointments: Hotel Dieu Hospital, St. Catherines, ON, Active Staff-Paediatrics 1953–58; Nova Scotia Hospital, Dartmouth, N.S., Staff Psychiatrist 1963–1965; Shaughnessy Hospital, Vancouver, B.C., Clinical Fellow 1978; Staff Psychiatrist OPD Psychiatry 1978.

Licences: British Columbia 1951; Ontario 1953; Nova Scotia 1963; Manitoba 1968.

DR. MARGARET JEAN HARDIE BECK

Jean Hardie was born in Vancouver, B.C., in 1927, the elder daughter of Rod and Dr. Margaret (Mardi) Hardie. She did her senior matriculation at McMaster University and medicine at University of Western Ontario, graduating in 1951 and interning at Victoria Hospital, London, Ontario.

Jean worked for the Metropolitan Health Service in Vancouver. She received the Diploma in Public Health from the University of Toronto in 1954 and returned to the Metropolitan Health Service until 1955.

Married to Dr. Richard (Dick) Beck in 1954, they have three children and four grandchildren. As the children grew, Jean studied part-time at the University of British Columbia taking a variety of courses, mostly in Linguistics, a field she thoroughly enjoyed. She now lives with Dick in Vancouver and Kelowna, continuing to enjoy her studies and spending time with her grandchildren.

DR. GLADYS STORY CUNNINGHAM
(1895-1972)

Dr. Cunningham was one of the nine Canadians chosen to write her story in the book, *Women Physicians of the World*, published in 1978, containing the autobiographies of ninety-one medical pioneers from twenty-seven nations who wereborn before 1912. The Medical Women's International Association, with Canadian Dr. Leone McGregor Hellstedt as editor, compiled and published the book. It was dedicated to the memory of Dr. Hellstedt who devoted several years to collecting the memoirs of prominent pioneer women physicians from many different countries.

Dr. Cunningham's story is copied from the book. Not noted is that she was instrumental in establishing the first family planning organization and clinic in Vancouver, B.C. She was honoured as a Fellow of the Royal

College of Obstetrics and Gynecology in London after obtaining membership in the Royal College earlier.

"I was born in Wawanesa, Manitoba, Canada, the third of five children of John James Story, a general merchant, and Hannah Story (nee Avison). My mother's ancestors were Scottish on her father's side and English from Yorkshire on her mother's side. In 1910, the Story family moved from Wawanesa to Vancouver, British Columbia.

"I took my matriculation in Vancouver in June of 1911. In the autumn of that year I became a freshman in the liberal-arts course at McGill College. This was a subsidiary in Vancouver, run and staffed by McGill University of Montreal, with the same examinations as in Montreal. After two years I went to Montreal to continue my studies and graduated in liberal arts in 1915.

"Since my early childhood I had wanted to be a doctor. My parents thought that I could satisfy my desire to be in the healing profession by becoming a nurse. Although I did not agree, I followed their wishes, and in the autumn of 1917 I became a probationer nurse at the Vancouver General Hospital. In the spring of 1918 I had my 'cap.' But I was firm in my desire to be a doctor, so I left the hospital and took a summer job teaching in a country school in southern Alberta to earn some money.

"In the autumn of 1918, I registered as a medical student at McGill University, with my parents' consent. That was the year of the great influenza epidemic. The medical school was closed, and the students were sent to do voluntary work in various hospitals. I began work in the hospital for infectious diseases. It was filled with very sick people, and unfortunately, I was soon a patient myself. The mother of a very good friend, a medical student, took me to her home. There, under the care of the family doctor, I gradually recovered, but was not able to do any more nursing. In the spring of 1919 I took second place in my class in the first-year examinations in medicine.

"Here I would like to interpolate a few facts about women as medical students at McGill. Women had not been admitted to the medical school as recognized students, but at the urging of Professor Ruttan, three female arts graduates of 1915 were allowed to enter, although not as recognized, legitimate students. However, one of these women, Jessie Boyd, took first place in her class the next spring. The authorities agreed to recognize the female students and in future to admit women on the same grounds as men.

Jessie Boyd was the first woman to graduate in medicine from McGill. She later married her arts classmate Dr. Walter Scriver, and became a professor of pediatrics and of internal medicine at McGill.

"My younger brother wanted to enter the university as a medical student too. Father said that he could not finance two of us at McGill, but that if I could switch to Manitoba, where fees and travelling expenses were lower, he could handle it. Sadly, I transferred. For the next three years my brother and I kept house together in Winnipeg, and then I spent the fourth year as an intern. Several scholarships and some summer jobs helped to finance us. On graduation in 1923, I was the first woman to win the prize in surgery.

"At no time during my medical studies at either McGill or Manitoba did I experience any discrimination on the basis of my sex. Indeed, at McGill the men students complained that the technician in charge of the specimens for dissection favoured the women students. In Manitoba, it was said that the professor of anatomy paid more attention to the women. Although the class began with ten women, most of them dropped out due to failure, disenchantment, or marriage. Marie Cameron and I were the only ones left. We were both given internships in the Winnipeg General Hospital—without question. Marie has spent her life in medical work in Costa Rica.

Although the class began with ten women, most of them dropped out due to failure, disenchantment, or marriage. Marie Cameron and I were the only ones left. We were both given internships in the Winnipeg General Hospital.

"In the autumn of 1919, I met Edison Rainey Cunningham while attending the opening student dance with my brother. I had heard the other girls talk about him as an outstanding athlete—hockey, football, and track captain. He was a Winnipeg man in fourth-year medicine, and that year he had returned to college a little late from a summer job. I went with him to a hockey match the next week, and in 1921, we became engaged. Ed had already decided to go as a medical missionary to western China, where his mother's sister Anna Henry was a doctor. After a year of post-graduate work he went to western China in 1922 under the auspices of the Methodist Church. I wished to have a degree before marrying. In the fall of 1923 I followed him.

"The day I arrived in Chungking, Szechwan province, where Ed met me, we were married by the Reverend George Sparling of the Methodist Mission. At that time there was war in and around Chungking between a warlord from Yunan, a province to the south, and a local warlord. The Yangtze River is very wide at Chungking, and during the fighting the only craft that could move on the river was an American gunboat which was stationed there to protect American commercial interests. The hospital, doctor, and most of the Mission were in the main city. Across the river were a large boys' school and also a school for occidental children. Parents were apprehensive because these children were cut off from medical care, so the Mission arranged for the Cunninghams to go across the river and stay there, studying the language and being available in case any of the children became ill. Two days after we were married, we crossed the river in the American gunboat—an odd honeymoon—and lived there with a Canadian family until the next summer. Our language tutor was a Chinese scholar of the old school. He taught us not only the language, but also the history and the customs. In the late afternoon we, along with another couple, walked about the surrounding country and sometimes climbed the ChunKing Hills, which are almost mountains.

The war planes came over the mountains from India, refueled, and proceeded form there to bomb the Japanese in eastern China. In retaliation the Japanese bombed Szechwan regularly.

"In the early summer of 1924, we went upriver with our tutor and across a valley to a summer resort where missionaries spent holidays to escape the hot, humid summer weeks. This place was on one of the lesser mountains below the 12,000-foot Golden Summit of Mount Omei, which is one of China's five holy Buddhist mountains. In October, we took a four-day journey by sedan chair to the city of Tseliutsing, where Ed had been appointed to work in the Mission hospital. In January 1925 the Mission council met, and Ed was moved to the city of Chengtu, the provincial capital and the side of the West China Union University, where we worked in clinical medicine and teaching until we left China in 1951.

"There were three hospitals in which the medical students of the West China Union University were taught—the men's hospital of the Canadian Methodist Church, the women's hospital of the Methodist Women's Missionary Society, and the Ear, Eye, Nose and Throat Hospital of the American Methodist Church. These hospitals and the West China Union University were partially staffed and financed through the United Board for Christian Colleges in China, which had its headquarters in New York. Thus, personnel of several nationalities and a variety of denominations worked together in a very healthy manner.

"In 1927, the first Communist rumblings hit Chengtu. The anti-foreign feeling was fairly bitter, and most of the missionaries were directed to leave, as the presence of so many occidentals was an irritant. After a short stop in Shanghai and then in Korea, we went to Peking, where we worked and studied in the Peking Union Medical College, a Rockefeller-supported institution, where some of the finest teachers in the world taught in rotation. Ed worked in Eye, Ear, Nose and Throat. I worked and studied in the Department of Obstetrics-Gynecology under Professor Maxwell of England.

"On returning to Chengtu in the spring of 1928 I was obliged to take over obstetrics-gynecology in the women's hospital, as the doctor who had been in charge did not return. This involved teaching medical students and nurses. I was also forced into advanced surgery and difficult abnormal obstetrics.

"In 1929, we returned to Canada for our first furlough. Ed went to England to study and acquire his diploma in ophthalmological surgery. I stayed in Vancouver and worked in the Salvation Army Hospital. There I learned to do direct blood transfusion. Later, I gave the first such transfusion in Chengtu.

"From 1930 to 1937 we spent our second term in China; we continued to teach in the Medical-Dental Faculty of West China Union University. During the 1937 through 1938 furlough I spent some time studying at John's Hopkins Medical School, then went to London, registered in the Post-graduate School of Medicine, wrote my examinations, and obtained my membership in the Royal College of Obstetrics and Gynecology.

"Our return to Chengtu for the stint from 1938 through 1945 threw us into war times. There was a large American airfield a few miles form the campus. The war planes came over the mountains from India, refueled, and proceeded from there to bomb the Japanese in eastern China. In retaliation the Japanese bombed Szechwan regularly. Since eastern China was overrun by the Japanese, whole universities moved with students, faculty, and equipment into western China. There were five universities operating on the West China Union University campus. Many thousands of civilians also came west. The capital was moved to Chungking, about 300 miles southeast of Chengtu.

"In 1945, just shortly before the war ended, with other Canadian and American families, we flew 'over the hump' into India, where we hoped to get a ship to Canada and the United States. Because of a lack of ships free to carry civilians, we were delayed in India from January to July. Then the governments arranged for the large numbers of civilians waiting in India to be taken to New York by the Red Cross Swedish ship *Griesholm*.

"Ed and I spent this furlough in Canada. The return to teaching in China in 1946 took us into an atmosphere of threat by the communists, who had made their Long March and were established in Yenan, to the northwest. In 1949, the communists took over the country, and on December 31, they marched into Chengtu. Within a few days they had taken over the West China Union University. Together with a few other occidental families, we stayed on to see whether we could work usefully under the new regime. It was an interesting and informative experience. However, it became apparent that we were an embarrassment to our Chinese colleagues, students, and friends. We left Chengtu on December 31, 1950, reached Hong Kong in March, and proceeded via Europe to Canada.

"Training Chinese doctors not only to practise but to reach and to administer hospitals had been the West China Union University's policy. By this time the deans of medicine and dentistry, the university hospital superintendent, and the superintendent of the outpatient department, as well as the heads of the various departments of the faculty, were almost all Chinese. They were men and women who had done post-graduate work in Canada, Britain, or the United States. The woman who took over obstetrics-gynecology sent a verbal message five years later, saying, "Tell Dr. Cunningham that we are carrying on the work she entrusted to us."

"In October of 1951, my husband and I set up our private practice in Vancouver, each having accreditation as a specialist. We enjoyed this period very much and were able to save a few dollars against an old age that is not too well

cared for by the church for which we worked. (Wives with the United Church missions, no matter what their work, get no salary.) At the end of June of 1962, we passed our records over to other doctors and retired. Since then we have travelled a little and engaged in other activities for which we did not have time before. I am fully occupied (aside from my role as homemaker) with my church, the YWCA, the University Women's Club, family planning, the Soroptimist Club, and general social and family activities. There is time to read and to enjoy the beauties of Vancouver.

"It has not yet been possible for us to have any contacts with former Chinese students and colleagues in mainland China. There are a number of them in Canada and the United States, but they do not have much direct contact with China, either. We hope that now, in the autumn of 1971, since Canada and mainland China have diplomatic exchange and mainland China has been recognized as "China" in the United Nations, these restrictions may be eased. Then perhaps it may become possible for us to be in touch again with the people and place where our hearts are."

Further information on Gladys Story Cunningham from her niece Mary Plant:

"My husband and I went to Chengtu while on a trip to China in October 1999. At that time we were fortunate to connect with two of the former students of Ed and Gladys Cunningham who were still doing some work at the university. We had made contact with Dr. Changan Deng beforehand through Carol Outerbridge, daughter of Dr. Ralph Outerbridge and his wife Margaret (author of the book *Beyond the Moongate*).

"We have not been in contact with Ellen Chu Ling, the wife of the other doctor, since February of 2000. Her husband is Dr. Hui-bin, a thoracic surgeon. Dr. Deng is a haemotologist. Both are over eighty now.

"Dr. Deng told us that after the Cunninghams and the other westerners had left Chengtu, life became increasingly difficult for the staff at the university and hospital, and during the Cultural Revolution, they were all sent to the countryside for three to four years. Eventually, they were able to return to the university because their skills were needed, as were the skills in English, which Ellen Chu-Ling possessed. They carried on with teaching, research, and operating at the university and in the hospital.

"Ellen Chu-Ling had very special memories of Dr. Gladys. She said that because she and her husband were very poor when she was pregnant, her diet was not the best. When it came the time to deliver her baby, she was in great difficulty, and she gives eternal gratitude to Dr. Gladys for giving her a beautiful daughter. The tragedy for them is that because of the forced move to the country, the daughter was not able to complete high school until much later, after their return. Then, because of her age she was unable to get into the university (from which both parents had graduated). She was later able to take a Dental Hygienist's course and was presently working for the Dean of the Dental Faculty at the university.

"The Communists entered Chengtu in 1949. The missionary doctors were forced to leave. The Cunninghams chose to live in Vancouver where Gladys' siblings and their families lived. Gladys had obviously been influenced by the Chinese medical model in Obstetrics where the patient is much more in charge. I realized this when she delivered our first two sons in Vancouver, and Dr. Eleanor Percival (recommended by Gladys) in Montreal delivered our next two solely in the Western style. I would say that Gladys was ahead of her time introducing and supporting the idea of "natural childbirth" to her patients who were interested in being awake for the birth of their babies. (Remember, I am talking about fifty years ago, when the fathers-to-be were sent home until the baby was born!)

"She and Ed were wonderful supporters of their young nephews and nieces as they raised their children, dropping in and doing whatever would help the young mother at that moment: washing dishes, folding laundry, or just providing a shoulder to lea n on. They brought the Orient to us in very special ways, from their wonderful letters home over the more than twenty-five years of their services in China, to their personal loving care upon their return to Canada. We will always cherish their memories and the 'Cunningham Treasures' in our homes.

"Dr. Gladys Cunningham died on September 8, 1972. She was seventy-seven years of age."

DR. TONKA (TONI) KAMBUROFF

I am a Bulgarian national, born in Preslav, Bulgaria, October 21, 1920, and I was the first daughter of Stoitcho Dobrev and Minka Dobreva.

At Preslav I completed four years of elementary school and three years of secondary (Progymnasium) school. I graduated with first class honours and then successfully passed the competitive examination in the National Gymnasium for Girls at Shumen, Bulgaria. At Shumen I finished the remaining five years of high school, following the course of semiclassical division of the above-mentioned Gymnasium. This course comprised five full years of the study of the following subjects: Physics, Chemistry, Natural History, Mathematics, Geography, Political Economy, Philosophy, Education, History, Hygiene, Citizenship, the Bulgarian, French, Latin, and Russian languages, Drawing, Sewing and Embroidery, and Physical Education. I passed the matriculation as a first class honour student in July 1939.

In October 1939 I went to Prague, Czechoslovakia, where I enrolled at the Czech University for Medical Studies. A short time later, this university was closed by the Germans, who were occupying the country. Since I was a Bulgarian national, I was allowed to continue my medical education at the German Karls University in Prague and completed the first premedical year (1939-1940). At the end of that year there were final examinations in only two of our courses, Physics and Biology, and I passed these with honours.

The next year, in order to improve my German language, I lived in Vienna, Austria, where I attended the University of Vienna, taking the second premedical year (1940-1941). I returned to the German Karls University in Prague in the summer of 1941. That year I passed final examinations in Chemistry (Inorganic, Organic, and Biochemistry), Histology, Anatomy including Neuro-anatomy, Embryology, and Physiology. I was awarded the degree of Candidate of Medicine.

In the early part of the year 1942, I began the clinic term in medicine at Karls, and finished my medical studies there in 1945. On the basis of my treatise "Resorption and Secretion of Sulfaguanidin," and the successful passing of the final exams, I was granted the degree of MD on February 3, 1945. The final examinations included the following subjects: Pathology, Psychiatry and Neurology, Ophthalmology, Otology, Rhinology and

Laryngology, Pharmacology, Medicine, Surgery including Orthopedics and Urology, Pediatrics, Obstetrics and Gynecology, Hygiene (Bacteriology and Immunology), Dermatology, Genetics, Physiotherapy, Preventive Medicine, Forensic Medicine, Radiology, and Dentistry.

In February 1945, I was appointed, upon nomination by the Head of the Clinic for Ear, Nose, and Throat Diseases of the German Karls University, as assistant to the auxiliary scientific staff of the said university, where I worked until the end of the war in May 1945 when the German Karls University in Prague was closed.

I then worked in private practice for a short time with a Czech physician, Dr. F. Shima, in Mnichovice near Prague. In April 1946 I left Czechoslovakia for Vienna, where I spent three-and-a-half years in post-graduate training in Medicine, working for the First Clinic for Internal Medicine of Vienna University, as a guest physician until September 1949. In close collaboration with Dr. E. F. Hueber, resident specialist of the clinic, I worked on special studies in electrocardiology, and was co-author with him of two publications on the subject: "Uber die klinische Bedeutung von Brustwand elektrokardiogrammen" ("On the clinical signification of chest leads in electrocardiograms"), von T. Dobreva und E.F. Hueber, *Klinische Medizin* Heft 12, 4, Jahrgang (1949), and "Uber das Elektrokardiogramm belm Herzmuskel infarkt" ("On the electrocardiogram in cardiac infarction"), von T. Dobreva und E.F. Hueber, *Weiner Zeitschrleft fur Innere Medizin*, Heft 30, 8, Jahrgang (1949).

My decision to come to Canada was mainly due to the upheavals during and after World War II and the devastation that befell my family. My entire medical study took place during the tumultuous war period which contributed to many difficulties and complications in my life. My story, "Odyssey," is very long. The following is only a small abstraction from it.

In September 1945, due to the new political conditions in Bulgaria, unexpected and worrisome events occurred. The Soviet Union suddenly declared war on Bulgaria (a monarchy and reluctant ally of Germany) and quickly occupied it. Germany promptly cut off all family communications and connections for the few Bulgarian students in Prague and we all feared the worst. I was in the midst of my medical exams. Fortunately, all students were allowed to complete their exams without any other interference. The

War's general devastation, the bombing, etc., continued. Later on I was called twice for interrogation at the Gestapo Quarters (the feared German secret Police), mainly regarding my communications with Bulgaria. On May 5, 1945, when the war was almost over and the Soviet Union had occupied Czechoslovakia, an atrocious Revolution erupted in Prague (the Czechs uprising against the Germans). The German universities, clinics, etc., were closed. All university professors, with the exception of the few who committed suicide, were arrested, loaded on trucks, and vanished. I, as a Bulgarian with no political affiliations, suffered no harm. However, I had no news of my family. I felt insecure and very concerned about my future.

I decided to move to Vienna in April 1946 where I received information from my parents not to return to Bulgaria. My future there was endangered. A close family relative, a naturalized Canadian, visited Bulgaria in 1948 and on his return to Canada informed me about the devastating situation of my family. The entire property of my parents was confiscated. They accepted the offer of this relative to help me emigrate to Canada and advised me to accept it. I was pleased to follow their advice. In the interim, my Bulgarian passport had expired. The Bulgarian Consulate in Vienna was taken over by the Communists. I was afraid to apply there for an extension of my passport and became stateless. Eventually my father was arrested and interned in a Communist concentration camp at an unknown location, not because of political activities but because he was a "capitalist." He was discharged a few years later, very ill and emotionally destroyed.

I left Vienna in September 1949 to come to Canada, invited by the close relative of my family, Mr. James Stojnoff Momoff, living in Hulatt, British Columbia, arranged with the aid of the Canadian Christian Council. I arrived in Quebec on October 3, 1949 after a long sea journey. I took the CNR train west to Vancouver with a small group of new immigrants from Europe who

I could not find Hulatt on the map but a CNR official arranged my transfer to another train which delivered me at 5 a.m. to Hulatt situated between Prince George and Vanderhoof, B.C. It was snowing heavily and I had the feeling I had arrived in Siberia!

were travelling to various destinations in Canada. The last of them disembarked in Edmonton. I was enchanted with the beautiful setting of Jasper. The Rocky Mountains were magnificent! I could not find Hulatt on the map but a CNR official arranged my transfer to another train which delivered me at 5 a.m. to Hulatt, situated between Prince George and Vanderhoof, B.C. It was snowing heavily and I had the feeling I had arrived in Siberia! My relative and his wife were very friendly and insisted that I remain with them for a while to learn English before moving to Vancouver in search of professional work. We had little knowledge of the difficulties I would have to overcome for the next several years. A major difficulty was that my university was not on the British Columbia list of accredited universities.

As required I had to do a rotating internship which took place at the Vancouver General Hospital from April 1950 to June 1951, and at the Royal Columbian Hospital, New Westminster, July and August 1951. In October 1951 I was granted an Enabling Certificate permitting me to take the Dominion Council examinations in 1952. I passed these exams in October 1952 in Winnipeg, Manitoba.

In Vancouver I met and married a recent immigrant from Bulgaria, Jordan Alexandrov Kamburoff, graduate in architecture from the Technical University of Vienna. He was in private practice and later the campus planner at the University of British Columbia. We shared many common interests, particularly in classical music and art.

From December 1952 to December 1955 I was employed by the Mental Health services, Essondale, B.C. January 1956 to May 1956 I spent in Paris, France visiting friends and attending two Psychiatric clinics: Neuro-Psychiatric et Neurologee: "Establissement National de Bienfaisance De Sain-Maurice," under Professor H. Baruk in February-March 1956, and Centre Psychiatric Sante-Anne, Clinique de la Faculte de Medecine Paris XIV under Professor Jean Delay in April-May, 1956.

I returned to Vancouver and entered service with the B.C. Provincial Government in July 1956. From November 1956 to November 1969 I was staff Physician at Woodlands School. While there I co-authored with Geoffrey Robinson, MD, FRCP(C), James Miller, PhD, Fred Gill, BSc: "Klinefelter's Syndrome with the XXYY Sex Chromosome Complex," which appeared in the *Journal of Pediatrics*, St. Louis, Vol. 65, No. 2, Pages 226-232, August 1964. From November 1969 to October 1985 (when I retired) I was an active medical staff member, serving as a general practitioner at the Riverview Hospital, Essondale, B.C. Sadly, my husband died in January, 1999.

DR. SHIRLEY BAKER THOMAS

In 1966, fourteen years after I graduated in Medicine at the University of Toronto, I wished to become a Neurologist. Why so long after graduation? Family (four children) intervened. During that time I kept in touch with medicine by working part-time at the Cancer Clinic, taking histories and doing physical examinations. This stood me in good stead later on, for I learned how to conduct such examinations and to dictate the results, all within the hour. I learned how to redirect a patient's flow of speech back to the subject without (usually) alienating them.

My post-graduate education included the obligatory year in Pathology which follows the junior internship. Then there was time at the National Hospital at Queen Square in London, England. This institution is the Mecca of Neurology. I also spent a few months at the London Post-graduate School at Hammersmith, learning more about medicine in general.

What, then, was the problem? And how did the Federation of Medical Women of Canada, B.C. Branch play a role? The problem was simple, the solution complex. In order to write the specialty examinations of the Royal College of Physicians and Surgeons, it is necessary to fulfill their preliminary requirements. These comprise carrying out an approved program at an approved centre, over a five-year period. For a few years I corresponded with Dr. James H. Graham, the secretary of the College, in an attempt to convince him and the decision makers at the College that consideration of part-time training over a more prolonged period would allow me to achieve the desired result, that is, competence in the field of Neurology. I was remarkably unsuccessful in this endeavour for at least two years. I also emphasized the fact that full-time training would not permit me to also carry out the household responsibilities of caring for a family. This latter point did not interest the College at all. My youngest child was three years of age and my eldest child eleven when I began writing to the College.

I was very fortunate in 1966 that the then Head of Neurology, Dr. D.J. MacFayden in the Faculty of Medicine, UBC, was sympathetic to my predicament. He was able to obtain funding for me to be taken on as a research fellow at Shaughnessy Hospital. This was most valuable as it enabled me to experience the ambience of a Neurology ward and to participate in the learning experience provided by patient examinations and frequent rounds by staff members. From January 1968, I continued at Shaughnessy Hospital as, "in effect, our senior house officer," to quote from Dr. MacFayden's letter to the College supporting my application. I had reapplied every year, telling them what I was doing in the field of Neurology. Dr. MacFayden went on to say that, "I have no hesitation in stating that her experience and subsequent increase in knowledge over the twenty-seven-month period (1966 and 1967) will be more than equal to a full-year's duty in a recognized Neurology program." This letter was looked on favourably for consideration by the College Committee.

On July 9, 1967, the Federation of Medical Women of Canada, B.C. Branch sent a letter to Dr. R.B. Kerr, the then President of the Royal College, signed by eight specialists and a General Practitioner. Here is the letter:

Dear Dr. Kerr,

We request the Royal College of Physicians and Surgeons of Canada to consider the accreditation of part-time post-graduate training. The current and expected future shortage of physicians has recently been emphasized, and yet the source, in particular of women physicians, has not been fully exploited. Many qualified women could, because of family responsibilities, fit better into a specialist field than into general practice, as the hours of work are better defined. However, it is difficult for such women to devote five years consecutive full-time work towards obtaining their specialist certification. We would like to see opportunities given, where individually merited, for physicians to receive credit for interrupted and for part-time training in major approved hospitals.

In January 1967, the College acknowledged the letter from the FMWC:

"The Credentials Committee reviewed your letter at a meeting held in the early part of December 1967. It was recognized that in the past there had been some opposition to the acceptance of part-time training. If such training is to be acceptable the committee felt that it would have to be taken in major teaching hospitals and under the approval of the chief of the service concerned. The Committee concluded by adopting a resolution:

"THAT in general the Credentials Committee would not be prepared to accept part-time post-graduate training but that the Committee would be willing to study individual cases, particularly where requests for approval of training are submitted in advance."

This resolution was approved by the Council of the College in January 1968. In March I again wrote to the College, cited my curriculum vitae, and referred to the above resolution. On May 15, 1968, my letter from Dr. James H. Graham stated:

"The Committee has stated that on completion on Dec. 31, 1968 of your current appointment as a senior house officer on the neurology ward at the Shaughnessy Hospital, you will require one year of approved full-time residency training in Neurology and six months of approved full-time residency training in Internal Medicine. On the satisfactory completion of the above training and providing the reports from those under whom you have trained indicate that you have demonstrated an adequate degree of competence in your specialty, you will have fulfilled the training requirements for the Fellowship examination in Medicine modified for Neurology."

In 1970, I wrote the examinations and carried out the oral examinations successfully. I feel, however, compelled to mention one last barb (I'm sure, unintentional) from the Royal College. In the mandatory letter of congratulations, Dr. James H. Graham stated: "A reception for New Fellows will be held immediately following Convocation; the wives and relatives are cordially invited to the Convocation and reception. Wives may also accompany their husbands to the President's Reception and the Annual Dinner on Saturday evening, January 23." Need I add I did not attend the Convocation, the Reception, or the Annual Dinner!

What was important was that my lengthy part-time training, rejected in advance in 1966, was accepted and acted upon in 1968. I owe a debt to those who supported me in what seemed to be a hopeless task, that is, a task of trying to get the Royal College to modify their views concerning such part-time training over a longer period of time than that required for full-time training. I believe that the Federation of Medical Women of Canada, B.C. Branch played a very important role in the softening of the approach of the Royal College. I am grateful to the women who signed the letter of 1967, most of whom I knew personally, but some of whom I did not. They supported the theme of importance of the concept of part-time training in order to accommodate family responsibilities of women doctors, a point of view which was then totally alien to the powers that existed in the Royal College. In May 1968, in the *Medical Post*, in Cleveland, the notion of part-time internships was brought into being for Residents in pediatrics, psychiatry, and child psychiatry. The theory was advanced that such training might even be "superior" to the classical training in that, with the longer period there was more likelihood of participation in seminars and other training scenarios.

To round out my story, I enjoyed over twenty-two years working in the private practice of Neurology. I had my own office and admitting privileges at a community hospital, Lions Gate Hospital, in North Vancouver. I shared on-call hours with another Neurologist for over ten years. The arrival of a third Neurologist reduced the on-call time. I retired from Neurology in 1992 after a very fulfilling and interesting career. I then studied Law at the University of British Columbia and was called to the bar in 1996. My husband, a Haematologist, now retired, supported me in every way. Our children have each developed significant careers, and our grandchildren are delightful. The family had to make adjustments because of my career, but I think that their lives were thereby enriched rather than deprived. My struggle to become a Neurologist was well worth it.

1953

DR. JACOBA (JULIA) VAN NORDEN

Dr. van Norden was named Jacoba after her grandmother, and was always known in Holland by her nickname "Toss." "Jacqueline van Vlissingen" was another name she used during the war when she was involved in the underground and working for the Red Cross. The name "Julia" was chosen when she started to work in medicine in Vancouver, British Columbia, so that the patients would know she was a woman doctor who shared a practice with her husband Dr. Herman van Norden.

Julia was born on February 8, 1919 in 's-Hertogenbosch in southern Holland. She was the elder daughter of Willem and Gerdina Damen Wouters. Her father was an inspector for the Postal and Telegraph and Telephone Administration of the Dutch government. Both parents were born in 1896 and brought up as Roman Catholics. They met at the time of the beginning of the First World War. Her father renounced the Catholic religion, and later her mother did the same. She could not agree with the edict that a married woman should be pregnant every year or two. Her own mother (Julia's grandmother) had twelve children, lived to be sixty-five years of age, and was known to have a great sense of humour. Her mother's sisters also had many babies, and Julia's mother was forever helping them.

The southern part of Holland was mainly Roman Catholic, but Julia's parents sent their daughters to a liberal school. They lived in a new house in the newer part of town. There were the usual confrontations between the girls from the liberal school and those from the Catholic school. The style of dress became frequently talked about amongst the girls: while the Catholic girls had to wear their longer skirts and long-sleeved blouses, others could wear their summery outfits. Julia's father was practical, honest, and straightforward. Whenever the girls were engaged in a minor misdemeanour, he taught his children that lying was worse than the offence. Julia remembers her elementary teacher as a kind and warm woman. In high school there were mainly male teachers. The principle had a daughter who was in Julia's class and they became close friends. The curriculum included mathematics, physics, chemistry, biology, geography, world history, and three foreign languages. Julia decided she eventually would study biology, medicine, astronomy, and theology, which she thought would answer all her questions.

By 1940, Julia was certain she wanted to study medicine. Madame Marie Curie was her role model. Her father preferred her to study law, but wanted her to wait for a while. She earned money for university by working in the Postal and Telegram departments and tutoring high school students. Her girlfriend also had to wait to go to university as her two older sisters and a brother were all attending university at the same time.

In September 1942, Julia began to study Basic Sciences at the University of Utrecht in the northern part of Holland. The Second World War was raging in Europe. On May 10, 1940, the Germans had invaded Holland. The universities were gradually taken over by the Germans, the Jewish professors dismissed and replaced by Germans. Ninety percent of the Dutch students boycotted the changes in the universities. The women students were sent to work in industries in Holland for the German cause, and the male students were sent to work in camps in Germany after the universities were mostly closed by February 1943, as there were so few students remaining. The Dutch people were forced to give all their silver, gold, and radios to the Germans. Julia's father hid one radio in an unused hearth and was able to follow the war news.

Before the war began the Dutch newspaper had written of the Nazi treatment of Germans who were anti-Nazi, sending them to camps and prisons, and of the disappearance of the Jews in Germany. Once the Germans invaded, the Jews of Holland were slowly disappearing. Of the 50,000 Jews, only 5,000 survived. Many of these were hidden and cared for by Protestant and Catholic families. Julia was determined to fight the Nazis, whom she called beasts. She and her friends decided to join the underground. She left home to protect her family and worked for a minister's family with six children. Her father had also joined the Resistance group.

A job which was ideal for Julia's activities became available at the International Red Cross Headquarters in Vught, a small suburb of 's-Hertogenbosch, in June 1943. The person who was the Head of the Red Cross was Charlotte van Beuningen, a wealthy, powerful Dutch woman in her seventies. She had joined the Oxford group in its early days and was a pacifist. Her family owned factories, coal mines, docks, and industries in Rotterdam. She lived in a villa on a large estate of farms and greenhouses. There were seven live-in servants, a chauffeur, and gardeners. The Germans had taken her cars, the work truck, and all her horses except one, two small ponies and a four-wheeled cart that had a secret drawer. In Vught, there was a holding camp in concentration style, and a small hospital of about twenty-five beds, with a former Professor of Obstetrics at the University of Utrecht as the Head of the hospital. The nurses and the doctor were inmates and were in a position to help in underground work.

Julia applied for the job of secretary to Mrs. van Beuningen and got it. The previous secretary, a man active in the Resistance movement, had been arrested (he later died in a concentration camp in Germany). Julia was given false identity papers and became Jacqueline van Vlissingen, a cousin of Mrs. van Beuningen, and was listed as a laboratory technician. She lived on the estate and had a room of her own and a phone. She was able to help with arranging safe houses and delivering messages from relatives of the prisoners in Camp Vught.

The women students were sent to work in industries in Holland for the German cause, and the male students were sent to work in camps in Germany after the universities were mostly closed by February 1943, as there were so few students remaining.

The Dutch population was united in giving help to the prisoners. Women volunteered five mornings a week to prepare sandwiches for the hospital. For the prisoners, clothing, wooden shoes, knitted socks, linen, medicines, vitamins, dressings, and soap were all collected and delivered by the Red Cross to the camp. In the secret drawer of the cart were medicines and messages for the prisoners. Many prisoners in the camp were Belgian officers. Lists of their names were obtained and sent via the underground to Brussels.

Julia had two girlfriends who were prisoners in the camp, Marta and Cjeke. They were forced to work under guard at the Michelin factory. Julia took a dangerous risk to arrange Marta's escape. She rode her bicycle to the factory, parked it against the wall, then climbed up onto the bicycle's seat and jumped over the wall. She then delivered a message that contained her family's address as a safe house for Marta. This was later found out, probably by the nasty wife of the Head Commandant Grunewald. The Second-in-Command, Unter Commandant Stoeker, originally a Swiss who knew Charlotte van Beuningen through the Red Cross activities and her secretary Jacqueline van Vlissingen, sent for Julia and warned her that a trap was being set for her. Bribed by the hope of release from the camp, a woman prisoner went to the home of Julia's parents, asked for help, and pretended that she was a friend of Julia. The way she parked her bike on the street roused the suspicion of Julia's father, and he told her that Julia had disappeared and he could not help her. Later, he saw a German army vehicle come to pick up the bribed girl. Cjeke, Julia's other friend who was a prisoner, was transported to the concentration camp Rabens Bruck, and was eventually set free by the Russian Army. Because Holland was not liberated yet, she managed to go to Sweden, and was diagnosed with tuberculosis, and was hospitalized there. After Holland's liberation, Cjeke was returned home and resumed her university education after a prolonged treatment there. Unfortunately, some other members of Julia's sorority had died in the camps.

There was a horrible tragedy at Camp Vught when twenty women prisoners were herded into a small room where the walls had been covered with sulfuric acid. All the women died. There was a huge outcry from the Red Cross and the Dutch population.

Julia had to go into hiding after an incident when a Dutch collaborator with the Nazis was mysteriously killed (presumably by the Resistance group in Vught). Julia was sent to Amsterdam by the underground to a safe house, where an apartment was rented by the underground contacts. There was a false wall in the apartment, behind which was a laboratory which falsified identity papers and food stamps for the underground. Julia kept busy cleaning the apartment, reading, and listening to music, as there were a lot of books and music records in the apartment. She was able to shop for her food since she could speak German. As she was blonde and blue-eyed, she was an "Edelweib" in the German mind and was not thought to be a suspect. She returned to Vught four weeks later. The killing of a Dutch traitor

was not of too much interest to the German military, so they did not prolong the investigation.

At Christmas time Mrs. van Beuningen planned to meet with Unter Commandant Stoeker to ask if the Red Cross could give presents and extra food to the prisoners. She was unable to go to see him and sent Julia with the message. The guard at the camp had expected Mrs. van Bueningen and when Julia arrived he examined her identity papers and said they were false. This was one of her most terrifying moments, but she insisted the guard contact Stoeker who came to solve the problem. Unter Commandant Stoeker agreed with the request of the Red Cross, but only on condition that the guards were to receive the same gifts. Julia had to make a decision. She knew the guards would steal the gifts if she did not agree with the Unter Commandant's proposal, so she decided she had to agree with him that the German guards were to receive equal Christmas gifts.

The war dragged on, but eventually the news came over the hidden radios that the Allies were getting closer. The Germans planned to move the prisoners to Germany. The Red Cross found out about this plan and offered to take over Camp Vught, but this offer was refused when Julia delivered the message to Unter Commandant Stoeker. Julia knew he had a Dutch girlfriend and she biked with a friend to talk to him. He was promised the protection of the Red Cross, but sadly, he said, he did not have the power to decide. He accompanied the two girls with their bikes back to the Red Cross Headquarters.

To save the prisoners from going to German concentration camps, the Resistance group decided to blow up the railway tracks so the transfer could not take place. They staged this with an ambulance and a pretend patient (as well as the hidden dynamite), which managed to pass the guards without raising suspicion. The railway track was destroyed as planned. Unfortunately, the Resistance group did not realize that there was another set of tracks, so the evacuation of Camp Vught took place. The Red Cross entered the hospital and found that the Germans had executed several prisoners and cremated the bodies. The very gruesome sight of the hospital bathtub full of bloody clothes was forever imprinted upon the minds of the Red Cross workers.

As the Allied forces moved closer to the border of Holland, the prisoners had been forced to dig trenches in preparation for trench warfare. The Red Cross supplied food for the prisoners, delivered by Julia and three others who took turns. A three-wheeled cycle with a large box containing food was covered by a white cloth with a bright "Red Cross" drawn on top. The Allied planes flew low and were firing. The German guards advised Julia and her partner who was pushing from behind to jump into the trenches with them. They refused and waved their arms, hoping the pilot would see their Red Cross sign. The shooting stopped! Julia said it was her luck that saved her again.

The Canadian Forces followed by the Dutch General Krull entered the town in September 1944 and liberated southern Holland. The enormous parade of Canadian soldiers and the noise of their vehicles would never be forgotten. The Canadians set up tents for 800 men on the van Beuningen estate, which was still the Red Cross headquarters. Julia, representing the Red Cross, was given permission to have a cab with a driver to travel to Brussels to deliver the names and messages of the Belgian officers who were now in German camps. On arriving back from Brussels she realized she had left her identity papers in the cab. A Canadian officer from Toronto offered to take her by an open jeep to the cab station. He wrapped her in an army blanket and drove her to the check point, and they were both promptly arrested by Canadian guards! Everyone was nervous as there was a counter-attack by the Germans very close by. Julia was thought to be a spy, and the Canadian an imposter. They were taken to the Canadian headquarters in a school to be interrogated. The Canadian had to describe in detail the city of Toronto. After fifteen minutes the cab with Julia's papers was located by the military police and the two were freed! They got a great welcome from those involved in the arrest.

The northern part of Holland was not liberated yet. Food and supplies were very scarce. Julia's sister was a nurse in a Red Cross hospital in The Hague. Julia got permission from the Canadians to visit her in a Red Cross van with supplies of food for the nurses who were badly malnourished. She was able to bring her sister back to their parents' home—both in their Red Cross uniforms. Julia's war experience had matured her; she had become more realistic, a better human being. When asked why she endangered herself, her reply was that she just wanted to help. At times she felt powerless to do so, resulting in a guilt complex and a great sadness. She admits she might have been more careful in certain circumstances and should have had more protection.

The war was finally over in May 1945 after the German capitulation. With northern Holland liberated, the four universities were opened in September 1945 for the students who had refused to co-operate with the Germans in 1943. Julia was determined more than ever to study medicine even though she was poor. Everything she had seen in the war convinced her to become a doctor. She returned to the University of Utrecht and graduated in medicine in 1949. After two years of internship she was licensed to practise.

Julia had promised her father that she would not marry until she graduated from medical school. She had met Herman van Norden, her husband-to-be, at a medical student assembly meeting in Brabant in October 1944 after the liberation of the southern part of Holland. He had found a chair for her and she thought how gentlemanly he was. She was in first-year medicine at Utretch and he was two years ahead of her in medicine in Amsterdam. Julia and Herman married in June 1949 after he had finished his internship. They had much in common, both having been involved in the underground activities.

To save the prisoners from going to German concentration camps, the Resistance group decided to blow up the railway tracks so the transfer could not take place.

With so many doctors now graduated and few jobs available in Holland, and with the loss of Indonesia, the need for Dutch doctors to work there was gone. Herman and Julia decided to leave Holland and emigrate to Canada. Herman had no family left in Holland; his mother had died in a concentration camp. His sister, sister-in-law, and her child had been on holiday on the coast of France when the war started, and managed to get to Indonesia where they were later imprisoned by the Japanese, but all survived. They had emigrated to New York. Julia's sister and husband and two children were now in Canada on Vancouver Island in British Columbia. Julia's parents eventually came to live with the van Nordens in Vancouver in 1960.

Julia and Herman obtained third-class tickets on a ship out of Rotterdam and landed in New York on December 12, 1951. After a visit with

Herman's sister in New York, they exchanged their train tickets for flights and reached Victoria, B.C., on Boxing Day. They decided to settle in Vancouver. They, as foreign graduates, were required to intern a year in a Canadian hospital in order to write the LMCC exam to practise in Canada. They both got jobs at Shaughnessy Hospital—Julia as a senior intern and Herman as a surgery resident. They were given living quarters and $150 a month each. (Vancouver General Hospital paid only $40 a month!) People at Shaughnessy were good to them. They successfully passed the LMCC exam and began their own general practice in Vancouver. They were busy, popular, kind, and compassionate doctors and helped many in need, including new immigrants, patients without money and medical insurance, and young pregnant women. They retired from private practice in 1993. Julia and Herman have three children and three grandchildren.

Julia was honoured by her country of birth by Queen Beatrix of Holland in 1993. She was awarded the Knighthood of the Orange Nassau (Queen Wilhelmina, Queen Juliana, and Queen Beatrix have all been grandmasters of this order). Julia was given the impressive medal for her distinguished services and activities in different fields.

(The information on Dr. Julia van Norden was collected from interviews with her and from a powerful videotape made by the Survivors of the SHOAH, produced in 1998, in which Julia told of her wartime experiences.)

1954

DR. JOYCE GOLDING CLEARIHUE

Curriculum Vitae

Born: March 10th, 1927, Victoria, B.C.
Marital Status: Single.
Occupation: Physician; Specialist in Dermatology.
Education: St.Margaret's School, Victoria, B.C.; Victoria College, 1943-44; University of British Columbia, 1947, Honours BA in Bacteriology and Zoology McGill University, MD, CM 1953; intern, Vancouver General Hospital, 1953-54.

Post-Graduate training in Dermatology: Montreal General Hospital, from January, 1955 to September, 1955; University of Pennsylvania, September, 1955 to July, 1956; Henry Ford Hospital, Detroit, July 1956 to June 30th, 1958; and in Allergy at the University of Illinois R and E Hospital, July to December, 1958.

Practice: In Private Practice in the Specialty of Dermatology in Victoria, B.C. from 1959 to January 1, 1986.

Professional Licences and Certifications: Licentiate of the Medical Council of Canada (LMCC), June, 1954; Licensed by the B.C. College of Physicians and Surgeons, 1954; Diplomate of the National Board of Medical Examiners, U.S.A., 1954; Royal College of Physicians and Surgeons Specialist Qualification in Dermatology, Certification, November, 1958, and Fellowship, September, 1972; American Board of Dermatology (U.S.A.), July, 1960.

Professional Career and Associations: Bacteriologist at the Provincial Health Labs, Vancouver, B.C., 1947-48; Active Staff, Royal Jubilee Hospital, Victoria, B.C.; Associate Staff, Victoria General Hospital, Victoria, B.C.; Past Chairman of Advisory Board, (1964–65), Gorge Road Hospital; Member, American Academy of Dermatology (U.S.A.) 1958; Canadian Dermatological Association, (Board of Directors 1974 and 1975); Pacific Dermatological Association (Vice President 1971–1972); Pacific Northwest Dermatological Association (President 1973); Canadian Medical Association, B.C. Division, CMA Section of Dermatology (Past Chairman 1968–1969); Victoria Medical Society (Chairman, Archives Committee 1974–1979); McGill Alumni Society, (Past President, Vancouver Island Section 1967–1969).

Community and Recreational Interests: Victoria YM–YWCA (Past President 1971–1972 and Board Member to1980); Victoria Science Fair (Judge 1974); Thetis Lake Nature Sanctuary; The Alpine Club of Canada, Outdoor Club of Victoria, and other hiking-skiing Clubs; Member of Advisory Committee, Community Education Services, Camosun College, 1974–1977; British Columbia Historical Association; Greater Victoria Civic Archives (Past Board Member); Craigdarroch Castle

Society (Past Board Member); University of Victoria Foundation (Member 1986–Dec. 1990); Friends of the Royal British Columbian Museum (Board Member for nine years to 1994); Canada 125 Anniversary Commemorative Medal, 1993; Lister Orator (Victoria Medical Society) March 1,1996; The Victoria Foundation (Honorary Governor, 1999).

Retired: January 1, 1986, having been the first female Dermatologist in Victoria and on Vancouver Island.

DR. JOAN FORD

Dr. Joan Ford is one of British Columbia's more famous doctors, having been made a member of the Order of Canada in 1991. Her citation reads: "Her compassion extends to the global community for although now retired from her full-time family practice in Burnaby, she continues to serve as a relief physician in isolated villages of Nepal. President of the Himalayan Aid Society, she is a shining example to others in her profession, and her selfless commitment to primary health care continues to have an impact on the lives of those less fortunate."

Dr. Ford practised general medicine in Burnaby for thirty-five years. Throughout the years she responded to the need for a doctor in isolated northern communities of British Columbia, often using holiday time to work there. She also did medical work in Dominica for several weeks in 1967 and again in 1969 under the auspices of the CESO (Canadian Executive Services Overseas). She worked in Nepal for six to eight weeks at Khunde Hospital in the Himalayas every two years from 1980 to 1990.

In the *Newsletter of the Federation of Medical Women of Canada* of February, 1981, Dr. Ford describes her first six-week locum in Nepal:

"To visit Nepal has been one of my priorities, but I did not want to go just as a tourist, so I could hardly believe my good fortune when Mr. Zeke O'Connor of the Sir Edmund Hillary Foundation took me up on an offer I had made several months before, and asked if I would like to do a six-week locum at the Foundation's hospital at Khunde, Nepal. Sir Edmund Hillary's briefing was simple: take a stethoscope and a pair of Adidas runners.

October 1980 I found myself on a plane to Kathmandu, then boarding a Twin Otter for the flight to Lukla. Here I was met by a young Sherpa man who accompanied me on the two-day walk to Khunde in the Khumba area of Nepal. It is not really that far in distance, but it is necessary to go slowly to acclimatize, as Khunde is at an altitude of 12,500 feet. When I arrived I had a warm greeting from Sir Edmund who visits his projects in this area once a year. Besides this hospital, the Foundation is responsible for village clinics and health workers, schools, and another hospital.

"My new practice was very different from my General Practice in Burnaby. The patients were mainly Sherpa people from the surrounding areas. There is a population of about 3,000. Some of these would be two or three days' walk away. There were also trekkers coming to trek to the Everest base camp from countries all over the world. The hospital was very well equipped with drugs and supplies, a small X-ray machine and a generator to power it, three acute beds, and six long stay beds. The patients' families were expected to look after them. Besides myself, there were two health workers with some medical training they had received from the resident doctor, and a cleaning lady. At times I would visit a neighbouring village and one of these workers would accompany me.

"Amongst the local people, the main problems were skin and chest infections, and with the trekkers it was usually altitude sickness or gastroenteritis. I was interested to see there was a demand for birth control, usually an IUD or DepoProvera. I was also called on to do dental extractions. This is an endemic goitre area and has been successfully combatted by giving IM injections of Lipiodol every five years. There was also a BCG program as TB is prevalent.

"The weather was very dry and sunny with a sharp drop in temperature at night, and the food supply was good at this time of year as these people live mainly on potatoes and rice, so there was not a great deal of sickness. The situation is not nearly so good in summer when the monsoon comes. There is heavy rainfall and the food supply is low.

"I had a four-day holiday at the end when the resident doctor returned, so Mingma, my interpreter, and I were able to trek to the Everest base camp and visit a British expedition who were planning on climbing the west face. The hospitality, kindness, and cheerfulness of the Sherpa people who have so little in the way of material goods, and of Sir Edmund Hillary and other members of the Foundation, made this an unforgettable visit."

Dr. Joan Ford was born in 1925 in Newcastle, Staffordshire, in England. She writes the following about her experiences: "My story begins in 1942, a sixteen-year-old girl in an English boarding school, at home for Easter holidays and a letter comes, the school has closed, commandeered by the U.S. Airforce for their headquarters. Too young for nursing or the services, I ended up at Sheffield University and so started my medical career. Looking back at my time in Medical School some memories come back vividly. A crowd of us students around a bed watching penicillin being given IV to a wounded soldier, one of the earlier cases of its use. Giving anaesthetics in the Emergency Department using a mask attached to a cylinder of nitrous oxide, seeing women coming in near death with septic abortions, and miners with crushed limbs, who showed such courage—'A bit of dirt fell on me, Miss.'

I remember seeing women coming in near death with septic abortions, and miners with crushed limbs, who showed such courage—"A bit of dirt fell on me, Miss."

"I graduated in 1948 and spent the next five years doing hospital appointments in medicine, pediatrics, and obstetrics, obtaining Diplomas in Obstetrics in 1951, and in Child Health in 1953. I then moved to General Practice which turned out to be a poorly-run practice and soon I found an ad for a job at the Children's Hospital in Vancouver, applied, and was successful. Late August 1953 I sailed on the Empress of Scotland to Montreal and then by train to Vancouver. With its mountains and seashore British Columbia seduced me to become a permanent resident. In no time I joined the B.C. Mountaineering Club, where I made lifelong friends, and even climbed Mt. Baker that Thanksgiving.

"I got my licence to practise the following June and went to do a locum at Bella Coola on the B.C. coast. My five years of hospital practice came in handy now as I was the only doctor, (no road in those days). No one had warned me I was the dentist as well. It was a toss-up as to who was more scared, the patient or doctor, when it came to dental extractions. I went back there for a second locum in the fall.

"Bella Coola had a single telephone exchange so the phone being called was identified by the number of rings. When the hospital phone rang there would be numerous clicks as people listened in. Our Mountie was aghast when he got orders to get his annual medical exam, as he realized he would have to come to me, and the locals were much amused to see when he would present himself.

"In November, 1954 I opened my own practice on Edmonds Street in Burnaby. I was surprised to find myself the only female GP on the staff of the Royal Columbian Hospital, but others soon came along. I worked part-time at school clinics for the first two years to get an income; after that the practice was busy. By 1959 it was too busy and driving me crazy, so I took on a partner and life became bearable again, and in 1962 another partner.

"Practice was very different from practice today. The GPs ran the Emergency Department and had to take turns a week at a time to care for patients who had no local doctor. The week before Emergency call there was police duty; any prisoner being transferred to Oakalla Prison had to be certified free from an infectious disease. There was no MSP medical insurance and we were often not paid for our work.

"In the 1960s I got the chance to go and work for two months on the island of Dominica. Several doctors from Surrey and New Westminster ran a partnership with the Dominican doctors. It was an island of extremes, magnificent beaches and desperate poverty, and a host of new diseases for me. The people were very friendly and cheerful in spite of having so few material goods. There was a sad lack of resources and medications. I vividly remember one home visit for a retained placenta. There was little furniture in the house and no light except for a candle. While concentrating on removing the placenta there was a smell of burning and I discovered to my horror my hair was singeing in the candle flame.

"I made a second visit two years later, but it was sad to see nothing had changed. Some public health measures would have eradicated yaws, typhoid fever, and many worm infestations. Shortly after my visit there was a backlash against white people and it was no longer safe to go there.

"I gave up practice in 1989. I had stopped obstetrics in 1980 about the time I first went to Nepal. I continued to do locums for several years. I was able to go to Dease Lake Clinic on two occasions, an interesting experience with a chance to meet the local Aboriginal community. I also went on a cyclone relief team to Bangladesh, a different learning experience, how not to send aid. We found there were plenty of local doctors who had a much better knowledge of the culture and endemic diseases, but I had a good lesson on life.

"I did my last locum in 1999. I was unable to keep up with all the new technologies and drugs, but I remain on the board of the Sir Edmund Hillary Foundation and keep in touch with my Sherpa friends."

Joan was a member of the Mountain Rescue Team for four years. This group was founded in 1956 in Vancouver, all experienced volunteer mountaineers. She was Director of the Save the Children Fund of B.C. from 1960 to 1990, and President on two occasions. She was also a Director of the Sir Edmund Hillary Foundation of Canada 1988 to the present, as well as a Director of the Trans-Himalayan Aid Society since 1980 and served as President. Joan is an active member of St. Albans Anglican Church and for years the Deanery representative to the St. Michael's Centre, Burnaby (an Intermediate and Extended Care Facility). A board member of the Western Society of Senior Citizens, she was also President of the B.C. Branch of the Federation of Medical Women of Canada, and National President of the FMWC for 1972–73. She was made an honorary Senior Member of FMWC in 1999.

In addition to the Order of Canada, her honours include the Canadian Medical Association Senior Membership in 1991; the Honorary Membership of the College of Physicians and Surgeons of British Columbia; and in 1991 the David Bachop Gold Medal of the British Columbia Medical Association "for contribution to health care in B.C. and other countries."

DR. ANNE LEES

"She's not a doctor, Mom," said one of my first patients as he returned to his mother, "she hasn't got pants on." The boy just expected a male doctor. After he had been hurried to the door by his embarrassed mother, I had a good laugh.

The boy obviously did not want to know that I had graduated from Liverpool University in 1949, served two years in several residencies and a year in public health, and done general practice before coming to B.C. After a year in Crippled Children's Hospital, I was eligible to take the B.C. licensing exams. Indeed at that time women were not completely welcomed, either by the medical profession or society, but here I was in Powell River, a thriving pulp and paper town with 6,000 population. I am grateful that the clinic gave me the opportunity to fulfill my duties and to break the ice for women who followed.

In the fifties the town boasted a well-equipped sixty-bed hospital, thanks in part to the generosity of the Powell River Company. There was an excellent sick benefit plan for employees and their dependents. The clinic had a senior partner near retirement and four other partners: a surgeon and three who had extra training in anaesthetics, internal medicine, and obstetrics. I was one of four assistants who shared hospital emergency calls as well as putting in a full day in the clinic. We also had a pathologist and radiologist who visited once a week. We all had lunch together, which was great for networking and case presentation, to say nothing of news from the city.

My first Saturday call included a powersaw injury of the forearm, an acute eye, and acute appendix. In between assisting the surgeon, I treated the normal run of lacerations, bites, fish hooks, allergies, and earaches associated with a summer weekend—not to mention the inebriates who had caused havoc to themselves or others. Not a dull moment!

I was soon accepted, and was able to start some prenatal classes for pregnant moms, which helped to reduce the fear in the case-room. The school medicals assisted me in getting help for the youngsters with ENT and eye problems, especially the recent immigrants whose parents had a language problem. The Indian children kept us busy in the children's ward.

I left the clinic after two years. My marriage and three daughters kept me busy for a few years.

In 1963, a visiting consultant suggested that I should think about a bit of work on Texada Island, which had a population of 1,000 and three industries—an iron mine, limestone quarry, and cement works. Why not?

So started an eventful but fun four years. The Island was serviced by a five-car ferry trip of forty-five minutes and a water taxi trip of twenty minutes. My husband was clever enough to find a car small enough to be the sixth car, but I mainly used the taxi. The crossing was often so rough that only the mail and I attempted the trip. I went over three times a week, seeing patients first in a room in the legion, then in a condemned schoolboard trailer. Evidently I was somewhat of an asset because after four months, a very functional suite was prepared for my use in the legion basement. I was to learn which cases I could treat on the Island and which needed transferring. I always appreciated the phenomenal support which materialized in true emergencies, and patients who came over as emergencies really appreciated the continuity of care when I admitted them to Powell River Hospital.

On one occasion I was escorted into the bush by a group of men concerned for a neighbour whom they felt should be admitted to Riverview. We duly arrived, and I was not reassured when they warned me I might be met with a gun, and they obviously had no intention of leaving the vehicle. Clutching my black bag, I went in. Whether it was the black bag or my skirt was open to question, but the man finally came with me like a lamb.

In the summer months I often camped with my daughters on the Island. On one Saturday night, an inebriated patient, who should have had a nasty eye injury rechecked in the morning, staggered out at bar-closing time and insisted the taxi driver take him to me. She could not persuade him otherwise. She started hoping he would settle, but no luck. He staggered down my trail to be met by a clothes-line of wet towels and bathing suits. He returned announcing I had surrounded myself with booby traps. That was the story that circulated around the Island!

Alas, all good things came to an end when the water taxi lost the mail contract, which propelled me into another change. I opened an office in Powell River and ran a solo practice for over twenty years. Life became more civilized but less adventuresome!

Looking back, I have had a happy, rewarding professional life with great colleagues throughout and many happy memories.

DR. LAINE LOO

Dr. Laine Loo was born in Estonia and experienced the horrors of war, with the Russians, and later the Germans, occupying her country. Dr. Jerry Richards of Victoria interviewed Dr. Loo for his series on physicians who took up the study of medicine because of their experiences in troubled times. This article was published by *The Medical Post* on December 3, 1991, and describes so well the difficulties and determination of a young woman in war-torn Europe, and how she became a very busy family practitioner in Vancouver after her eventual arrival in Canada. The article is printed as published in *The Medical Post*, under the title, "Nobody knows the troubles she's seen," written by Dr. Jerry Richard in 1991:

"Dr. Laine Loo looks to be a typical West Coast pensioner as she walks vigorously through the forests around her Pender Island home, halfway between Vancouver and Victoria. In fact she is a woman who took her degree in medicine during an air raid, and later had to qualify twice again in countries and languages that were foreign to her native Estonian.

"Given what lay ahead, it was as well she got her start in medicine at an early age. Her mother was a nurse-midwife in a twenty-bed hospital serving the needs of a factory community on the west coast of Estonia. Their family apartment was attached to the hospital, and Laine, as a young girl, became as familiar with the goings-on in hospital as at home.

"The hospital was a model of efficiency, with one physician and one nurse for a community of 2,000 people. The staff consisted of a pharmacist, a cook, a cleaner, and a man to keep the woodstove going. If an operation had to be carried out, the pharmacist acted as assistant while the cleaning woman handled the instruments.

"All the nursing and much of the medical care was given by the nurse-midwife, as often as not under her daughter's youthful eyes. When Laine finished high school one of her teachers persuaded the family to put her name down for the Faculty of Medicine at the University of Tartu. Had it not been the war, she might have become a seventh generation nurse-midwife.

"When Laine had finished two years of study, the Germans swept across Western Europe and the Russians seized the opportunity to occupy Estonia. From then on Estonian students were obliged to study Marxist-Leninism and encouraged to learn Russian.

"The worst blow of all was that the importation of German or English textbooks was forbidden. Then 20,000 Estonians were deported to labour camps in Siberia, many of them never to return. Laine's fiancé Heino, who was studying engineering, narrowly escaped being taken away with them.

"Young Estonians soon formed themselves into a resistance movement. Laine signed on as first aid worker. One day, as a diversion from their duties, she and two other young women went out to gather strawberries in a field that lay between the warring sides. All they wanted was to get enough berries to make jam for their soldiers. But the Russians started shooting. The three unarmed girls returned the fire with their only weapons, clods of dirt, which they hurled with angry shouts. The Russians, either out of amusement or embarrassment, held their fire and the girls went on with their picking.

"In the summer of 1941, the Germans attacked Russia and in a rapid march to the east occupied Estonia. Life became slightly easier for the Estonians after that because the Germans left them alone as long as they did not make trouble. But the Wehrmacht began recruiting the resistance fighters into its ranks. Laine decided it was time to go back to school.

"Going back to the university from her post of duty near the Latvian border was not easy, especially since a Nazi official had stamped her travel documents "Not Allowed to Travel by Train." The train was little more than a cattle car with benches, but it was better than walking. Determined to get on with her education, she took a rug to the station and persuaded some travellers to roll all five feet of her in it and stow her under a bench. Hiding there, she was at least warm if not comfortable. The trip covered 200 kilometres and was slow, typical of one of the wartime conditions, but she eventually reached her destination undetected.

"Once back at university, she married Heino, who had now found a job as engineer in the city. He was allowed an hour off, no more, for the ceremony. The little family set up housekeeping on slender resources, getting barely enough food for one meal a day. Fortunately, they did not smoke and were able to trade their cigarette rations for books and food. Three cigarettes was the going rate for an egg.

"In 1944, the fortunes of war turned and the Russians, now on the offensive, began fighting their way back into Estonia. Laine was now pregnant. A month after the baby arrived, she finished her medical studies. By that time fighting was going on close to the university. Her graduation ceremony was marked by the Russian bombers overhead and loud explosions outside. The official whose job was to administer the Hippocratic Oath to the new graduates hastily handed out copies. "Don't read it," he urged. "Just sign and get out of here." The students scribbled their signatures and ran for the safety of the basement.

"In the midst of these excitements Laine's husband became seriously ill with tuberculosis and was sent to a sanatorium. Laine retreated with her new baby to the home of her parents, and took over the practice of a local doctor who had fled the country. Her patients paid her with what little food they could spare. She felt lucky on the occasions when she got milk or eggs, because she could give some to her baby and send the rest to the sanatorium for her husband. In time when the Russians reached the region of Heino's sanatorium, Laine had managed to save a quart of alcohol from her medical supplies, and traded it for enough gasoline to enable one of Heino's friends to bring him away to safety.

"Glad as she was to have her husband home, she was dismayed at the prospect of having to continue his treatment herself. Heino, however, looked at it as an easily solved problem in engineering. He put together a pneumothorax machine out of milk bottles and rubber tubing, and instructed her in the technique of keeping the affected lung properly collapsed. Her part was to insert a needle into his chest and allow air to run in until he cried 'enough!'

Her graduation ceremony was marked by the Russian bombers overhead and loud explosions outside. The official whose job was to administer the Hippocratic Oath to the new graduates hastily handed out copies. "Don't read it," he urged. "Just sign and get out of here."

"But the Russians were approaching and soon were on the doorstep. Heino was not in good condition for travelling; nevertheless, the family decided to flee. Laine stuffed as many diapers into a pack on her back as she could and put the baby into a pram while Heino loaded a few precious belongings into a suitcase. Thus organized, they set off to walk the ten kilometres to the nearest beach. From there some friends took them by motorboat to an island where a fishing schooner was preparing to sail for Sweden. Along with 200 other fugitives, they piled on, even though they knew conditions on board would be close to impossible. The vessel contained no food and almost no drinking water. Fortunately, the captain's wife was expecting a baby at any minute and took Laine into her cabin to give whatever obstetrical care might become necessary.

"Only one seaman was on board. He chose a few passengers as crew, gave them some rudimentary instructions, and then the little vessel sailed. Fortunately, a good wind set in from the east, which was unusual in the Baltic, and soon was pushing them steadily along in the direction of Sweden. After twenty-four hours they saw lights ahead. Assuming they were approaching the coast of Sweden, they started a signal fire on deck. But the lights proved to be those of a German naval convoy and what they got in return was gunfire. The schooner was headed straight for the convoy, but the man on the tiller, reluctant to lose the advantage of his favourable stern wind, kept resolutely on, merely giving orders to douse the lights. By good luck some Russian planes arrived on the scene and distracted the German gunners.

"Twenty-four hours later, with its passengers safely escaped from Russians and Germans alike but almost mad with thirst, the vessel arrived in the heavenly peace and plenty of a Swedish port. Laine hurriedly obtained some milk and was amazed to see her baby, who had been exclusively breast or bottle-fed, taking a cup in her tiny hands and draining it almost at one gulp. The Swedes settled the family in a refugee camp. Laine was recruited to help the camp doctor as interpreter. She soon demonstrated her abilities by showing him that the patient was suffering from diphtheria, not from a mere sore throat as he had assumed.

"Heino did further studies in engineering (now in Swedish) and got a loan to help establish a home for his family. It was just as well he did so because Laine was rejected for a licence to practise on account of her youthful appearance. She was, in fact, twenty-four, but had no way of getting proof of qualification because her university was now firmly inside the U.S.S.R. For the time being she found work as technical assistant in a hospital radiology department. In the end and chiefly because she quickly mastered Swedish, she was given a temporary licence to practise on the condition that she had to work in a northern mental hospital. Ironically, many of the patients awaiting her spoke not Swedish but Finnish. While thus employed she kept her hand in general practice by sometimes acting as district medical officer, even going out on skis to make house calls.

"After the war Heino learned his parents had been sent to Russian concentration camps where his father died under mysterious circumstances. His mother was released after seven years and allowed to return home. Laine's parents had escaped safely to Sweden.

"Laine was eventually accepted for an internship, and at the end she would be allowed to write examinations that gave her an unrestricted licence to practise. Having gone that far, however, she and her husband decided to leave, mainly because his aunt in Canada offered to sponsor them as immigrants. And so with their children, now seven and two, they set out on the sea again, this time for the new world.

"Almost immediately after arriving in Canada, Heino found a job with a Vancouver engineering firm. While he was settling into his work, Laine, for the third time in her life, began jumping through the hoops that would gain her a licence to practise. She had to write the basic science examinations again—this time in English—do the clinical examinations, and complete a year of internship. At last, ten years after her graduation in medicine, she gained a licence to practise in British Columbia.

"She established a general practice using her home as an office, and began interviewing patients in the five different languages she had mastered. As her reputation grew she became busy—too busy she now thinks—working up to ninety hours a week, making house calls at all hours, and visiting patients in three hospitals. Heino, who was fully occupied in designing bridges and public buildings, complained she rarely got a good night's sleep. During one particularly bad stretch she was called away from her bed every night for three weeks in a row.

"On the day Dr. Loo retired from practice her office resembled a funeral home more than a medical centre, so full was it of flowers from her patients. With her husband she moved to the peace of Pender Island in the Gulf of Georgia. There she practised part-time for a few years, but she and Heino preferred to spend their summers in the garden and their winters in Mexico. Looking back on the wartime days they were amazed to think how little attention they paid to the dangers they were passing through. As for Estonia, they hoped it would someday become completely independent."

Addendum: Heino Loo died in 1992, and did not live to see his home country,

Estonia, gain its independence. After Estonia's freedom, when the two Loo children celebrated their fiftieth birthdays, Dr. Loo accompanied each to Estonia where they were introduced to their relatives.

(Kind permission was given by author Dr. Jerry Richards of Victoria, and by Mr. Rick Campbell, Editor, Medical Post, *to include Dr. Loo's story in this book.)*

DR. PATRICIA A. RADCLIFFE

I was born and raised in Vancouver. When I was twelve, I was walking down to the Tennis Club with my sister, who was then twenty, and she asked me what I wanted to be when I grew up. I replied, "Either a nurse or a teacher," to which she responded, "Why don't you become a doctor?" And that was when my decision was made. I didn't have any close connections to Medicine, but my mother had gone to a woman physician for years. She herself always wished she could have become a lawyer, so she had no objections to my wanting to do this. My father never quite understood why any woman would want to become a doctor, although he expected all his children to go to university, but he never objected in any way.

I would be remiss if I didn't mention other influences that affected my choice, even at the risk of being politically incorrect in this day and age, where to admit to being a Christian is often frowned upon. My belief in a merciful and loving God became a defining part of my life, and I believe a great influence for whatever good I have been able to do. My parents were not church-goers, but I attended Camp Artaban, the Anglican Church camp on Gambier Island, from the age of ten. My sister and brother had gone to camp before me, so it was natural for me to go too. I was influenced by a group of wonderful women, and when I was fourteen I chose to be baptized and then confirmed. The church has been an important part of my life ever since.

My church attendance and teaching at Sunday School also led to my relationship with Rolly, the other most important influence in my life. He lived just three blocks from me, and on the route to the church on one Sunday morning in September, he appeared and walked to church with me. He had just returned to UBC after several years as a Navigation Instructor with the Commonwealth Air Training Command and was treasurer of the Sunday School. I was in Grade 12 at the time and we started going out together.

I finished high school the next spring and won a University Entrance Scholarship for the princely sum of $175, which was a year's tuition at UBC at that time. After two years in Pre-Med I was accepted into first year Medicine at Queen's University in Kingston, Ontario, which was then the only medical school left in Canada which had a six-year course (after Grade 13 in Ontario). All the others (and there were only eight) had converted to four years, usually after an undergraduate degree. Many people have asked me why I didn't continue at UBC, and the answer, of course, is that UBC didn't have a medical school at that time. In fact, there had been a recent study done by Dr. Dolman, the professor of Bacteriology, in which he stated categorically that B.C. didn't need a medical school, and wouldn't for the foreseeable future! So students from B.C. were forced to apply to all the other Canadian schools and to those in nearby states in hopes of being accepted. As it turned out, UBC did open its medical school in 1950, so the first class graduated in 1954, a year after we finished.

Rolly had finished his BA that same year and applied to a number of medical schools, but had not been accepted. However, he insisted that I should take the opportunity and go to Queen's. He stayed at UBC and did his MA in Experimental Zoology and Psychology, and was then accepted into the University of Oregon Medical School in Portland.

I registered at Queen's on my twentieth birthday, September 22, 1947. Our class of sixty-six consisted of sixty men and six women, and when we graduated in 1953, there were fifty men and six women. We were the fifth class at Queen's to have women in the modern era. Queen's had first admitted women in 1881, but discontinued in 1894 (because the male students and some of the professors made life miserable for them), after which women students went to the Women's Medical College in Toronto. Our class was almost evenly divided between ex-servicemen, many of whom were married, and those right out of high school in Ontario. Two of the women were nurses who had served in the forces, two were from Ontario schools, and the other besides myself was also from B.C. None of us were what you would call militant feminists, but rather normal, intelligent women who wanted to become doctors. We were accepted by the men and participated with them in all the normal activities, including running the intramural "Harrier," a long-distance run from the university campus out to the penitentiary (in what was then Portsmouth but is now part of Kingston) and back. I think we all finished in the top half of the class. We all subsequently married and had children, and all but one practised, with three of us becoming specialists.

Our first year was really a Pre-Med year, so there was quite a lot of repetition of what I had already had at UBC, with inclusion of English with required public speaking in the class, Biology, Chemistry, and Physics. Second year we started the pre-clinical Medical courses, including Radiation Physics, Histology and Embryology, Organic Chemistry, and the first of two years of Anatomy. Anatomy took up three afternoons, starting with at least an hour's lecture done with slides in a darkened lecture hall. Needless to say, it was often difficult to stay awake! Third year was more of the same, with Physiology, Biochemistry, Bacteriology, and Pharmacology. In fourth and fifth years we got all our clinical subjects with lectures, clinics, and Pathology labs. Sixth year was all clinical, with half spent in Ottawa at the Ottawa Civic Hospital and half in Kingston at all the hospitals there. We did get to do a few things, including two deliveries, but it was mainly clinics and observing others.

I registered at Queen's on my twentieth birthday, September 22, 1947. Our class of sixty-six consisted of sixty men and six women, and when we graduated in 1953, there were fifty men and six women. We were the fifth class at Queen's to have women in the modern era.

We felt we were fortunate in that the majority of our lectures were given by the head of the departments, so there was a consistency about them. For instance, all our Ob-Gyn lectures were given by Professor Edwin Robertson, who was a dapper little Scot and a very dynamic lecturer, to say the least. He demonstrated the passage of the fetus through the pelvis by ducking under the table at the front of the lecture room and coming out the other side—something we never forgot. Professor Dermid Bingham gave all our General Surgery lectures, which were spiced by quotes that I still remember, like from Sir Frederick Treeves: "If you see a bird on the roof, it is more likely to be a sparrow than a canary."

The first two years I was home for the summers, working as a telephone operator the first, and as a stenographer at the Cancer Clinic the second, where I learned a lot of medical terminology and also met Drs. Margaret Hardie and Lucy Ellison. I came home after third year and started work at the Cancer Clinic again, but other plans intervened. Rolly and I had been going out together for six years by then, and had been formally engaged for one year after he was accepted at Oregon. Queen's was looking for someone with research experience for a project in Obstetrics, so he was able to transfer to Queen's. We got married on July 12, 1950, and left for Kingston immediately after the wedding. So we did our final three years together. This made life much more pleasant for both of us. We were also very fortunate to have Rolly's mother, a widow, come to Kingston and basically do the shopping, cooking, washing, etc., for us. She had been born in Vancouver and although she had been to California, had never been east of the Okanagan, so she quite enjoyed the change of scenery. She had a room up the street from our apartment and came down every day to look after us, which was a great help to me.

Other than the first summer after we were married, Rolly and I did some work on the Obstetrical research project, so we both got experience in the field and it essentially paid our way through the rest of medical school. We were working with the Reynold's tocodynamometer, which was a precursor of the present day uterine monitors, and we published a paper with Dr. Gordon Mylks, an Associate Professor in the department, at the end of it.

The Dean of Medicine, Harold Ettinger, was Professor of Physiology and also the uncle of my closest friend among the women in our class, which was very helpful, as we knew him well. So I got the job of filling in during the summer vacation periods for his secretary in the Physiology department. Rolly and I also did the pregnancy tests while the regular technician was on holidays. These were the old Ascheim-Zondek (A-Z) tests done on rabbits, injecting a sample of the patient's urine into a vein in the ear, waiting forty-eight hours, then anesthetizing them with ether, opening their abdomens, and looking at the ovaries to see if there were any developing follicles—a far cry from today's simple tests!

After graduation we came back to Vancouver to intern at St. Paul's Hospital, along with a group of our classmates, as seven of the fourteen interns at St. Paul's that year were from Queen's. We were paid $50 a month, plus room and board. This meant fish every Friday, so everyone not on call tried to go out that evening. The Sisters of Charity of Providence still ran the hospital at that time, and there was a Sister in charge of each floor and each department. I believe they had one female intern before me, but no married couples, and at first they put me in the nurses' residence and Rolly in the interns' quarters. Needless to say, we weren't very happy with this arrangement, so we got a room in one of the old rooming houses a block from the hospital. It was noisy and smelly and not very private, so after a week of trying this out we more or less presented Sister Superior with an ultimatum: let us have a room together in the hospital area where the doctors-on-call slept, or we would go elsewhere. This she did and it worked out well for us.

It was a very busy year. As I recall, we spent three months on each of Medicine and General Surgery and one month on Obstetrics, Gynecology, Pediatrics, EENT, Orthopedics, and Emergency. We were on call every other night, and every night for the month on Obstetrics, as there was no Senior that year. I got to do seventy-five deliveries the month I was on Ob, even several deliveries from Dr. E.B. Trowbridge, who was head of the department and Chief of Staff. He had the reputation, deservedly, I might add, for being rather nasty if he didn't like you. Fortunately he liked both Rolly and me, and so we got along very well with him. He was a superb Gynecological surgeon and a very skillful Obstetrician and we learned a lot from him. He later delivered all our children.

I'll never forget the feeling I had the first few nights I was on call in Emergency when I'd hear a siren going by on Burrard and wonder if it was an ambulance and if I'd be able to handle whatever it was. However, we found that our training at Queen's was at least as good as all the others, and we got to do more and more as the year wore on. Even in those days we had to occasionally deal with obstreperous patients in Emergency, and one female drug addict was quite regularly bodily carried out by the police, screaming her head off.

One of the duties none of us liked was being on Surgical Day Call when Dr. Lyon Appleby, the chief of Surgery, was operating. "Ap" liked his patients put to sleep with Sodium Pentathol in their room before they were transported to the OR, and with virtually no Anesthesia training, we were all scared to death! One of our fellow interns unfortunately gave a patient a little too much one day, and that practice was discontinued, for which the rest of us gave a great sigh of relief!

One night Rolly and I wandered through Emergency on our way into the hospital just in time to help try to save a man who had been stabbed in the leg by his girlfriend. She had managed to cut the femoral artery, as we subsequently learned. About half a dozen of us were working on him by the end, but he had virtually exsanguinated before they got him to the hospital. I remember shoving a needle into the vicinity of his heart and injecting Adrenaline, to no avail. We lacked the sophisticated resuscitation methods and equipment (and knowledge) available today. We all got called as witnesses in the subsequent murder trial— our one and only court experience, thank goodness. (She was acquitted on the basis of self-defence.)

There were few women on the Medical Staff at that time, but Josephine Mallek was the one that took the most interest in me and the several other women that came during my three years at the hospital. She invited us to many gatherings of the Federation of Medical Women, so we met some of the other women in practice at that time. There were several women Anesthesiologists on staff, one of whom, Mary Mate, I had known slightly at Queen's (she was three years ahead of us), and also a few others who had staff privileges at the hospital. In those days it was easy to get Visiting Staff privileges in any of the hospitals, but not so easy to get Associate or full Staff.

I had decided I wanted to specialize in Obstetrics and Gynecology, and Rolly thought he'd do Orthopedics. I had hoped to stay at St. Paul's in Ob-Gyn, but they only had one "senior intern" (no organized residency program in those days). The only other applicant was a man who was a Roman Catholic, so he got the job. No one had applied for the position in General Surgery, so I was able to get it. I vividly remember the first day, assisting Dr. Appleby who wasn't feeling very well. "Ap" was a very fast surgeon, and he got the thyroidectomy done very quickly and then told me to

These were the old Ascheim-Zondek (A-Z) tests done on rabbits, injecting a sample of the patient's urine into a vein in the ear, waiting forty-eight hours, then anesthetizing them with ether, opening their abdomens, and looking at the ovaries to see if there were any developing follicles—a far cry from today's simple tests!

close! Here I was with a rather bloody gaping hole in the front of the neck, not knowing quite what to do at that stage! Fortunately the Sister in charge saw my predicament and called one of "Ap"'s associates who came and bailed me out. Other than that experience, I really had a very good year and learned a lot, especially from several of the doctors who let me do a considerable amount (under their supervision) as long as the follow-up was done and progress notes were written every day. I accumulated a series of one or two of various procedures, including one gastrectomy and one abdominal-perineal bowel resection. I assisted on the first ilio-femoral endarterectomy that was done at St. Paul's, which took about ten hours—I was given enough time off in the middle to have lunch. The majority of the surgeons accepted me without any problem. One man was quite testy at times when you were assisting him, and of course the only time I nearly fainted in the OR so that I had to stop assisting was with him—I was about four months pregnant at the time.

Here I was with a rather bloody gaping hole in the front of the neck, not knowing quite what to do at that stage! Fortunately the Sister in charge saw my predicament and called one of the associates who came and bailed me out.

The following year I stayed on in Ob-Gyn, in the middle of which our first son was born. I was due October 9, which was the Sunday of Thanksgiving weekend. One of the lady anesthesiologists had the women house staff to dinner the Saturday evening, so I was looking forward to sleeping in the next morning. However, I woke up about 7 a.m. with abdominal cramps which I misinterpreted at first. Then I realized they were coming every five minutes, and my uterus was getting hard with them, so I decided I was in labour. I finally woke Rolly up and told him. His reply was: "You can't be. It's your due date!" Nevertheless, I was. The Case Room nurse started giving me the daily report when we walked in, but I assured her I wasn't interested that day! Our son Charles was born several hours later, and Dr. Trowbridge nearly didn't get there in time. I took a month off after he was born, the only "sick time" I took in the whole three years I spent at St. Paul's, so I was a little upset when my next paycheque was considerably less than I expected. However, I was able to convince Sister Superior of this fact, and they paid me my whole stipend—which was all of $150 per month, with no room or board. We were fortunate to have Rolly's mother to look after the baby, with some help from my mother, or we would have had much more difficulty doing what we did.

After interning, Rolly went to UBC as a Teaching Fellow in Anatomy and then to the Vancouver General as a first-year resident in General Surgery, preliminary to doing Orthopedics. But he decided there were too many sore backs in Orthopedics. So the next year he went back to St. Paul's and Ob-Gyn. I spent that year doing General Practice as an employee of Dr. L.A. Patterson who had a very large practice spread all over Greater Vancouver. At that time the hospitals weren't nearly as fussy about qualifications of doctors who operated, and Dr. Trowbridge vouched for me, so I was able to do major Gynecological surgery in both St. Paul's and the old Grace Hospital. It always seems to be the first case that is the most difficult, and this was certainly true of the first one I booked at the Grace. She was a patient I had diagnosed as having large fibroids in her uterus, which she certainly had. But she also had old Pelvic Inflammatory Disease and all of the pelvic organs were stuck together! So instead of taking about one-and-a-half hours, I think it took me about four. However, she did well post-op except for one minor bleeding episode the day after she went home. I learned a great deal about looking after patients that year, and often made rounds anywhere from Burnaby Hospital to St. Paul's and those in between, and house calls from the North Shore to Burnaby or Richmond at times.

We were concerned about where we could go for the additional two years necessary to complete our specialty training as required by the Royal College of Physicians and Surgeons, as we thought it would be difficult to find a place that would take the two of us in the same field at a senior level. However, we were very fortunate in that Dr. Trowbridge knew Dr. Howard Taylor, who was head of a new department of Obstetrics at the Cleveland Clinic, having trained with him in Cleveland. He phoned Dr. Taylor and found out the Clinic was looking for residents in Ob-Gyn and that they would welcome us.

So off we went to Cleveland. We were able to do the final two years of our training there, at the third year and senior resident level. I believe I was the first woman resident in a surgical specialty at the Clinic. We lived in an apartment over the boiler house just across the parking lot from the Salvation Army's Booth Memorial Hospital and Home for Unwed Mothers, which was five miles (and twenty stop lights) straight down Euclid Avenue from the Clinic. We alternated calls at Booth for deliveries, and also gave numerous saddle block anesthetics for the private patients over the two years we were there. (This is what they used for so-called "natural childbirth" there! We had been used to using pudendal blocks and continued to do so on most of our own patients.) One of us was always on call. The six months of each year that we were on Obstetrics we looked after and delivered the resident patients at Booth, and also those at the Florence Crittendon Home for Unwed Mothers which was just two blocks from the Clinic. These latter patients, some as young as twelve or thirteen, were delivered at the Clinic with minimal supervision, although we always had back-up from a staff man (or the chief resident in the first year) whenever needed. Whichever one of us was on Gynecology saw private patients in the office setting, especially for Dr. Jim Krieger, who was the chief of the department and didn't do any Obstetrics. We would see the patients, take their history, present them to him, and examine the patients with him. This way we got to see a lot of complicated cases, as the Clinic had referrals from a wide area. We assisted him in surgery, as well as alternating night calls at Booth. In our final year we often operated under his supervision. We also assisted on the Gynecological parts of several pelvic exenterations for treatment of advanced cancer—not something we ever expected to do ourselves!

As part of the requirement of our Senior Residency we had to produce a research paper, and I did mine on Urinary Fistulas. This was turned into a Clinic Exhibit which was displayed at the Annual Meetings of both the American Medical Association and the American College of Obstetricians and Gynecologists, both in Atlantic City that year, so we got to go with the display.

Grandma Radcliffe was with us to take care of Charlie, who was almost two when we went to Cleveland, and to cook the meals, do the shopping, etc. These were two very interesting years, and we got a tremendous amount of experience that stood us in good stead later on. Even at that time the Clinic had a reputation as one of the best facilities in the U.S., and as we were classified as Fellows of the Clinic we were paid $400 per month the first year and $450 the second year, tax-free, which we thought was great.

We returned to Vancouver in the summer of 1959 with the idea of practising there, and rented office space from Dr. Tom Masterson, a general surgeon, on Broadway between Pine and Burrard. We passed our Royal College certificate exams as specialists that fall, and that was an experience in itself, as the examiner from Toronto was very nasty. He kept asking me about a sixteen-year old with menorrhagia, and no matter what I said, he replied, "OK. So she goes on bleeding—what do you do next?" Not what one likes on an oral exam!

We were able to make ends meet, mainly from referrals from Dr. Patterson, but it soon became obvious that it would take too long for Rolly to be busy enough to be happy. He could have become a member of the Associate Staff at St. Paul's if we had stayed, but there was enough discrimination still against women that I'd have had to wait longer. Rolly did several locums for Dr. Gordon Blott in Nanaimo, who was on the Council of the B.C. College of Physicians and Surgeons, and Gordon asked him to join him and that was how we happened to move to Vancouver Island.

Rolly started work with Gordon on August 1, 1960, and the rest of us, including Grandma Radcliffe, moved on Sept. 9, 1960. We had had a very difficult summer as Charlie had spent most of it in hospital after having an acute abdomen, thought at first to be a retrocecal appendix, but which turned out to be an acute obstruction of the right kidney pelvis by an aberrant artery. An attempt was made to relieve the obstruction through the original appendiceal incision and insertion of a ureteral catheter. The catheter was left in place for several weeks and then removed, at which time the obstruction recurred, and he was operated upon again through a proper kidney incision. With all of this, and some subsequent infections, he was in hospital for six weeks of a hot dry summer. I was very pregnant at the time, and shortly after we finally moved to Nanaimo, I returned to Vancouver to stay with my parents until our daughter Patricia was born three weeks later.

When we arrived in Nanaimo there were just over twenty doctors and I was the first woman, or, as Rolly liked to put it, I was the first doctor who happened to be a woman. In fact, I believe I was the first woman doctor north of the Malahat.

When we arrived in Nanaimo there were just over twenty doctors and I was the first woman, or, as Rolly liked to put it, I was the first doctor who happened to be a woman. In fact, I believe I was the first woman doctor north of the Malahat, and there were only a handful in Victoria at that time. There were two clinic groups: the Hall-Giovando Clinic (which is now the Medical Arts) had seven or eight members, including a General Surgeon and the only Pediatrician and Orthopedic Surgeon, as well as Dr. Mervyn Thomas, an Ob-Gyn; and the Browne Clinic (now Caledonian) also had about the same number, including a General Surgeon and Ob-Gyn's Drs. Jim Howey and John Dickson. The latter had taken his specialty exams at the same time we had and moved to Victoria several years later. In addition there were the "independents": Gordon Blott, who although not certified, confined his practice to women; one Internist; one certified Anaesthesiologist, although he did general practice as well; one Radiologist; one Ophthamologist (for the whole of upper Vancouver Island); as well as three independent GPs—now Rolly and myself. There were four doctors in Ladysmith, two in Chemainus, three in Parksville, and the brothers Macdonald in Qualicum. The hospital was the old building on Kennedy Street which is now Malaspina Lodge, a private intermediate care facility, but construction had just started on the present site, which was opened in January 1963. It has been the main upper Island hospital ever since, and while it has had several additions and renovations, at present it has about the same number of acute care beds as when it opened, in spite of a tremendous growth in population in the Hospital District and the whole upper Island.

Our office was located in a small downtown building beside what was then the only liquor store, but we soon moved into the new Madrona Building, still in the downtown area. We were there until 1976 when we moved into a new office complex across from the hospital, which was much more convenient if we got called for a delivery or some emergency in the middle of office hours. Things were much more laid back than now, and the doctors often sat around in the Doctors' Lounge after making rounds in the morning and settled the affairs of the world. It's not like they do now—rush in, see their patients, and rush off to the office!

At the time of our move to Nanaimo I was more into having babies than delivering others, so I did very little Medicine the first few years. However,

because Rolly and I were in the same field, I never lost touch with what was going on. I was there if needed to assist if Gordon or Rolly were away, and I remember lumbering into the old hospital to help Rolly with an emergency Caesarean when very pregnant with our second son and being greeted by a nursing supervisor who didn't know me and who tried to direct me to the Labour Room—we still laugh about it. I started going into the office on Monday afternoons, which was Gordon's day off, and initially might see one or two patients, but this gradually increased over the years and I began to have more deliveries and some surgery. In the meantime Rolly had become very busy, doing most of the consulting work for Ladysmith, Chemainus, Parksville, and Qualicum, and going over to Port Alberni one day a week where he operated as well as seeing patients in consultation. In Qualicum, Dr. Thomas left the Medical Arts Clinic and I was asked to be their consultant until they could obtain a new fulltime Ob-Gyn. This I did for six months until John Wood arrived to take over. This meant seeing patients in their office who were referred by their GP's, and subsequently operating on those that needed surgery and being called for complicated deliveries. Up until that time Dr. Larry Giovando really didn't know who I was, and I remember him walking down the hall in the OR one time with Alan Hall and whispering "Who's that?" after Alan said hello to me. But after he had assisted me when I operated on one of his patients, I became one of his best friends.

There was a rapid influx of doctors to the area in the few years after our arrival, and Nanaimo had most of the specialists on the Island outside of Victoria for some time, and still has more than the smaller cities on the upper Island, as our hospital is the major regional hospital on upper Vancouver Island. At first a number of specialists came up regularly from Victoria, but this decreased as more and more of the specialties were represented here. The only ones not represented, and not likely to be for a while, are Cardiothoracic and Neurosurgery and some subspecialties. Several of the doctors left, for varying reasons. It was six years before another woman doctor arrived to stay, and that was Frances Horner, a Dermatologist who is still practising. Paddy Mark was the first woman GP and she came in 1970. Somewhere in between we had a Pediatrician who was with the Caledonian Clinic, but she moved back to the Lower Mainland to get married after only a year or two. Since then there has been a gradual increase in the number of women, in conjunction with the increase in the number of women Medical students, who now make up one-third to one-half of most classes. In last year's B.C. Medical Directory there were forty women doctors in Nanaimo-Lantzville, out of 179 total. A few of these do only locum tenens.

My practice gradually increased as our children grew up and became independent. In 1978 I was asked to go to the Parksville Medical Clinic one half-day a week, which I did until we retired. During that time I saw a lot of patients in consultation for the doctors in the area, including quite a few from Port Alberni. I also saw many of their maternity patients in the last trimester and subsequently delivered them, as the doctors found it too difficult to get to the hospital in time, since there is no hospital in the Parksville-Qualicum area and most patients come to Nanaimo. Dr. Gordon Blott retired in 1980 and I then spent Monday and Wednesday afternoons in the office and Tuesday mornings in Parksville. Thursday was our regular operating day, which usually meant a full day in the OR, although we often had extra surgeries on other days, and Friday was our day off. However, as long as we were in town we were on call for our patients or for emergency consultations twenty-four hours a day, which meant a number of night and weekend calls. We also saw patients without referrals, including a lot of nurses and others who considered us their primary caregivers.

In the early 1980s we made the decision to retire when the office lease was up in 1986, which we did. In the meantime we were able to recruit a young Ob-Gyn to join us in the office and take over when we finished. He only stayed a few years after we retired and then moved to the U.S., but in the meantime a number of others arrived. One of them is a woman, Janet Hamilton, but she has been having babies and now only does assisting in the OR.

I can honestly say that I experienced very little discrimination either in medical school, during my hospital training years, or while in practice. In part I think this was because I expected to be treated as any other physician and I didn't expect any special considerations. I remember my first day as an intern being told by a Neurosurgeon that he didn't approve of women in Medicine, and for quite valid reasons: many, if not most, women do not practise full-time the way most men do, and medical education is very expensive. However, he didn't hold it against me, and was never nasty. There was one English surgeon who fancied himself a "ladies' man" and I guess I was not admiring enough! The man in charge of the interns' schedule was also miserable at times, such that my schedule as a junior intern was harder than some of the others, which only meant that I got more experience.

We retired earlier than many doctors do, and with no regrets. We were among the last specialists in the area willing to take calls at any time, and this becomes wearing after a while. Rolly was five years older than I, and there would have been no point in him retiring without me too. And, quite frankly, we were both getting fed up. Medicine was no longer enjoyable, but had become a chore. The practice of Ob-Gyn had changed dramatically since we had started in practice, both in the so-called technological advances, and in the attitude of patients. There was a lot of satisfaction in accomplishing a difficult delivery, which was what we'd been taught to do, and mothers were grateful. Maternity patients on the whole were happy and looking forward to their babies. There were the unfortunate cases where the babies died, usually from unavoidable causes like premature separation of the placenta, or a true knot in the umbilical cord, but luckily there weren't many of these cases. There were also a few goofs, such as undiagnosed twins that surprised everybody, and unusual cases, such as a twin-to-twin transfusion occurring in a doctor's wife who was referred to Vancouver where she was successfully delivered and both babies did well. Another was a twin pregnancy with hydramnios where one twin was an anencephalic. Rolly and I between us did a number of amniocenteses and managed to allow the normal twin to develop to near term and be successfully delivered. There were some astute clinical diagnoses as well: for instance, a nurse from the Nursery was referred to me because of extreme pelvic pain at four months pregnant. I was able to determine on examination that she had a large ovarian cyst lodged in the pelvis, so the uterus was sitting on top of it and being stretched as it grew. I was able to successfully remove the cyst and she continued to term and delivered a healthy baby girl.

I remember lumbering into the old hospital to help Rolly with an emergency Caesarean when very pregnant with our second son and being greeted by a nursing supervisor who didn't know me and who tried to direct me to the Labour Room—we still laugh about it.

However, when patients started coming in with their "Birthing Plan" and their demands for how the delivery was to be conducted and wanted the doctor to sign it specifying that they would not be given any medication, no episiotomy, etc., it got to be a bit much! If midwives want to take the risk of delivering babies in patients' homes, they are welcome to it. A so-called "normal delivery" is in retrospect only. There is really no such thing as a "low-risk" pregnancy.

Most of the Gynecological cases requiring surgery were straightforward, but as with any surgery, once in a while one gets fooled. The worst one I had was a patient that had been examined previously by another Gynecologist elsewhere who advised immediate surgery because he felt there was a significant possibility of cancer. From what I could feel on examination, I agreed, and I operated on her shortly after. (This was before the days of ultrasound.) There was absolutely nothing wrong with her pelvic organs, nor her bowel, but even after her routine pre-op enema, her bowel was loaded with hard little rocks of stool! So it was a good news-bad news story she had to be told after the laparotomy: no cancer, and I admitted I had made a mistake. But at least someone else had thought the same way about what we were feeling!

There were of course a few cases of pelvic cancer of one sort or another. Ovarian cancers in general have a poor outlook, as they so often cause no symptoms until late in the disease and have spread widely before they are discovered, especially in young women. I remember one girl I saw at age sixteen with a tumour about the size of a six-month pregnancy. I operated within six weeks, and it had by then grown to near term size. The Pathology report called it a borderline malignancy, and there was no gross nor microscopic evidence of any spread, so after consultation with the Cancer Clinic, nothing further was done. She remained well for about five years and then developed symptoms of spread and subsequently died. Another patient in her forties refused to have a pelvic exam although she continued to see me for ongoing abdominal and pelvic symptoms. By the time she allowed a full examination and the diagnosis was confirmed, it was too late to do anything except try to keep her comfortable. Uterine cancers are fortunately usually diagnosed early because of bleeding, and I only had one patient that went on to die from it, as she was an older lady who had ignored her bleeding for a long time. We saw a lot of in-situ cancer of the cervix, thanks in large part to our Provincial screening program. Any female beyond menarche who was having sexual intercourse had a Pap test whenever we did a pelvic examination. This allowed us to treat it, usually with a cone biopsy only, which preserved the uterus and thus her fertility. Dr. Krieger in Cleveland had been one of the earliest proponents of this procedure. The so-called "sexual revolution" with early intercourse and numerous partners has had the effect of causing increasing changes in the cervix which lead to cancer, which a lot of young women do not seem to realize. Fortunately patients with full-blown cervical cancer, such as we occasionally saw in the early days, especially in Cleveland, were very rare, and they were referred to the Cancer Clinic in Vancouver, mainly for radiation therapy, which was the treatment of choice.

However, clinical skills in both diagnosis and treatment were gradually replaced by more and more complicated tests, which in many cases cost much more but give very little more information. Caesarean section rates went from about five percent to nearly twenty-five percent now, for a number of reasons: babies are bigger—on average nearly a pound, from what we were taught in medical school, presumably due to better nutrition; fetal monitoring scares people into intervening sooner; patients' expectations of labour are often unrealistic, and the presence of the husband (or significant other) hovering around watching the wife's suffering doesn't help; less homogeneous populations with mixed marriages and mismatched pelves; and last, but not least, the spectre of a potential lawsuit if everything is not perfect. To illustrate the latter, Canadian Medical Protective Association fees were $25 per year when we started and for many years after. They then went to $200 for everybody, but with the increase in suits and escalating awards, doctors were divided into categories according to the risks of getting sued, and Ob-Gyn's are in the highest category, along with Anesthesiologists, Neurosurgeons, Orthopedic, and Cardiac surgeons. Our fees went to $2,000, then $5,000, and finally $8,000 the year we retired, and I don't know what they are now. We had our share of complications, as any surgeon must admit that no matter how careful one tries to be, occasionally things will go wrong. However, we were fortunate in never having a post-op death or being sued, which was a blessing.

There was great satisfaction in accomplishing a complicated delivery and getting a healthy mother and baby. Our generation of Ob-Gyn's were trained to do forceps rotations and breech deliveries, which was one reason the Cesarean Section rate was so low. I was sometimes referred patients when they had been told they had to have a Cesarean. One I remember was a nurse who had moved to the Lower Mainland from Nanaimo after her marriage. She was a tall, well-built woman, but the baby was a breech, and she was told she would have to have a Section. She said "no" and came back to Nanaimo and I was able to deliver her without any difficulty. There was also one who had a footling breech. It was her second pregnancy and she had had a rapid and easy delivery with her first. She had been told of all the risks by another Obstetrician who said she must have a Caesarean, and I repeated them when she was subsequently referred to me, but she was adamant that she wanted a vaginal delivery. So I somewhat reluctantly agreed to deliver her. Shortly after, I got a phone call in the middle of the night that she had arrived fully dilated with a prolapsed cord! I don't think I have ever moved so fast in all my life. Fortunately we lived just ten minutes from the hospital, so I threw on some clothes, woke Rolly to call the Pediatrician, and was at the hospital in less than fifteen minutes. No time to change or scrub, just grabbed a gown and gloves, and the baby was safely delivered and handed over to the Pediatrician as soon as we got the patient into the Case Room. That child is now an adult—I still run into the mother periodically.

In addition, we were not trained to do such things as colposcopy or laparoscopy, the latter being mainly used for tubal ligation in those days, before the development of its use for extensive "key-hole" surgery as done by many General Surgeons as well as Gynecologists today. We could do a tubal ligation in ten minutes, skin to skin, through an incision less than one-and-a-half inches long below the pubic hair line, as day-care, so could see no reason to take the time and effort to learn to do the other, which took considerably longer to do. It is one thing to learn a technique in your training years, and another to learn something major in the later years of your career. Several of our confreres made the effort, and more power to them. But with younger doctors in the area who had been trained to do some of these things, we just referred patients when necessary.

Also now, with the "New Directions" in Health Care, with Regional Health Boards, all politically appointed, which the New Democratic Government brought in, I'm very happy to be out of it. Patients in general became much more demanding and less trusting of our judgment, and no matter how well informed people are, it is difficult to explain complicated medical matters in the relatively short time one has with a patient, no matter how hard you try.

And there was the matter of abortions. When we started out, the only abortions talked about, especially at St. Paul's, were spontaneous ones, known to the layman as "miscarriages." Indeed, it was even illegal to prescribe any method of birth control, although this was ignored by most doctors long before the law was changed in 1967. Unmarried women who got pregnant usually went through with the pregnancy and gave the baby up for adoption. Some (even married women) were so desperate that they had "backroom" abortions, and many of these ended up in hospitals with bleeding or severe infections, which often led to infertility or sterility, and some even died. When we were in Cleveland a few truly "therapeutic" abortions were being done, but only in those cases where the life of the mother was clearly at risk by continuation of the pregnancy. After we came to Nanaimo, they could only be done with the agreement of a consulting doctor who did not himself do abortions, and very few were done. But as we all know, once the law was changed abortions have become commonplace, and unfortunately are sometimes used as a method of birth control. Believe me, in spite of the impression given by those opposed to any abortions, no doctor who does them likes doing them. By necessity they must be done urgently, and take up considerable office and OR time. While the procedure is a lot simpler than it used to be, it is not without difficulties and potential complications, and should never be considered an alternative to adequate birth control, especially at this time when there are a number of very good contraceptives, and easy methods of sterilization for one or other partner.

We had our share of complications, as any surgeon must admit that no matter how careful one tries to be, occasionally things will go wrong. However, we were fortunate in never having a post-op death or being sued, which was a blessing.

So we stopped seeing new patients at the end of February, 1986, stopped delivering babies at the end of April, the last patient I delivered being one of the ICU nurses. Charles, our older son, was married on May 3, and we took off after the Victoria Day holiday on a cross-Canada camping trip in our then new Volkswagon camper van. We returned in early July and finished up any remaining booked surgery by the end of September. Rolly had been Medical Chief of Staff at the hospital for several years, and he retired from that at the end of the year. He was also on the Council of the College of Physicians and Surgeons for sixteen years and he carried on with that until his term expired in 1989.

We had very little social life when we were in practice, as we always had to be near a phone until the last few years when we had a pager. Most of our outside activities centered on our family, including yearly camping trips all over B.C. as well as up the Alaska Highway into the Yukon and Alaska, and into Alberta and up as far into the N.W.T. as Yellowknife. There were also church-related festivities as well as Kiwanis dinners and conventions (Rolly being a long-time Kiwanian), and a few Medical occasions. We made a point of going to a large Medical meeting or post-graduate course, usually in the U.S., about once a year in order to keep up with changes in the specialty. Our main escape otherwise was an occasional weekend cruising in our sailboat, when we had someone to cover for us, and this we did even in the winter, when possible. I joined the University Women's Club shortly after we moved to Nanaimo and have kept up my membership over the years, although not very active during my later working years. We had seasons tickets to both the Vancouver and Victoria operas, and I still have for Victoria, and I keep in touch with several of my friends from school in Vancouver.

Since retirement we have been busy having grandchildren, our other two children having married in 1987. Each of the three have two children, so I do quite a bit of baby-sitting. As well we did a lot of camping in our van, more sailing in local waters, gardening, and generally puttering around at home. In 1990 I was asked to run for the Hospital Board as a member of the Hospital Society, which I did successfully. When I was on the Board we had a very good group who all had the best interest of the community at heart, which hadn't always been the case in the past. I was elected Chairman in 1992 and this took up a lot of my time, especially with the increasing restraints, and all the changes talked about in health care at that time. I retired from the Board in 1995, and all Hospital Boards were done away with when Regional Health Boards were appointed.

For the most part, we really enjoyed the practice of Obstetrics and Gynecology. We always felt that we had the "Golden Years" of Medicine, having started in practice shortly after universal hospitalization came into being, but before Medicare was brought in, and thus having seen the "before and after." Today's doctors don't realize what it was like to get paid for those patients who had some medical coverage, which paid ninety percent of the Minimal Schedule of Fees. The total Maternity fee, including pre- and post-natal care and delivery, was $75, which meant we got $67.50. If they didn't have any insurance, we might get paid by half of the patients, except for SAMS (Social Assistance Medical Services) patients for whom the Government paid only about forty percent of the Minimal Schedule every three months. I remember Dr. Appleby talking about receiving the occasional chicken or garden produce in lieu of pay by some patients he operated on during the Depression, but things were never quite that bad for us!

I am very happy to have lived in Nanaimo and to have brought up our children here, but it is changing rapidly, and not always for the better. Unfortunately Rolly died in July 1999, but I am lucky to have Charles, a lawyer, and his family living here, and our daughter, Patty, a veterinarian, and her family in Port Alberni, so I see them often. I try to see Tom, our younger son, a physicist, and his family who are in Kingston, Ontario, at least once a year. Having lived in Nanaimo for forty-one years, I have a lot of friends from all my past activities who keep life interesting, and there is always plenty to do to keep me busy.

1955

DR. MARGOT BOOTHROYD

I was trained at the University of London in the Royal Free Hospital. After graduation in 1950, I did a variety of junior hospital appointments in

England, and in 1953, I married a surgeon who, at that time, was applying all over the country for a consultant position. Jobs were then very hard to come by, as often there would be a hundred applicants for each opening. Therefore, it was not difficult to make the decision to emigrate. Luck was on our side as Lawrence was, most fortunately, turned down for a job in Zimbabwe (South Rhodesia then). It was then a toss-up between Canada and Australia—and Canada won!

We came to B.C. in 1955, and during my first pregnancy I got a sessional job with the North Shore Public Health Authority, doing school health examinations and working for Well Baby Clinics. For the next seven years, I stayed at home with four young children and returned to the sessional work when the youngest was three. I really enjoyed this escape from the domestic scene as I continued to work for Well Baby Clinics until my retirement in 1993. And I only realized how long I had been with the North Shore Health Unit when I started to give shots to the children of many of my former clients!

From 1975 until 1990, I established my family practice in West Vancouver, receiving many elderly patients from an older doctor on his retirement, and a fair number of women patients who were looking for a female doctor. There were not too many of us around in those days. My practice was pretty relaxed, therefore I had time to talk to the patients, which for me was a big plus. Now ten years after retirement, I still meet a number of them shopping in Safeway and most of them look healthier now than they did under my care. There is a message here, I am sure!

Looking back, I know I never achieved great things in my medical career, but I gained the trust and support of my patients. And most importantly, I did enjoy my diverse lifestyle. So life has been good to me.

DR. MADELINE (HUANG) CHUNG

Dr. Madeline Chung was one of the first certified women specialists in Obstetrics and Gynecology when she began her practice in Vancouver in 1955. Born in 1925, Madeline spent her first five years in Shanghai, China. Her father, a mining engineer, graduated from the Colorado School of

Mines and went to Butte, Montana, to prospect for copper. There he met and married his future wife, and both returned to China. They had three daughters, Madeline being the eldest.

When her father became the transport superintendent for the Burma Road, he moved his family to Guangzhou (Canton), then to Hong Kong, a city which he considered more cultured, as Madeline was ready for high school. Her mother became an English teacher while Madeline and her sister, two years younger, attended the True Light School. Madeline graduated about the time when the war with the Japanese in Hong Kong took place. After her graduation, she was accepted by the Yale Medical School in Shanghai. She admits she was a serious student, regimented in her studies and learning of the piano.

When the British surrendered to the Japanese in December, 1941, Madeline's mother had both teenaged daughters' hair cut short and dressed them as boys for safety's sake. There was a gun emplacement nearby, and as the Japanese soldiers approached their home, they escaped through the back door, with their mother's leg injured, and eventually crossed over to mainland China. (The mother had developed osteomyelitis and was not cured until penicillin became available.) The Yale school in Shanghai had to be evacuated

When the British surrendered to the Japanese in December, 1941, Madeline's mother had both teenaged daughters' hair cut short and dressed them as boys for safety's sake.

because of the war, and through his work, Madeline's father was able to release transport trucks to carry the equipment to western China. Her mother travelled in the truck, but the students walked a good part of the way, overnighting at farms and sleeping on straw mats. They managed to arrive in Guilin just before the Japanese and hurried to Kweiwong and finally Changsha in Hunan province where the medical school was set up.

There were fifty medical students, half of them girls. Some of the male students left to become interpreters for the allied forces in Chunking and elsewhere. The instruction was in English. Madeline graduated in 1948 from Hsiang Ya Medical College, Hunan, which was part of Yale—in China Medical School.

Madeline survived an exhausting ordeal to reach the Medical School and then four years of studies under wartime conditions, such as food scarcity and cramped quarters. She speaks of this phase of her life without complaint or bitterness. In Chunking her father entertained and became friends with some of the members of the American armed forces. These friendships helped Madeline get the sponsorship to do her internship in Tacoma, Washington, after her graduation in Medicine. Her parents eventually moved to the United States after their retirement; her sister, who was two years younger, first studied Medicine, then went into Chemistry at Northwestern University.

During her training in Tacoma, Madeline met a neurosurgeon from the Mayo Clinic who urged her to do her specialty training in Obstetrics and Gynecology. She applied to Mayo and received a fellowship for three years (1951–1954) in Obstetrics and Gynecology. Afterwards Madeline did another internship at St. Joseph's Hospital, Vancouver, B.C., and then went to Montreal for further training. She met her future husband, Wally Chung, a fourth-year medical student from Victoria, B.C., at McGill University.

Madeline wrote the LMCC exams and was certified as a Specialist in Obstetrics and Gynecology. Wally Chung did post-graduate work in General Surgery and Vascular Surgery. Shortly after they were married, Madeline and Wally went to China, but decided not to stay there as they found the Communist atmosphere very constraining. They returned to Canada and started their practices in Vancouver. They had two children—a daughter, now a geriatrician, and a son, a transplant surgeon.

Madeline found practice slow to build up for the first few years. Competition was fierce as many European women doctors had arrived in the 1950s to practise in the city. Fortunately, the large Chinese community in Vancouver appreciated her, and by 1996 she had delivered 6,500 babies. Although the investigation of sterility was her favourite research project, she had little time to pursue her research as she became very much in demand in practice and in teaching.

In 1988, she suffered a terrible accident while driving home after doing a caesarean operation at Grace Hospital. She had fractures of the right arm, leg, and ankle. Many of her medical friends expected her to retire, but before long she was back to work, continuing until 1996. While remaining active in the medical community and busy pursuing her other interests, Madeline car-pools her five grandchildren on appointed days; and from the number of tricycles and toys in the car park, she and Wally must now do a lot of babysitting.

Teaching appointments: Active staff of Grace Hospital (now B.C. Women's Hospital), 1956; Clinical Instructor, UBC, 1957; Clinical Assistant Professor, UBC, 1981; Clinical Associate Professor, 1989; Clinical Professor Emerita, 1990.

Honours: Fellow of the Royal College of Obstetrics and Gynecology, 1967; Best Undergraduate Teaching Award, 1991; Senior Membership, Canadian Medical Association, 1993; Prince of Good Fellow, Vancouver Medical Association, 1998; Honorary Life Member, B.C. College of Physicians and Surgeons, 1999.

Other Community contributions: Founding Member of the True Light Chinese School in Vancouver, 1981. Served as Superintendent for twelve years. In 1999 the enrollment was over 1,000.

Present: Has given numerous lectures and seminars to the Chinese community on health problems affecting the female.

Madeline participated in two evangelical missions to backward areas in China (with the Evangelical Medical Aid Society), near the inner Mongolian border, populated mostly by Moslem people.

She is also a member of the Mayo Foundation for Medical Education and Research, the Northwest Pacific Obstetrics and Gynecology Association, the Society for Obstetrics and Gynecology of Canada, as well as the Board of Directors of the Chinese United Church of Vancouver, the Chinese Culture Centre, and the Soroptimist International Club, and chairing her church congregation.

DR. HELENA BOZENA HALE
(1891–1977)

Dr. Helena Bozena Hale was educated in Austria and Czechoslovakia, and received her degree in Medicine from Prague in 1937. She did post-graduate work in Psychiatry in Germany, England, and Canada. The Certificate of Psychiatry of the Royal College of Physicians and Surgeons of Canada was granted to her in 1955. She practised Psychiatry in Victoria, B.C. for many years.

Dr. Hale died on November 12, 1977 at the age of eighty-six years.

DR. SARAH LOUISE (SALLY) HEMMING

I graduated in Medicine from Glasgow University, Scotland and did six months of medicine and six months of surgery from 1956–1957. I came to Canada in July 1957 and hoped to do six months of obstetrics and six months of anesthesia, but was told by D.L.E. Ranta at the Vancouver General Hospital that I had to do a junior rotating internship to sit the LMCC exams, which I did. This I found out later was not strictly true!

I was married and my husband was also an intern so I had to stay in the women's residence on Heather Street and my husband, Fred, had to stay across the street. Both places were carefully guarded by custodians! We found an apartment (which wasn't easy on $100 per month) and we also had a beagle that, with the help of friends, we used to sneak into the hospital when we were both on call. The "apartment" was really a room with a shared kitchen in a house on Heather, which later became the Speech Therapy Clinic and was eventually demolished. As most of the tenants cooked on electric frying pans, it was quite common to see all of us escaping over the low wall when we all plugged in at once and blew the fuse, much to the irritation of the landlord.

In 1958 we went to Salmon Arm, B.C. to join a practice with Drs. John Alexander and Ralph Williams. Ralph was the reason we came to Vancouver. We met him in Scotland when he was recovering from a near fatal bout of staphlococcal pneumonia while I was surgical resident there. My husband had thought of going to Rhodesia as he had been there with the Royal Air Force during the war, but Ralph extolled the beauties of British Columbia, especially the fishing, so here we were. On his return to Canada Ralph had joined Dr. John Alexander in general practice and we joined them later.

We built a house on Mara Lake in Sicamous, but in those days there was no ambulance service, so my husband taught first aid to the local Kinsmen and they became the ambulance service. At first I gave all the anesthetics for the practice but as I began having a family it became difficult to whip into Salmon Arm for emergencies so finally I had a part-time practice with my husband after we split off from John and Ralph (the separation was friendly). After the Rogers Pass opened in 1963 life became very difficult. In the winter there were road accidents and in the summer a swelling population of tourists, boating accidents, and drownings, and it was nineteen miles to the hospital. I have great sympathy with the doctors in Northern B.C. who still face seven days on call. In our day there were no specialists in Salmon Arm so we either had to get surgeons from Vernon or Kamloops or ship the patient out. Not easy with the Dominion (train) going through at midnight and bad weather preventing us from flying people out.

I do remember that our senior partner was quite upset because I refused to fill in for the office staff on occasion. He would not have asked the male doctors. Most of the patients thought I was a nurse as I stitched them up! When I came to Canada, I was surprised to find very few women in medicine. In the year I graduated in Britain the ratio was one woman to five men. I remember having a heated discussion with a friend's son, a resident in surgery, who was angry that the University of British Columbia was admitting so many women in the 1970s, as he thought they would marry and leave medicine.

In the 1960s my husband went into aviation medicine, so with four children in tow, we left Sicamous, and moved to Toronto. While I was pregnant with my fifth child and after the urging of my husband's friends, I took the Diploma in Public Health course, as my husband's new field of medicine meant we would move to Ottawa. I worked the day I delivered my fifth child and I went back to work three weeks later. I was the Medical Health Officer for Peel County in Ontario for one year and when my husband was moved to Ottawa I did locums and some school health there. I remember phoning to enquire about a job in a general practice. The man I talked to asked all the questions, not unacceptable, as to sex, marital status, number of children. He said there was no way they could accept a married woman with children as she would not be available seven days a week. For doctors whose practice closed on Thursdays for golf and who all had unlisted phone numbers, they should have tried Sicamous where people would wander into the house if the doctor wasn't in the office. (My children had their share of illness there, partly due to the number of people arriving with a sick child who promptly vomited on the hall floor.)

When my husband returned to British Columbia as the Medical Officer for CP Air, I applied for a job in Boundary (as advertised by the *Province*), and I was advised that they did not employ women as they might have affairs with the Health Inspectors! I then applied to the City of Vancouver and was also told women were not desirable. I guess they had quite a few working part-time and wanted a balance. I worked at Riverview for a year and thought I would be doing medicals, but was in charge of a ward. I got used to dealing out large quantities of drugs and when I demurred at ECT, I was informed that everyone took turns, or else.

During my time in Vancouver I was certainly not the first woman doctor; people like Dr. Agnes Black and Dr. Reba Willets were there before me, but after the war there very few. And for several years, as the *Province* stuck to "men only," there was only me.

I must say one of my great pleasures before I retired in 1992 was to go to medical meetings and see some very bright women at the top of the profession. I'm sure it's still very difficult to combine a medical career with a family. I have two sons in medicine, one an anaethetist and one a transplant surgeon, and I can see by watching their hours in residencies that things haven't changed.

DR. MARGARET MAIER HOEHN
(1930 – 2005)

Professor Margaret "Peggy" M. Hoehn, MD, FACP, FRCP(C), age seventy-four, died on July 16, 2005.

Dr. Hoehn was born in San Francisco, received her BA from the University of Saskatchewan, and her MD from the University of British Columbia, Vancouver. A pioneer from an early age, she was one of three women chosen to join the first class of medical students at the University of British Columbia in 1950. After completing her Residency and Teaching Fellowship in Neurology in Vancouver, rotations as a Clinical Assistant in Neuroradiology in the National Hospital for Nervous Diseases in London,

England, and Chief Residency in Neurology at the Veteran's Hospital in Boston, Dr. Hoehn accepted an academic appointment in Neurology at Columbia University in New York.

Dr. Hoehn is known for her work in Parkinson's disease. She was the first person to create a rating scale for neurological examinations of Parkinson's patients and collaborated in the creation of the Hoehn and Yahr scale, used internationally to measure the stages of Parkinson's. Dr. Hoehn continued to conduct groundbreaking research on the effects of various treatments for Parkinson's disease and, between 1958 and 1996, published over 193 scholarly articles. She lectured world-wide on her research throughout her career.

Later in her career, Dr. Hoehn was the Director of the Parkinson's Disease and Movement Disorders Program at the Colorado School of Medicine in Denver, and in addition, conducted numerous clinical trials to test the efficacy of various treatments for the disease. She continued to evaluate and treat patients until her health prohibited it. She was beloved by her patients for her dedication to improving their conditions and her approachable and caring manner. She was known for her good heart and passionate love of life.

Peggy was a loving mother of two children, Bob and Eve. An inexhaustible world traveller, she scuba dived in the Red Sea and explored Southeast Asia and China in her last decade of life.

DR. MARJORIE E. DUPONT JANSCH

I was born in California on May 6, 1928. My family moved to Canada in 1935 and tried farming in northern Alberta. After a few nasty Alberta winters, we moved to Metchosin on Vancouver Island. I graduated from Victoria High School in 1946 and went on to Victoria College, which was at that time located in Craigdarroch Castle.

I had always dreamed of going to medical school. With financial help from my parents, I registered at the University of British Columbia, and began my third year as an undergraduate in the Arts and Science Program in the fall of 1948.

In those years, a sudden wave of veterans swelled the ranks of students working towards their higher education. Residences and training facilities were built to create more spaces for the already overcrowded campus: "Army Huts", the long, rectangular portable buildings that served as classrooms and laboratories were seen everywhere.

As an undergraduate, I enjoyed UBC very much and relished most of my courses. Biology and zoology were my real loves, but I had trouble with organic chemistry. The eeriness of my biochemistry experience was enhanced by the fact that we had our labs at night and the Chemistry Building was designed in a gothic architectural style. Eventually I felt at home with corpses, and picked vertebrate zoology and invertebrate zoology as my elective classes. The lady I boarded with didn't mind that I was a medical student, but drew the line at me washing the dishes to get the odour of embalming fluid off my hands.

The UBC campus was quite pretty. In the spring, the lawns were dotted with students taking in the air while they studied. I was happier than I had ever been and dreamed of a bright future.

First Years of Medical School, 1950–1952
I passed my final exams and received a Bachelor of Arts degree in Biology and Zoology in 1950. I was accepted into the first class of the School of Medicine at UBC.

I met Ted Jansch at our second biochemistry lecture when we both arrived late to a locked door. Since we seemed to have missed our chance to go to class that day, we went out for coffee instead. Ted was from Chemainus and had served as a Corporal in the Medical Corps in London, Ontario, during the war. We discovered that we had both gone to Victoria College at the same time. We became friends and began studying together. Ted was a natural at chemistry with a real knack for explaining things, and he started coaching me. The chemistry was right between us, too, and we soon became engaged.

It was a policy for the first graduates of the School of Medicine to produce a doctoral thesis. In the second year, we were expected to begin. For my thesis, I planned to work on a survey of Schistosome Dermatitis that was found in the lakes of British Columbia. I arranged a job collecting data at Cultus Lake and Kelowna for the summer under the supervision of Dr. Jim Adams, the UBC Professor of Parasitology. While Ted was tutoring me in biochemistry, he put together a diagram for me to study, which showed the interrelationship of the biochemical cycles in the human body. This diagram became the basis of his doctoral thesis.

Summer, 1952
As I was preparing to leave for my summer work in Kelowna, Ted and I were staying in the dormitories at UBC. We had our meals in the cafeteria where we met a student who was just getting over a bout of mumps. The next day I took a bus to Kelowna with Don Edwards, with whom I was to share the work of the survey.

Don and I introduced ourselves to the Department of Public Health, and arranged our equipment for the Schistosome Survey. Later that day I became ill. The doctor at the Public Health Unit confirmed mumps and sent me home to my rooming house for ten days in isolation. I was provided with a telephone and daily visits from the Public Health Nurses who brought me food, books, and work. Sometimes I climbed out the window onto a small ornamental balcony to avoid the heat.

The Schistosomes we studied caused a painful itch on the skin of some people after they swam in fresh water. This was commonly called Swimmer's Itch and was a real blight for resort owners on the lakes. Through a grant from the Department of Public Health, we were hired to find ways to prevent this rash. Don and I collected freshwater snails from various parts of Cultus, Okanagan, Skaha, and Osoyoos Lakes. Since I had sensitive skin, I was used as the human tester to see if the species produced an itch. I put a drop of water containing cercariae on my inner forearm. I could tell very quickly that I was being penetrated because as the drop was drying, the prickling started. The next day I had fluid-filled papules spreading on my inner arm. We used a mixture of copper sulphate and carbonate to treat areas of the lake that were close to swimming beaches.

The landlady who owned the boarding house in Kelowna was a Jehovah's Witness and was suspicious of doctors. When she realized that I wanted to become a doctor, she became very disagreeable and turned off the water when I ran a bath. A kind health nurse finally lent me her tub. Luckily, the schistosome survey was done by the middle of August. During that summer, Don and I discovered two new species of schistosome. These discoveries thus became the basis of my doctoral thesis.

Third Year of Medical School, 1952–1953
Ted and I were married on August 23, 1952 in Metchosin. Peg Dobson, one of the three women medical students in my class at the time, was my bridesmaid. Her future husband Al Cox was my high school classmate and in the same class at Medical School as the rest of us.

For our honeymoon, Ted took me to a resort on Thetis Island. I should have known better than to marry an avid sport fisherman. We set off to Porlier Pass in an old wooden boat that seeped water and had an engine that wouldn't run. Ted spent the first couple of days of our honeymoon working on that motor on the dock or cleaning fish and delivering them across Stuart Channel to his mother's freezer in Chemainus.

We started our married life in a trailer in Acadia Camp #1 on the UBC campus. There were three places to study in the trailer: the table, the small desk, or the sofa bed. When exams were approaching, I would take the potted plant off the table and all three areas would be used in rotation.

The material that we studied in third year was preclinical. We did public health, neuroanatomy, pharmacology, physiology, pathology, and bacteriology. After the Christmas break, we had some preclinical courses at Vancouver General Hospital. To prepare for our exams, Ted and I alternately quizzed each other on the material.

Our class would be the first to graduate from the UBC School of Medicine, and about fifty percent of the students were war veterans. They had their share of riotous parties. Everyone drank and celebrated the good moments.

Our biochemistry lab courses were at best boring. The students found a way to alleviate this problem. Sometimes students would go to the supply lab to get ethanol in open glass beakers and throw a party under the trees. Ted and I were usually so absorbed in our work that we didn't notice the whereabouts of other students. Eventually, the faculty was informed of the failing biochemistry experiments that required absolute ethanol by the drum. The ethanol was then rationed and if students left the lab early, they were not allowed to return to the building because the inebriated students might induce harm upon themselves when they worked with Bunsen burners.

Before the end of the 'free ethanol,' some of it found its way back to the homes of Acadia Camp, and we were invited to parties to sample the Acadia Camp Cocktail. This was a dangerous concoction of canned grapefruit juice and ethanol.

There were also formal parties. Sometimes faculty members would invite a few of their students or the entire class home for scrumptious buffets or sit-down dinners. Ted and I really enjoyed these parties as we rarely had delicious food at home on our student budget. Our faculty was drawn from Canada, the United States, and Britain. Many of the U.S. faculty had come to Canada to get free of the McCarthy commission that targeted "Communists." Certain beliefs and points of view were considered suspect. Intellectuals were often targets.

The Annual Medical School Ball was at the end of the school year. It was the social event of the year. It was a formal event for the staff and students held at a downtown ballroom like the one at the Hotel Georgia. If a student was too broke for the ticket, one of the clinical doctors would find one. There was no excuse to stay home. At the Ball there were a large number of affiliated medical doctors. I think that every doctor in the Vancouver area was considered a member of the faculty, since the general practitioners would allow medical students to obtain office experience at their clinics in the summer.

Fourth Year of Medical School, 1953–1954
At the beginning of our fourth year in 1953, we had only a few lectures at UBC. Most of our work was done at Vancouver General Hospital and the smaller St. Paul's, which is closer to the city core. VGH had a maze of underground tunnels full of scurrying people. During the two years that we were there, they were constantly renovating. Departments were shuffled around in the buildings, so we often had trouble finding where we were supposed to be. Examinations of hearts and lungs with a stethoscope were difficult with the pounding of jackhammers and falling bricks. I don't know how the patients endured.

In the hospitals we met a new lot of clinicians who became our teachers. We studied subjects like obstetrics, pediatrics, and pathology in the stuffy old basement lecture halls. Distractions included a student who would habitually snooze in class. To our amusement, he fell out of his chair several times.

We were also able to see patients in the hospital. Wearing short white coats upon which our names were pinned, we followed the clinicians hastily through the surgery and pediatrics departments. We felt quite conspicuous in our short coats when all the 'real doctors,' the interns and resident physicians, had lab coats that came down to their knees. One doctor took us to see a patient with asthma in a plastic oxygen tent. He was trying to demonstrate to us how harsh you had to be with difficult patients. He was nasty with her, thereby setting off a horrendous asthma attack. This doctor was not well-equipped to teach us good bedside manners!

We also had to put in our time at Essondale Mental Institute. The mental institute was absolutely repellent to me. In those days, schizophrenics were treated with electrical shocks. Next to the old Vancouver General Hospital was the polio and tuberculosis unit where patients were confined to Iron Lungs, the enormous machines that breathed for the patients.

Our budget was very tight, although Ted and I shared many of the expensive textbooks. Because most of the students living on campus were as poor as we were, we noted that their clotheslines flew green pajamas that strikingly resembled the hospital greens!

During our last year of Medical School we felt this awful doom looming at the end: our final exams. We were to be given oral and written tests. The oral examiners would choose one subject to test us on—if it wasn't a good subject for you, or if you had never heard of it (it has been known to happen), then you were sunk. We had to study hard. We all felt like chased rabbits looking for the correct hole to dart into, fearing that we may have missed the most important one.

Preparing and defending our doctoral thesis was a nuisance. But we worked hard on ours nonetheless, mostly gathering information and typing. Later, it was decided that the medical students would no longer be required to write theses. Ted and I both won prizes on our theses.

At 1954's Medical School Ball, dinner was good and the music was grand. Early in the evening the MDs were an affable bunch. A social occasion like this seemed to signal the liberal use of alcohol and the acceptance of drunkenness. This ball was no exception.

We survived the ball and passed our final exams. The year was 1954 and we were proud to be the first graduating class of the School of Medicine!

Internship and Motherhood, 1954–55

Ted and I applied for a one-year internship at St. Paul's Hospital and were accepted. St. Paul's was run by the Sisters of Providence, nuns who used their rosaries and crucifixes often. With great reluctance they let Ted and I have cots in the same room.

We were busy all the time. We each had turns in the surgery, medicine, pediatric, maternity, gynaecology, and emergency areas. It was hard work as we worked days and were on call all the rest of the time. The emergency rooms were small and very busy. I was relieved to see the mentally ill patients treated with new drugs. It was a gentler treatment, to use Thorazine to sedate violent patients instead of restraining jackets.

I became pregnant in the winter of 1955. This made the nun's eyebrows raise. My white uniform became tighter and tighter until an anesthesiologist who had had twins took pity on me and gave me a maternity uniform.

I became pregnant in the winter of 1955. This made the nun's eyebrows raise. There were uncomfortable moments in morning surgeries when I felt quite ill. My white uniform became tighter and tighter until an anesthesiologist who had had twins took pity on me and gave me a maternity uniform.

As our internship was ending, Ted found a position in Quesnel in the central region of British Columbia. Fortunately, we arrived in Quesnel before the baby was born. The morning after our arrival, Ted left for the hospital to see patients and took me with him. The maternity ward was full of babies and mothers, so I was put in a side room by a stairway. It was a very public place with faces peering through the window. Dr. Thompson delivered our son Philip on July 5, 1955—five days after I completed my internship.

I had a chance to return to Vancouver Island to cover for Dr. Howie McDiarmid for a month in Tofino on the west coast. Ted remained in Ucluelet. Mom Jansch came with me to look after Philip. There was a hospital in Tofino as well as a clinic in Ucluelet. This was my first try at general practice and I had a busy schedule. Later, when Dr. McDiarmid decided to go away for an extended period, we took the opportunity to cover for him. Ted travelled to Tofino to begin work while I stayed in Chemainus and gave birth to my daughter. Dr. Gordon Heydon, a former classmate, delivered Patricia in March 1957.

Ted treated many injured loggers as it was a dangerous profession, but the First Nations people in the area were most needful of our services. Many drank heavily and often the women were physically abused. The women and children came in with head lice, anaemia, and the wounds of domestic violence. There was little access to birth control so I delivered plenty of babies.

Financially, we did well in Tofino. We paid off all our large debts, including our student loans. We were wary about Tommy Douglas from the Federal Government bringing in socialized medicine. We did not see how it would benefit general practitioners. We planned to move to the U.S. when it happened.

We bought a practice on Salt Spring Island that included a house with a gorgeous view of Ganges Harbour. It also included an office that was under a maple tree full of noisy crows. On Fridays, Ted or I would make rounds at the small clinics on the outer Gulf Islands—Pender, Saturna, and Mayne. We took the water taxi in the winter and our sixteen-foot aluminum runabout boat in the summer.

USA, 1966–1978

Ted had always been interested in pathology, so he accepted a Residency at Rhode Island Hospital in the U.S. We moved in 1966. I got a job in the Child Development Center at Rhode Island Hospital and also did laboratory studies in Cytogenetics.

In 1970, when Ted finished with his Residency, he accepted a job in Fort Wayne, Indiana. I worked at the Fort Wayne State Hospital and Training Center with mentally-challenged children, then did genetic research at St. Joseph's Hospital.

I volunteered in several clinics in the worst parts of the city. There were many poor people in Indiana, and not everyone could access the welfare system. I saw a thirteen-year-old who was married with two children. She looked like she was thirteen going on thirty, haggard and worn out—what a life for a teen! There was a little girl who had blisters on her toes because her parents didn't have enough money for food much less for shoes. There was a prostitute that had such severe gonorrhoea that she ended up in the

hospital with IVs. I began to think that the Canadian socialized system was not so bad after all—the poor patients get care and the doctors get paid.

I obtained a position as an associate director with the Fort Wayne Red Cross and worked in the blood bank's Pheresis Department. In 1976 Ted and I separated. Two years later, I was invited to live with friends, Martin and Marian Petersen. This was the beginning of a twenty-five-year long living and working partnership. In 1978, I travelled to U.S.S.R. with a group of geneticists. We were one of the first tour groups allowed to enter the newly-opened border of Communist Russia.

Oregon, 1979–2001

I accepted a position sharing a general practice with the elderly Dr. McCandless in Roseburg, Oregon. The business of medicine was not easy. Payment that came from insurance billings took a long time to arrive, but expenses were unrelenting. A pipe in the ceiling burst and flooded the office, so we moved to a new one. Our practice got busier and busier.

In March 1980, when I had only been with Dr. McCandless for seven months, he had a stroke and passed away. It was sudden but not surprising. I missed him and felt that he still had a great deal to teach me as he had had fifty years of practical experience. In spite of my initial uncertainty, I began my own practice and did quite well.

In 1985, I accepted a partnership with Dr. Lott and moved into his attractive, modern office. Dr. Lott was extremely relaxed and good to work with.

I retired in 1991. I loved the Oregon coast, and as the Petersens and I spent much of our time there, we built a home in Waldport in 1995. I enjoyed retirement. There was time for long walks on the beach hunting for agates and fossils after winter storms. I enjoyed spinning and weaving. We travelled up the Alaska Highway with an Airstream trailer. I sailed with my daughter Pat and her husband Rob Castle in Johnstone Strait, Mexico, and Fiji.

In 2001, I returned to Canada to be closer to Pat and Rob, and I am sharing a home with them. I have slowed down and if I hadn't written my story several years ago, I might have forgotten it all by now.

DR. RUTH ROFFMANN

I was born on April 6, 1917 in Cologne, Germany. It was a Good Friday, and I have always felt that this was a good omen, accompanying me through the high points and low points of my life, enabling me to always come out on top of situations. Due to my father's job, we moved a lot, and finally ended up in Konigsberg, our easternmost province, where I spent my formative years, finishing school and starting medical school in 1937. It was the university where Kant taught and Helmholtz demonstrated the ophthalmoscope. We were encouraged to visit as many universities as possible to get a well-rounded picture of different views and methods in medicine. So I managed to go to Freiberg (Black Forest / Rhein), Berlin, and Breslau in Silesia, where I graduated in 1941.

The war was well under way, and more and more of our male students dressed in uniforms. Some were called up for active duty. Since WWI, there had always been a good number of female students in medicine. Now we really increased the percentage noticeably. As long as I can remember there were always female middle-aged MDs in town, both in general practice and as specialists.

I was interning in a hospital right inside the Siegfried Line, opposite the Maginot Line, when one late evening we got orders to evacuate the hospital. We had two ambulances which went back and forth for the rest of the night. I was scared to death to travel with two patients who had head injuries, one very quiet and the other a bit restless. Fortunately nothing happened. We were dumped into a spa way into Black Forest where we enjoyed a few peaceful days, taking the waters, etc. But I kept thinking of my bike which I had left behind. In those days, it was considered a precious commodity.

So when the ambulance had to go back to save more equipment, I hitched a ride and, incidentally, on the way back saw for the first time an abandoned town. Oh, that silence! There were signs which read, "Please feed my cat, milk my cow, look after the chickens!" I pedaled like blazes to get away from there. The war caused me to be cut off from my family for weeks. With Poland being so close to my home province and all that bombing and shooting, I was also cut off from getting my monthly allowance. So

many fellow students took pity on the "poor girl" from East Prussia. I did not want loans, and non-payable loans flowed in. I made it to Berlin where I continued my studies until I took my last plunge to Breslau.

More interning. I do not know why the MDs had such faith in me and asked me to cover one weekend when a man with the DTs came in. Since he was rather wild, I had him locked up in the padded cell. Alas, it turned out that he was the local dentist! What an embarrassment in a small town. I was happy that I did not have to cover any more.

On October 15, 1941, our group graduated. We celebrated that night, and the next day I was on the train heading for home. I had had enough wandering. I wanted to be with my family as the war got worse. A job awaited me in the surgical department of the City Hospital. Gradually we were introduced to war surgery, like removing shrapnel from civilians, due to the increasing air raid. We also had to look after the police who served near the front and came home for further treatment. We found out what maggots could do: cleaned festering wounds, even though the sight was not really elating. I should mention that all this happened before the use of penicillin. We had Sulphonamides as the utmost helper then.

Food was getting scarce, and we were hungry after many extra hours at work. In the hospital cafeteria they served one dish made of dried prunes in an evil-looking sauce. One day the internists were threatening to do away with that dish before we surgeons had a chance at it. One of the boys said, "Doesn't this look like the empyema that we just treated?" The internists fled, and we had a good fill. So war was not without humour.

In 1944 a rural hospital asked for replacements for the boys who had gone to the front. I was chosen to fill the position. I did not like the thought of leaving my family again, but there was no choice. It was a beautiful summer, with the harvest in full swing. I had a room at the top floor with a full view of the country below and beyond.

In rural hospitals we had limited service, and my chief sent me with an infant to my hometown for specialist treatment. The hospital could not accommodate the baby, and after treatment they sent us home. How was I going to feed that baby on rationed milk? Then I had an idea: Why not go to my old hospital and admit the baby? My friend quietly put it into a crib in the children's ward, and I went home to visit my family. That night we had the first truly massive air raid. We were saved, but what about my hospital and the baby? I had to find out!

Raging fires and the accompanying fire storms made me take detours, extending a walk of fifteen minutes to two hours. My old hospital was safe and the baby too! They gave me a bottle, and we fed the baby with sugar water at my parents' place. I was on the first train back into the diaspora the next morning.

My room allowed me to watch what was going on outside. Fortifications were dug in the neighbourhood, and a never-ending trek of refugees came along the road from the east. Trainloads of wounded civilians arrived at our little town, from the place where my relatives lived. Imagine bending over a stretcher and wondering if your uncle or aunt was on it. I was saved from this experience, but we learned quickly how to deal with a massive influx of patients. Mother Superior and I seemed to have a knack for this, while our elderly chief was only in our way. We sent him home and did our thing. In a few hours we had everybody in a bed or on a stretcher, or at least on a mattress in a hallway. Next day the real work began: changing dressings and maybe casts. We were fortunate to send a number of those patients out by train to the west before we were enclosed by the enemy. From then on we kept essentials like valuable documents and a change of clothes in a rucksack, just in case. One night we were kept awake by the biggest air raid on my home town. We went to the flat roof and saw a "magic carpet" of fire weave up and down in that direction. Next morning I told my chief that I was going home to see what had happened to my relatives. He was not pleased, but even if he had forbidden me to go, I would have left anyway. What I found next to the railroad station was not encouraging: ruins, with some still smoldering. During the forty-five minute walk to home, I saw many houses that were destroyed. But ours wasn't! So I went back to work on the next train.

It was obvious that we were losing the war. One day a surgeon from the army visited our hospital. His Standard hospital had just been reduced to a Field hospital, and he invited us to take a look. I wished I never had. Soldiers came in right from the battlefield near us, wild-eyed and desperate. The worst was a man with pneumothorax whose injured rib cage flapped wildly with each breath, and his eyes were wide in desperation and agony. So this was war at a close-up. That surgeon asked the chief why there were still women at his hospital. In the same afternoon three nurses approached me and told me they were leaving. Was I going to join them? Imagine the agony between your oath and reality. Staying meant death or the salt mines in the Urals, rape or death by starvation. For years afterwards I suffered from the decision to join the exodus until a friend who was in the Royal Air Force and had bombed Hamburg, put me at ease: "What good would your sacrifice have done to mankind? Staying alive allowed you to save more lives."

So we took one piece of luggage, the rucksack that contained the papers and the clothes, and entered the ambulance which took us just so far. Then we joined a hospital train that was going nowhere. That train was ill-equipped. There was nothing to fight gas gangrene, nothing to change dressings. We finally quit the train loaded up with letters from the soldiers to their loved ones, to line up for crossing the "Haff," a huge bay of the Baltic Sea, but not before some army doctors had tried to retain me for services.

That crossing! There were places marked that were not safe to enter on the brittle ice. Horses and wagons had gone down the night before. We made it to the peninsula and to the place where they shipped wounded soldiers and some refugees to safety.

Nurse Leni had secured a number of vials of morphine, enough to kill us in case the enemy overtook us. And we had a conference discussing how to deal with them. By then we were relatively safe, but the soldiers were in agony, so the morphine went quickly. And we had to go back to the peninsula. It was -20° C, the ground was covered with snow. There was a crowd of people surrounding something. Leni went to investigate and soon motioned us to come too. A woman was giving birth on the snow. We asked the crowd to step back, and the nurses spread their capes for privacy. Leni delivered a lusty baby boy. Who knows what became of that child.

We finally made it on board a navy ship destined for Stettin. It was a

Nurse Leni had secured a number of vials of morphine, enough to kill us in case the enemy overtook us. And we had a conference discussing how to deal with them.

hospital ship, and it had everything: medications, dressing material, and food! There was a small OR, and soon we were involved in changing dressings, opening abscesses, etc. We had so much to do, and the OR table did not allow us to change patients quickly enough, so for less severe cases, we invented the "stand-up anaesthesia": we propped the soldiers up against something, gave them a whiff of ether, did what had to be done, and returned them to their beds. And it worked! We were glad we were kept busy because the day before we left Gustloff, a ship full of refugees had been torpedoed. Although we were escorted by frigates, they could not protect us from suffering the same fate. When the ship's siren howled, we dug deeper into abscesses, cut casts quicker, and tried not to think of the lurking dangers.

Once in Stettin, we jumped off the ship, literally. I never knew before that I could jump so high and far! The nurses helped me to get a foothold on dry land. We ended up in Thuringia, which was to become East Germany after the war. I joined the practice of an ailing colleague for almost two years. Luckily I got a request from a family friend to do a locum in the Rhein/ Ruhr valley. After finally joining a GP in what was to become East Germany, I went to the west, doing locums in the Rhine/Ruhr valley and ending up in Hamburg in the surgical department of a large children's hospital where my sister worked as a nurse. She had the brainwave to emigrate. Canada accepted us, and here I should say, "Canada, here we come!"

The Indian moccasin telegraph seemed to cross the Atlantic. The first shock came with the news that there were no midwives in that far-away country! Like most Europeans, my sister and I were delivered by midwives who had to undergo rigorous training and were guided by the "midwife law." I could deliver a breech and remove a retained placenta, but had never conducted a normal delivery. Fortunately, I received help from the small community ward, which was part of the children's hospital designed to give student nurses a chance to learn about the care of the newborn. Every free hour I spent with the two midwives who let me observe but did the actual job. From them I learned patience

Next came the language problem. We studied plenty of English in school, reading *King Lear* and *The Forsythe Saga*. But we soon realized that we did not even know how to ask for the bathroom or how to shop, so we read *The Egg and I*, hoping that this would get us down to earth. Alas! We knew all about chickens, but not much about daily life. We just had to rely on good fortune. Fortune alone did not prepare us for the Canadian pronunciation nor for the American one which I needed in an interview with Dean Weaver. We finally agreed that before I answered his questions verbally, he would write the questions down. I was then put on the list of applicants for the next meeting of the College of Physicians and Surgeons of British Columbia. At that meeting I met a few other Europeans who hoped to make Canada their future home. We finally wrote our basic sciences and failed wholesale—GPs and Specialists alike. The second try had us pass, and then came the introduction into the real medical world of Canada: internship at the Royal Columbian Hospital in New Westminster.

Now I suddenly realized that there were very few women MDs in western Canada. Just one Canadian girl and a Dutch one were lodged at the Nurses' Residence where we could not have any visitors in our rooms. We had to receive them in the lobby. I was thirty then and had been used to an independent life-style for years. Well, eventually the Interns' Residence was deemed "safe" for all of us. And we did have great sessions in the European sense. My adult colleagues had no problem with me. I was useful and experienced. Then came the exams, the LMCC or Council exams. When I got that letter with the news that I had passed, I started to rush to New Westminster to celebrate. Alas! Outside the hospital I met one of the surgeons who told me to hold my horses for a real good party. Only two of us foreigners had passed the exams, and the other ones were preparing for their retreat back to Europe. What a letdown!

We studied plenty of English in school, reading King Lear *and* The Forsythe Saga. *But we soon realized that we did not even know how to ask for the bathroom or how to shop!*

Sometimes the language barrier could create lots of misunderstanding at work. One time as an Intern I was asked to do a "cut down." "Cut down on what?" I naively asked the attending nurse for an explanation, only to look into wide-open disbelieving eyes. I must explain here that they had just unveiled a fake MD in Halifax, and the nurse saw another imposter in *this* female. She opened the tray for me and left to inform the head of the interns about this incident. Meanwhile I proceeded happily, knowing from the instruments that I was supposed to do a venesection. An angel arrived just in time to connect the IV for me, and I easily passed the test. Otherwise I had no trouble with the nurses, who were glad to have a female doctor in the hospital.

About my social life at that time? There were invitations and there was the annual dinner of the New Westminster Medical Association. I was invited, but had heard that females got the official invitation only to decline it dutifully. My thinking was that if I was good enough to work with the boys, I was good enough to "play" with them! I asked one of the trustworthy seniors if I was too forward. He replied, "Go, girl, go!" The first time was rather tame, with me sitting in the room where ladies were allowed in the Westminster Club. For the second time there were younger, more progressive boys around. They wanted me in the 'inner sanctum.' Two of them pulled my arms, two others pushed me. At the door of the 'holy grail,' the butler stepped in front of us and sternly stated, "No women allowed past this door!" One colleague shouted, "This is no woman. This is a DOCTOR!" And so I crashed the gender barrier! One fact still bothers me: the butler died of a coronary a few days afterwards. Coincidence? Here I get a bit ahead of myself. I joined a group of GPs in Surrey after my exams. Two of us branched out after a while, and together with a few more family MDs, several dentists and a pharmacist, we built our clinic in a pretty U-shaped building with a lawn inside and flowering bushes and a tree in the courtyard. I mention this because the contrast was so great when I moved to 100 Mile House where the choice of office space was very limited. We ended up building our facility there too, and so 100 Mile House had their first clinic.

Gradually things changed around New Westminster and Surrey. Younger MDs took up practice. St. Mary's was rebuilt; The Royal Columbian got a new Emergency; Surrey Memorial Hospital came into being. Two lady doctors arrived from the U.K. and the first husband and wife MD team settled in the area. I came to know a few more female doctors once I started

At the Flying U there was a cute head wrangler who herded the horses and us dudes. It was love at first sight, and I took every opportunity to sneak up to that place.

to practice. Dr. Ethlyn Trapp and Dr. Olive Sadler visited Royal Columbian Hospital to administer radiotherapy before the Cancer Clinic took over. They were well respected for their professional acumen and their warm-heartedness. I am sure I owe it to them that I was also accepted easily by my male confreres.

And now to the Cariboo in general and 100 Mile House in particular. My original fascination was absolutely non-medical. In 1957 my sister and I were finally in a position to go for a real holiday with horseback riding and no cooking! We found such a place at the Flying U Guest Ranch on Green Lake in the 70 Mile area. At that time 100 Mile House barely existed; there were only a few houses, a garage, and a gas pump. I am not even sure if the hotel was built then. There was an Auto Court and a grocery store. If you wanted to shop, you went to Clinton. What a contrast now! At the Flying U there was a cute head wrangler who herded the horses and us dudes. It was love at first sight, and I took every opportunity to sneak up to that place.

Finally in December, 1963, on the shortest day, the longest night, we got married in Prince George where my sister and family gave us a wonderful wedding. His name was Jake Reinertson, and he was generous enough to let me keep my maiden name as a business name until my retirement. In those days this was not common and sometimes led to funny situations. I once overheard the mailman asking about this Reinertson living with two women in the same apartment. The explanation from the superintendent was: "She is one and the same, just having two names like a movie star." The next test came when I filed my first tax return at 100 Mile House. Under furious blushing my accountant mumbled that only married couples could claim each other. It took some explaining. Now we had to find a place close enough to 100 Mile House where Jake could raise livestock and I would be within reach of the hospital which was then in the planning stage and soon to be built.

It was in full swing when we moved into our spanking new home at 90 Mile, twelve miles away from the village. We brought with us a small herd of cattle, a good number of horses, a cattle dog, and a cat from my brother-in-law's place across the street.

I applied for staff privileges at the hospital and met with stiff resistance from one member. However, 100 Mile was all for progress and wanted a lady doctor. I joined Dr. Fischer in his practice and soon was well away. By now I was fifty years old. I keep telling people who reach this milestone that the old saying is wrong: Life starts at fifty!

What a different life was out in the boondocks. At that time we had six MDs and a surgeon for a short time. There came the time when the men from the U.K. left the area and we were reduced to two lonely souls. I mention this in light of the present plight of rural MDs. It was no fun to take calls every second night, especially since my patients hated him, and his patients hated me! (Dr. Fischer had passed away by then.) And there were the maternities who wanted to be delivered by a female. I cannot remember how long this difficult time lasted, but when my husband offered to sell our place and move on, I contacted the B.C. College of Physicians and Surgeons and asked them to find someone to fill my position. In the end, they found a semi-retired colleague from the coast who found another MD wiling to come along. Suddenly life turned normal, and when I asked half-jokingly for a two-month holiday, the new MDs thought it was a good idea. From then on I always took July and August off.

New to me was caring for the Indians. Originally things were pretty grim at our reserve. The priest started a program to dry them out. Others, especially a nurse, continued the work. Finally the Indians wanted to be clean. Now they go to university to become teachers, accountants, etc. They were wonderful patients full of humour and story-telling, and they liked to test you from time to time. If they were found to have lied about the cause of an accident, they broke out in a peal of laughter. The older generation was finally convinced to have their babies delivered in the hospital. We supplied them with a bell button to let us know when they felt like pushing. Yes, they rang the bell, and we lifted the covers, and often there would be a baby with the placenta duly delivered without us! The next generation was a bit more difficult.

Here I have come to a quick end of the story. I semi-retired at age sixty-five, and was no longer on call. Next I gave up maternities. That was hard but necessary. At age seventy I had to quit the office hours as well. The people of 100 Mile House gave me a great send-off, which I will always remember.

Just a quick note on our private life. My husband had been living in this country since 1936 and was well liked. So we had quite an extended social life which had been hard to maintain as a single person. We had our cabin on Green Lake, a romantic place to escape when we had our days off. The great-est joy, however, was riding the range with my husband. Apart from checking on the cattle, we saw an abundance of wildlife. Black bear, moose, deer, and coyotes were still plentiful in those days. We once observed the mating dance of a pair of sandhill cranes, and during hunting season we were often followed by ravens in great numbers who hoped that riders would shoot an easy meal for them. We did not mix hunting and range riding on the same day.

My husband passed away in November, 1992. Life has not been the same for me, but I am still surrounded by nature, with Canada geese coming back every year to nest and moose visiting in the winter, trying to get at the hay for my only remaining horse. Deer can be seen close to my place. Marmots whistle the alarm whenever a coyote travels through. I am grateful for the small joys of life.

When I look back on the eighty-three years of my life, I must say I was blessed by wonderful people who walked along with me: my parents and my sister who made many sacrifices to help me through medical school, and later my sister who 'dragged' me to Canada, a move which I never regretted, and finally my numerous friends, co-workers, and acquaintances who always popped up at the right time to help me along. Maybe coming into this world on a Good Friday was a good omen indeed. (*Dr. Roffmann died July 14, 2006*)

DR. BLUMA TISCHLER

Dr. Bluma Tischler, the youngest of three children, was born in Baranowicze, Poland, which lies near Minsk and just south of Lithuania. At the end of the Second World War, Baranowicze was absorbed into the U.S.S.R.-Russia. Following the collapse of the U.S.S.R., Baranowicze became part of the independent Republic of Belarus. Bluma's father, an accountant, and her mother, a dentist, were Jews who grew up in pre-revolutionary Russia, survived the First World War, and settled into a middle-class life in the newly created state of Poland.

While still in high school in September 1939, she and her mother went on a brief trip to Warsaw. During their stay Hitler invaded Poland, and Warsaw began to go up in flames under the onslaught of German bombers.

Bluma and her mother headed home. What would have been a one-day trip in peace time became an ordeal of many days through a country whose transport and communications had suddenly been turned over to the task of mobilizing against the invasion. When they finally reached home, Bluma's father welcomed them back as if from the dead.

Her father feared the arrival of the Germans, but almost immediately it was the Red Army that swept in, claiming the eastern part of Poland that had been promised Stalin under his agreement with Hitler. From then on Bluma, who already spoke Yiddish, Polish, and French, was obliged to continue her schooling in Russian.

She saw a particularly haggard young girl walking painfully along the path. "Look at that poor girl!" she exclaimed. "How thin she is!" As the girl approached, Bluma's mother realised that the poor, thin girl was none other than her daughter, who had been evacuated to a collective farm in Uzbekistan, a neighbouring republic of Tadzhikistan.

In June 1941, the Germans, having overrun most of Western Europe, attacked U.S.S.R.-Russia. Bluma's family, knowing how the Nazis were likely to treat the Jews, fled to the east. They did not have time to collect her older brother and sister who were studying engineering in Lwow, but set out immediately, travelling at first by horse and buggy, later on foot.

Stumbling along in the dark one night, the family got separated. Bluma's father, she later learned, cast about in desperation for ten hours looking for his wife and daughter. He was never seen again, presumably having been shot by the oncoming Germans.

Knowing nothing of her father's fate, Bluma and her mother continued their painful march to the east, wearing out their shoes and going barefoot a good part of the way. Bluma remembers becoming so tired that she would gladly have died rather than taking another step. After they had gone about 600 miles and reached Voronezh, her mother called a halt.

Bluma took up her interrupted high school education, studying now in Russian. Her mother, in between trips to the railway station in search of the rest of her family, practised her profession of dentistry as best she could in order to find sustenance for herself and the one child she had left to her.

Then, restored for a time, they moved on, now in the cold of oncoming winter, through northern Ukraine and on to the Ural Mountains. From there they angled southward into Central Asia until, having travelled a total of 2,300 miles, they were able to stop in Stalinabad, the capital of the Tadzhik Soviet Socialist Republic (now Tajikistan).

This Republic lay north of Afghanistan and was utterly foreign to Bluma and her mother, but it had the merit of being far from the advancing Germans in a relatively warm climate. Bluma went back to high school, still studying in Russian, but now having to learn the language of the local Tadzhiks as well.

Meanwhile, her mother found work as a dentist in a military hospital. Although they were hungry and living in a corner of a squalid house whose mud floor had been partitioned off to allow space for five families, they were safe, at least for the time being.

Bluma's mother resumed her daily trips to the railway station, looking for news from her family. One day when she was walking with an acquaintance near the railway track, she saw a particularly haggard young girl walking painfully along the path. "Look at that poor girl!" she exclaimed. "How thin she is!" As the girl approached, Bluma's mother realised that the poor, thin girl was none other than her daughter, who had been evacuated to a collective farm in Uzbekistan, a neighbouring republic of Tadzhikistan. This daughter had received word that her mother was in Stalinabad and set out to find her. Bluma's brother also turned up, but his stay was interrupted when he was drafted into the Red Army. Later, he was wounded in the bitter fighting around Leningrad.

Somehow the family managed to get by. Bluma's mother was able to occasionally salvage scraps of hospital food to take home to her family. While she was wasting away and her legs became grossly swollen (nutritional edema), a doctor discovered that she was giving what little food she had to her family and eating nothing herself. The doctor warned her she would die if she did not start eating half the food herself. With her mother eating again, Bluma finished high school and was accepted as a student in the medical faculty that had been evacuated from Leningrad and taken up residence with the existing faculty in Stalinabad.

Bluma's classmates were almost all women and all had been warned that when they finished their studies they would immediately be sent off as medical officers to the Red Army, where they would help in the struggle for survival against the Germans. In the meantime, they would have to learn to handle small arms. Bluma learned to strip and assemble a rifle, reflecting that she would willingly fight the Nazis if it came to it, but she hoped it would not. Meanwhile, she sought what comfort she could find in the intellectual pleasure of study and peace in the medical library, where there was at least enough light to read by.

In time she was joined in her studies by a young student, Isaak Tischler, a wounded soldier of the Red Army who even possessed a medal. He was one of the few young men left in sight and therefore a rare catch. For his part, he was attracted to Bluma because he recognized her accent when she correctly answered a question that had stumped a half a dozen others in the class. Isaak realized that she was not only a compatriot, but exceptionally smart into the bargain. It might be worthwhile getting to know her.

Bluma and Isaak began studying together. When the Russian army at last drove the Germans back and reoccupied Poland, they resolved to return together and continue with their education in Lwow. They eventually did and both succeeded in being accepted into the medical school there.

Isaak and Bluma did not want to stay in U.S.S.R.-Russia permanently and knew that they must marry before they could resume the further years of travel that would inevitably lie ahead. Not only was marriage required by Jewish custom, but there were the conventions of the day to reckon with. Under the prevailing Communist regime they became husband and wife in a cursory civil ceremony. But that was not good enough for Bluma's mother. She had not brought her daughter up properly and dragged her halfway across Europe and Asia to see her living in sin. Only a proper wedding would do.

Isaak set out to find a rabbi. Before the war there had been about fifty synagogues in Lwow. One alone was now left standing and it had escaped destruction only because the Nazi German army had used it as a garage. With the restoration of peace, it was struggling back to its feet and its rabbi, who had been hiding throughout the war, had emerged to minister to the spiritual needs of any surviving Jews he could find.

Together Isaak and Bluma went to the synagogue. The rabbi was suspicious. He did not believe their story. They looked and sounded more like Russians than Jews, he said, directing a particularly skeptical look at Isaak, who was wearing a Russian army greatcoat several sizes too big for him and a Siberian hat. A busy rabbi had no time for triflers.

But Bluma and Isaak had encountered obstacles before. They were not easily put off. How, they asked one another, could they persuade this rabbi to do his duty by a couple of bona fide Jews? They knew that for a man who had lived through exceptionally dangerous times he was only being properly cautious. It had not been long since people lost their lives when they put themselves forward as Jews. They put their heads together and began conferring in Yiddish. The rabbi listened, skeptical at first but gradually persuaded by what he heard coming from the mouths of the couple that a few minutes earlier had seemed like imposters.

In the end, he accepted them, provisionally at least, as genuine. But he raised another objection. He had no wine and a marriage would not be solemnised without it. That was the ancient tradition. Isaak went out, determined to make sure the ceremony took place. The essentials of life were hard enough to come by in Lwow, and for the likes of a poor medical student, wine was indeed a luxury. Once again, Isaak demonstrated his instinct for survival. He found some kvass, a drink made of fermented bread. Its alcohol content was nothing to speak of and it could not even remotely have been classed as wine, but after he had added a little juice from a bowl of borsch it was at least red. All obstacles were overcome at last, and the rabbi conducted the ceremony. He raised an eyebrow when he tasted the red liquid that Isaak had handed him, but he had not survived the war without learning to compromise, so he went on until the ceremony was completed.

Isaak and Bluma spent their first year of married life in Lwow. When the

One day the Sister Superior, working beside Isaak, confided to him that Jews were rumoured to be killing Polish children. Next day, in a further spasm of anti-Semitic rage, some citizens of a nearby town fell on those Jews who were left over from the Holocaust and began slaughtering them.

war at last ended, they decided to move west again, this time heading for Breslau, a part of Germany that had, under the rearrangement of post-war boundaries, become part of Poland. Both already were Polish citizens; they enrolled for another year of university in Breslau.

A Catholic hospital took them on as undergraduate interns while they continued their studies. One day the Sister Superior, working beside Isaak, confided to him that Jews were rumoured to be killing Polish children. Next day, in a further spasm of anti-Semitic rage, some citizens of a nearby town fell on those Jews who were left over from the Holocaust and began slaughtering them. The Polish police stood by, and order was restored only by the intervention of the Red Army.

Isaak and Bluma, now regarding themselves as having no homeland where they would live in peace and without fear, decided to flee. In company with other migrants, now called "displaced persons" in post-war jargon, they crossed illegally into Czechoslovakia and again illegally into Austria. In their travels, they were guided by other young Jews who knew the lay of the land and did not hesitate to get the border guards drunk or otherwise distracted while smuggling their charges from one country to another.

In their travels, they were guided by other young Jews who knew the lay of the land and did not hesitate to get the border guards drunk or otherwise distracted while smuggling their charges from one country to another.

When they finally reached Vienna, Isaak and Bluma were housed in one of the Rothschild mansions, a house of many splendors, and later in a former prisoner of war camp near Llnz. From there they made their way to Munich, Germany, where they applied to the university for admission to the final year of medical studies. The German university authorities, a few of whom had been opposed to the Hitler regime and were conscience-stricken over what it had done to Jews, immediately accepted Isaak and Bluma.

Meanwhile, an American Jewish aid society awarded them bursaries on which to live. Isaak had learned German in high school and fit easily into the routine of lectures. Bluma had studied French. She sat through the first hour of lectures by a renowned professor and understood only two words. That night she wept inconsolably. Had she gone this far, mastered five languages, learned to handle a rifle, studied under deplorable conditions, lost her father, all her aunts and most of her high school classmates, only to be defeated by a strange language in which the verb came only at the end of sentences so long that the beginning was forgotten before the end was reached?

Next day, Isaak bought a two-volume textbook of medicine written by the very lecturer whose words, at least when spoken, had defeated Bluma, and together over the next two months the two of them translated every sentence. When she reached the end of the book, Bluma not only had a good grasp of internal medicine, but knew enough German to become not just a passable student but a good one. After graduation, she wrote her thesis for the degree of MD on a subject in pediatrics. Isaak, now beginning to take an interest in neuropsychiatry, as it was then called, wrote on an aspect of syphilis of the central nervous system.

After they finished their researches and internships, they resolved to migrate to Canada. They made their way to Bremerhaven and took passage on a German ship that had been captured by the Canadian navy. Having no money, they had to work their passage across the Atlantic by doing the most menial of shipboard chores, such as cleaning toilets. However, they were still left owing the balance of their fare, $250 a piece. Nevertheless, the Canadian immigration service took them on a good faith with the understanding that they would eventually repay the debt. In fact, when they were eventually able to start repayment, the service told them to forget about it.

One night, in the mid-Atlantic, the ship's doctor called Isaak to help him operate on a young Ukrainian girl for acute appendicitis. Isaak interviewed the patient in her native Ukrainian and soon showed the doctor that his diagnosis was wrong and an operation was unnecessary. The doctor, vastly relieved that his meager surgical skill was not going to be put to the test, took Isaak into his cabin and poured him a drink, and asked him to be his assistant. No more cleaning toilets!

Bluma's sister had managed to reach Canada before them and was able to help them as next of kin through Canada's then difficult immigration system. Isaak and Bluma eventually arrived in Montreal and settled in to take

English lessons from an unlikely source, a Protestant sect. Meanwhile, they applied to innumerable hospitals for positions as interns. Their challenge was to find two enabling certificates that would allow them to write the examinations of the Medical Council of Canada.

Isaak applied for a certificate in Quebec, but was refused because he could not speak French. Resourceful as ever, he scraped up all the money he could find and went to Toronto. There he received a sympathetic reception from the registrar of the College of Physicians and Surgeons. After he had found Lwow and Stalinabad on the map, the registrar was happy to oblige. Soon Isaak had the precious certificate in his hand. But he could not leave yet. He explained that his wife needed a certificate too. When asked why she did not come with him to Toronto, Isaak replied, "We only had enough money for one train ticket," and he had earned the amount by giving nursing care to a patient with general paralysis for which he earned $3 for a twenty-four-hour shift. The registrar was a kind man and looked over Bluma's credentials and, without actually setting eyes on her, filled out her certificate. In time Isaak and Bluma were accepted as interns by a Catholic hospital in Montreal and there the Sister Superior, on learning that they were a married couple, provided them—out of her hospital's own funds—with a small apartment nearby.

The two immigrants finished their internships and passed the licensure examinations. They resolved to study further, Isaak in psychiatry and Bluma in pediatrics. After four years of training they passed their specialty examinations, and were ready to start practising medicine in British Columbia. They have two sons, one a doctor and the other a lawyer. They live comfortably and look back on their early experiences without dramatising them.

It was hard going, they admit, but many had suffered more.

(This article was written by Dr. Jerry Richards for the two issues of Medical Post, *October 2 and 9, 1990, under the title: "The Road to Medicine: Fugitives." Dr. Richards and Drs. Isaak and Bluma Tischler have given permission to include the story in this book. Editor of* The Medical Post, *Mr. Rick Campbell, also has given permission.)*

On September 18, 1992, Dr. Bluma Tischler was the honoree at the Pioneer Dinner and Dr. Henry Dunn was the speaker to give tribute to her at this testimonial dinner, describing her struggle in Europe and great dedication and success while working at Woodlands School. Dr. Tischler addressed the Pioneer Dinner following Dr. Dunn's tribute to her:

"Many thanks for selecting me as your honoree at the Pioneer Dinner. I confess that when Volker Ebelt approached me I was ambivalent. Limelight is always tension-producing. When Volter mentioned that Henry Dunn would 'roast' me I could not help but accept. And when the Academic Day program came out listing Harvey Levy, Cheryl Greenberg, and the many friends I worked closely with I knew it was the right decision. I would like to thank you for the excellent presentations and for bringing metabolic disorder into focus for the Pediatric community.

"Henry outlined my involvement in mental retardation. You may be interested in knowing how I first became involved. This is a question many pediatric residents who rotated through Woodlands also asked me.

"After my training in Pediatrics in Montreal, I arrived in B.C. in October 1954. I had a letter of introduction from Dr. Allan Ross, who was the Head of the Department of Pediatrics at McGill University, to Dr. Jack McCreary who was the Head of the Department of Pediatrics at UBC. I planned to go into private practice. Dr. McCreary suggested that I should become the senior resident at St. Paul's hospital, which would help acquaint me with the local pediatric scene.

"My husband Isaak, who is a psychiatrist, had arrived in B.C. ahead of me to take a position at Essondale Mental Hospital, now Riverview. Dr. Gee, who was the Director of the Provincial Mental Health Services, noticed in Isaak's application for the position that his wife was a pediatrician. He suggested that I could also work for the MHS. Isaak was surprised and emphasized that I was a pediatrician and not a psychiatrist. Dr. Gee repeated the offer. Isaak raised the volume of his voice, thinking Dr. Gee, who was about

He explained that his wife needed a certificate too. When asked why she did not come with him to Toronto, Isaak replied, "We only had enough money for one train ticket," and he had earned the amount by giving nursing care to a patient with general paralysis for which he earned $3 for a twenty-four-hour shift.

sixty, was hard of hearing. 'Yes, Dr. Tischler, I hear you,' said Dr. Gee. 'We have a place called Woodlands School which is a residential setting for the mentally retarded.'

"A week or so later I visited Woodlands School in New Westminster. It made a tremendous impact on me, and very little in my pediatric training prepared me for what I saw. A few days later I went back to Dr. McCreary. I decided to work in Woodlands for one year based on practical considerations. We lived in New Westminster; I was pregnant, and could not drive at that time—my son says I still can't drive. I had the impression Dr. McCreary was surprised with my decision. He told me not to isolate myself in Woodlands and to stay in the mainstream of pediatrics. He arranged for me to spend half a day a week in the Outpatient Department of the Health Centre for Children, and Dr. Dunn to spend some time at Woodlands as a Fellow in Pediatrics.

With the rapid movement towards de-institutionalisation in the last decade we will need more pediatricians, psychiatrists, and family physicians in the community properly trained in the field of the mentally handicapped.

"Over the years I came to appreciate this advice. Our careers have been helped by teachers and leaders who care, like Professor McCreary did, about pediatricians as individuals and about the delivery of service to children. I was the first pediatrician in Woodlands School and my intended stay of one year stretched to more than thirty years.

"In the mid '50s there was tremendous excitement in the field of mental retardation. In 1954 Dr. Bikell in Germany, in 1955 Louis Wolf in England and Armstrong in the U.S.A. reported the successful treatment of PKU with a diet low in phenylalanine if started in early infancy. In 1959 Lejeune in France and Jacobs in England reported an extra twenty-one chromosome in Down Syndrome.

"Many prominent scientists and clinicians were suddenly drawn to the field of mental retardation. In 1955 we surveyed the population of Woodlands with the FeCl test and the following year one-half of the group identified as PKUs (having phenylketonuria) were placed on the diet low in phenylalanine. The other half was the control group. The two youngest, aged eighteen months and six years, improved.

"Woodlands School became one of the two official centers for PKU in the province, the other being at the Children's Hospital under Dr. George Davidson. Both centers, which had always worked closely together, were amalgamated four years ago when I retired from Woodlands.

"At Woodlands, we established a number of positions for pediatricians, psychiatrists, and family physicians. The challenge for us was enormous. In the '60s the population of Woodlands was 1,400. Now it is around 150. In the audience today there are a number of physicians from Woodlands who helped make Woodlands a progressive institution. With the rapid movement towards de-institutionalisation in the last decade we will need more pediatricians, psychiatrists, and family physicians in the community properly trained in the field of the mentally handicapped.

"Today, even after so many years of involvement, to follow the normal development of a child with PKU on dietary treatment still remains tremendously gratifying. Retarded PKUs who were never treated or who were treated late continue to remind me of the impact of our advances. Maternal PKU, an area in which I remain actively involved, is a problem born of our success. And we are facing new challenges.

"In my research I worked with many gifted individuals at the Children's Hospital and UBC. Let me mention some of them: Derek Applegarth, Patricia Baird, George Davidson, Henry Dunn, Edith and Patrick McGreer, Jim Miller, Margaret Norman, Geoffrey C. Robinson, and Sydney Segal.

"I'd also like to pay special tribute to Tom Perry whose contributions are well recognized in B.C. and internationally, and to Dr. Clarissa (Lory) Dolman, neuropathologist and an exceptionally gifted teacher who made the clinicopathological conferences at Woodlands a special event. Both passed away recently.

"Throughout my professional life I was involved in different facets of medicine—clinical, research, and administrative duties. While now one is trained in administration, my generation grew into it. Specialised goals and objectives for the upcoming year are a recent innovation. We certainly have more structure now, but I am not sure that there is any more commitment.

"I would be remiss not to say a few words about parents. While we encounter some very demanding parents, we also meet many parents of multi-handicapped children who rise to the challenge of not only improving services for their own children, but also for those with similar disabilities. The progress in the delivery of services to mentally handicapped children is greatly due to their efforts.

"Let me finish with a few words about the physician's families. From recent discussions with female residents it is clear that child care still remains a major problem often associated with guilt. The change in the present generation, however, is that they speak about it openly without fearing that it will mar their careers. This is healthy and will improve family life for both women physicians and men as well.

"I had to adjust to a rigid system. I am pleased to see the system is starting to adjust to the requirements of the family, and recognizes biological imperatives such as pregnant physicians and those with young children. As a pediatrician, I especially welcome the change.

"Many thanks again and I appreciate that the roasting did not burn me. Henry, you were kind. Thank you."

From the Curriculum Vitae of Dr. Tischler; her University of British Columbia Medical School Appointments included:

1962—Clinical Demonstrator
1965—Clinical Instructor
1972—Clinical Assistant Professor
1978—Clinical Associate Professor
1985—Clinical Professor
1989—Clinical Professor Emerita

Dr. Tischler is a Fellow of the Royal College of Physicians of Canada and a Fellow of the American Association of Mental Deficiency. Her Honours include: On the occasion of the retirement of Dr. Bluma Tischler in 1988, a book was published by Woodlands in her honour: *Bluma Tischler, MD, FRCP, FAA, MD: A Life Retrospective of a Woman Physician*. In 1977, she was awarded the Queen's Jubilee Medal for her work in mental retardation. On May 8, 1978, during the third Session of the thirty-first Parliament of the Province of British Columbia Legislative Assembly, she, accompanied by her husband and son Fred, was honoured; an announcement was also made that the Government had undertaken to establish a graduate fellowship in biochemical genetics, the Dr. Bluma Tischler Postdoctoral Fellowship, with an award of up to $20,000 a year for graduates of medicine and allied disciplines. And on May 18, 1978, in recognition of her outstanding contributions in the field of mental retardation which has earned her an international reputation, Dr. Tischler was honoured by the American Association of Mental Deficiency in Denver, Colorado. The association, which is the only recognised international interdisciplinary professional and scientific organization dealing with mental retardation in twenty-two countries, has selected Dr. Tischler as the winner of its 1978 research award on mental retardation. By 1978, Dr. Bluma Tischler had thirty-six publications on mental retardation.

Special notes to my colleagues:
Since the horrors of World War II there has been tremendous progress in all spheres of human endeavour. Sadly, however, we have yet to eradicate war, hunger, poverty, and many other plights on human existence. As women and physicians we now have both the capacity and the opportunity to greatly diminish such suffering. I hope that, in a small way, I have been able to make a positive difference over the course of my career.

My professional life has been dedicated to working in the fields of developmental and neurological disorders. I entered these fields in the mid 1950s during a very exciting time when we were just starting to understand some of the etiological factors of these disorders. Throughout my career I have worked to enhance the understanding of biochemical and genetic disorders with a special emphasis on phenylketonuria (PKU). I have also fought to enhance the delivery of services to the mentally handicapped, both in residential settings like Woodlands as well as within the general community.

The medical profession has a wide array of areas for one to pursue one's interests, abilities, and concerns. Within that broad spectrum each of us should be able to find the niche we are best suited to. But an effective and well-rounded physician must have a solid grounding in both the sciences and the humanities. And with the present lack of discrimination against

We have yet to eradicate war, hunger, poverty, and many other plights on human existence. As women and physicians we now have both the capacity and the opportunity to greatly diminish such suffering.

female physicians, coupled with the growth of group medical practices, it has become much easier to combine professional life and family life. While quality care and compassion are critical components of a first-rate physician, we should not focus ourselves so single-mindedly on our own profession that we neglect our families. I, myself, am the mother of two sons, an ophthalmologist and a Crown Counsel, and a grandmother of three grandchildren.

1956

DR. FRANCES FORREST-RICHARDS

Frances Forrest was born in Saskatchewan in 1924. Her family moved to Calgary, Alberta in 1929 where she had all her schooling until graduation in 1941. She enrolled at the University of Alberta, Edmonton, in the combined BSc, MD program in 1945, taking the first year at Mt. Royal College in Calgary. She earned a B.Sc. degree in 1949 and MD in 1951. Her internship was at the Minneapolis General Hospital. She resigned from a Fellowship in anaethesiology at the Mayo Clinic after two months. Unable to decide on an alternative specialty, she worked as a general practitioner at the Rochester State Hospital for two years.

Frances, as a second-year student, had married a third-year student, A. Gerald Richards, in 1949. They had their first child in 1954. That year they moved to Cambridge, England where Jerry continued his training as an internist and Frances worked at a USAF base hospital at Wimpole Park, again as a general practitioner. On their return to Canada, Frances worked at Riverview Hospital, Essondale. She returned to work there again after the birth of their second child in 1956. She resigned in 1957 when pregnant with their third child due to a shortage of housekeepers who seemed not to be willing to take on the care of three children. Frances registered in post-graduate courses at the University of British Columbia in 1961 and was accepted into their

residency program in psychiatry in 1962. She wrote her certification exam in 1964. This was upgraded to a Fellowship in 1972.

Her professional career as a psychiatrist included part-time work, again at Riverview Hospital, consulting appointments at Burnaby Mental Health Centre and Student Health Service at UBC and finally as Assistant Head, Department of Psychiatry at Shaughnessy Veterans Hospital.

A move to Victoria due to her husband's work meant a new start in 1973. After helping to organize the opening of the Day Hospital Program at the Royal Jubilee Hospital, she opened an office for the private practice of psychiatry and, for some years, found herself the only woman psychiatrist in Victoria. There were also brief consulting appointments at CFB at Esquimalt and the Memorial Hospital for Veterans.

Professional associations included memberships in the CMA, CPA, APA, and the Victoria Medical Society; past-president of the Federation of Medical Women of Canada (National and B.C. Branch), past-president of the North Pacific Society of Neurology and Psychiatry, past-president of the Western Canada District Branch of the APA, past-vice-chair of the Section of Psychiatry, British Columbia Medical Association, and its Social Issues Chair and Alternate Delegate, BCMA Volunteer work included membership in several community organizations and government boards.

Travel has been a favourite pastime for Frances since her first trip to China in 1977 which inspired her to study Chinese and Japanese at the University of Victoria. A trip to Russia in 1989, to Yugoslavia in 1990, and to Cuba in 1997 stand out. Of no less interest were courses in French at Laval University in Quebec, Tours in France, and Lausanne in Switzerland; and trips to London for opera and theatre. Recent trips have been reduced in distance, to Vancouver for opera and theatre, but have inspired an interest in music as both a volunteer and donor.

None of her children chose medicine as a career. All are married, and to date there are five grandchildren.

DR. JOYCE MAVIS TEASDALE

Curriculum Vitae

Born: May 6, 1925, Liverpool, England.

Citizenship: Canadian, immigrated to Canada in 1951.

Education: Leeds University Medical School, 1943–49; MB, ChB, Leeds, 1949; Diploma Child Health, Royal College of Physicians & Surgeons of London, 1951; LMCC, 1953; CRCP(C) Paediatrics, 1955; FRCP(C) Paediatrics, 1970; Leeds General Infirmary Professional Units Medicine & Pediatrics, 1949–50, MB; Queen Elizabeth Hospital for Sick Children, London, England, 1950–51, Diploma of Children's Health; Assistant Resident, Pediatrics and Pathology, Vancouver General Hospital, 1951–52; Resident, Medicine, Leeds Regional Thoracic Centre, Leeds, England, 1953–54; University of Leeds Medical Scholarship, 1943–48.

Qualifications: MD 1949, DCH 1951, FRCP (C) Pediatrics 1970; Emeritus Associate Professor of Pediatrics, University of British Columbia, 1990; President, St. James Social Service Society, 1992–97; Honorary Staff, Children Hospital; Board of Directors, Cooper Place Long Term Care Facility; Board of Directors, B.C. Bereavement Foundation; Board of Directors, English-Speaking Union in Canada.

Academic Activities: Head, Division of Pediatric Hematology and Oncology, University of British Columbia, and Children's Hospital, 1977–90; Investigator, National Cancer Institute of Canada; Principal Investigator, Children's Cancer Study Group (U.S.A.), 1972–87.

Professional Activities: Professional Care Committee, B.C. Division, CMA; Past President, Vancouver Pediatric Society; Past President, B.C. Branch, Federation of Medical Women; Consultant in Pediatric Cancer to CCABC in Vancouver and Victoria.

Public Service: Youth Education Committee, Canadian Cancer Society Board, Camp Goodtimes, Canadian Cancer Society, Founding Member & Director of Ronald McDonald House Board, Family AGAPE Centre for Women and Children Trustee, St. James Anglican Church Board, St. James Community Service Society, 1992 (serves Downtown Eastside) President, St. James Community Service Society, 1992–97.

Professional Employment Record: Teaching Fellow, Department of Paediatrics, Faculty of Medicine, UBC, 1955. Demonstrater, Department of Paediatrics, Faculty of Medicine, UBC, 1956–57. Clinical Instructor, Department of Paediatrics, Faculty of Medicine, UBC, 1956–58. Instructor II, Department of Paediatrics, Faculty of Medicine, UBC, 1958–59. Assistant Professor, Department of Paediatrics, Faculty of Medicine, UBC, 1959–1964. Associate Professor, Department of Paediatrics, Faculty of Medicine, UBC, 1964–90. Responsible for organization of Third Year Paediatrics Teaching, UBC,1960–1974. Member of First & Second Year Curriculum Committees, UBC, 1970–1974. Member of Third Year Curriculum Committee, Faculty of Medicine, UBC, 1970–1974. Member of Paediatric Educational Advisory Group, UBC, 1970–1976. Head of Division of Paediatric Oncology, Department of Paediatrics, UBC, 1977–90. Leave of absence: March-June 1974 (paid).

Memberships in: Canadian Paediatric Society; Vancouver Paediatric Society (Past President); Western Society for Paediatric Research; North Pacific Paediatric Society; Canadian Medical Association, B.C. Division; Association of American Medical Colleges Federation of Medical Women: Chairman, Education Committees, Past President. American Society of Clinical Oncology, Canadian Hemophilia Society. Award for Services in the Cause of Hemophilia: April 1980. Principal Investigator Children's Cancer Study Group, U.S.A., 1972 to present. Member Special Studies Committee of that Group. Paediatric representative to the Clinical Trials Committee of the National Cancer Institute of Canada from the Cancer Control Agency of B.C. Study Chairman—Clinical Trials in Relapsed Leukemia of the National Cancer Institute of Canada 1980. Trial activated 1981. Pediatric Consultant to the Cancer Control Agency of B.C., 1981–90. Visiting Pediatrician Royal Marsden Hospital London, England, 1974. Visiting Pediatrician Cancer Clinic Royal Jubilee Hospital, Victoria,

1975. Pharmacy and Therapeutic Committee of the Cancer Control Agency. Medical Director, Haemophiliac Clinic of B.C., 1979–82. Member Medical and Scientific Advisory Committee of the Canadian Hemophilia Society, 1980. Co-Chairman Bone Marrow Transplantation Committee, Vancouver General Hospital, 1980–81. Emergency Services Committee, Vancouver General Hospital, 1970–82. Chairman Advisory Committee of the Emergency Services Committee, Vancouver General Hospital, 1971–82. Blood Transfusion Committee, Vancouver General Hospital, 1979–82. Child Care Committee of the B.C. Division Canadian Medical Association, 1969–73. Member, Youth Education Committee of the Canadian Cancer Society, 1981. Member, Medical Advisory Board, Hemophilia Society of British Columbia. Member, Speaker's Bureau, United Way. Director, Ronald McDonald House, 1981. Trustee, St. James Church, Vancouver, 1984–87. Board, Family AGAPE Centre for Mothers & Children, 1984.

Research and Professionally Related Scholarly and Creative Activities: Clinical studies in the treatment of childhood cancer with the major children's cancer study group of the U.S.A. I was appointed as Principal Investigator of these studies and as a Pediatric Representative to the Clinical Trials Committee of the National Cancer Institute of Canada. I was a member of the Special Studies Committee, Children's Cancer Study Group, 1975–79. Chromosomal anomalies in patients with cancer. Clinical investigation into childhood cancer treatment—Vancouver Foundation, 1973–1978. National Cancer Institute of the United States, Grant Number 5 UIO CA29013-02; Clinical Trials in Children's Cancer Treatment, 1981–83. National Cancer Institute of Canada National Trial Induction & Maintenance of Second Remissions in Childhood Leukemia, 1979–81 (Grant applied for 1982). Supervisor, Canadian Cancer Society Student Project on Long Term Effects of Cancer, May, 1980, Stephen Ng.

Other Relevant Information: Dr. Teasdale has published many articles in journals, including the *B.C. Medical Journal, Canadian Hemophilia Handbook, Canadian Medical Association Journal, Canadian Journal of Genetics*, and *New England Journal of Medicine*.

1957

DR. MARGARET (DOBSON) COX

"You have been accepted as a member of the First Year Class in Medicine which will begin instruction on September 7, 1950."

This message signalled an exciting day in my life; UBC was opening its Faculty of Medicine, sixty students were to be admitted, and I was one of the three women in the class. The others were Marjorie Dupont and Margaret (Peggy) Maier.

After immigrating from Britain in 1947, I registered at UBC for the pre-medical course, completing an undergraduate degree in 1950. A group of practising women doctors in Vancouver regularly invited female medical students to their homes, where they entertained us and answered our questions about possible careers. This friendly mentorship was very valuable.

Although the temporary huts where the medical school was housed were not impressive to look at, the excellent teachers recruited by Dean Myron Weaver made our curriculum vibrant with their enthusiastic leadership. The members of our class got to know each other well during intensive study time together, and we also organized the first Medical Ball at the Hotel Vancouver in 1951. In the microbiology lab we were seated alphabetically so I was next to Pete Devito, whose neighbour was Al Cox. Pete got tired of us talking across him so he let me take his seat!

The summer break from May through August allowed students to earn next year's tuition fee of about $800. In successive years I worked as a nurse's aide at the Provincial Mental Hospital in Coquitlam and a lab technician in hematology at the Royal Jubilee Hospital in Victoria.

Halfway through our second year of studies we were introduced to clinical studies at the Vancouver General Hospital. We wore our first white coats and walked the wards with our new stethoscopes. Divided in groups of five, we were trained by volunteer city physicians and surgeons. We learned to listen, take case histories, and perform physical examinations. Our lectures were in the Willow Chest Centre, which was attached to the other buildings by one of many underground tunnels. I remember our first pediatrics lecturer, Professor Jack McCreary, who bounced into the auditorium with a baby under each arm, and proceeded to mesmerize his audience with the wonders of infancy and early child development.

While I was working in the summer of 1953, I was found to have a minimal pulmonary tuberculosis infection, which meant I would have to rest for several months, postponing my final year and MD graduation. This was a bitter disappointment as I would not graduate with my classmates, and my marriage to Al Cox would be delayed.

In September, I was admitted to the Willow Chest Centre, from whose windows I could see the fourth-year students walking between the hospital buildings. I felt well, but had to submit to complete bed rest for three months. Fortunately, I benefited from three very effective medications—streptomycin, para-amino-salicylic acid (PAS), and isonicotinic acid hydrazide (INH). I buried myself in reading and listening to the radio. My fiancé Al, my parents, and my friends helped a lot, and the experience of being a hospital patient changed my perspective on medical care and communication. The sometimes hurried visits of the attending doctor made me realize the importance of clear and empathetic conversation.

By Christmas I was home on an increasing exercise program. Al and I got married in May, and he graduated with the first UBC MDs. In the fall I resumed my studies and completed my degree in 1955. I had to continue medications for eighteen months, but had no further illness.

During the year I interned at the Vancouver General Hospital where Al was then a resident in internal medicine, I realized the difficulties every married couple had to face when maintaining a balance between professional and home lives. Our days off and nights on call seldom coincided and there were no married quarters, so we shared an apartment with another couple, Wally and Madeleine Chung, who were residents in surgery and obstetrics. As house staff pay was low, Al was in the RCAF Reserve as a part-time medical officer, working one or two evenings a week. This led to a summer relief job on a Canadian airbase in West Germany in 1956, after which we began a year in London, where Al had a British Council scholarship to study, and I got a job with the North London Blood Transfusion Service. London rewarded us with a learning experience and a rich cultural life. Our daughter Sue was born just weeks before we returned to Canada. I found the midwife system very supportive, backed up by house and attending staff as a team. Our voyage home was marked by fog and icebergs in the Atlantic. Our baby also received lots of attention as she was the youngest passenger!

We settled into new work in Vancouver, with Al becoming a resident in pathology, and later promoted to chief resident in internal medicine. I worked part-time with Vancouver Metro Health as a medical officer in schools and well-baby clinics. My mother enjoyed looking after Sue on my work days, and I had the advantage of being a mother most of the time, keeping up medical work with children, and being able to attend rounds at VGH to keep in contact with events there.

Since my husband wanted to specialize in cardiology, in 1959 we moved to Seattle where at the University of Washington he gained experience through research, cardiac catheterization, and the early use of the computer in medicine. We spent three months in Salt Lake City where a pioneer analogue computer was so big that it occupied a whole room and the attention of an engineer. I found part-time employment in the Pediatrics Department of University Hospital doing data research on congenital anomalies and the follow-up of high risk newborns. On our return to Vancouver in 1962, this experience led me to a research project with Dr. Henry Dunn's long-term study of the sequelae of low birth weight, involving nursery and home follow-up of premature babies until they entered school. Several other married medical women shared in this research, working part-time or full-time as our families grew. It was an ideal situation for us; we learned about detailed infant and child neurological and developmental evaluation, and became experienced writing reports and giving papers at scientific meetings. This interdisciplinary

During the year I interned at the Vancouver General Hospital where Al was then a resident in internal medicine, I realized the difficulties every married couple had to face when maintaining a balance between professional and home lives.

research eventually led to the publication of Dr. Dunn's book *Clinics in Developmental Medicine* in 1986.

With three children we settled our home in Vancouver in 1969. Yet during the same year, my husband was appointed the first Professor of Medicine at the new faculty of Memorial University of Newfoundland, St. John's. It was difficult for us to leave Vancouver, but the decision to go was influenced by the attraction of being a part of a new school after our own background of being students in the first class of medicine at UBC. We drove the 5,000-mile Trans-Canada Highway with a tent trailer and moved into our new home. Like UBC, the first class of medical students attended their classes in temporary buildings on campus until the completion of the Health Sciences Centre in 1974. The gradual influx of new faculty members came mostly from Canada, the U.S.A., and Britain.

The survival of very small premature babies still meant a number had cerebral palsy and sensory and developmental difficulties.

I began some voluntary work with a preschool program, where my mentor Dr. Norah Browne and I worked together examining children in an urban renewal area. The program provided enriched learning experiences for both preschoolers and their parents (later, the medical school opened a family practice clinic in the same district). My volunteer work subsequently led me to a locum job directed by Dr. Clare Neville-Smith, in the school health system in St. John's, who helped me in getting established. Dr. Browne then invited me to join her in a clinic she had started at the Janeway Child Health Centre which helped children with communication and development problems. She had also organized a cleft lip and palate clinic team. The clinics were in the outpatient department of the children's hospital, and families came from all over the province by boat, bus, taxi, or plane.

In 1972, both Dr. Browne and I were made Clinical Associates in pediatrics, training medical students, interns and residents, and participating in the lecture program on Growth and Development of the second year at the medical school. We also made videotapes with parents and children who had visual and hearing problems, learning difficulties, and developmental delays. There videotapes were used in telemedicine conferences via satellite, a system initiated by Dr. A.M. House at Memorial University. In Newfoundland and Labrador, doctors were scattered in communities separated by long distances, and public health nurses and outpost nurses were then heavily depended on in delivering care. The telemedicine system enabled links to hospitals which could tune in and participate in rounds and conferences with larger centres. The system became useful also to other community groups, workers, and first-aid personnel on oil rigs offshore.

The provincial education department took an interest in a research program conducted through the university's telemedicine office which facilitated the preschool home training of severely deaf children. Many of these children were deaf because of prenatal rubella or for genetic reasons. Parents were taught auditory training to benefit their children's language learning years before school so that they were better prepared for education at the school for the deaf in St. John's. Each family received videotapes and visits from an itinerant preschool teacher of the deaf. Standardized assessments before and after the program showed significant language improvements, and both teacher and equipment became a regular part of the education department afterwards.

Our clinic staff was involved in early child learning and daycare centres which helped preschool children with developmental difficulties. In 1973, the Early Childhood Development Association presented a brief to the provincial government urging better standards and licensing of child care centres, and a training program for preschool caregivers.

In 1974, Al became Dean of Medicine at Memorial University, which meant more opportunities for me to meet faculty outside the pediatrics discipline. The Janeway Child Health Centre remained some distance away from the university campus and Health Sciences Centre, even though the children's hospital and tertiary care neonatal intensive care nursery later moved to the campus site.

In 1980, the Provincial Perinatal High Risk Program opened under the direction of Dr. Ann Johnson, a neonatologist. We began neurological studies of low birth weight and other high risk newborns in the intensive care nursery and at follow-up clinics. Outcomes were improved over those for babies born in the early 1960s due to advances in technology and care, but the survival of very small premature babies still meant a number had cerebral palsy and sensory and developmental difficulties. As many of their families lived far from St. John's, these babies were transported by air to the site of the tertiary care nursery. Our teams therefore needed to make follow-up visits by travelling to Cornerbrook, St. Anthony, Goose Bay, and other distant sites. Flying into the northern airstrips on small craft was always a novel experience! I benefited from attending professional meetings such as the Canadian Ross Conference on Neonatal High Risk Follow-Up, and our perinatal high risk team presented papers at both Canadian and U.S. conferences.

At the same time, I also served on the Boards of Directors of the Newfoundland Medical Association, the Canadian Pediatric Association, the Daybreak Parent and Child Centre, and the St. David's Group Home.

I began to arrange ambulatory education for students and house-staff in 1985 under the encouragement of Professor Rudi Ozere. Some of them elected extra rotations in developmental clinics or special topics for presentation at research forums. I was an Assistant Professor of Pediatrics at the time, and co-ordinated the Growth and Development course for the undergraduate second year, took part in clinical skills tutorials, and learned to evaluate both written and oral exams. Although I had never expected to become a teacher, I found much reward through the experience.

In 1987, my husband retired as Dean of Medicine and we took a sabbatical leave. We spent most of our year in Boston, where Al enrolled at the Harvard School of Public Health and I worked as a Research Fellow in Developmental Pediatrics at the Children's Hospital. We travelled around Massachusetts and other New England states. I learned much from the interdisciplinary teams directed by Dr. Allen Crocker and participating in their clinics. From June to July of 1988, we travelled to New Zealand and Australia, visiting medical schools at Hobart in Tasmania, Adelaide, and Melbourne, where I had the privilege of presenting a paper of Newfoundland Perinatal High Risk data at the Royal Children's Hospital.

In 1988, we returned to Newfoundland, where Al became Vice-President of Memorial University. On our retirement in 1991, we moved to B.C.

to live in Cobble Hill on Vancouver Island. It was not easy leaving our two sons, grandson, and friends whom we had known for twenty-two years. After we moved to a log house on three acres just north of Victoria (where Al grew up), we maintained some medical linkage: Al as Co-Chair of the National Co-ordinating Committee on Postgraduate Medical Training and I as Co-Chair of a Ross Conference on the Health of Disadvantaged Children. We volunteered at therapeutic horticultural and riding programs, took courses in gardening and writing, and I got involved with a Child and Parent Daycare Program. Al began growing vegetables in an extensive organic garden, particularly garlic. For several years we sold about twenty varieties of vegetables at the Farmers' Market in Duncan—such an enjoyable experience! Encouraged by my writing group, I write poetry mostly about the cycle of rural life, and have taken up piano lessons again. Al and I are both active members of Sylvan United Church in Mill Bay.

We continue to enjoy our retirement. Reflecting on the past, I realize how our careers have intertwined from the time Al and I met in medical school through our travels, studies, and work in Europe, the U.S.A. and Canada. My own medical career was influenced not only by pediatric interests but also by my family. Thus I could not write a reminiscence about myself without mentioning us as a medical couple. Memorial University of Newfoundland and Labrador kindly summed this up by giving us, on our departure, a plaque inscribed: "In recognition of their . . . contributions to the Faculty of Medicine . . . for more than two decades, the Albert and Margaret Cox Annual Lectureship in Medical Education is established . . . 1991."

Public health nurses and outpost nurses were then heavily depended on in delivering care. The telemedicine system enabled links to hospitals which could tune in and participate in rounds and conferences with larger centres. The system became useful also to other community groups, workers, and first-aid personnel on oil rigs offshore.

I AM NEWBORN

I am newborn—
Gaze at me
And I will follow you
With my eyes.

I am newborn—
Hold me,
And I will feel
Your strength

I am newborn—
Warm me
And I will
Be comforted.

I am newborn—
Feed me,
And I will move
With grace.

I am newborn—
Play me music,
And I will
Listen.

I am newborn—
Sing to me,
And I will coo
To your voice.

I am newborn—
Heed my cry
And I will trust you
With my mind.

I am newborn—
Comfort me
And I will
Quiet.

I am newborn—
Stroke my hand
And I will
Grasp your finger.

I am newborn—
Talk to me
And I will learn
From you.

I am newborn—
Love me,
And I will love you
With my heart.

I am newborn—
Pray with me
And I will find
My Soul.
—*Peg Cox, 2000*

(Published in Pediatrics and Child Health *in January 2002.)*

DR. AILSA THURGAR
(1911–2000)

Ailsa Thurgar was born in England in 1911. She trained as a physiotherapist and practised this profession for twenty years until she decided in her late thirties to change course and pursue a career in medicine. She graduated as a physician in London in 1955 at the age of forty-four. Ailsa boasted that she was so destitute as a student that she was forced to give up smoking, but unfortunately slipped back into the addiction shortly after receiving her first paycheque.

Dr. Thurgar immigrated to Canada and started her 'third' career with a residency in pediatrics for one year at Vancouver General Hospital in 1959. This was followed by a move to Rumble Street in South Burnaby, where she practised until 1978, caring for a small, devoted, and mainly elderly population. She lived happily in a basement suite and was genuinely disinterested in financial remuneration. Her patients were her friends, and she spent many of her leisure hours visiting elderly patients for tea or coffee and a chat. She suffered a stroke in 1985 that prevented her from driving, but not from continuing to ride a bicycle. Dr. Thurgar died in the year 2000.

Ailsa was something of a remnant from a bygone age, but her passing is another sad milestone in the transition from family physician to walk-in clinic and "client" anonymity.

Her obituary was written for the In Memorium column of the *BCMJ* by Dr. M. J. Goldberg of the editorial staff.

1958

DR. EILEEN NASON CAMBON

I was born a Maritimer and I am an eighth-generation North American of my father's ancestor who landed on the New England coast in 1639 from England. My great-great-great-grandfather was a seafaring man and found his dream spot along the Saint John River in what is now New Brunswick. He and his family settled there before the Loyalists arrived. My mother's ancestors arrived in N.B. from the British Isles in the early 1800s. I was born in Saint John in 1926 and spent most of my childhood in a beautiful little town, Saint George, on the Magaguadavic River, with Lake Utopia a couple of miles in one direction and the Bay of Fundy in the other.

There were four of us, two boys and two girls, in our family. My older brother and I were one year apart and in our first small hometown, Fredericton Junction, I was allowed to enter Grade 1 with him as I had no other playmate nearby. School was easy for me and despite being the youngest child, I led all grades except Grade 4 when my brother led for me! That year at the age of eight after having whooping cough I was ill with lobar pneumonia with a lung abscess, long before penicillin was available. Both parents believed strongly in education for girls as well as boys, and had several generations of teachers in their families. My mother was one until her marriage. In those days married women were not allowed to continue teaching.

While attending high school during World War II our little town of Saint George lost many young men in Europe. There was an army base at Utopia and a Commonwealth Air Training School at Pennfield Airport close by. My father, a World War I veteran, kept reassuring my mother that the war would be over before my brother reached enlistment age. How wrong he was.

I was only sixteen when I finished high school, and it was decided I should attend Grade 12 in Saint John High School, which then was equivalent to first-year university. My family had moved twenty-five miles from Saint John and I commuted by train. I was again the class leader and was offered three scholarships from three universities. I chose the University of New Brunswick as it was closer to home. My brother was now overseas with the army and I felt I could offer some emotional support for my parents during weekends at home.

I was admitted to the second year at the University of New Brunswick and in 1946 I graduated with a Bachelor of Science degree in preparation for my long-time plan to study medicine at McGill University. Young male students were leaving to join up and some were returning injured from the war to become students again. By my fourth year there was a huge influx of returning veterans which began the rapid increase in student population at UNB compared to the UNB of 500 students when I began. I had a variety of summer jobs, one as assistant agent for the CPR; I was 'promoted' to night operator the next summer, clearing many of the troop trains heading for Halifax. I also worked as a librarian's helper at UNB. I enjoyed university life.

Dr. William Argue, a graduate of McGill, was my biology professor. Near the end of my graduating year he had a long talk with me as he knew of my plan to become a medical doctor and knew my scholastic record was very good. He wanted me to realize that my application to McGill might not be successful and he advised me to consider alternative training. He informed me that Canadian medical schools limited the number of women students, that returning war veterans had priority for medical training, and there was a limited quota of students accepted from the Maritimes. I could not believe what he was telling me. He insisted I have a second choice, just in case. He advised me to apply for a scholarship to do a Master of Science degree in Biology, and his preference was the program at Vassar College in Poughkeepsie, New York. How right Dr. Argue was! Having never been treated differently because I was a female student, I was heartbroken when I was not accepted at McGill, and especially so when some non-vet men were accepted. I did receive the Vassar Scholarship, but it did not console me. However, I got my act together and went off to Vassar, worked very hard, and at the end of the year (June, 1947) received an MSc degree. The year proved to be a good one. Everyone was kind and helpful, and I made life-long friends. I spent weekends in New York City with classmates, and had trips to the mountains in my Ecology course. And I was finally accepted into McGill Medical School for the fall class of 1947.

My class at McGill had 111 students, including sixty-nine veterans both Canadian and American, and eight women. Of the women three were nurses (one a married woman of forty who had worked with Dr. Wilder Penfield at Montreal Neurological Institute and another who had been

Having never been treated differently because I was a female student, I was heartbroken when I was not accepted at McGill, and especially so when some non-vet men were accepted.

overseas in the Forces), two American women, the remaining three from Quebec, Ontario, and myself from New Brunswick. One nurse, after a few months, found the work overwhelming and left.

Medical school was hard work and very interesting. As with most medical students there was a great feeling of accomplishment when we finally dealt with patients, and knew in our hearts that we had chosen the right profession. We had excellent teachers at McGill and in the hospitals. We women cringed at some of the jokes, but on the whole the male students were gentlemen. A veteran student from New York claimed a woman studying medicine had penis envy! We women did not approve of his theory, but he was later to become a good friend. We all were terrified we would fail first year and this fear united many of us from the beginning.

I met my husband-to-be in medical school, Kenneth Cambon from Quebec City, a veteran who had been in the army for six years. His regiment had been sent to Hong Kong; he survived the battle and was taken prisoner of war by the Japanese, and was in prison camps in Hong Kong and Japan for forty-four months. He was the youngest in his regiment, having lied about his age in order to join the army after finishing high school. On the way back to Canada he was informed that the Canadian Government via the DVA was offering veterans who wished to go to university an allowance to cover tuition and room and board. I have heard him say that it was the smartest thing the Government could do for them. After two years pre-med the veterans were allowed to enter medical school. We were married at the end of our second year of medicine and his allowance increased from $60 per month to $90! We managed with the help of our families and with both of us working during the summers at hospitals and labs. We had lots of company, as many students were living on the DVA allowance, and some had children. And we all knew things would eventually get better. We both graduated in 1951, the first couple to marry as medical students and graduate together in medicine at McGill. I must admit that during my third and fourth year oral exams I did not wear my wedding ring (I had kept my maiden name) as there were a few professors on the Medical Faculty who were still against women in medicine. McGill had always discouraged all medical students from marrying, but with the already-married veterans in the post-war classes the rules had to change.

When it came to discussing salaries, my husband was offered $200 a month more than I who was expected to do the same amount of work! We told the officials we couldn't accept such discrimination.

After graduation we were faced with the problem of procuring internships at the same hospital. We had decided to have a change of scenery and planned to go west, so we applied to the Vancouver General Hospital and to the Royal Jubilee Hospital (Victoria). There was no space at the VGH as the medical students from British Columbia at McGill were given priority. The Jubilee accepted my husband, but would not accept another woman because the female intern had gotten pregnant the previous year and left. We were very disappointed. Dr. Harold Griffith, of the curare fame in anesthesia, was in charge of hiring interns at the Queen Elizabeth Hospital in Montreal. He heard of our predicament and invited both of us to join his intern staff. It was a great year, especially for those intending to go into general practice. The interns did a lot of surgery, obstetrics, and general medicine with supervision. We were paid the magnificent sum of $50 each per month and were given room and board.

We had planned to do general practice in a small town in Quebec. My husband met an Alcan Company executive while he was on medicine rotation caring for the executive's wife. Alcan was looking for two doctors to go to their subsidiary, the Demerara Bauxite Company, in Mackenzie, British Guiana (now Guyana) in July 1952. We were intrigued despite objections from our fellow interns who said we would return jobless after the two-year contract and would be two years behind the times. We were interviewed at the Alcan headquarters in Montreal. When it came to discussing salaries, my husband was offered $200 a month more than I who was expected to do the same amount of work! We told the officials we couldn't accept such discrimination. They must have been desperate for doctors at their mine in the jungle as they finally gave in to us.

On our trip down to the West Indies we had to stop in Trinidad and planned a couple of days there. The first morning at breakfast we were horrified to read the headlines in the local newspaper that the Pan American plane we had travelled on the day before, while continuing on to Venezuela, lost two passengers after the rear door blew open and they were sucked out over the Venezuelan jungle. I was not a relaxed passenger when we had to continue on to British Guiana via the British West Indies Airline. We were met in Georgetown, B.G. by the Company launch for the trip up the Demerara River to the town of Mackenzie. This was my first exposure to the jungle, and to the heat from being so close to the equator.

In Mackenzie the Company hospital had 100 beds. The chief medical officer was Dr. Charles Roza, a Guianese, and an excellent doctor trained in Edinburgh. The first week of clinical work was exhausting, as the whole population of the town seemed to arrive with any pretense of illness to try out the new doctors. We were not used to working a few degrees from the equator and it took time to acclimatize. The matron at the hospital was a Canadian nurse, a widow, who managed to keep the hospital in top-notch shape. There were an equal number of black and East Indian nurses, all trained in the capital city, Georgetown. There was an X-ray machine, a good technician who was also the pharmacist, and a laboratory. The emergency nurses could assess and treat a variety of injuries and illnesses. One was superior, a big, very black male nurse who could calm an excited or drunk patient, and with his assistance I sutured many a lacerated scalp in the middle of the night.

Everyone was welcoming. I was never fearful in Mackenzie, and the people there were respectful and helpful. The staff had their own club with a swimming pool. We were living in the area when the company allowed the black and East Indian staff to become members of the club and have homes in the former white staff village of Watooka. We had two weeks of holiday every year. Our first year of holiday was spent in Trinidad and Tobago where we learned to snorkel. The second year we went via the freight plane to the Rupinuni district of B.G. near the border of Brazil where we travelled in the back of a truck to the ranches and rode horseback for fun. Returning by air from Lethem, Rupinuni, we had to sit on wrapped sides of beef from recently slaughtered cattle going to the market in Georgetown. We each had trips to the famous Kaiteur Falls where we checked on the Geological Survey workers and their families. We had great fishing weekends (when both of us were not on-call) on the Essiquibo River, reached via a railway scooter. I caught the biggest lukanani (a perch-like fish) one year, and it was common to see piranha (perai) sometimes biting through the hook.

To be a doctor in such a country was very satisfying. We looked after the company employees and their families, as well as the people along the Demerara River, many of them Amerindians. We were amazed at how literate the people of B.G. were and realized that wherever the British colonized there was education of the inhabitants. The variety of illnesses was fascinating. Of course, there were the usual run of colds and coughs, worm infestations, anemia, filariasis, amoebiasis, and typhoid as in many tropical areas. Malaria had been fairly well controlled with DDT spraying. We treated the botched abortions from across the river, the ectopic pregnancies, and the high incidence of gonorrhea, hydrocoels, and hernias. I was called the local Rabbi, as once the East Indian mothers heard there was a woman doctor who could do circumcisions, they defied their priest who used a split bamboo stick for the procedure, and brought their baby boys to the hospital. As the word spread, when I entered the staff club, some of the smart-aleck staff men would clutch their crotches! I was in charge of the Maternity Clinic in the town, as well as the Baby Clinic. The babies were beautiful from the day of birth, smaller than those I had delivered as an intern in Canada, and of course without the pallor of our white newborns.

The two years passed quickly. We had decided we would like to do more training in one phase of medicine for a year and then return to general practice with more expertise in that one area. I was accepted to attend the course in Ophthalmology at the Institute of Ophthalmology in London and my husband was accepted to do a year in Ear, Nose, and Throat at Grey's Inn Road and Golden Square Hospitals in London. Alcan Company asked us to extend our stay until replacements arrived in mid-August, and in return gave us an open-air ticket to Canada when our courses were finished. We agreed. We had mixed feelings leaving British Guiana. We had become

I was called the local Rabbi, as once the East Indian mothers heard there was a woman doctor who could do circumcisions, they defied their priest who used a split bamboo stick for the procedure, and brought their baby boys to the hospital.

very fond of our patients who were so appreciative of our work with them. As the boat, the *R.H. Carr*, was preparing to take us to Georgetown, the dock was filled with the people of Mackenzie who came to say goodbye and wish us well.

After our European tour we reached London to start our respective courses. I found the eye clinics at Moorfields Hospital exciting. My group consisted of post-grad students from Hong Kong, Australia, Egypt, Pakistan, India, U.S.A., and England. I saw as much pathology during the ten months in London as I did in my first ten years of practice in Canada. Clinicians in the hospital and the professors at the Institute of Ophthalmology were inspiring. We began to consider seriously the idea of becoming specialists, and certainly with my choice of Ophthalmology I could control my work hours when and if we finally had children. We sent off applications to university hospitals in the U.S.A., mainly in the southern states as we wanted to experience that part of the world and travel to Mexico on holidays. Again my husband was accepted by most, and I was informed there were no facilities for women surgical residents! At last we got word that the University of Texas: Medical Branch in Galveston would accept both of us into second year of specialty training. Apparently, the operating room nurses in Texas did not mind sharing their changing rooms with women surgical residents, and to my great delight, the Chief of Ophthalmology was a woman!

Living in Texas was quite a change for us from poor post-war England. As residents we were paid $200 a month each and were supplied with an air-conditioned apartment for $200 a month. We had been living on savings from our work in British Guiana, so now we were 'financially stable.' The so-called staff clinics were charity-based and very busy. The chief resident was a navy veteran and the junior resident a man from Columbia. The next year I was made chief resident which did not make the work load easier, but we and the new junior resident worked well together. Under supervision of skilled surgeons on staff, the chief resident did most of the eye surgery of the clinic patients who came from Texas. At that time patients were kept in hospital ten days after intraocular surgery. In my final year I did part-time teaching in the clinics, and research sponsored by a McLaughlin Fellowship grant. We had two weeks of holiday a year and had trips to Mexico, the first one by train from Nuevo Laredo to Mexico City, and then on to Cuernavaca, Taxco, and Acapulco. We continue with our love for Mexico.

After eight years of marriage and childless, with lots of advice for me to take a year off to relax, I became pregnant during the most exhausting year of my life. I was chief resident, and the second-year man had contracted infectious mononucleosis and was ill for three months. The junior man and I covered the clinics and on-call during that period, and I was doing most of the surgery. Fortunately, I was well and able to work. We had a beautiful baby girl on the last day of February 1957. I was given six weeks maternity leave. Obtaining a nanny was not a problem in Galveston, with so many warm, loving Afro-American women available. After our very busy year as chief residents in our respective specialties, we were given a month vacation and we drove to eastern Canada to show off our child to our families in Quebec and New Brunswick. My final year of part-time teaching and research on whether viruses exist in the conjunctiva of normal eyes was much less hectic. We loved the Texans, the friendliest people in the world. Galveston's beaches were inviting and the little city was entertaining. Our fellow residents became good friends, and later a few came to Vancouver to visit us. The staff had hoped we would remain in Texas, but we always intended to return to Canada to finally live in the west (after our first attempt in 1951).

We packed our Ford station wagon and headed for British Columbia in July, 1958, with our little Texan, a good traveller. I was booked to have the oral exam of the American Board of Ophthalmology in San Francisco on our trip north. Having passed the written exam in January, and with medical friends in that area to help baby-sit, I survived the oral sessions and passed successfully. We had chosen Vancouver as our home base and knew if we did not succeed there we could always go back to Texas. My husband had been in communication with Dr. Gordon Francis, the Head of the Department of Ear, Nose, and Throat at Vancouver General Hospital, and was given a warm welcome in that department. He was able to cover a practice for another ENT man who was ill. We set up a temporary office on Broadway, waiting for a new office building to be completed at Broadway and Pine. We found a house to rent, bought second-hand furniture, hired a lovable Scottish nanny, and enjoyed the hottest summer Vancouver had experienced in years.

I had applied for staff privileges and clinical work at Shaughnessy Hospital and began to work in the Department of Eye, Ear, Nose, and Throat in September, 1958. It was then a DVA Veterans Hospital, and the Chief, Dr.

Eddie Alexander, and the ward nurses gave me a warm welcome. When I worked at Shaughnessy I was in charge of one or two clinics a week for twenty-eight years, and performed eye surgery on WWI veterans from my clinics. I continued at Shaughnessy after it became a community hospital, and I could admit my private patients for surgery. In addition I had visiting staff privileges at Vancouver General Hospital and Children's Hospital. I was the first woman ophthalmologist to start private practice in British Columbia. It was slow going. I covered for established eye specialists, Drs. Jim Minnes and Bill Wilson, on some weekends and they would send me their 'overflow' patients. Gradually, and mainly by patients' word of mouth, I became busy. I received the Specialty Certification in Ophthalmology from the Royal College of Physicians and Surgeons of Canada in 1959.

Having worked for Alcan Company as general practitioners, we were invited by Alcan and the Medical staff at Kitimat, B.C., to do the consultations in our specialties. We travelled at least twice a year to do clinics there for fifteen years. Terrace doctors requested the same service for their patients rather than having them travel to Kitimat to be examined, since we had to land at the Terrace Airport on the way to Kitimat. The doctors in Smithers decided they needed us too! Ken and I initially travelled together up north by plane, but after a tragic air accident when four children were left orphans, we changed to flying separately. We worked long hours in those northern towns for nine to ten days, covering the three areas. The patients and doctors appreciated our efforts. I was able to do surgery for strabismus there, but of course those with any intraocular problems requiring surgery had to travel south. I joined the Children's Hospital Travel Clinic in the 1960s which organized clinics twice a year in Dawson Creek, Chetwynd, Fort St. John, Fort Nelson, and Cassiar. The Travel Clinic consisted of Orthopedic, ENT, Pediatric, and Ophthalmology specialists and two nurses. In later years we had clinics only in Fort Nelson, as more private specialists covered the other areas. I thoroughly enjoyed the northern clinic trips, the friendly people, the work, and hoped that I had accomplished something worthwhile over the years.

We had another beautiful daughter in February, 1962, welcomed by her big sister and a six-year-old foster child, an aboriginal boy. This little fellow had been in the Health Centre for Children at VGH waiting to be discharged after a bout of ear problems. He was under my husband's care. Ken became fed up with the bureaucracy of the various Children's Societies and offered to bring him to our home. And he did! The child's parents both had tuberculosis, were in hospital, and no one came for him. We were told that within two months he would be placed in a home with his siblings. The two months stretched to eighteen months from June 1961 until Christmas 1962. He was lots of fun and a real challenge—just what I needed! Fortunately, I had excellent help at home at that time.

I became active in the Federation of Medical Women of Canada and was the President of the B.C. Branch in 1964. I was the National President of FMWC from 1973 to 1974, which was the fiftieth anniversary of the Federation. From 1977 to 1987, I was the National Corresponding Secretary for the FMWC with the Medical Women's International Association. I attended MWIA Congresses from 1974 every two to three years as a delegate for FMWC, travelling to many countries. I was one of several FMWC members who were awarded the Queen's Jubilee Medal in 1977. I thoroughly enjoyed the MWIA Congresses and was constantly amazed at what women doctors have accomplished in so many countries.

I was the first woman ophthalmologist to start private practice in British Columbia. It was slow going. I covered for established eye specialists on some weekends and they would send me their 'overflow' patients.

A great sense of humour in my partner was a real bonus for me. My husband knew when we met that I had every intention of practising medicine, and that I hoped for more out of life than many of the women of my generation were destined to have. My husband was a great help with our children, and very supportive of my work and ambitions.

In the late 1980s I reduced my hours at work and gradually restricted my practice to my former patients in the 1990s. I retired in late 1995, at nearly seventy years of age. In 1986, I was honoured by my first university, the University of New Brunswick, with an Honorary Doctor of Science degree, to celebrate the 100th anniversary of the first woman student admitted to UNB. In 1991, I was made a Senior Member of the Federation of Medical

Women of Canada. In 1999, I was given the honour of Senior Member of the Canadian Medical Association; in 2000 the College of Physicians and Surgeons of British Columbia granted me Honorary Membership; and in 2001 the Medical Alumni Division of the University of British Columbia presented to me an Honorary Alumnus Award.

We have two grandchildren, a girl born in 1984 and a boy in 1988—the delights of our old age. I love to travel and have persuaded my reluctant-tourist husband to accompany me for most trips. We have travelled to China and Japan several times, as our younger daughter studied and worked in China and is Mandarin-speaking. In 1995, the whole family travelled to Tokyo for Ken to launch the Japanese edition of his book *Guest of Hirohito*. Our older daughter teaches high school English on the Sunshine Coast and is the mother of our grandchildren. Our daughters have different personalities; both are bright, interesting, musical, beautiful, and fun.

We have practised medicine in the best of times, during the years when physicians were respected for their accomplishments, and were able to be in control of their own profession. General practice is the backbone of medical care and I would push for every graduate to do at least a year or two in this field. I have often said that medicine is by far the most interesting and best of careers, at least for me. I liked the discipline of practising medicine, the variety of patients of all ages, the challenges and the camaraderie with colleagues in hospitals and meetings. My final advice for future women medical doctors is that you must make decisions early to organize your life and career to avoid becoming stressed out trying to raise a family as well as being a busy practitioner. It is also important to have a partner who respects a woman's ambition and career, who gives her the support she needs with the ever-present ups and downs of family life.

DR. DOROTHY M. (SIMPSON) GORESKY

The first day of spring—that bodes well for beginning this autobiography of my medical career and also the fact that I received my medical degree exactly fifty years ago. Life is full of beginnings, endings, and new beginnings.

My beginnings were on a farm near Battleford, Saskatchewan. Though I received no indication from my immediate family that women were less favoured than men, my experience in the wider world was just that. First of all, the only careers for women outside of marriage seemed to be teaching, nursing, or secretarial work, none of which held any great appeal for me. Second, when I applied for a Queen's University scholarship and tied with a boy, it was awarded to him. And third, when I applied for nurses' training at the Regina General, the specialist there insisted that prior to admission I must have sinus surgery, which I declined.

Throughout my life, however, seeming misfortune has often proven to be fortuitous. While waiting to apply to a nursing school elsewhere I started work at the Saskatchewan Mental Hospital. One Thursday I received a call from the new principal at the high school from which I had just graduated. It was to invite me to accept the Governor General's medal I had been awarded. In that brief interview he opened to me the possibility of medicine as a career, and after his consultation with the university on Friday, I resigned from the mental hospital on Saturday, washed and packed everything on Sunday, and enrolled in the University of Saskatchewan's two-year Pre-Medical course on Monday.

The School of Medicine had facilities for just the first two years of medical training and accepted only twenty-four students from Pre-Med, with the requirement that they sought admission for their last two years at other medical schools across Canada. The war had just ended so there were many veterans returning to civilian life and vying with the rest of us for the twenty-four coveted positions. Seven of these veterans and three women, including myself, were eventually admitted to medicine.

Probably our hardest work took place in the anatomy lab under the slanted glass roof of the Field Husbandry building, but here we also had our most frolicsome times. Veterans lacked the competitiveness of their younger classmates and delighted in setting them up for amusing situations. Two of the top students were fittingly chagrined when they discovered two vets seemingly puzzled by a problem and they offered their superior knowledge to help identify muscles of the lower leg. It was at a point in the dissection where the knee was disarticulated. It took a long time before the pranksters revealed they had turned the lower limb front to back, creating a most confusing relationship.

Clinical sessions made medicine come alive. On one memorable occasion we were asked what examinations were required in addition to those already noted by the clinician. It was agreed that a rectal exam should be done. There was a lengthy pause before one brave fellow stepped up.

The student approached the stretcher first from one side, then from the other. He cautiously lifted a corner of the sheet with one hand and introduced his other underneath. After a short time in which he was obviously uncertain how to proceed, he lifted the sheet high, put his head underneath, and pulled the sheet back over his head. Just what went on under there we would never know, but the class had to be complimented on waiting to break into laughter only after the patient had been wheeled away.

My final years of medicine were in Edmonton where I met and married Walter Goresky. It was poetic justice that the hospital we interned in had refused me for nurses' training. Accommodation for women interns was in the nurses' quarters which had a curfew, consequently we married women chose to double up in single beds with our husbands when on duty and rented places off site which bit into the great sum of our $75 a month salary.

The majority of doctors at the time I graduated, even though they might plan to specialize later, often went from their one-year internship into a general practice in a small town. This was true for Walter and me who by then had our first child. The house we bought was both home and office with the front hall serving as a waiting room and a ground-floor bedroom becoming the office. Number two and number three children were added to our brood before we left Neudorf. My practice was mostly limited to giving all the anaesthetics and caring for the office for three afternoons when Walter serviced two other villages. Two dollars was charged for brief office visits and five when a full examination was indicated. Urinalyses and CBCs were routine office procedures.

Like many small towns in Saskatchewan at that time, Neudorf had a twelve-bed hospital. These hospitals had accommodation for nursing staff, a kitchen to provide full meals, and a small operating room.

My anaesthetic training during internship was limited to intravenous Pentothal which we rarely used, or a hand-held mask for administering open-drop ether. The only piece of anaesthetic equipment was a suction machine.

Late one evening we admitted a man with acute appendicitis. All was readied by the nursing staff for the surgery, but when I checked our equipment I discovered the machine was not working. Walter decided to call on the local blacksmith, Chris Hauser, who was also his close buddy. Chris was no ordinary blacksmith. If he was presented with a task for which no ready-made tools existed, his innovative mind and skilful hands produced whatever was needed. Although Chris acknowledged on his arrival that he had never seen a suction machine before, much to our relief he soon had it working.

"Would you like to stay and watch the operation?" Walter asked.

"Jesus, Doc. You mean it?"

In a few minutes Chris was outfitted with gown and mask. We had some concern that there might be a risk of an unwanted patient in the OR. However, he eagerly listened as Walter explained everything. As the operation proceeded, Chris leaned closer and closer to the table and eventually uttered one of his classic observations: "Jesus Christ, Doc. That looks pretty simple. I think I could do that!"

The druggist and his wife became our great friends and confidants. Among the locals about whom he gave information was a Mr. S. whose house was described as a small shack with a dirt floor and apple boxes for furniture. His first two wives had died and his twenty-odd children were cared for by a third wife. "If ever he needs your care, Walter, he will pay you promptly."

Accommodation for women interns was in the nurses' quarters which had a curfew, consequently we married women chose to double up in single beds with our husbands when on duty and rented places off site which bit into the great sum of our $75 a month salary.

It was winter. Walter had gone to the hospital. I was doing dishes at the kitchen sink when suddenly I was aware of a presence behind me. I turned to find the doorway filled with an enormous figure dressed in a great buffalo hide coat. There was no need to ask the identity of the man whose gruff voice announced, "I'm here to pay for the babe." It was likely that Walter was still delivering the placenta!

We had read about psuedocyesis, but rather doubted its existence. Such doubt was removed by the entry into our care of a tall, heavily-built woman in her late thirties. History revealed she had three children and menstruated regularly, though recently with very scant flow, and she claimed a doctor in a neighbouring town agreed with her own diagnosis of a four- or five-month pregnancy. Being unable to confirm this by physical examination, I ordered a rabbit test, which came back negative. She made monthly visits with an ever-increasing abdomen, but never a hint of foetal presence. Eventually she arrived at the hospital 'in labour' and only when X-rays were taken and she did not deliver a child was she convinced she had never been pregnant.

We had been taught in medical school that fifty to seventy percent of people seeking medical help would have no demonstrable organic illness, yet never were we given any suggestions for treatment other than reassurance that they would get better.

In 1955 we moved to Kansas where Walter studied psychiatry. One had to be an American citizen in order to practise in that state, so I was totally away from medicine for most of three years except for having my fourth child and a brief practice in a public clinic when they were unable to attract an American doctor. Legal conditions were met by all prescriptions being countersigned by a licensed doctor.

On return to Canada Walter had still to fulfil a fourth year at the great monthly sum of $350, so I worked mornings for the Burnaby Metropolitan Health Clinic. Once Walter was established in a practice I chose to stay at home with the children until the youngest started school. Despite the fact that I felt a degree of incompetence by my years away from medicine, I would never have traded the joy of personally experiencing my children's first crawling, first standing, first steps, and so many 'first discoveries' they made. Nevertheless, it was gratifying for me to make my re-entry via the Student Health Service (SHS) at UBC in 1965 as the first woman physician there, with the convenient hours initially of 10 a.m. to 3 p.m.

In time I wanted to know more about what was at the root of those seeking medical care who had no demonstrable organic illness. We had been taught in medical school that fifty to seventy percent of people seeking medical help would fall into that category, yet never were we given any suggestions for treatment other than reassurance that they would get better. My first step was to write Dr. Hans Selye who generously granted me a personal interview about his research on stress. Interesting as was the interview, it did not lead to any approach to treatment.

The entire field of stress management, both within and outside of traditional medicine, has since burgeoned, but at that time I found no ready sources of help or training. Left on my own I ventured into courses on hypnosis, autogenics, therapeutic touch, yoga, meditation, visualization, relaxation techniques, and techniques now termed 'cognitive therapy.' Eventually in 1980 I made contact with Joe Neidhardt, a general practitioner interested in using similar techniques and hoping to answer a major problem for GPs both then and now—that the time consumed for stress management receives inadequate remuneration. I entered a research study under Joe with about forty other physicians, nurses, and social workers using a series of booklets he had produced.

Because of this particular interest, nurses directed students to me and in addition to individual care. On Friday afternoons I held two-hour sessions for groups of five to ten students for a series of six classes. Briefer courses were given to students in several faculties and also to several community organizations. I felt rewarded, but also somewhat jealous that books like Herbert Benson's were being published with great acclaim, discussing procedures I regularly used.

Many ordinary, informative, sad, and fun things happened during my twenty-three years at the SHS with a particularly dedicated, well-trained staff of doctors, nurses, and secretaries. Contraceptive care and counselling regarding pregnancies, particularly for the unmarried, became an accepted part of our practice. A comment made by one of the nurses soon dubbed a regular clinic for pelvic examinations and Pap smears as, "The Primrose Hour"! Native women and single mothers with children who had extra burdens to carry were always extremely appreciative of our care. And it was significant to me that many of the gay students sought women doctors rather than men. The service was moved from Wesbrook in 1980 to become the first active section in the new University Hospital Acute Care Unit. Initially receiving little recognition from the wider medical community, the SHS has now become known for the excellent service provided to students.

As I was anxious to pursue other interests, in 1988 I retired from practice a couple of years before age sixty-five. Life has had its share of personal ups and downs, including divorce in 1975, but I would not choose to have missed out on any of the cards dealt to me.

My major current interest is alerting people to the devastation being caused by transnational corporations through the Multilateral Agreement on Investment and now through the World Trade Organization and the International Monetary Fund. The problems afflicting our planet are enormous, and public action worldwide is gradually emerging. We live in challenging times.

My Role in the Antinuclear Movement
The six–year-old stood fascinated as light streaked across the desert sky. "What's that?" he queried.

"It's a missile," answered his father.

His parents' conversation about missiles and the weapons they could bear whirled around the boy as the Nevada night-time sky continued to be lit by the man-made objects. Then quietly and thoughtfully his words intervened: "I'm glad that Grandma's doing something about it."

When invited to contribute to these memoirs, I was encouraged to include some of the talks I had given on nuclear war. I have chosen, rather, to relate what inspired me to become involved. I believe it was Schweitzer who said, "When the knowledge in the head gets together with the feelings in the heart, then true wisdom is born."

My feelings in the heart are deeply rooted in my childhood experiences of life on the farm. There I was surrounded by the sights and sounds, the sunlight and shadow, and the scents of the Saskatchewan prairies. I was under the spell of changing seasons, each bearing its own special gifts and its own particular problems. I was keenly aware of changes in weather, each adding to or detracting from anticipated harvests. Thus prairie-born and prairie-bred, I grew up with a deep recognition of our dependence on Mother Earth, with a deep sense of the interconnectedness of all life. It is this, and the wish that my grandchildren might inherit a kinder world, which has spurred me to action when knowledge on particular issues has come my way.

So what knowledge led to my participation against nuclear weapons? While attending medical school I saw a film on the devastation of Hiroshima and at that time incorrectly assumed that nuclear bombs would be banned so there could never be a recurrence of such unspeakable horror. The fallacy of that assumption was revealed to me in 1981 when a group of young physicians returned to Vancouver from a conference in San Francisco on "The Medical Consequences of Nuclear Weapons and Nuclear War." It was like a physical blow when I saw that all there was left of the city was its burned-out, rubble-strewn streets with shadows on the walls. But while I was experiencing an overwhelming sense of sadness, I recognized that such sadness was not for people, for my children, nor for me, but for Earth—the Earth which had nourished me as a child. I knew then, however small a contribution I could make, that I must be dedicated to its preservation. That night I joined with two Vancouver physicians to form a steering committee, and later became founding president of what was to be one of the major chapters of Canadian Physicians for Social Responsibility. This organization subsequently became known as Canadian Physicians for the Prevention of Nuclear War (CPPNW) and still more recently as Physicians for Global Survival (PGS).

Raising awareness on prevention of nuclear war involves knowledge of different facets of nuclear weapons. The one presented most frequently and having the greatest impact on audiences is "The Medical Consequences of Nuclear Weapons and Nuclear War." Other topics for the numerous presentations I made to conferences, service organizations, churches, colleges, medical associations, and many community groups included the nature of nuclear weapons and their delivery systems, Canada's part in their production and testing, and how even a fraction of world military expenditures could provide clean water for everyone in the world and could control major diseases.

But the topic I was most drawn to was the psychological damage to Hiroshima survivors and the psychology of war-making. In addition to providing information on how the worldwide military machine has produced weapons of mass destruction, it seemed to me to be of equal importance to explore with others the reasons why such obscenity occurs, and to discover ways in which a paradigm shift might occur away from war-making nations toward peace-making nations.

In 1989 I spearheaded the Vancouver Lanterns for Peace ceremony on Hiroshima Day, organizing doctors and veterans to make presentations to over 4,000 school children and instructing them how to produce shades for the lanterns. The beauty and meaning of those ceremonies remain one of my most poignant memories.

My involvement with the prevention of nuclear war led to membership on the National Board of Directors (of CPPNLW) from 1982 to 1988 and the National Presidency from 1985 to 1987. In addition I was one of the Canadian delegates to the International Physicians for the Prevention of Nuclear War (IPPNW) for its 1983 congress in the Netherlands and 1987 congress in Moscow. I was with our Canadian delegation when the IPPNW was awarded the Nobel Peace Prize in Oslo in 1985. In 1992 I gave the first lecture and was honoured to receive the Tom Perry Peace award, which was set up by CPPNW in memory of Dr. Perry's invaluable dedication to peace. For two years I sat on the Special Committee for Peace for Vancouver City Council, and editions of the *BCMJ* and *Canadian Doctor* carried articles on my participation.

Because of my conviction of the rightness of Schweitzer's statement about the head and the heart, I felt no reluctance to always include references to the heart whenever I spoke. In order to make people understand why I was so driven to preserve the Earth and fight for peace, I often liked to mention an experience in 1982 at the Fraser River—a place where I received spiritual nourishment:

"The sky was suffused with one of those beautiful sunsets bequeathed us by the eruption of the Mexican volcano earlier in the year and the poplars were still clothed in their clear, bright, crisp yellows of fall. There had been strong winds the previous week and I had to scramble over and crawl under the trees blown across the path. As I emerged from under one of the trunks, I found myself totally bathed in brilliant, golden light. The sky, the leaves, and I had become one. It is this unity of all that exists on our planet which brings true meaning to my life."

DR. MARGARET (PEGGY) MANSON (MOUAT) JOHNSTON

Born: August 14, 1928, (sixth child of six), Ganges, Saltspring Island, British Columbia.

Ambition: Wanted to become a doctor since at least the age of twelve; not sure why except one male relative told me that medicine was not a profession suitable to a woman.

Primary and Secondary Education to Grade 12: Saltspring Island.

Undergraduate: Victoria College, and University of British Columbia, BA, 1948.

Medical: McGill University, MD, CM, 1952.

Rotating Internship: Queen Elizabeth Hospital, Montreal, Quebec.

Medical Residency: One-year residency at Vancouver General Hospital.

Dermatology Residency: Three-year residency at Henry Ford Hospital, Detroit, Michigan.

Specialist Qualification: Royal College of Physicians and Surgeons of Canada, 1959 Certification, and Federation of the Royal College of Physicians (FRCP).

Medical Practice: Dermatology, Nanaimo, British Columbia, for five months. Vancouver, B.C., from the fall of 1959 to 1989.

Hospital Appointments: Active Staff, Vancouver General Hospital; Active Staff and Head, Division of Dermatology, B.C. Children's Hospital; Courtesy Staff, St. Vincent's Hospital.

University Appointments: UBC Faculty of Medicine (1960–1989); UBC Department of Medicine, Division of Dermatology from 1960 as Clinical Instructor to Clinical Professor; UBC Department of Pediatrics, Associate Professor.

Medical Associations: Canadian Medical Association; B.C. Medical Association; Canadian Dermatological Association; Federation of Medical Women of Canada, and B.C. Branch President for one year; American Academy of Dermatology; Society of Pediatric Dermatology.

Since retirement I have held only the usual retired or life memberships in the Canadian Medical Association, B.C. Medical Association, Canadian Dermatological Association, and the American Academy of Dermatology.

Husband, Children, Post-graduate Medical Training, and the Practice of Medicine
I first met my husband Albert Johnston when I was so young that I don't remember, but he did and reminded me when we met again at McGill, working together as externs at the Provincial Mental Hospital during the summer of 1951. We married in 1952 when I was interning and Al was a fourth-year medical student. After Al's internship and my residency year at the Vancouver General Hospital, we went to Detroit, Michigan—Al to attend Wayne University (Ophthalmology) and I to spend an enjoyable year with our first child, Kathleen. We went on to three years of our respective Residencies. Late in my second year of Residency, our son Jim was born. We were blessed in having a wonderful, loving Afro-American nanny.

We returned to British Columbia where Al accepted an Ophthalmology locum for a year in Nanaimo, B.C. I made up the Residency time I had missed during pregnancy, and in a few months joined Al in Nanaimo. I became the first practising Dermatologist in Nanaimo, and stayed five months before returning to Vancouver, our offices now ready. I took a couple of months off work to have our second son, Bill (now a practising Ophthalmologist in Nanaimo). Five years after our move to Vancouver, our fourth child, Tom, was born. Al and I were involved in a busy, happy social mix, and my husband contributed enormously (without changing more than two diapers in a lifetime) to the home, our country retreat, and family upbringing with all those soccer, hockey, and rugby games.

We practised for over thirty years in our respective specialties and loved Vancouver, a great place to practise medicine and raise a family. All the other Dermatologists were male; I was the first woman Dermatologist in Vancouver. Roberta Ongley became the first female Resident in the Vancouver Dermatological Residency program, and she was a great one.

I loved my practice and the association with the Vancouver Dermatologists who were friendly and co-operative, and practised a high calibre of clinical Dermatology. Apart from losing one patient who bolted from my office without even seeing me, mumbling, "I didn't know it was a woman," being a female never presented a problem. In medical school our male classmates were often somewhat protective of the six girls in my class.

Until more recent years, much of the teaching of the Residents, medical students, and family physicians was done by part-time clinical teachers. Teaching Dermatology was entirely dependent on part-time initially, and continued to be so to a large extent during my years in practice. My special interest gravitated towards Pediatric Dermatology.

When the new B.C. Children's Hospital was opened in the late 1970s, we acquired a full-time Resident there. Before long I was spending more and more time at the Children's Hospital and found myself dividing my time equally between the hospital and my office. Dermatology had no formal space at the hospital, but my Pediatric friends, especially Dr. David Smith of the OPD and Emergency, pitched in and lent me space and support to develop general Pediatric Dermatology clinics. Various other members of the UBC Dermatology staff lent their time and expertise to the sub-specialty clinics. Dr. Bill Stewart, then Professor of Dermatology at UBC, helped to establish a formal Division of Dermatology at the hospital (within Pediatrics) during that time.

The B.C. Children's Hospital was and is a wonderful place to work, and I felt very privileged to be there and to have the opportunity to associate and share care with so many great Pediatricians and Sub-specialists. I was happy to retire knowing that Dr. Julie Prendiville would soon arrive to be the first full-time Pediatric Dermatologist at the B.C. Children's Hospital and UBC.

After years of two busy practices, teaching, and raising four lively children, Al and I now enjoy a much quieter life. We live in Richmond, B.C. during the winter months, but otherwise spend most of the time at our long-time family retreat and home on Salt Spring Island. We are proud of our wonderful children and their spouses, and three grandsons whom we enjoy so very much.

My only question is: "Where did all the energy come from?" I would do it all again if I had the chance.

DR. JUDY HORNUNG (MRS. FRANK KALLA)

I was born in Czechoslovakia in 1934. In 1939, my family left on the last outbound train to escape the Nazi invasion. We landed in England where my younger sister and I were to grow up.

My father, who had medical degrees from Prague and Vienna, had to study in Cardiff for two years to qualify for British licensure. Once qualified, he worked as a locum in a small town in Lancashire. In the meantime, I attended a series of boarding schools in London, Cornwall, Yorkshire, and Cheltenham—all over England. After the war, our family settled in North London, where my father bought a family practice.

Throughout my childhood I always thought, "When I grow up I am going to be a doctor." Dad relished his profession, and he was much loved and admired by his friends (who frequently consulted him with their medical problems) and his patients. He was a wonderful role model for his two daughters and other family members. My cousin, a very prominent physician in the U.S., claims that my father inspired her choice of career.

English schools promote sports for all students. Although I was not particularly athletic, I did learn to love many sports, and to this day I continue to play and enjoy tennis, skiing, and swimming. When my children were growing up, I made sure they learned to play hockey and tennis, swim, ski, and skate. I introduced them to sailing, though it never appealed to them. But I have wonderful memories of weekends spent at the United Hospital sailing club during my years at medical school. London was such a great city to live in as tickets for wonderful concerts and operas were all sold at inexpensive prices or even free (unsold tickets were frequently donated to the medical schools on the day of the performance). In retrospect, I am extraordinarily grateful to both my parents and the schools I attended which introduced me to art, music, and sports.

In 1958, I graduated from St. Mary's Hospital Medical School in London, England. I was one of fifteen women in a class of sixty. It was unusual at that time that twenty-five percent of our class was female. A few years prior to our admission, the University of London had dictated that each medical school was obliged to take a minimum number of women. St. Mary's had not met this requirement because they viewed every female admission as a loss of a potential super rugby player. The university policy finally caught up with them in 1952, and as a result, our class had an exceptionally large number of women.

Since my only travel experience at that point had been summer holidays to other countries in Europe, after graduation I decided to pursue an internship as far away as possible. New Zealand was my first choice, but they were not interested in taking more doctors. Canada seemed a good place to go, and I found British Columbia to be especially appealing. After my internship arrangement at VGH, a classmate and I travelled by ship to Montreal and by train to Vancouver. VGH had four female interns that year. We lived in a residence separate from the men (who were in the building which later became the residence for nurses). As all interns did (and still do), we worked hard. But my memories of that year are happy ones. I feel we were treated fairly; I was unaware of any gender discrimination. Any negative experiences were shared equally. For example, when assisting hip pinnings, the junior intern stayed in the OR holding the leg of the patient, but all others left the room as X-rays were taken. (Orthopedics was not a popular rotation.) Other memories include: learning about the strange game of football while sitting in the OR lounge, and adjusting to the informality of addressing staff men by their first names—a practice unheard of in England.

During my first year of practice, I served as a paid assistant to a very busy GP in New Westminster. It was wonderful training for me, since he was a knowledgeable and experienced doctor who covered all aspects of family practice. The only difficulty we had was when he tried to impart his surgical skills to me. I was not a good pupil, and finally he realized he would never turn me into a surgeon. The medical staff at the Royal Columbian Hospital were very friendly and helpful, so it was never a problem to find support and advice for difficult cases, and during my internship year most patients seemed to have difficult problems. There were not many women on staff, but I only remember feeling well-accepted by male colleagues. Although we worked long hours, we managed to find time for social life. Or at least, enough time for me to meet and marry my husband, Frank.

Frank had come from Hungary and his qualifications were not as easily accepted as mine had been. Therefore, he had to do several years of residency and write all the exams, including the basic sciences. Once Frank had received his licence, we decided to enter practice together in Vancouver.

We found a location to our liking, hired a nurse, and hung out our "shingles." Building up a practice from scratch wasn't easy, so we both took other jobs: working in the health department, the venereal disease clinic, and student health services at the University of British Columbia. Our practices gradually grew and became increasingly rewarding. The first patient to come through our door was still with us when we retired in 1997. One of the local GPs was particularly kind and helpful, often sending people our way and dropping in on us from time to time with advice not found in any textbook. For instance, he taught us that if we only had two patients, we had to make sure that they were booked close together so they would see each other. At first my practice consisted almost entirely of women and children, whereas Frank would see both men and women. Gradually, men did start to come to see me, not only for sore throats, but also to let me treat their more major medical conditions. But it did take some years before a significant number of male patients had chosen me as their family doctor.

During our first year of practice, I especially enjoyed the freedom to be fully in charge of patient care, doing obstetrics and newborn care, admitting and treating many patients in hospital, and being involved in surgery as an assistant. In fact, my husband was able to do many of the surgeries, as he had trained and been certified as a surgeon in Hungary. At that time, general practitioners who were considered competent were given surgical privileges to perform various operations, including appendectomies, hernia repairs, varicose veins stripping, and even cholecystectomies. We were on staff at St. Paul's Hospital, the only hospital we attended, except on the rare occasion when a woman chose to have her baby at the Grace or a sick child was admitted to Children's. Since most inpatients were in one location, there was less time spent on the road and more time on the ward. The mornings were always spent in hospital or doing home visits. Office hours were in the afternoon. This allowed us more time with colleagues in coffee rooms or corridors. Prior to retirement, I spent much more time in my office and would only make hospital rounds in the early mornings or in the evenings after work. Rarely did I have time to talk to colleagues who were equally rushed if we happened to bump into one another.

When our own children started to arrive, I dramatically decreased my working time to about four hours per week, as I had difficulty finding good child care and we did not want live-in help. When my oldest son was two years old and the second boy six months, we were so grateful to find the most wonderful woman to care for them while I went to work. She was a friend of my mother-in-law; it was love at first sight for her and the children.

After we hired a nanny, I readily increased my working hours to three or four hours per day, but not every day. Luckily, Frank could cover for me at other times. I did not return to full-time work until our youngest (third) son was in first grade. Our nanny stayed with us until they were all school-aged. To this day we still see each other. In her nineties, she is still a very loving, bright lady who is always a pleasure to visit. My grandchildren love to spend time with her as much as their fathers did.

Building up a practice from scratch wasn't easy, so we both took other jobs: working in the health department, the venereal disease clinic, and student health services at the University of British Columbia.

Once the boys were in school I started to work regularly, but still not full-time, as I liked to be home after school and needed to do the chauffeur duties. I could not take after-hours call, since I needed to be available for after school activities and to look after the boys, so my long-suffering husband covered calls for both of us. It never occurred to either of us to switch roles. Today, I realise many couples would have had a different strategy. For me there seemed to be no choice. I loved my "job."

I have never been a huge professional hockey fan, but I did enjoy the kids' minor hockey games. And it was wonderful, on a sunny spring day after school, to ski Grouse Mountain. It was very important for me to be involved in the children's lives in those elementary school years, so even after returning to the practice almost full-time, I would still book out if there was an important event. However, I was sorry not to be able to regularly volunteer for field trips, etc. At that time, there were few "working" mothers, so parent-teacher conferences were always scheduled during the day. It was difficult for my husband and I to attend, but I usually managed, and then reported the good or bad news to their father.

By the early seventies we had moved into a new office, which we shared with another GP, Shirley Rushton. This turned out to be a wonderful partnership. We were able to cover for each other's holiday relief and to consult one another on difficult situations while sharing the amusing ones, like the time a patient asked if I had received her autopsy result. We were also lucky to have pleasant, friendly, and helpful staff. It was a pleasure to work in that atmosphere.

When my sister, who worked as a public health physician, left Vancouver for Toronto, I decided that I would apply for part-time work with the same department, rather than put in extra hours in the practice. For ten years I did two half-days a week with the health unit. I never regretted that decision. The work was so different and it was a new experience being a "team player." Working in the schools with children, teachers, social workers, and various professionals was a great learning experience for me and it increased my respect for these people. I took great reward in the students, offering health education in the classrooms and assessing physical and psychological problems. At that time I became interested in scoliosis. With great help and encouragement from Fred Bass, the MHO of our unit, and pediatric orthopedic surgeon Steve Treadwell, I started a scoliosis screening pilot study for Grades six and seven children in my schools. This was exciting because we were able to identify some children with scoliosis early and refer them to their family doctors for further treatment. Public health was a terrific experience. I learned a great deal and met some wonderful colleagues in many professions, some of whom remain good friends.

In the mid-seventies, my partner Shirley Rushton decided we should write the College of Family Practice certification exam. At that time there were still relatively few certificants. And it meant dedicating several hours of study time to refresh and learn. I know I am eternally grateful to the audio digest tapes, which provided an ideal learning tool for a very busy mother with a full-time practice. I played them in the car, while making the dinner, and at any other suitable moment. In fact, I thoroughly enjoyed the experience of being a student again. After passing the exam, I returned to Calgary for several years as an examiner. This decision proved to be very interesting and rewarding. I also became a member of the College Board and was honoured to represent B.C. on a committee which met regularly in Toronto. I was impressed by my colleagues on that committee, and I enjoyed the discussions and work involved. The College of Family Practice was still young at the time; it was exciting to play even a small role in its evolution.

In the eighties, when St. Paul's hospital grew into a much larger institution, we decided to move our hospital privileges to St. Vincent's. It was much smaller, and we appreciated the chance to be involved in a way that we had not at St. Paul's: active on committees, attending teaching rounds, and so on. There was also a strong sense of camaraderie amongst the medical and other staff. Many years later, two of our sons have also become active at the same hospital. Another activity I found very satisfying was my involvement in the department of family practice. Teaching first-year students is a wonderful way to reconnect with my own memories of those early years.

I retired from my practice in 1997 when I was fortunate enough to find a very good physician, Vivian Paul, to take over. I still miss my former patients who in many ways felt more like friends. I know that might not be politically correct, but after knowing someone for so many years, he or she truly feels like a friend. I still meet many of my former patients in the neighbourhood, and I am always eager to hear their news.

Nowadays I do occasional locums and spend time with my wonderful grandchildren, but that's another story.

DR. DORIS KAVANAGH-GRAY

On balance, I think that a lifelong inability to spell has been a blessing. It's true that it is a bit provoking when colleagues snicker while reading one's on-call progress notes, so I have usually carried one of those small computer dictionary things when accuracy is preferable, but in general I've considered this defect a minor flaw, sharing Mark Twain's "contempt for the man who can only spell a word one way," and I just don't do spelling. This attitude, honed by maturity, was not always so. In childhood and at my father's insistence, I strove to conquer this imperfection. Father was an avid reader and a believer in the principle that anything is achievable if one works hard enough, and he struggled diligently to overcome this handicap in me, the eldest of his two daughters. Night after night, after the dinner dishes were cleared, we would sit side by side at the kitchen table while he instructed, drilled, and oversaw the writing out of long wavy columns of corrected, previously mis-spelled words. During these lengthy, but to me secretly enjoyable sessions (did I appreciate the extra attention?), I absorbed many of my father's values—his respect and love of books and learning, and the virtues he made of industry, perseverance, and organization—attitudes that have proven invaluable in life.

An idea born of my father's attempts to indoctrinate proper spelling habits was to deduct a penny from my weekly twenty-five-cent allowance for each mistake. It took no time at all to appreciate that an honest answer to the question, "How many spelling mistakes did you make today?" would result in a serious negative cash flow. So another skill acquired during these spelling lessons was the ability to stretch the truth—actually, to lie—and I became quite accomplished. The secret, you know, is to first convince yourself that the story is true, then you are most persuasive. This skill has served me well. Through the years I have been able to entertain friends and dinner companions with amusing anecdotes (my performances occasionally marred by a surprised and painfully honest husband who doesn't always recognize the altered facts). In addition I have saved myself much inconvenience: "An inch of lie is worth a yard of explanation."

My mother was, and at eighty-six, is still the ideal mom, providing a secure and loving environment in which my sister Leneen and I throve. We never were aware of the existence of such abominations as child neglect and abuse. No matter how tainted my spelling errors or blemished with white lies, I believed myself to be the centre of my mother's universe, and that is heady stuff with which to feed the growing ego. So, armed with the love of reading and learning, the virtues of industry and perseverance, plus the ability to tell a pretty good tale, and bolstered by a strong ego, I set out to make my mark in the world.

During high school I had spent the summer months working at odd jobs, fruit-picker in Grimsby, filing clerk in Ottawa, etc., and I came to appreciate that being in charge of something was infinitely preferable to being taken charge of, so during my last year at Lisgar High in Ottawa, I filled out and dispatched applications to every Canadian University requesting admission to Law and Medicine. This was 1947. War Veterans were flocking back to universities in large numbers. Vacancies in Law or Medicine were scarce and no one seemed much interested in a seventeen-year-old, non-spelling female blessed with nothing more than a high school certificate. Only the University of Ottawa granted me an interview, and though this interview went quite well I thought—a pleasant chat with Father Danis, the somewhat austere Dean of Admissions (looked a little like my father!)—I heard nothing further.

By late August I was becoming more and more desperate to escape the filing room of the Metropolitan Life Insurance Company. I requested another interview with the Dean. On this occasion I tried very hard to impress the good Father of my great

Vacancies in Law or Medicine were scarce and no one seemed much interested in a seventeen-year-old, non-spelling female blessed with nothing more than a high school certificate.

desire to study medicine, and the more I pleaded, the more passionately did I believe that Medicine was the only life for me. All thoughts of a career in Law vanished or never were, and, "Oh fabulous joy," I GOT IN! What elation. I later learned that Harold Sachs and I were the only two accepted without a prior university degree. Why accept us at all? The reasons were unclear, in the nature of an experiment perhaps, but I got in and it was one of the best things that every happened to me.

The other best thing was John Gray. On registration day as we first-year med students were uncertainly milling about, one student stood out: John Gray, tall, handsome, forceful (did everyone look a little like my father?). Without speaking a word I decided then that I would marry that man. And six years later I did.

Medical school was fascinating. Everything delighted and excited me. I couldn't get enough of facts, concepts, attitudes, postulates, etc. The professors, largely drawn from war-devastated European universities, were admirable men and remarkable teachers. I absorbed everything—the facts, the figures, the attitudes and the skills; methods of teaching from our formidable Polish Professor of Medicine, Dr. A. Fidler; ease in dealing with patients and families from our jovial Irish Professor of Pediatrics, P.J. Maloney; the ability to make precise anatomical drawings from our austere German Professor of Anatomy, Dr. Auer, etc. etc. There were captivating lectures in English Literature by a witty academician, Emmet O' Grady. Our faculty possessed a wild and astonishing array of accents, made all the more incomprehensible by our ignorance of medical jargon. And in addition, after years spent at The Convent of Notre Dame for young ladies, I was in an entirely new world, a world of men. Ishbel Currier and I were the only two women in the otherwise masculine environment. To be precise, there was one woman, a robust, competent, from-the-farm woman, and me, an uncertain, eager-to-please, seventeen-year-old girl. Ishbel, completely confident and comfortably at ease, never tried too hard to fit in. To my great admiration and secret delight, and despite obvious professional displeasure, she habitually knitted during lectures, placidly and persistently, producing a steady stream of large, somewhat drab socks, sweaters, and caps, the recipients of which were a mystery. In my anxiety to be 'one of the boys,' I dared not engage in such feminine pursuits, though in the end, it was I who indulged, and publicly at that, in the ultimate of female activities—pregnancy.

Ishbel and I could not have imagined more splendid men and better comrades. Never did we experience the slightest prejudice (or were we too naive to recognize its presence?). My classmates were intelligent, funny, and supportive. From the first day when we were assigned our specific locations until the day we graduated, we unwaveringly occupied the same alphabetical space at lectures and clinics—Ishbel Currier front row to the left next to Maurice Babineau, and I, Doris Kavanagh, second row to the right between John Gray and Beverly Kelly.

Initially our male colleagues treated Ishbel and me as amusing curiosities—but always with courtesy. Of course, there were the usual pranks, especially in gross anatomy—why was it suddenly my turn to dissect when we reached male genitalia? I had expected facial muscles. Ishbel too was

assigned 'the naughty bits,' when by alphabetical rights she was slated for the brachial plexus. Still, the jests were generally clever and never malicious, and Ishbel and I joined in the laughter as cheerfully and easily as did our so-called tormentors. By second year most of the games were over. The curriculum was extensive, we were studying hard, and life became more serious. We blended into a large, sometimes unruly but mostly affectionate family, with Ishbel and I only two more members of the class of '54.

The sixth year was to consist of an internship at the Ottawa General Hospital under the watchful eyes of our clinicians, which was to culminate in national examinations and (God willing) an MD degree. John Gray and I could see financial light at the end of the education tunnel, and given six years of alphabetical proximity, planned to marry at the end of the fifth year. Our world was informed.

As expected, our fellow students responded enthusiastically with congratulations, cheap bottles of wine, and even a pre-wedding shower of sorts. The faculty, as we were to discover, were also far from disinterested, and I was summoned to the office of the Dean. What would he want with me? I never skipped classes, my marks were good, my histories up to date. Dean Richard was not smiling when he received me into his inner sanctum and commanded me to sit. With few preliminaries, he informed me that news of my forthcoming marriage had reached his ears. It was his duty to admonish me and to catalogue the inherent dangers of this plan. Marriage, I was told, was a contract most solemn and most grave, fraught with risks and hazards not immediately obvious, but which it was his duty to itemize. Was I not planning post-graduate training? Did I not realize that residency positions for women were scarce—and for married women practically nonexistent? Were I to marry, the doors to higher education would close. Assuredly, I must postpone and preferably abandon this idea of marriage. The thought was ill-conceived, ill-advised, injudicious, and intolerable! Of course I agreed—and of course dismissed altogether this advice.

Nor was John spared prenuptial counselling. Father Danis, our designated student preceptor, invited John to his rooms. As advisor and friend, he proposed to discuss practicalities, for example the possibility of issue arising from the consummation of marriage. If such issue were forthcoming, further training would be jeopardized. Offspring would prove expensive and insurmountable hostages to fortune. John later told me that he reassured the good Father that pregnancies were not planned, that we had paid the strictest attention to the all too few lectures on birth control and understood every nuance of the rhythm method, the only contraceptive method taught and available to the practising Catholic. No, there would be no children until our four years of residency training were complete, until we were financially prepared. John also told me that Father Danis did not appear to have the same faith in the rhythm method as our teachers on OB-GYN apparently did, but then, Father Danis was a cleric, albeit a seemingly worldly and sophisticated cleric. His views were not as reliable as those of the medical profession—and we chose to ignore his advice as well.

And so, having satisfactorily disposed of these trifling details, we wed, and moved our books, clothes, wedding gifts, and my parents' spare couch to a two-room attic suite on Nepean Street. We settled down to married life. Most nights either John or I, or both, were on-call. Any sleep to be had, was had at the hospital—on separate beds, in separate rooms and separate buildings—John in the interns' quarters and Ishbel and I across the street in the nurses' residence. But (and it was a delicious "but") every fourth or fifth night we slept in our attic room, on our couch.

Despite all the assurances to the contrary, the rhythm method of birth control proved unequal to the strains of our on-call schedule. Without a doubt, I was pregnant, and my due date determined for mid-April. Internship was to end in mid-May and exams in June. There was no question but that the schedule was a bit tight though not impossible, and my only real concern was to avoid the gloating "I told you so's" likely to be voiced by authority. My classmates were intelligent, funny, and supportive, and they all rallied around, switching schedules and rotations at my request, taking my occasional night call, my assists with long hours at surgery exchanged for morning blood-drawing duties, etc., even providing me with ever larger Lab coats as my "condition" became more and more apparent, from size eight to eighteen. The Dean was unaware of my "condition" until one spring day, I found myself on a collision course unable to avoid him. Dean Richard thundered, "Dr. Kavanagh! What is this? This is a fine state of affairs. Did I not warn you? Did I not advise you? I take no responsibility for this!" The best I could summon was, "No sir, I assure you, you are not responsible."

After a few days of quiet, I received a written invitation to join Mother Superior for tea in her bureau to discuss "les affaires." Mother Superior, Director of the Ottawa General Hospital, was in her way as awesome a figure as the Dean. Tall, austere, elegant, aristocratic, with, it was rumoured, such a tongue as to reduce even the proudest staff man to stammering little boy status when displeased. After tea was served Mother Superior explored with delicacy the practical aspects of my impending delivery: Who was to be the accoucher? Who was to pay for the delivery room, the hospital bed, and the medicines? Then she urged me not to distress myself further and assured me that le bon Dieu would provide.

After a few days I was summoned to the office of Mother Bursar, the one who prowled the corridors patrolling for financial leaks. I was informed that all students are insured on entrance to medical school. "But Mother, that's for an accident. This a preg. . . ." An icy stare from Mother Bursar, who then asked, "This is not an accident? This is a planned event?" I had to concede—she had a point. "So it is settled."

And so it came to pass that while I was on-call on the OB service, on April 19th at 6 p.m. baby Cynthia was born—Dr. De St. Victor was in attendance and John administered the anesthetic (alphabetical rotations persisted and he was on-call). For the remainder of the intern year (May) my classmates took my calls with never a protest of complaint. Two months after Cynthia's birth we wrote the final exams and graduated in June. I was Gold Medalist of the class, notwithstanding the high school diploma, spelling errors, and baby Cynthia.

We moved to Detroit, Michigan for post-graduate training in internal medicine for me and in surgery for John, at the Henry Ford Hospital. Those six years in Detroit were the hardest six years of my life. Two more children were born, our son Jay, and then our second daughter Andrea. We had very little money, and the hospital days were long. Memories of those years in the late '50s are still achingly vivid and are largely memories of fatigue— absolute,

Father Danis did not appear to have the same faith in the rhythm method as our teachers on OB-GYN apparently did, but then, Father Danis was a cleric, albeit a seemingly worldly and sophisticated cleric.

profound fatigue. I recall one summer evening about 10 p.m. driving into our back yard after a post-work-day shopping trip to Sears (shoes for the children) and the Black Bear Supermarket (the week's groceries). John parked the car, the kids were asleep among the piles of groceries in the back seat, and I was *so* tired. The effort needed to get out of the car and the thoughts of the duties which lay ahead—bathing the sleepy children, tucking them into bed, sorting and storing the groceries, and then preparing my presentation for the next day's hospital grand rounds, was overwhelming. I could hardly make myself move. The option of everyone just staying where we were was very seductive. Absolute stillness—such an ultimate luxury! And I often see that same exhausted look on some of our women residents and I worry. We were told that the long hours, the fatigue, etc., were necessary, the 'fire that tempered the steel,' and I suppose there is some truth to that, but surely that same fire can warp and destroy other equally valuable materials.

Memories of those years in the late '50s are still achingly vivid and are largely memories of fatigue—absolute, profound fatigue.

In 1959 John drove back to his hometown of Vancouver in the hope of finding a position on the surgical staff of St. Paul's Hospital (where his father Edward Gray once had been chief of staff). Meanwhile the children and I remained in Detroit where I was a fellow in Pediatric Cardiology. During those months as a 'single mother' (the modern term applied to a somewhat sad lifestyle), I sat for my American and Canadian Specialty exams, and wrote letters to various Vancouver hospitals inquiring into possible positions in Cardiology.

Three months later in October of '59, when I joined John in Vancouver, I was interviewed by a pair of remarkable men at St. Paul's Hospital, Dr. William (Bill) Hurlburt, chief of Medicine, and Dr. John Sturdy, chief of Pathology. These gentlemen, with the blessing of the then-owners of the hospital, the Sisters of Providence, were in the progress of changing the focus of the hospital from surgical to a more balanced medico-surgical facility and were actively searching for young sub-specialists in medicine to establish a variety of divisions. I came at the right time and with the right training and was hired at $300 a month as the first geographically installed

physician with a mandate to set up a Division of Cardiology. In quick succession, more sub-specialists were added to the staff—a hematologist (Bill Ibbott), a gastroenterologist (Stan Stordy), an endocrinologist (Tom Davis), respirologist (Bill Young), and neurologist (Ken Berry). These were all very bright and enthusiastic young men with great plans and ideas, and nurtured by Dr. Hurlburt, the plans came to fruition.

Every work day most of the GIFTS (geographically installed full-time staff), as we called ourselves, would lunch together at Ruebin's on Granville, mostly on liver paté and lemon pie. These lunches were stimulating, eclectic affairs. Ideas would be paraded and challenged, plans hatched, and initiatives launched, all the while interspersed by joking and laughter. It was largely at Ruebin's that the divisions were organized.

I was given a generous free hand at organizing my division. Dr. Dwight Peretz joined me in 1962, and his mandate was to develop and manage an ICU; and shortly thereafter Dr. John Boone came to serve as liaison with the Pulmonary Division and later to attend to the electrophysiological aspects of cardiology.

Gradually a surgical team was gathered and trained, and open heart surgery was launched using Dr. Harold Rice's home-made pump oxygenator. Dr. Robert Gourlay, a most able surgeon (though in the field of cardiac surgery, largely self-taught), performed our first OHS in 1960—the repair of an atrial septal defect in a twelve-year-old charmer from Kelowna named Elizabeth Ann Lavery. Later Dr. Al Gerein was recruited for valvular surgery and Dr. Bob Miyagashima for the congenital heart repairs.

Meanwhile the cardiological practice grew steadily. After setting up the cardiac catheterization and angiographic laboratory with Dr. Rice's mechanical and organizational talents and energies, money donated by the Heart Foundation and the P.G. Woodward Foundation, and space provided by the surgical department, we were off and running. At the time, there was a long waiting list at the Vancouver General Hospital for cardiac catheterization studies on young patients with congenital heart defects. Dr. Morris Young, chief of Pediatric Cardiology at the VGH, suggested that I might perform some of these studies to whittle down the list. I leaped at the opportunity and was soon studying four children a day. With this exposure, the lecture tours around the province, and the encouragement of the Department of Continuing Education of

UBC, I began to receive consultations in my own right. In the early days it was common to have a surprised patient of either sex exclaim on arrival, "But you're a woman!" Later it softened to, "You're a woman, but my doctor says you're very good." Now, of course, this has all changed. No patient surprise! No qualifying comments! More frequently, patients and referring MDs actively seek a woman consultant, but not in those early days.

Still, there was very little hostility or prejudice. The only overt sexism I encountered was from the mouth of babies. St. Paul's Hospital boasted an active pediatric department at the time, and many of the in-patients were native aboriginal children, patients of Dr. Coddington, known affectionately as the "Indian Doctor." One morning I was auscultating the chest of my own little patient, while in the next crib Dr. Coddington's patient, a solemn, six-year-old black-eyed beauty, was scowling and watching intently. As I removed my stethoscope, I smiled at my young audience, and was rewarded with a deeper frown and the disdainful query, "Why for you using Dr. Coddington's 'tethoscope? You just a mudder!"

The early days of cardiac surgery were exciting times. The field was exploding with new information and technologies. Innovative operations were solving age-old mechanical problems, and driven by the surgeons' demands for more accurate diagnoses, sophisticated investigative tools were becoming rapidly available. Novel and potent medications with potent side effects and elegant mechanical devices demanding unfamiliar expertise were presented at each new international cardiac meeting. Cardiac defibrillators, Beta blocking drugs, pacemakers, coronary angiography— it seemed that we were awash in new intelligence, and that the knowledge painstakingly acquired in training was not obsolete. We learned on the job.

We performed much congenital heart surgery in the sixties, and always, one of the medical staff, usually the anesthetist, surgeon, or I would stay twenty-four to forty-eight hours 'worrying,' and adjusting the rate of IV drip here, the concentration of O_2 there, drawing blood gases, monitoring urine flow, etc. We half jokingly believed that the post-operative complication rate was inversely proportional to the level of physician anxiety expended. And we learned a lot at those bedside vigils; we came to understand the causes of cerebral edema, the significance of acidosis, the ominous message in decreasing urine flow, all the while building a powerful rapport with our nursing colleagues and developing a heart-breaking sympathy for the parents of our small charges.

Fuelled by patients' need, the Divisions of Cardiology and Cardiac Surgery flourished. Surgery expanded from two cases a week to five a day, the number of cardiologists grew from one to eleven, sub-specialty areas multiplied, and now the Division is the Centre of Excellence for Cardiology in British Columbia. I am enormously proud of my colleagues and of the Division.

In 1997 I retired from practice, and felt a little anxious with the closing of a door, but I was tired and, I thought, growing cynical. When one night I realized I would rather not get up to attend to yet another patient in cardiogenic shock (what was the use? They all seemed to die anyway), I decided it was time to quit—leaving the field to younger, still enthusiastic and more capable hands. And this I did. Our three children are grown and have left home. The eldest, Cynthia, practises OB-GYN in Ontario and has four perfect (of course) children. Our son, Jay, lives in Whistler and works in the taxi business and has two equally perfect children, and our youngest, Andrea, lives on her own here in Vancouver and works in the mail room at St. Paul's Hospital.

As I removed my stethoscope, I smiled at my young audience, and was rewarded with a deeper frown and the disdainful query, "Why for you using Dr. Coddington's 'tethoscope? You just a mudder!"

John and I live a happy, contented life, travelling a bit, skiing and biking a lot, and have become quite proficient ballroom dancers. I frequently lecture the public, usually on the topic of Women and Heart Disease or Gender Differences in Cardiology, and in this capacity (and often under the auspices of the Heart and Stroke Foundation) travel a lot around B.C. and the Yukon. There I frequently meet former patients and the meetings are always sweet and moving. Recently, in Kamloops, a stunningly beautiful, strawberry blonde young woman sought me out after the presentation. Did I remember her? She was accompanied by an older woman and a small red-headed girl. I remembered the mother from thirty-three years earlier, looking much like her daughter did today, but terribly worried; rushing to hospital in the wake of her newborn 'blue baby' flown down earlier by air ambulance. It was 6 p.m., the tiny infant was scarcely alive, limp, and deeply cyanotic. The babe was quickly studied, a diagnosis of pulmonary valve atresia was entertained, and by seven she was in the OR and anesthetized. I was present when Al Gerein pressed open the minute pulmonary valve with a Brock Dilator. We held our collective breaths as we witnessed a miracle—as this tiny blue bit of life turned pink before our eyes. And this was she. This was baby Megan, all grown up and magnificent, and being a mother as well. This was an emotional reunion. Megan's mother began to cry, Megan to sob, and the bewildered little girl to wail, and tears filled my eyes as well. With the joy of the moment, with the tears, the hugging and squeezing, I remembered the happiness the practice of medicine has given to me. I've loved all of it.

I think I've been a 'good doc.' Patients still call two or three times a week to inquire after me, to get some reassurance, and maybe bring a smoked salmon or a jar of homemade jam. For this joyful life, I am forever grateful: to Father Danis, who opened the doors of medical school; to Bill Hurlburt who provided the environment and freedom to build; to my husband John, always supportive and proud of my accomplishments; to my mother and her unconditional love; and to my father, though he did fail in his attempts to impart spelling competence.

DR. LOIS MACKENZIE-SAWERS

I was born in a log house in the Peace River country in 1924. There was no doctor in Spirit River at the time, so my mother was attended by a friend who had been a nursing sister in WWI, as had my mother. I attended the classic one-room country school with my older brother. When it became time for high school, I was in the same grade as my brother, which was rather handy, since we had to live in town during the week. Spirit River High School also consisted of one room in those days.

My brother enlisted in the Royal Canadian Air Force (RCAF) as soon as he graduated from high school. I was only seventeen at the time, so I spent a year going to Normal School (teacher training) and teaching. The training was about three months and I taught school for six months. In the fall of 1942, I enlisted in the RCAF and spent all my service time in Ontario, working as an equipment assistant. This involved handling all varieties of supplies except food, vehicles, and aircraft.

When the war in the Pacific began winding down, I spent a lot of time thinking about what I was going to do after discharge. Having tried teaching, I did not think it was for me. One day I suddenly had the idea of going to medical school and becoming a psychiatrist. That pinned down my future for the time being. There were a few obstacles to this plan, however, one of which was not having taken courses in high school that would qualify me for a science entrance into university. So I spent a year teaching and upgrading my math. After that, I was allowed to enter pre-med and was one of five girls in our class of fifty at the University of Alberta in Edmonton (the Calgary Medical School was still far in the future).

The Medical School at the U of A was still operating under the wartime accelerated program, which consisted of two years of pre-med and four years of medicine. We received our BSc after the first year of actual medical school. My class was the last one mostly composed of war veterans.

After graduation in 1953, we were firmly told by the Dean that we were to intern in Alberta because there was a great shortage of house staff. I spent two years of rotating internship at the Royal Alexandra Hospital in Edmonton. Once again the question arose, "What shall I do next?" I had lost the desire to do psychiatry quite some time ago. I decided pediatrics would be an interesting speciality, probably because the only people I liked among the attending staff at the Alex were pediatricians.

Because I was late looking for a job in Peds, I ended up going to the Children's Hospital of the East Bay in Oakland, California. The McCarthy era was just ending and the U.S. did not attract me at the time. I had the impression the U.S. was filled with kooks or worse. Fortunately, I found that most of the people I met were just like Canadians, and I had two very good years in Oakland. In 1957, I went up to the Vancouver General for my final year in Pediatrics. I also got married in 1957 and my husband and I both agreed that Vancouver was a great city to settle down in.

In 1958 and 1959 I worked as a Fellow following the development of low birth weight infants. When this became a part-time position, I opened a pediatric practice in 1959, after writing and passing my Certification of Pediatrics.

Later in the year I got pregnant. Diaphragms were very inefficient at that time! The thought of night house calls *and* a baby exhausted me already—before the baby had even arrived. I was not making any money at my office anyway, so I got out of a very loosely written lease and started doing baby clinics and public health in the schools. I continued working part-time in public health with two additional babies (diaphragms did not get any more reliable) for fifteen years. By that time, I was bored out of my gourd and since my kids, theoretically, did not need as much attention, I returned to the Vancouver General for a retraining year in pediatrics from 1974 to 1975.

This was not an easy year. The changes in clinical medicine over the past fourteen years both astonished and horrified me. My near vision was also poor, but I did not realise this until the end of the year, which explained why I had such a terrible time with IVs. My stress level was very high and the minute a group of house staff sat down for instruction or discussion, I would drop off to sleep. This, of course, made a great impression! Things at home were not great either. Our two younger daughters were skipping school in large chunks and had varied other problems. Nevertheless, I survived the year, but I can remember feeling sorry for some of the eager young girls who were actually going to study medicine.

After I recovered a few months later, I became interested in medicine again. It was clear that I would have to do another pediatric year if I wanted to make a living as a pediatrician. After turning down this option, I decided to do some GP locums and see how things would turn out. First, I had to do a two-month obstetrics-gynecology rotation to learn how to do vaginal exams! This little thing was one thing I had never been trained to do during my rotating internship in obstetrics after graduating from medical school. We had done rectal exams and no outpatient work at all.

Happily, I did enjoy doing GP locums and continued my education at the expense of my patients.

In 1978 I bought Alisa Thurgar's practice in Burnaby and practised there as a GP until 1997. I enjoyed my years in Burnaby. The hospital was a pleasant place to work and I made many friends among the staff. And, except for the very occasional time, I enjoyed and liked my patients.

Since 1997, I have continued to do locums for my friends and they have not stopped asking for me yet.

DR. MARGARET TREMBATH

The second daughter of a United Church clergyman and his second (ambitious and over-protective) wife, I graduated from the University of Toronto's school of Medicine in 1947—the last class to be "accelerated" due to World War II. I had lived a somewhat controlled and certainly protected life, thus my university education was a 'liberating' experience. Learning had always been easy for me, and I had never been forced to develop any discipline regarding studies. I cannot lay claim to a very bright academic result—I was too busy as a delayed adolescent—having too much fun. Junior Internship was done in Regina. This decision was in part to maintain independence from 'home,' but largely because a stipend was offered by these hospitals. One of my classmates and I split our year between the two general hospitals, each spending a half-year at Regina General Hospital and the other half at the Grey Nun's Hospital. Each hospital had services not present at the other—Isolation at the General (and in the midst of a polio epidemic, I became really slick at spinal taps!) and Oncology at the Grey Nun's. I remained in Regina for a couple of years doing a practice in Pediatrics under the tutelage of the city's resident specialists, then returned to Toronto to take up an internship in Pathology at The Hospital for Sick Children for the magnificent sum of $100 per annum. I became a Resident in Bacteriology at "Sick Kids" the following year, and then with my husband in his first year internship, found it necessary to 'stay home' to look after our first daughter. Funds were very limited (married DVA allowance was something like $60 per month) and I did a couple of months of locum tenens in general practice, and went back to Regina to do a summer of locums at my old clinic. We moved to British Columbia after my husband's senior internship. After the arrival of our second daughter, we settled in Mission, and my husband started to work with a clinic group in General Practice. I had still some hope of completing my training in either pediatrics or laboratory medicine, but the difficulty of commuting to Vancouver while trying to care for a young family was too intimidating for me. I preferred to care for my children myself—any mistakes made in their upbringing would be my own.

We moved into a new area in Surrey. My husband started his own practice which required my assistance. I changed my 'professional' name to my married name (good advertising he thought) and worked with the Public Health doing health checks at a number of schools. I also did the office 'scut work' of immunizations and well-baby clinic sessions.

None of these duties was very demanding, but I felt that I had been out of the loop so long that I was not up to a true practice. We added a third daughter to our family, and by this time I was truly behind the times as far as medicine was concerned, and would have needed a full refresher course to bring me up to speed. Despite feeling very guilty about not using my education, family considerations took first place, and I did not attempt to return to practice. My husband began to enroll me to do insurance physicals, pilot medical exams, and to do surgical assists in the three 'local' hospitals—Surrey Memorial, Royal Columbian, and St. Mary's. By the time he was ready to take an early retirement, he had developed a heavy program of aviation medicine, working with both large airlines (TCA & CPA as they then were) as well as doing his own practice in this field. All the assisting work was thus left up to me. We assistants worked in all the major surgical specialties, and this gave one a broad experience. Over the years, a cadre of such 'assisting specialists' grew and is, I believe, ongoing. As skills and knowledge increased, we were much appreciated by surgeons. Seeing surgeries from so many different specialties gave us the experience to sometimes recognize 'tiger country' before it was seen as such by the operating surgeon; an assistant is not only an extra pair of hands, but a pair of noticing eyes as well. This particular little 'specialty' was one I quite enjoyed and continued to work in until my own retirement in 1996. It was interesting to be part of the changes in Surgery over a twenty-five-year period—from early arthroscopies to laparoscopic surgeries.

A visiting Med Student was horrified and disgusted by the thought of any graduate in medicine wasting an education to such an extent as to be doing only surgical assists. I had never quite felt that strongly about it, but no doubt he has a point.

DR. BERNICE WYLIE

Somewhere in early childhood, I knew that I was to be a physician, not a surgeon, nor a nurse, but certainly a front-line worker. It was deep inside me, unshakable even by my concerned parents, irrevocable despite other opportunities and passionately desired, but quietly so. This choice was not welcomed by my family and friends. Dissuasion, though tried vigorously, was useless. I knew and that was that. Even now, I cannot unravel how this came to be.

School was fun for me, the work easy, and so I revelled in a large array of extracurricular activities—art and music, competitive swimming, and all the sports available—even baseball, which I truly disliked. Basketball and volleyball were my favourites. Music was pursued at every opportunity—symphonies, choir, and of course, piano—with exams and competitions throughout.

University, once entered, wrapped me into its busy life. Beyond the halls of the medical school, the Women's Undergraduate Association and the Medical Undergraduate Association were the university women's athletics in which I was active.

During any spare periods (and some not so spare), I life-guarded, clerked at a night school, worked in the Post Office, cashiered at Eaton's, and, of course, spent the summers 'up North.' The ideal compromise was always to land the best paying camp job at a top quality summer camp. I did well in that, and I spent two summers in Temagami as girls' waterfront director, then two in Haliburton as junior camp director, and as girls' camp director. What wonderful experiences they all were.

By third-year medicine, I was ruminating more and more. Was I really studying all this material for the right reasons? Doubt had struck deep into my head and heart. What should I do? Maybe this childhood dream was off mark.

The Trudeau Sanatorium at Saranac Lake, New York advertised a six-week externship. I was accepted and my life changed. Nestled in the Adirondacks, Trudeau Sanatorium was a chest disease investigation and treatment hospital. A small cadre of top physicians, radiologists, pathologists, and bacteriologists worked side by side to hone the finest team possible to address the key chest problems of the day. The leading problems were: Tuberculosis (with the new drugs streptomycin and PAS available, along with Phrenic Nerve Crush, Lobectomy and Wedge Resections, Pneumothorax, and Partial Thoracotomy), Histoplasmosis, and the industrial diseases, Silicosis and Berylliosis. To achieve success, the patient had to recover and return to active living in society (i.e., students to school / university, mothers back to family life, careers mended). In addition, they were to do even better than before the illness. To this end, there were special Arts and Crafts programs, music and entertainment, and opportunities to practise careers. Half a century ago, the goals of holistic medicine were being achieved at Trudeau without fanfare, but with genuine hard work and respect.

Back in Toronto for the final year of medicine, clinical work took on a new hue. I could not learn enough fast enough or in depth enough, for I had found out my own secret. Patients were very happy to be seen by me, treated by me, and in fact they did well. What a relief. There was a place in Medicine for me and I was going to find it. The clinic work and the rotations through Obstetrics and Neurology left indelible memories. The last year was a whirl of activities, working part-time, studying when I could (in streetcars mainly), and attending undergraduate meetings (including the University of Toronto Student Council).

The Canadian medical student / hospital program matching system was an enigma to me. Through this system, your future life was cast—you are allocated to go somewhere in this vast nation. I landed in Vancouver.

Coming off the train after four days and five nights of travel, I unloaded my trunk and self at the Women's Residence. Reporting to the Administrator right away, I was, to my great dismay, piloted down the hall to the Emergency Room to start work then and there. The uniform assigned to me did not fit (they expected a man). The telephone numbers were unfamiliar, but the patients had the same types of problems. I survived and quickly gained confidence.

Periodically during internship, one sees daylight outside—depending on the rotation and the kindness of the Senior Resident. Getting out to buy groceries or a dress was wonderful. Since we earned $150 for the full year, we knew how to be frugal, particularly as travel costs were to come out of this. The vast underground passages of VGH became our second home in summer and winter as they connected all the separate hospital building structures north and south of West 12th Ave, Heather to Laurel Streets. Before one could settle in, applications for the next year were due. With little real experience to our credit yet, this was a difficult time.

The magnetism of Vancouver was already at work. I stayed for a senior residency in Medicine, then Pathology, and then entered the Shaughnessy Military Hospital Resident Program for the final years. Here, once again, I found the concern for patients extended far beyond mere medical treatment—with assistance and training to re-enter community living and help for families too. In this superb atmosphere, learning medicine really evolved into learning life and learning where medicine could offer help in this bigger scene. Most staff members offered their assistance to everyone equally and generously. Not only did we learn, we grew up in a caring, sharing environment.

Once exams were over, the true test of capabilities started. Would I practise as a junior in a medical group or would I strike out on my own right away? With very little in the bank, but with youthful enthusiasm, the door of the office at Oakridge was opened, and I waited to see if I could survive the first three months before cash ran out. The vision of weeks on end reading journals and newspapers until patients arrived was quickly dispelled. I was very busy within two weeks and soon looked for quiet time to write up reports. Clearly a female physician practising in internal medicine was needed in Vancouver in the 1960s. Soon community activities, events of the Federation of Medical Women, and children, all became embroidered into the intricate pattern of medical practice, teaching, and more learning. Holidays were spent at the family cottage in Muskoka where my brother's children romped and played with ours.

Throughout the years, I took all my day and night calls with reciprocating holiday relief. Weekend call exchange came much later and was much welcomed. Even so, I was on twelve days and nights of every fortnight. Winter holidays were exceptional and few.

Reporting to the Administrator right away, I was, to my great dismay, piloted down the hall to the Emergency Room to start work then and there. The uniform assigned to me did not fit (they expected a man).

"Get a Gimmick" was a phrase used by many colleagues who advised me to have a "super specialty." I resisted this recommendation for I did love General Internal Medicine. Yet, certain areas emerged as special interest areas, each in their own ways. One evening, I received a call from a senior physician stating that I had been selected to initiate a rehabilitation program at a local convalescent hospital. Not only did I protest my unsuitability, I did not even know where the hospital was located or what it did! My protests were soon put aside for I was to do it, and, of course, I did, because I dared not fail or let him down. It was great work; the staff was keen, the team responded, and rather quickly Holy Family Hospital emerged as a viable rehabilitation unit.

Dr. Brock Fahrni also deployed me into Rehabilitation and Geriatrics at Shaughnessy Hospital. Working directly under him, I gained excellent experience. Even more important was the insight I gained into a very broad concept of medicine. I learned the value of applying techniques of rehabilitation broadly in medical practice. Approached again to do specific rehabilitation of stroke and multiple sclerosis patients, I joined the G.F. Strong Rehabilitation Centre.

Likewise, for Diabetes, it was the direct approach of Dr. Fred Bryans and Dr. Molly Towell, two senior physicians in the UBC Department of Obstetrics, who urged me to work with their diabetic pregnant patients. This triggered the development of the Diabetes and Pregnancy Clinic in the 1970s—first at VGH, then at the new Grace / B.C. Women's Hospital. Through my practice years, many of my community activities were related to these special interest areas.

Now that I am detaching myself from the daily rumble of medical activities, I appreciate the opportunities to sleep through the night without a call, read without interruption, or start a task with a hope of finishing it. In fact, it is very refreshing to enjoy ordinary things—a film, dinner out, a trip to the island without arranging call, or not being attached to the pager. Medical practice has been the most enjoyable and rewarding career choice and a privilege of the first kind. Certainly, I shall miss the great friendships and collegial times. At present, I am enjoying watching the world more carefully, thinking about many human issues, learning more, and re-establishing old friendships.

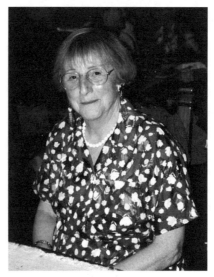

Dr. Mary Hallowell, 1950

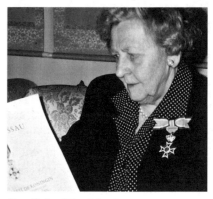

Dr. Julia Van Norden, 1953

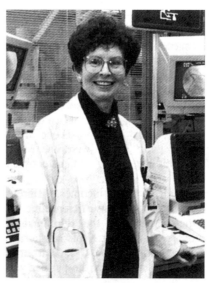

Dr. Doris Kavanagh-Gray, 1954

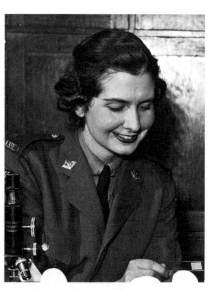

Dr. Evelyn Fox, 1945

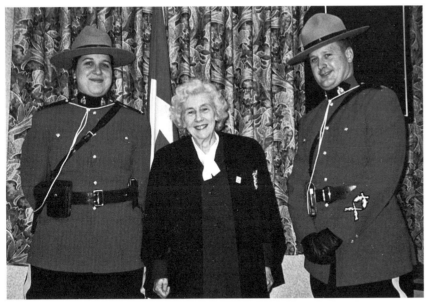

Dr. Joan Ford (1954) as a judge

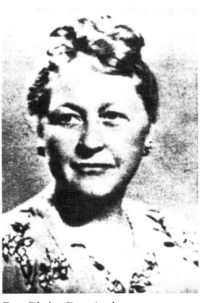

Dr. Gladys Cunningham, 1954

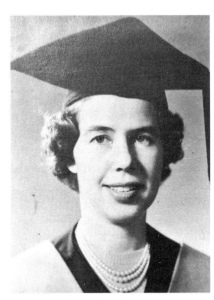

Dr. Marjorie Ellen Jansch, 1954

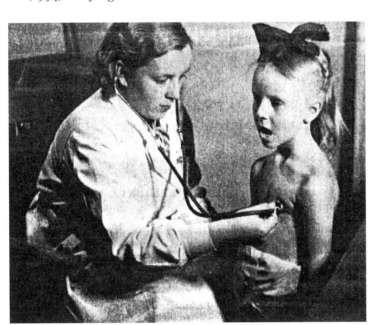

Dr. Laine Loo, 1954

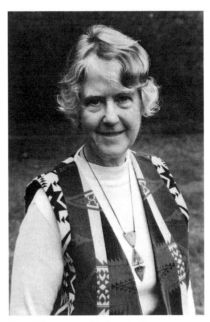

Dr. Margaret (Dobson) Cox, 1955

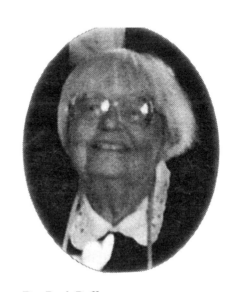

Dr. Ruth Roffmann, 1954

Notes from VMA JOURNAL 1950–1959

January, 1950 This *Bulletin* consists of many articles.

February, 1950 Population of Vancouver 385,000: Chinese 6,877, Hindu 133. Infant Mortality was 19.5.

April, 1950 Epidemics of rubella, measles, and mumps occurred. Dr. Elizabeth Nora MacKay, Saanich Health Officer has been transferred to Creston, B.C.

May, 1950 Dr. Ludmila Zeldowicz wrote an article on "Headache." Dr. Lois Crawford, interne at Vancouver General Hospital, will undertake post-graduate anesthesia training at Shaughnessy Hospital.

Dr. Helen Martin, interne at VGH, will enter General Practice in Prince Albert, Saskatchewan. VMA Summer School May 29 to June 2 had an attendance of 224 which has been the usual number for the last few years. Dr. J.S. Kennedy and Dr. Ruth Kennedy will practise in Climax, Saskatchewan. Dr. Ardeth Robertson will do Staff Medicine at Tranquille, B.C.

September, 1950 BCMA Golden Jubilee Annual Meeting dates are September 26–29. Dr. Maud L. Menton, who has until recently been Professor of Pathology at the University of Pittsburgh and at the Children's Hospital in Pittsburgh, is carrying out a research project at the British Columbia Medical Research Institute on a grant from the B.C. Branch of the Canadian Cancer Society.

November, 1950 There is an urgent problem of hospital accommodation for the sick of British Columbia, especially of Vancouver. The population of Vancouver has doubled in the past 20 years, and the number of hospital beds available has hardly risen at all.

December, 1950 Dr. Elaine Stefanelli, formerly Dr. Elaine MacLean, and her husband have begun practice at the Williams Clinic in Trail.

January, 1951 The infant mortality in British Columbia during the first quarter century has been the most favourable of any of the provinces of Canada; during the same period the infant mortality has been reduced by over 50%. The Crease Clinic opened in January, 1951.

February, 1951 There is a shortage of hospital beds because the construction of hospitals has lagged for a great many years. The population of the Vancouver area has almost doubled.

March, 1951 Population of Vancouver in 1949 was 385,500 and in 1951 was 397,140. There were epidemics of chickenpox and influenza in March, 1951. Recently, MSA altered its plan of payment of accounts and is paying ninety percent of the account instead of 75% to 80% as formerly. On April 5, 1951 the British Columbia Medical Research Institute will be opened.

May, 1951 Vancouver General Hospital internes, Dr. Shirley Patterson is now in general practice in Vancouver, and Dr. Helen McKibbon is now at the Mayo Clinic for further training. Dr. Winifred Wilson, former Public Health Officer of North Vancouver, wife of Dr. C.B. Wilson, has twin daughters. Dr. Isabel Day gave her report on the VON Advisory Board.

June, 1951 Dr. George Saxton of the Membership Committee reports there are 1,713 medical doctors registered in B.C.; 1,400 are in private practice. The Canadian Medical Association has 918 members from British Columbia. The VMA Summer School registration includes Drs. Doreen Davidson, Irmla Kennedy-Jackson, Elda Lindenfeld, Josephine Mallek, Susan McMaster, Elaine Peacock, Olive Sadler, Margaret Sylling, Reba Willits, and Lola Zeldowicz.

July, 1951 Epidemics of measles, rubella, and chickenpox occurred in July.

October, 1951 The opening of the Academy of Medicine of British Columbia took place in Vancouver.

November, 1951 Dr. Ethlyn Trapp continues as a member of the committee on Cancer. Dr. Gladys Cunningham and her husband, Dr. E.R. Cunningham, former missionaries in Chengtu, China, have opened a joint practice in Vancouver.

December, 1951 Drs. Estelle and Arnott Stevens are practising in Campbell River, B.C.

January, 1952 Another epidemic of measles and chickenpox has occurred.

February, 1952 Dr. Margaret A. Kennard of the Department of Neurological Research, Faculty of Medicine, University of British Columbia, is a senior researcher in Mental Health. Her article "The Use of the Electroencephalograph in the Diagnosis and Treatment of Epilepsy" was printed in the February *Bulletin*. Dr. Polina Zdanowcz married Mr. Paul Pariseau in Victoria.

March, 1952 Recent publication by VMA members: Mallek, Josephine; Kanee, B.; and Zack, J: "ACTH and Cortisone in Pemphigus Erythematosis." *CMAJ* 65; 564–566, Dec. 1951. Dr. Josephine Mallek of Vancouver has received Certification in Internal Medicine (for Endocrinology). The VMA Osler Lecturer for 1952 is Dr. Ethlyn Trapp. Her topic is "Modern Alchemy." She is the first woman to give the Osler Lecture to the Vancouver Medical Association. There were epidemics of scarlet fever and measles in March. Dr. Doreen Walton is practising in Trail.

October, 1952 Opening of the new British Columbia Institute by the B.C. Cancer Foundation took place in October, 1952. VMA sponsored a refresher course in Malignant Disease. Lecturer included in the program: Dr. Ethlyn Trapp, "Treatment of Cancer of the Corpus Uteri"; Dr. Margaret Hardie, "Treatment Results of the B.C. Cancer Institute" and "Radiotherapy"; and Dr. Lucille Ellison, "The Role of Hormones." Dr. Josephine Mallek spoke on "Endocrine Therapy in Childhood" at a VMA lecture series. Registry for voluntary registration of handicapped children in B.C. was organized during 1951. In 1952, the Division of Vital Statistics will automatically register all newborns who showed a birth injury or congenital malformation would be registered automatically. There are 1,325 B.C. doctors who are members of the B.C. Medical Association. Dr. Laura Coleman has returned to the British Columbia Provincial Mental Health Services after two years' post-graduate study in London, England, and is now on staff of the Child Guidance Clinic, Vancouver, B.C. Dr. Elspeth

Evans married Dr. Donald Walker, and both are practising in Vernon, B.C. Both were internes at the Vancouver General Hospital.

December, 1952 Population of Vancouver is 344,833. By October, 1952, there were 1,071 births. Infant mortality was 17.1.

January, 1953 Dr. Elizabeth Mahaffy, Assistant Medical Health Officer for the Victoria-Esquimalt Board of Health, has been granted a bursary for a year's study at University of California to work for her MPH degree.

February, 1953 In November, 1952, the infant mortality rate was 11.1 per 1,000, and in December, 1952, the rate was 27.2. The newly reconstituted B.C. Division of the Canadian Medical Association has its first anniversary. A free diagnostic and screening service is available at the Cytological Diagnostic Laboratory located at the B.C. Cancer Institute, Vancouver.

March, 1953 There were epidemics of mumps and chickenpox from November, 1952, to March, 1953. In March there were 476 cases of mumps. The number of cases of gonorrhea continues to be very high. Population in Vancouver was estimated to be 390,325. (The population from March, 1953 is listed in the *Bulletin* as total population without listing Asians separately as previously.) Dr. Helen B. Zeman is now Resident in Pediatrics at the Rosedale Hospital in New York.

April, 1953 Dr. Evelyn Gee, on the staff of Tranquille Sanatorium, attended two courses at the University of California, San Francisco, one on Cardiovascular Disease and Electocardiography, and the other on Pulmonary Function. Dr. Margaret Kennard gave a report with pictures to the Section of Neurology on the "Ablation of the Cingulate Gyrus in Cats."

May, 1953 The VMA meeting discussed Health Insurance as part of Canada's developing Health Plan. Dr. Doreen Davidson of Vancouver is doing post-graduate work at the Royal Hospital in Wolverhampton, England. Dr. H.J. van Norden and his wife, Dr. Julia van Norden, will begin a joint practice on May 1, at 2021 East 41st Avenue, Vancouver.

June, 1953 Dr. Gladys Cunningham of Vancouver has been elected as a Fellow of the Royal College of Obstetricians and Gynecologists in London, England, in recognition of her work in China as a missionary.

July, 1953 From the Statistics of the Vancouver Health Department in April, 1953, infant mortality rate was 43.9 per 1,000. Dr. Jean M. MacLennan of the Metropolitan Health Service was recently certified as a specialist in Pediatrics.

August, 1953 The *Bulletin* is now listing the names of newly-registered doctors in British Columbia. Dr. Isabel Day, a very respected Vancouver physician, died in August, 1953. She served for many years on the Advisory Board of the Victorian Order of Nurses.

September, 1953 The population of Vancouver is 390,325; Burnaby 61,000; North Vancouver City 16,000; North Vancouver municipality 16,000; West Vancouver 14,250; Richmond 19,186; University Area 3,800; University District Lot 172 1,469; for a total population of 522,030. The population of British Columbia in 1953 was 1,230,000, an increase of 32,000 over the previous year. In 1953, sixteen percent of the population of B.C. was over 60; in the rest of Canada it was eleven percent over 60.

October, 1953 There were 95 cases of poliomyelitis in 1953, 64 in the metropolitan area to August, then a gradual decline in number. In the VMA Annual Report, the VMA Summer School had 180 registrants. There were several Vancouver doctors as speakers. Dr. Norman MacKenzie, President of UBC, was the guest speaker at the luncheon.

December, 1953 There were 25 newly-registered doctors with the College of Physicians and Surgeons of B.C., including Dr. Polina Pariseau of Victoria and Dr. Amy Wong of Edmonton, Alberta. The College of General Practice of Canada will soon be brought into being.

January, 1954 At the end of their term the graduating class of the UBC Medical School will spend a month with General Practitioners of Vancouver on a preceptorship basis. Dr. Pauline Gould commenced post-graduate training at the University of Toronto in September, 1953. Elinor Black MD, FRCS (Canada), FACS, FRCOG, Chairman and Professor of the Department of Obstetrics and Gynecology at University of Manitoba and the Winnipeg General Hospital, was guest speaker at the General Practice Scientific Session of B.C. Division of CMA. Dr. Elda Lindenfeld received specialist qualification in Psychiatry in the recent Royal College exams.

February, 1954 Dr. Mary Leath is resident in Pathology at the Royal Jubilee Hospital, Victoria. Dr. Margaret Jean Hardie is on leave of absence from the Metropolitan Health Committee of Vancouver to study for the DPH at University of Toronto. Dr. Irene Morrison is training in Psychiatry in Massachusetts and hopes to return to British Columbia later.

March, 1954 Dr. Susan McMaster's article in the *Canadian Public Health Journal* of February, 1953, showed that of the 244 cases of pertussis studied in 1950, no case occurred in any child who had received four doses of the vaccine and followed up with the usual booster dose. Dr. Clarissa Aszkanazy and Dr. Margaret Hardie received Specialist Certification from the Royal College of Physicians and Surgeons of Canada. New registrants included Dr. Elsie Ritch, Vancouver, and Dr. Erna Keddis, Port Alberni.

April, 1954 The first graduating class of the Medical School of the University of British Columbia has 54 graduates. The ceremony will take place on May 17, 1954. There are two women, Mrs. Margaret Guest of Regina, Saskatchewan, and Mrs. Marjorie E. Jansch of Metchosin, B.C., in the graduating class of 1954.

May, 1954 Congratulatory letters to the first medical graduates of UBC were received from the Minister of National Health and Welfare, Paul Martin, and from the Provincial Minister of Health and Welfare, Eric Martin.

June, 1954 There was a case of diphtheria in a 14-year-old girl, diagnosed by Dr. Agnes Weston of the Metropolitan Health Service. Vancouver Medical Association has 750 members, with 505 active members.

July, 1954 There is now a replacement of the Kahn test by the VDRL (Venereal Disease Research Laboratory) test, developed by the U.S. Public Health Services.

August, 1954 VMA is sponsoring a Symposium on Geriatrics on October 20, 1954, with six speakers from Canada, United States, and Scotland.

September, 1954 The Health Centre for Children was opened by the Duke of Edinburgh. The Centre has 155 beds and plans for 240 more in a few years. There are 14 certified pediatricians at the Health Centre. Dr. Barbara Kraft is in practice in Kitimat, B.C. Public Health in proposing fluoridation of water, recommended the adoption in 1951 and reiterated this stand in 1954. British Columbia has 94 hospitals with over 25 beds each. Accreditation of Hospitals was originally done by the American College of Surgeons. In 1952 the accreditation was taken over by the Joint Commission on Accreditation of Hospitals which is Canadian and American, and by a Canadian Commission on Hospital Accreditation.

October, 1954 In the fall of 1954, a Medical Education Series meeting was held in upper Vancouver Island. The speakers were Dr. Kay Belton and Dr. Frank Turnbull. Public Relations: There is a radio program broadcast from Vancouver CJOR weekly on Thursday nights, on medical subjects. A second program was added for housewives. Each Saturday the *Daily Colonist* newspaper of Victoria, and the *Daily Province* paper of Vancouver publishes a medical column written by one of the VMA members. Public Forums are held almost at monthly intervals in Vancouver and Victoria and are very popular. The B.C. Division of the Canadian Medical Association in 1954 had 1,090 paid members, plus retired doctors and seniors making a total of 1,212, which makes B.C. the second largest division in Canada. At the General Assembly meeting it was suggested that MSI (Medical Services Incorporated) be instituted to cover those not eligible for MSA, i.e.: individual members and small firms.

November, 1954 Dr. Joan Ford is in General Practice in South Burnaby. Dr. Agnes Weston is now with the South Burnaby Health Unit.

December, 1954 The number of Infectious Hepatitis cases in B.C. increased from 10 cases in 1949 to 789 cases in 1953. The City of Vancouver had 305 cases in 1953 with six deaths. Births in 1953 were 7,776. Infant death rate was 23.7.

February, 1955 Dr. Laura Coleman is currently employed by the Department of Psychiatry at the University of Toronto in the capacity of Research Assistant.
Communicable Diseases Statistics for 1953 and 1954:
Bacillary dysentry increased from 172 cases in 1953 to 305 in 1954.
Infectious jaundice decreased from 303 cases 1953 to 173 in 1954.
Measles increased from 1,196 cases in 1953 to 2,470 in 1954.
Poliomyelitis decreased from 207 cases in 1953 to 58 in 1954.
Scarlet fever decreased from 662 cases in 1953 to 495 in 1954.
Typhoid remained the same, three cases in each year.
Whooping cough increased from 169 cases in 1953 to 290 in 1954.

Sixty-eight years ago the Salvation Army Hostel for unmarried mothers, Maywood Home on 8th and Alder, was opened. In 1927 Grace Hospital was built and 747 patients were cared for when Vancouver's population was 168,360. In 1954 Grace Hospital cared for 3,590 patients when Vancouver's population was 400,000.

At the Congress of the Medical Women's International Association (MWIA) held in Italy in 1954, Honorary Membership in MWIA was conferred on Dr. Ethlyn Trapp for exceptional service to the medical profession. Dr. Trapp of Vancouver was one of two Canadian women to receive the honour.

June, 1955 On June 28th, 1955 the Poliomyelitis Pavilion at the Pearson Tuberculosis Hospital in Vancouver was officially opened by the Honorable Eric Martin, Minister of Health. The Pavilion has 55 beds in the single storey.

September, 1955 Dr. Lois Dorothy Crawford has received Specialist recognition in Anesthesia. Dr. Madeline Chung has begun a practice (Obstetrics and Gynecology) in downtown Vancouver. Dr. Maartje Helena Cuylits is now with the Metropolitan Health Service in Vancouver.

January, 1956 Statistics from the University of British Columbia Drug Addiction Research Group (approved by VMA): 289 men and 111 women addicted to heroin; 146 men and 41 women addicted to morphine; and a few addicted to cocaine.

February, 1956 A testimonial dinner was given for the long-time editor of the *Vancouver Medical Association Bulletin*, Dr. J.H. MacDermot. All Osler speakers were invited. Dr. Ethlyn Trapp, the first and only woman Osler speaker, attended the dinner. Dr. Jane Randolph and Dr. W.A. Davies are now practising in Torrance, California. Dr. Rosarina Maria D'Amico is assisting Dr. M.K. Weare in his practice in Smithers, B.C.

March, 1956 Dr. Barbara Kraft of Kitimat, B.C. was elected to associate membership of the Vancouver Medical Association. In 1954 and 1955 there were rubella and scarlet fever epidemics, and also many cases of measles and whooping cough. The British Columbia government accepts the Federal Health Insurance Plan, as a Province-administered health insurance scheme.

April, 1956 The Senate Committee of the University of British Columbia talks about a University Hospital on site at UBC. The BCMA Section of Neurology and Psychiatry had a dinner meeting honouring Dr. Margaret Kennard who spoke on "A Survey of Neurophysiology of the Last 25 Years."

May, 1956 Dr. Laine Loo was elected to membership of the Vancouver Medical Association. Born in Estonia in 1920, she attended medical school there and received her MD in 1944. She practised medicine for a short time in Sweden and Estonia, then she came to Vancouver in 1954 where she engaged in General Practice. Dr. Loo is married and has two children. Dr. Doris Elspeth Mackay was elected to membership of the Vancouver Medical Association. Dr. Mackay was born in Calgary, Alberta and she attended the University of Alberta, receiving a BSc in 1945 and MD in 1948. She obtained certification in Anesthesia in 1954 and registered to practise in British Columbia in 1955. At present she is an anesthetist at St. Paul's. Dr. Mackay is married and she is a golf enthusiast.

June, 1956 Dr. Madeline Huang Chung was elected to membership of the Vancouver Medical Association. Dr. Chung was born in Shanghai in 1925 and she attended Yale Medical School at Hunan, China, and later did a Fellowship in Obstetrics and Gynecology at the Mayo Clinic, Rochester. She registered to practise in British Columbia in 1955 and is engaged in the Specialty of Obstetrics and Diseases of Women. Dr. Chung is married to Dr. Wallace Chung.

July, 1956 Dr. Audrey M. Mandeville is practising in New Westminster with her husband, Dr. A.F. Mandeville. Dr. Jean Ure will continue in Obstetrics at Vancouver General Hospital. Dr. Betty Chin is now working at Tranquille. A new five-storey building at Broadway and Granville opened its doors in June. It is called the Vancouver Medical Building. Dr. Helen Johnson is now Associate Pathologist at the Royal Columbian Hospital. Dr. Lee Kornder and Dr. Thais Hall of British Columbia were married this spring and will interne at St. Paul's Hospital.

September, 1956 Dr. Maria Bryant has gone to Children's Memorial Hospital in Montreal for post-graduate training.

October, 1956 "Practice for Sale: General practice, suitable for a woman doctor, with equipment and office furniture. Location Victoria. Available on short notice." Apply to Publisher of *Bulletin*, VMA, 675 Davie St. Vancouver. [First notice in the *Bulletin* specifying a woman MD.] Dr. Geraldine Kent is practising in Vancouver, B.C.

November, 1956 Dr. Lila Scott is practising in New Westminster, B.C. The Vancouver Medical Association is in favour of a Department of Dentistry at the University of British Columbia.

December, 1956 Dr. Doreen Steele is working at the Nanaimo Indian Hospital. Polio vaccine is now available and 200,000 children, with parental consent, have had at least one dose of vaccine. In 1957 vaccine will be free to all pre-school children two to five years of age. In Canada there are now 17,000 doctors; 11,000 are members of the Canadian Medical Association.

January, 1957 Dr. Margaret Kennard is now with the Mental Health Services in the United States.

April, 1957 Doctors receiving their Specialty Certification from the Royal College of Physician and Surgeons of Canada in January and February: Dr. Agnes B. Weston, FRCP, Public Health; Dr. Pauline Hughes, Psychiatry; and in June: Dr. Elsie Ritch, Anesthesia; Dr. Maria Bryant, Pediatrics; Dr. Charlotte Mahaffy, Public Health; Dr. Sarjit Kapoor Sidoo,

Pediatrics. Dr. Alice McDonald has opened a practice in Physical Medicine in Harrison Hot Springs Hotel. Dr. Doris Mackay has begun practice in Anesthesiology. Dr. Dorothy Stillwell is now practising in Colorado.

July, 1957 Basic Training School for Medical Laboratory Technologists has been established in the University of British Columbia Medical School building at Vancouver General Hospital, under the direction of the Department of Pathology of the UBC Medical School and the Vancouver General Hospital. The Nursing Staff at the Penticton General Hospital has taken strike action.

August, 1957 Dr. Jean Izatt is practising in Prince George. Dr. Ruth Kennedy of Vancouver is working at Essondale.

October, 1957 Dr. A.C. Gulliford and Dr. Eva Gulliford are now practising in Salmon Arm, B.C. Dr. Enid Tredger is working at Woodlands School in New Westminster, B.C.

November, 1957 Dr. Peter Lehman became President at the Annual Meeting of BCMA in September at the Hotel Vancouver. Dr. Betty Chin is in practice with Dr. D.B. Ryall at McBride, B.C.

December, 1957 Dr. A. Hardyment is the President of the Vancouver Medical Association for 1957–1958. Dr. Maria Mate is now married and is practising anesthesiology privately in Vancouver.

January, 1958 Dr. Florence Brent has started a practice in Vancouver in the Specialty of Gynecology.

March, 1958 Dr. Bluma Tischler received her Specialist Certificate in Pediatrics from the Royal College of Physicians and Surgeons of Canada. Dr. Honor Kidd gave reprints of her article "Pioneer Doctor John Sebastian Helmecken" to the VMA Library for the Historical Collection. VMA member, Dr. Elda Lindenfeld has had an article, "Emotionally Disturbed Children, A New Approach in B.C.," printed in *CMAJ* 78: 287, Feb. 15, 1958.

May, 1958 Dr. J.H. MacDermot continues as Editor of the *VMA Bulletin*.

June, 1958 The number of doctors served by the Vancouver Medical Association is 946 or fifty-three percent of the doctors in B.C., 877 in Vancouver, 13 in Richmond, and 56 in Burnaby.

July, 1958 There are 1,830 doctors registered and living in B.C. Members of the Canadian Medical Association, B.C. Division number, 1,461.

August, 1958 VMA with its active membership of 500–600 realizes it cannot financially continue its functions of the Library, the *VMA Bulletin*, and Summer School, plus cost of maintenance personnel. The British Columbia Medical Association with its larger membership is the only alternative association to take over functions which the Vancouver Medical Association has carried out for 34 years. Dr. Ethlyn Trapp has given a gift to the VMA Historical Collection of material relating to the establishment of the medical school in British Columbia. B.C. Division, CMA Annual Meeting will be in Kelowna, October 7–10. Dr. Margaret Hardie will be one of three speakers at a Round Table discussion on "Cutaneous Malignancy."

October, 1958 Dr. John Dick's report on the Library of the Vancouver Medical Association suggested that the Council of the College of Physicians and Surgeons be asked to give a grant for the creation of an overall library plan for the whole Province, the source being an increase in the annual dues of every practitioner in British Columbia. The only women doctors mentioned in the B.C. Division Annual Reports were Dr. Rebs Willits of the Child Care Committee and Dr. Margaret Mullinger of the Nutrition Committee.

December, 1958 This is the final issue of the *VMA Bulletin*, which began in 1924 and lasted 34 years. Dr. W. Keith has written on the history of the Early Canadian Ships' Surgeons, of the Trans Pacific Service and the C.P. Steamships Limited. On the January 1, 1959, *Vancouver Medical Association Bulletin* will cease to exist and the *British Columbia Medical Journal* will be established.

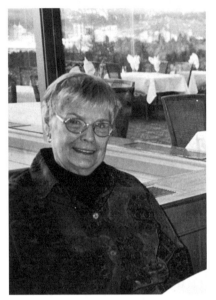

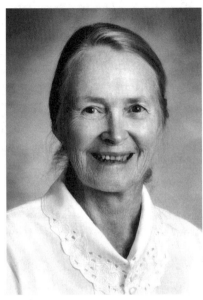

Dr. J. Mavis Teasdale, 1956

Dr. Eileen Cambon, 1958

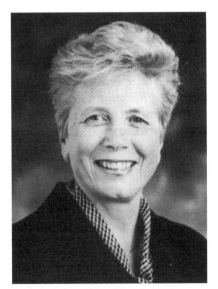

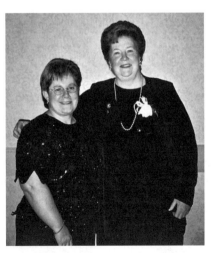

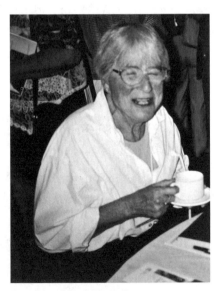

Dr. Peggy Ross, 1958

Dr. Shelley Ross (1974) and Dr. Bernice Wylie (1959)

Dr. Lois Mackenzie-Sawers, 1959

Stories from 1960 – 1969

There were 180 new registered women doctors from 1960 to 1969.

1960
Dr. Yvonne Elizabeth Duncan
Dr. Mary Hallowell
Dr. Roberta J. McQueen
Dr. Shirley Rushton

1961
Dr. Barbara Allan
Dr. Janet Halley
Dr. Violet Larsen
Dr. Magdalene Sara Schmidt Laszlo
Dr. Joy C. Longley
Dr. Anne (Patty) Vogel

1962
Dr. Nelly Auersperg
Dr. Yang-Shu Hsieh
Dr. Patricia Kirkwood Johnston
Dr. Betty Wood

1963
Dr. Danica Maria Beggs
Dr. Beverley Tamboline

1964
Dr. Patricia A. Baird
Dr. Margaret Elizabeth (Love) Patriarche
Dr. Betty Poland

1965
Dr. Pamela Aldis
Dr. Vivien Elisabeth Basco
Dr. Victoria Bernstein
Dr. Margaret Shirley Neave
Dr. Irene Puetz

1966
Dr. Margaret Carlson
Dr. Anne Derks
Dr. Kathleen A. Elliott
Dr. Louise Jilek-Aall
Dr. Patricia Rebbeck
Dr. Mary Alice Sutter

1967
Dr. Marlene E. Hunter
Dr. Mara Love
Dr. Sue Penfold
Dr. Eve Rotem

1968
Dr. Erica Pia Crichton
Dr. Elspeth Davies
Dr. Irmgard Elisabeth Hermesh
Dr. Patricia (Paddy) Mark

1969
Dr. Betty Huggett Chan
Dr. Barbara Robinson

DR. YVONNE ELIZABETH DUNCAN

Notes on University Days

Pre-med was only a one-year program. I was in a class of over 200 students, with a large percentage of veterans who were financially subsidized by the Canadian Government's Department of Veterans Affairs (DVA). Six subjects were mandatory. There were no spare periods and few of the laboratory classes could be allotted full-time. We were asked to imagine what our results would be if we were to mix such and such ingredients together. In the first month of our classes all pre-med female students were interviewed by the Dean of Women. She told me I should register in another class as my chances of getting into medicine were too slim. I was female, not from Manitoba, and veterans who obtained a sixty percent average were guaranteed a position in medicine. It was not a 'fun' year. I worked and worked, or studied and studied!

First year medicine was a world of difference from pre-med. There were sixty-five students in our class, one-third veterans and amazingly seven women, the largest class at that time and for many years. We quickly established a congenial bond with one another. Although none of us were athletic, we had a keen interest in physical activity to compensate for the hours we spent sitting, listening to lectures, and studying. We signed up for team play and university competitions in volleyball, basketball, bowling, and on sports days with relay racing, dashes, broadjumping, curling, and swimming.

An amusing predicament befell the university in my fourth year. The head girl in the Sports Department phoned me to verify my participation in most of the events. I had racked up more points than any other woman at the university and therefore qualified for a special prize. However, the obvious intent of the call was something else. I had not excelled in any of the sports, and there was a woman in the university who had achieved great acclaim. The general consensus was that this true athlete should receive the coveted award. I heartily agreed! As consolation, a white coat-sweater with a big M was delivered to me. It resides for posterity in the bottom of a trunk in our crawl-space to this day.

Intern Days

The intern year was considered as part of the university medical course—the fifth year after the four years of medical school. We earned no salary for the year; indeed we paid tuition of $110 to the university for the privilege of interning. The hospital provided us a basement suite—which consisted of a small kitchen, sitting room, and bedroom with two cots—for Brenda Devlin and myself, the two women accepted at the General Hospital that year. An additional two women, both doctors, joined the year's rotating internship; one was from China and the other Hungary, both fleeing political unrest in their countries. The Chinese doctor and her husband and young son had to leave everything behind in Shanghai, including her medical documents. The two foreign doctors were required to do an internship before licensing.

We received two uniforms, each a two-piece suit-like affair. We were lucky if we got through one day without having to change, so we resorted to wearing the green operating room pajama-like suits for much of the week. Laundry service was once a week. This change of outfit led to my being called before the administration to explain the use of the operating room attire by the female intern staff. When the situation was explained to the said officialdom, we received an order for two more uniforms to me made for each female intern. The male interns had been given four uniforms at the beginning of their internship as there was a ready supply of used ones from past residents.

Eating arrangements were also remarkable. Female interns ate with the nurses in the nurses' residence. The menu of the nurses was very different from the one the men received. The men's residence refrigerator was stuffed with meat and vegetables and desserts at all times for snacks and missed meals. Ours was not stocked ever. The women interns missed many meals because we could not free ourselves from work at the one-hour, four allotted meal times. We resorted to eating bread and butter or jam and toast from the ward refrigerator. At times we even asked private ward patients if we might sample their food packages, brought in by relatives and placed in near-by refrigerators. This regular carbohydrate diet resulted in added poundage, much to our embarrassment. Over Christmas the male interns invited us to partake of their festive repast and of course we accepted. However, on Christmas morning the administrator informed the men their plan was not acceptable. In response the men, unbeknown to the administration, brought their meal to our small apartment and we all enjoyed the feast.

In third year medicine Doug Dundee had joined our class from Saskatoon. His medical school had only the first two years, so the students had to transfer to another medical school to finish their training. By intern year Doug and I had fallen in love, and had an understanding that we would probably marry after internship. Because of this possibility we were not allowed to intern in the same hospital! Other couples in the past had respected this unwritten ruling. Fortunately, Doug preferred to do his internship at St. Boniface Hospital in Winnipeg.

Our intern year was complicated by the onset of the polio epidemic which started in the spring. Six interns from each of the two teaching hospitals were to spend two weeks at the infectious disease hospital, until such time when the epidemic was over. As a result, all of the interns had little free time. As for allotted holiday time at the General Hospital, there was none. We only had one day off for our graduation exercises!

The polio epidemic stretched into the fall of 1953. All interns spent time on the polio wards. The mortality and morbidity were worrisome. Respirators were flown in from all over the world, and we had quick lessons in how to use all of them, especially when the electricity failed and we had to manually operate the machines. Electrical storms were common that summer and the hospital's wiring was sorely tried, with so many machines operating full-time. We made rounds every hour, and at least once on the hour someone was in extreme difficulty, requiring resuscitation, suctioning, or bronchoscopy for mucous plugs. Babies were being born in short order, while the mothers were pulled out of the respirators for short periods. There were few time tables for any of us. We worked as long as we could stand it, then grabbed a few hours of sleep if possible. Routine laboratory work, spinal punctures, and tap examinations were all done by the junior interns once we became accomplished in emergency procedures. Gamma globulin was given to all of us; so many cc's injected into our buttocks was not something you forget in a hurry. Back at the General Hospital seemed tame by comparison.

Theoretically, we were each supposed to be off-call every other evening when we were not covering Emergency once every sixteen days, or for a sick colleague. There was always routine laboratory work to be done for the 'public' patients. Many evenings were spent pipetting and sloshing blood and urine samples about, and setting up sedimentation tests.

Our many veteran classmates had a particularly hard time adjusting to our work load, as most were married with small children and saw little of them. We single souls covered for these men for a few hours a few nights a week. This led to embarrassing times when I discovered the missing interns were on urology rotation and passing a catheter was a frequent necessity on that ward.

Orthopedics was my final rotation in the last month at the hospital. My chief was noted for his expertise in back surgery. My main duty in the operating room as a second assistant was to hold the patient's leg straight in dorsi extension using both arms and hands for two to fours hours at a time. Perhaps it was exhaustion or postural hypotension, I woke up four mornings in a row in the surgical recovery room. Such an embarrassment! For the remainder of the month, I was assigned to less vigorous and less boring chores, such as assisting with casting, setting up tractions, and the like.

General Practice Days

Following graduation I joined my older brother, Don, in practice in Norquay, Saskatchewan. It was a small town of 400 people in northeastern Saskatchewan, a farming community, with most of the people of Swedish origin. The ten-plus bed hospital was a typical cottage hospital, with appropriate staffing with registered nurses, nurses' aides, and a laboratory technician. General medicine, paediatrics, minor surgery, and obstetrics could be adequately practised for the times. Surgery requiring the presence of three doctors was performed in the nearest, next level hospital in Canora, some thirty miles away. The trip to Canora was made by the two of us. During the winter months the roads were hazardous because of snow drifts and white-outs. In the spring the pot-holes in the gravel road could envelop two car wheels at any time. Other times in the middle of the night one of us would fall asleep and the car would slide off the road. Fortunately, the ditches were shallow, and little bodily harm was done.

Within a week of my arrival home in Canora to live with my widowed mother and brother, Don left for a course in Seattle, Washington for one eek. He had not had a holiday for years. Within a few days I was having second thoughts about the practice of medicine. My first emergency was a young man with an acute incarcerated inguinal hernia. On my second attempt to reduce it I succeeded, but not before I sweated a bucket or two. Fortunately, the reduction lasted until Don returned and could deal with the surgery electively.

The following day an attractive, blonde, blue-eyed eighteen-year-old Swedish farm wife presented in labour with a placenta praevia. A gentle rectal exam confirmed the diagnosis to my satisfaction, but I was left with a dilemma. This was her first baby, contractions were strong and three to five minutes apart, haemoglobin was six gms. The road to Canora was pot-holed and thought to be very difficult if not impossible to navigate. There was no other doctor close-by. We had a sterilized Caesarean bundle for just such emergencies. We had a very intelligent head nurse and a willing practical nurse. The lab technician was on holiday, and the Red Cross had collected blood from all our known doctors. We had to proceed as best we could. I anaesthetised our patient with an induction of chloroform and deepened with open drop ether (the only anaesthetics available at the time). Once anaesthetised, the head nurse kept the patient asleep with ether, and the practical nurse and I scrubbed. I did a classical mid-line incision, and had the baby out very quickly. The baby cried lustily right way, music to my ears! And we sewed up the incision without further ado. The mother wakened shortly after, and was joyful to have a beautiful newborn. The mother's stomach did not even rebel against the ether. The mother's low count of haemoglobin was a worry to me, especially if she should bleed heavily post-partum (ergotamine was used sparingly then). I did a major cross-match on my own blood and that of the patient and found it compatible. I had the nurse draw off a pint of my blood, and we administered it to the mother as soon as possible. The mother did well and continued to

Most bachelor homesteaders preferred to administer their own medication in the local hotel pub before presenting themselves for [tooth] extractions.

thrive. I wrote reams of notes on the care she had for my brother and possibly future doctors, should other such pregnancies occur. Years later I spoke to the doctor covering the area and learned that this patient had gone on to have four more pregnancies, all delivered vaginally without difficulty. Caesarean operations had been planned for each subsequent pregnancies, but precipitated labour and delivery occurred each time! Patterns of practice do change, as we all discover. One hesistates to criticize any one doctor for any one occurence . . . you had to be there.

One of the many advantages of small town practice is that the doctor has the privilege of developing a close rapport with all the citizens, but in particular the local ministry and the RCMP. In my first winter in my Norquay practice, the RCMP local constable brought us a motorized toboggan they were developing in hopes that it would be useful in finding people off the beaten track, people stranded, or sick in isolated areas. It was a large tobog-gan, the same shape but a little longer and wider, perhaps twelve feet by two. It was uncovered, had a motor in front, a firm seat in the middle, and a storage area at the back. My brother went on a trial run with it and the officer, and made a house call as well. It was not too impressive because it was tippy and exposed riders to the elements, the wind especially. This version of a winter vehicle never materialized, to my knowledge, but undoubtedly it was a precursor of the snowmobile in use today.

My brother introduced me to dentistry and its ramifications. Dentists were in short supply in all prairie towns and Norquay was no exception. The closest dentist was in Canora and hence not accessible to many people who shopped in Norquay. North of Norquay there were no established communities, but there were a number of homesteaders who lived mostly off the land and came to the nearest town only twice a year for supplies and to touch base with civilization. There were also a number of Indian reservations surrounding Norquay, and they too were content to obtain their needs in Norquay. Saturday mornings and afternoons were for ordering and packing supplies, and the rest of the day would be spent socializing before setting out for home in the evening or Sunday morning. Visiting the doctor or having a bothersome tooth attended to were left until all the other activities were completed. I was given a few lessons on how to do a total nerve block with local anaesthetic, then how to pull a large tooth or a small one, and which implement was best suited. Pain-killing and/or extraction were all we could offer, but our services were in demand just the same. Most bachelor homesteaders preferred to administer their own medication in the local hotel pub before presenting themselves for extractions. Of course our services were offered free of charge, so this salved our consciences somewhat regarding acting as dentists and the recipients seemed grateful.

General Practice in Whitewood, Saskatchewan
In June 1955, I joined my new husband, Dr. Douglas Dundee, in his practice in Whitewood, a town of 800 people, a mixed farming community in the southeast corner of the province. It boasted a ten-bed cottage hospital. A larger, better equipped hospital of twenty plus beds and surgical capability at Broadview was run by the Catholic Church and an amiable group of nursing and administrative sisters and nuns. We had admitting privileges at their hospital also. The long-time resident doctor at Broadview, Andrew Campbell, or Andie, acted as handy consultant and surgeon or anaesthetist whenever we had need of another helping hand or a curt piece of wisdom.

Whitewood proved to be a fantastic learning ground for us. The townspeople took us into their embrace and we soon became acquainted with everyone, and lasting friendships resulted. We were particularly fortunate in having an intelligent and compassionate hospital staff. The cook was a local person with no formal dietary education, but she was a natural cook and provided exceptional menus, suitable for all dietary needs. The aromas from the kitchen alone, I believe, healed a lot of ailing souls. There were no complaints about the food, unlike many hospitals today.

In the early spring of 1956, I was very pregnant with our first baby when the young doctor in the nearest town, Wapella, had a heart attack. We were asked to cover temporarily if possible. I agreed to cover for emergencies, and to be available in their doctor's office three days a week. It proved to be an interesting venture and a great chance to see more of the countryside. Wapella had an older community population which necessitated house calls, often to quite remote areas. Several times I was transported by sleigh and two- to four-horse teams. I hospitalized a number of the elderly with pneumonia in our Whitewood hospital.

My first clinic day in Wapella was a memorable one for me as I arrived with much trepidation, not knowing anyone and wondering if they would accept me, this highly pregnant doctor. I walked into the waiting room and found it to be full of men, fifteen of them. I thought it was a welcoming committee or a joke. It turned out that they were patients who heard about me and came for medical attention.

One patient on the first day was a young man who had been wheelchair-bound for four years. He had been seen by specialists in Regina, but the diagnosis was unclear. He presented that day with a rash and as I had no idea what it was, I took his blood and urine samples and did a tuberculin skin test, a routine test which had been drummed into us during our intern years. Much to my surprise, the serology test results came back to me from Regina by return mail. I plied my new patient with massive does of penicillin and to my great joy, within a week my patient's wheelchair was shed! Unfortunately, results such as that are not a common occurrence in a doctor's life, but they help to make up for the discouraging cases which occupy so much of a physician's time.

Obstetrics in an isolated area proved to be more of a challenge than we had ever imagined in our intern year. Rural areas seem to present more complications than the textbooks would have you believe were possible. Much of this was of course due to the lack of education in the rural population, and regular prenatal care was not thought necessary. A case of note that brings shivers to me even today was when one wintry day a woman, nine months pregnant in an advanced labour with a sixth child, showed up at the hospital with her husband. She had planned to have the baby delivered at home with the help of a neighbour, but after hours of strong labour, she decided to come to the hospital by horse and sleigh as their road had not been ploughed. We could not detect a foetal heart; she was obviously exhausted and her cervix was not fully dilated. We administered analgesics, and reassessed her at short intervals. The head presented and was low enough for delivery, yet there was little progress. The patient's condition became more disturbing when we noted the presence of a Bandl's contraction ring in the mid-abdominal area. We had to deliver the best we could. I administered an anaesthetic and gave her phenobarb. Yet, nothing happened. We allowed her to wake up and gave more and move oxygen. There was no lessening of the severity of the ring. Again we gave anaesthesia and this time the ring relaxed, and with the aid of outlet forceps we finally delivered the baby. However, the small infant was not resuscitable. Following the delivery a steady haemorrhage occurred which did not respond to IV fluids and ergotamine. We had no access to blood for transfusion as the Red Cross blood bank had just taken blood from all the donors. We had to consider taking our patient to the nearest, fully equipped hospital at Moosomin some thirty-five miles away. At this point the only way to stop her from haemorrhaging was to apply fist pressure vaginally while compressing the uterus with a second hand on her abdomen.

Imagine the scene . . . a blustery, cold wintry afternoon. A patient bundled in warm clothing with an IV in one forearm, with me . . . one hand in a sterile glove inserted deep in her vagina, and my other hand on her abdomen firming up a post-partum turgid uterus. The patient was shifted from the hospital bed, to stretcher, and to the back seat of our car with me crouching on the floor while maintaining my anti-haemorrhaging duties! The head nurse held the patient's head in her lap while holding the IV bottle in an elevated position. My husband drove the car as best as he could, and we slithered and slid our way cautiously to Moosomin. Moosomin Hospital was a thirty-bed facility with three resident doctors and a surgeon, and a full laboratory service. Blood transfusions were started and within a few hours we were able to leave our patient in capable hands. Our patient remained in the hospital for five weeks, as she had developed deep vein pelvic thrombophlebitis. She was treated with anticoagulants and antibiotics, and eventually made a full recovery. Fortunately, she refrained from having further pregnancies.

Veterinarian Efforts

In rural areas, requests for veterinarian services were not uncommon. There were fewer dentists and vets in smaller towns. Fortunately, we had a *Merck's Manual for Vets*. On several occasions, we were pressed into doing something for fractured legs in dogs rather than putting the animal out of its misery. Once we had to put a plate in and screw it into the hind leg of a large German shepherd. The hospital's garage served as an operating room; and I was the anaesthetist, the Matron the assistant, and my brother

the surgeon. The dog survived the ordeal and managed to put in more able years on his four legs. On another dog, a large Heinz variety pooch, we did a closed reduction and cast on a front leg. When he awakened from the anaesthesia he was lovingly taken home where he crawled under a bed. He began howling in the middle of the night and couldn't get out from under the bed. The bed had to be taken apart and the dog carried outside where he relieved himself. Several weeks later he decided he could remove the cast himself and did so by biting it off bit by bit, to the great relief of his doctors.

Further Medical Training in England

We spent the years from August 1957 to December 1959 in England. Our experiences prior to this time prompted us to seek further training and expertise in surgery and obstetrics and gynecology; particularly as we believed we wanted to continue in family practice where the need was the greatest, in relatively isolated areas. Doug obtained his primary fellowship in surgery in London in the fall of 1957, and following this training he did residencies in Colchester and Derby. As a woman physician with a child, I had difficulty obtaining a position in the same hospitals as Doug and in the branches of medicine I was most interested in. However, once I got a job and proved myself, the opportunities improved.

Of course there were many things to adjust to in a different country with different customs. There was no denying the vast amount of experience one could attain at this time, and there were many memorable ones. I'll mention one as it was somewhat humorous in retrospect.

One morning at about three o'clock, while on emergency service but not actually on duty, I was wakened by a very apologetic nurse. There was a patient in a car outside of the emergency who was in need of a doctor, but who refused to come in unless she could be seen by a female doctor. I rushed down to the emergency area and out to the car park where a grateful gentleman introduced me to his wife in the back seat of his car. There was blood all over the seat, and a very overweight, middle-aged, tearful, and embarrassed lady related her story. She told me that because she found it a particularly cold night, instead of going to the washroom downstairs, she decided to use the commode, rarely used, but tucked away under her bed. She pulled it out and, as she tried to sit herself awkwardly on it, the commode shattered in many places, sending shards of porcelain into her buttocks. Poor soul! This lady was then transferred to a stretcher, given analgesic and relaxants, and was placed on her abdomen to be sutured.

Kitimat, British Columbia

I gained tremendous experience during my practice in Kitimat from December 1959 to August 1969. My brother Don had been in a solo practice for three years when Doug and I joined him. Kitimat, a community of 12,000, has an Alcan Aluminum smelter site, seaport, Indian village, and a nice mix of professionals (mostly engineers and medical staff for a ninety-bed hospital), and pot-line workers from all over the world, mostly Portugal, Greece, Italy, Germany, Quebec, and smaller numbers from the rest of Canada. A plant at Kemano supplied the necessary power for Kitimat's smelter, and the community of Kemano depended on Kitimat's resources for its supplies and medical care.

During most years there were six to seven family physicians in residence, a general surgeon who also acted as the Alcan medical officer, and a full-time anaesthetist, Dr. Barbara Kraft. Dr. Evelyn Fox was the first female family physician in Kitimat, arriving with her engineer husband in 1956. She remained in full-time practice until illness necessitated her retirement.

The hospital, built in 1960, was a treat to work in, as it was fully equipped with first-rate facilities including operating rooms, delivery rooms, and laboratory and X-ray services. It was granted full accreditation with the first available assessment. This was accomplished with a great deal of effort on the part of every physician, as this required each of us participating in at least two to three of the hospital committees including records, medicine, surgery, pediatrics, etc.; keeping acceptable records on every patient upon their admission; attending monthly or bimonthly general staff meetings; running an educational program with visiting expert physicians; and so on. Consequently, our visits back home to Saskatchewan became shorter and shorter.

There was a need for family physician anesthetists to cover Dr. Kraft's holidays and when the two operating rooms were busy. Instruction by Dr. Kraft on the use of the gas machine was given freely, and in addition Dr.

Paul Woollacot and I attended three four-day courses sponsored by the hospitals in Vancouver. This chore was probably the one that I disliked the most in all the years I spent in general practice. There was something inherently difficult in intubating our Native Indian population. Native children were so prone to upper respiratory infections that tonsillectomies seemed to be a necessity in most of them. Their parents, too, were difficult to intubate, as generally they had shorter and stouter necks that had less flexibility. This difficulty was agreed upon by my fellow intubators, and eventually we became better at intubating, but I was always happier to be elsewhere than at the head of the operating table.

Emergency evacuations out of Kitimat were occasionally a problem. Our closest airport was Terrace which was twenty miles away. As luck would have it, the need to fly a patient out invariably occurred in the winter months, and often when the weather was socked in and no plane could fly. The next best bet was to seek a float plane from Comox to land in the Douglas Channel to meet a motor launch that carried the patient as close to the shore as possible, then transferring the patient via stretcher. On one occasion, we had to bring a ten-year-old child, who was ill with tuberculous meningitis and otitis media, on the journey. The plane circled the channel seeking our boat at the appointed hour, and landed near us in a choppy sea. The wind was fierce and we shivered and teetered trying to keep the boat steady. Our patient, wrapped in wool blankets and with hot water bottles and an intravenous drip, was kept as comfortable as possible. After several attempts, the transfer successfully took place. Fortunately, the trip from then on went smoothly, and the patient and her mother arrived safely at the Vancouver hospital, and the anti-tuberculosis medication was continued. A month later, our patient came back to Kitimat fully recovered.

Another obstetrical nightmare for us happened in Kitimat when my brother Don was on a summer vacation. The afternoon he left, a young primipara of his went into labour. She delivered uneventfully within the expected time but continued to bleed. The placenta had been slow to separate but appeared intact. In spite of the use of drugs, fundal pressure, and vaginal packing, the patient continued to bleed excessively. We administered blood and did a D and C after a careful examination for a retained cotyledon. The scrapings were moderate, but the uterus appeared to have contracted adequately. Again after another hour had passed further bleeding was experienced, and a blood transfusion was ordered. Next we consulted a Vancouver specialist while we packed the uterus. The advice was to proceed with a hysterectomy if the packing failed to produce results. With much trepidation, through the night we did just that. Our patient behaved and no further alarms were raised. On the pathology report we later discovered that the placenta submitted for examination was likely a placenta accreeta, which definitely was not a good thing to have!

Cruiseship passengers with curious ills were at times brought to Kitimat. Cruiseships did not stop regularly at Kitimat because the town is situated some forty miles up the Douglas Channel. However, they occasionally did come to us as the channel could accommodate all sizes of ships and our hospital was known to be well-equipped. We had seen patients with fractured hips, pneumonia, and one with a subdural hemorrhage. It was not possible to transport the patient with the head injury out by plane, so again under the guidance of a Vancouver specialist in neurosurgery with telephone consultation, burr holes were performed, but unfortunately, the patient did not survive.

Post-mortems were expected to be done by rural physicians at that time. The RCMP asked for them when the circumstances of death were suspicious. No physician was keen to do these cases, so a rotation schedule was set up. This was one obligation I could not bring myself to carry out. I prevailed upon my husband to do my share of autopsies in return for house calls he disliked to do. I know I got the better deal!

Friends as Patients

Having your friends as patients can be very upsetting at times and is usually not undertaken, but in a rural practice many friends do grow to become your patients. You are obliged to continue to treat, but resort to consultations as much as possible. One memorable misfortune in a family of a head nurse (our friend) occurred when two of her five children died of acute leukemia. The second child developed this condition in Kitimat when she was five. She spent some time in Vancouver, receiving initial treatment there, and returned to Kitimat for follow-up and continuing chemotherapy. I had the task of administering Methotrexate intrathecally at regular intervals,

something we all dreaded doing. One time her treatment date was scheduled in November, shortly after 11 a.m.; while injecting the medication, an orderly came into the room and announced that President Kennedy had been assassinated. A few months later, the little girl and her mother returned to Vancouver to see Dr. Mavis Teasdale in consultation again, and shortly after she left us for a better place.

Time For a Change

After ten years in Kitimat, B.C., we realized that we were unlikely to keep up our hectic lifestyle of constant on-call work and very little time for family and social life. We were missing too much of our two children's formative years.

We headed for Toronto, as Doug was accepted in a radiology residency at the Toronto Western Hospital, and I found a job in the Family Practice Clinic at Wellesley Hospital as a clinician and clinical instructor at the University of Toronto Medical School. Four years later the pull of British Columbia mountains and sea saw us back in B.C., with Doug adding a Certification in Radiology to his previously obtained in London, England, Fellowship in Surgery. I had completed a Certification in Family Medicine while in Toronto. We chose the Vancouver area, living in West Vancouver where I started a practice again, and Doug joined a radiology group in Vancouver.

Comparing urban and rural practices is difficult, as there are so many variables and the passing of each decade produces changes in modes of practice. In the city there is relatively easy access to specialty services of every kind—diagnostic and therapeutic. I had privileges at Lions Gate Hospital in North Vancouver, a fully accredited hospital. I could enjoy and participate in regular ward rounds in nearly all of the main specialties, with input from all the sub-specialties. The four hundred beds (later drastically cut) accommodated patients from the North Shore of Burrard Inlet and communities north and inland to Whistler. The physician staff, just over two hundred members, was small enough that we were on a first name basis with most. We therefore were able to share many enjoyable, regular, information exchanges in hallways or consultations and debates in a coffee room.

Rural practice was much more demanding with constant commitments to patients, more frequent life-and-death decision-making, more frequent dealings with emergencies in the office, home, and hospital settings, and performing more minor medical and surgical procedures.

Urban practice was less hectic but had its own stresses; especially in the 1990s when the government introduced cutbacks and reorganizations. Time and money constraints created problems and tension for so many young people and families. Stress-related diseases were becoming more common. Recommended therapies were often disappointing in their applications.

The greater work load of urban practice seemed to also create a greater number of chores that were required to be done in out-of-office hours. Patients' hospital records needed admission and discharge histories; hospital committee meetings were scheduled during lunch hours or early evenings; and a greater deluge of forms and letters needed to be completed and addressed to different people and different organizations, such as the Workmen's Compensation Board, the insurance companies, to employers for reasons of absence from work, compassionate leave, post-partum leave for mothers (or fathers), and to lawyers, and more lawyers with regular updates (probably fifty percent of the legal requests related to whiplash injury).

In spite of all the difficulties, the practice of medicine remains a treasured privilege and experience for me. I truly enjoyed it, warts and all! However, I could not have done any of it without the ever-loving and tireless support of my brother, Dr. Donald Duncan, in my first year of practice in Saskatchewan, and later in the Kitimat years, or without the support of my husband, Dr. Douglas Dundee. We have been tuned into each other for over forty-five years now with an addition of our four years of courtship, and the infatuation goes on! In later years, while in my own practice, when my work time extended to twelve to sixteen hours a day, Doug would take on most of the shopping and cooking tasks if he arrived home before me. This commitment has continued into the retirement years, complete with breakfast in bed!

We have been fortunate to have two great sons who are very special. They received degrees at the University of British Columbia—one in Law, and the other in Commerce. We also have a darling granddaughter. I am truly blessed. I have had a good run and cannot ask for anything more of life!

Curriculum Vitae

Born: January 11th, 1931, Brandon, Manitoba.
Family: Two children, David born in Regina, Saskatchewan, March 31, 1956, and Michael born in Kitimat, B.C., July, 1960.
Education: Primary in Canora, Saskatchewan; Secondary: Yorkton Collegiate Institute, Saskatchewan; University of Manitoba, Winnipeg, Manitoba, Pre-med 1948–49; University of Manitoba Medical School 1949–1953.
Internship: Winnipeg General Hospital 1953–1954.
Experience: 1954–1955: General Practice with brother, Dr. Don J. Duncan, at Norquay, Saskatchewan; 1955: Married, May 25, to classmate Dr. Douglas Dundee; 1955–1957: General Practice in Whitewood, Sask.; 1957–1959: Post-graduate training in England, in London, Colchester, and Derby (Emergency and Gynecology); 1959–1969: General Practice in Kitimat, B.C.; 1969–1973: General Practice in Wellesley Hospital, Toronto, Ont.; 1973–1975: General Practice at Hanna Medical Clinic, Burnaby, B.C.; 1975–1994: Solo practice in West Vancouver, B.C.

DR. MARY HALLOWELL

With the degrees of MB, ChB, DCH, and FRCP (Edinburgh), I became weary of making slow progress up the 'consultant' ladder in the British National Health Service. I disembarked from the *Corinthia* in Montreal at 2:30 p.m. on October 4th, 1960, took the LMCC exam in Winnipeg, and subsequently travelled to New Westminster, British Columbia. I had been invited to join a surgeon and an obstetrician-gynecologist who were trying to establish a group practice. This proved to be an abysmal failure. Local doctors stressed that New Westminster needed a paediatric consulting practice. On a return trip to Winnipeg in 1961, I gained my Certification in Paediatrics and this enabled me to bill the full consultation fee. Prior to that I could only bill the general practice consultation fee.

There were two other paediatricians in New Westminster who were interested only in primary care. Consequently, I was usually on call twenty-four hours a day, seven days a week. It was at times very exhausting, but also very satisfying. I certainly needed the knowledge and skills I had acquired in the previous two-and-a-half years in the Birmingham Children's Hospital. I treated very sick children with gastroenteritis, respiratory infections, meningitis, nephritis, nephrosis, leukemia, and complications of infectious diseases, as well as many sick neonates. In winter a child severely dehydrated with gastroenteritis seemed to arrive in the Royal Columbian Hospital Emergency almost every night.

Before immigrating I had carried out approximately eighty duodenal biopsies and I continued to do these as the indications arose. My name appears as a joint author in the *Quarterly Journal of Medicine* on this work.

I was granted privileges at the Royal Columbian and St. Mary's Hospitals, and was soon appointed to the active staff of both hospitals and made Chief of Paediatrics. Having little idea of the duties the job entailed, I found it difficult to get information regarding my responsibilities. However, I knew that I was in charge of putting on paediatric rounds once a month, which was a very pleasant task. The other two paediatricians (both male) were characterized by their absence at these rounds—"You can't expect me to come to your rounds."

It was the internists who became my friends and warned me of the pitfalls of Consulting Practice in a tightly-controlled general practitioner city. I was warned that general practitioners would make non-complimentary remarks about specialists in their hearing, but I would just have to ignore them. How true this statement proved to be. On the other hand, I did experience one very amusing incident shortly after my arrival. I was invited to the New Westminster Doctors' Annual Christmas Tea. One general practitioner probably assumed that I was a doctor's wife and started to tell me about a new paediatrician in town who had treated one of his very sick infants with severe dehydration and hypernatraemia with a solution containing sodium. All my attempts to give him a talk on electrolyte balance,

dehydration, and water intoxication failed as he slowly realized that I was this strange paediatrician. I think he was just too shocked to absorb anything further. I might add that the baby made an uneventful recovery.

Initially most of my time was spent in the hospitals. Over the course of the next decade, children's general health improved with the introduction of Medicare and increased immunization rates. Other paediatricians arrived in New Westminster and Paediatric Wards opened in hospitals in the Fraser Valley. I gradually did less work in the hospitals and more in the office, and I took up the study of Allergic Diseases. My practice became largely a consulting office practice, which I retired from after twenty-six years. Then I took a year off and spent the next twelve-and-half years doing part-time work in a walk-in clinic.

My first home in New Westminster was a small apartment on the top floor of a frame building facing the south-west. The first summer I discovered why no one wanted to rent it: it was incredibly hot. A colleague suggested that I should join the New Westminster Tennis Club as it possessed a telephone and I could be on call there. At this time there was a medical telephone answering service, but no pagers or answering machines. The idea appealed to me as tennis was the only school sport I had enjoyed. Little did I realize at the time how much enjoyment and how many amazing opportunities this sport would eventually bring into my life.

I purchased a "dollar forty-nine" racquet at the Bay, and arranged tennis lessons at 7 a.m. once a week. The tennis pro had a psychopathic personality and appeared for only about half the scheduled occasions. On fine summer evenings I went to the tennis club between finishing at the office and carrying out night rounds in the hospital. My tennis remained mediocre, but started to improve when I retired from full-time practice. However, I did not become a Senior Canadian National Champion until the age of seventy-three, when I was a winner in the seventies doubles. I have been the President of the British Columbia Senior Women's team for many years, and on two occasions played on the Pacific North West Sectional Teams in the States. In 1997, I played on the Canadian team sent to the International Friendship Cup in Suzuka, Japan.

In my early years in practice, vacations were few and far between and of short duration. On a brief visit to a friend in San Francisco, I became acquainted with the American Tennis Association, and subsequently the World Medical Tennis Association was formed. This organization holds a week-long meeting with medical lectures, a tennis tournament, and social activities in a different country every year. I have attended many of these meetings, playing with physicians from thirty-nine countries, and have had some exciting adventures along the way. In 1992, the meeting was in San Remo, Italy. The half-day trip with "local flavour" was an excursion to climb to a quaint old village at the top of a mountain. We set off on a glorious sunny afternoon, but having made the climb to the village square where dinner was about to be served, darkness suddenly fell and a severe and prolonged thunderstorm started. We sheltered in the village church and when the lightning eventually ceased, it was still pitch black outside; we took the candles from the church to light our way down the steep narrow alleyways to the main road at the foot of the mountain. Buses were waiting to take us back to our hotels.

I have enjoyed my life in Canada and feel very fortunate to have practised medicine at a time when there was easy access to hospitals and no interference from hospital administrators so that patients could be speedily investigated and treated.

DR. ROBERTA J. MCQUEEN

I am a first generation Canadian and, coming from a medical background, the third generation of doctors. My father was born in Scotland and immigrated as a young boy. He entered Manitoba Medical School, graduating in 1909 at the age of twenty. He had to wait until he was twenty-one before he could begin to practise. During his first few years he was also the Superintendent of the Winnipeg General Hospital.

In 1914, my father enlisted in the Canadian Medical Services of the Army and went overseas. He returned to Winnipeg in 1915 to form the 11th Field Ambulance Unit which he took overseas to serve in France and Flanders. In 1917 he returned to England to become the Superintendent of the Canadian General Hospital at Bushey Park in England. Dr. J.D. McQueen received the Distinguished Service Order for his services during the war.

On his return to Canada, my father spent several years in New York City in postgraduate training in obstetrics and gynaecology. He returned to Winnipeg and married a nurse who had been a community nursing sister. She became active in the Victorian Order of Nurses, latterly serving on the local and federal Board.

I was born in 1922 in Winnipeg, and from an early age, was exposed to all aspects of the health care system. In my early years, the practice of obstetrics and gynaecology comprised pre- and post-natal care, including six to eight weeks post-natal care at home. Thus I had time to spend with my father while he made his calls. During the depression years, this type of practice continued. However, payment was very limited, and much of it was in produce. I had to learn the meaning of confidentiality, to answer the telephone and to ask questions regarding pains, frequency, breaking of waters, etc., then to locate father and pass on the message.

From about the age of eight years, I began to talk about going into medicine. Both of my parents tried very hard to dissuade me, especially as our local medical school openly discouraged females and few were accepted.

From about the age of eight years, I began to talk about going into medicine. Both of my parents tried very hard to dissuade me, especially as our local medical school openly discouraged females and few were accepted.

The Medical School of the University of Manitoba, in my time, required two years of pre-medical studies before applying. I was accepted into the Medical School in the fall of 1941. Because of the war, our year was the first to be accelerated. In the end, we were the only class to graduate early, and then we only gained six months! The class graduated in November, 1945.

Our class was made up of sixty people (four women and fifty-six men). All first-year students were interviewed by our Dean (who happened to be Professor and Head of Psychiatry as well) who did the psychiatric assessment. He was very hard on the women. He told me that I would be a failure since I would be married before I finished, and that there would be no favours because my father was a Professor of the Medical School. This was my introduction to the first year.

In our first year, all students received a physical assessment, and those eligible were accepted into the Army Medical Corps with their way through school paid. Each received all benefits. I did not pass the exam because they found a healed adult TB lesion, so I was not eligible for the Army.

The four women in our first year were always being teased. We were not permitted to live in the same quarters as the men, nor share meals with them. We lived in a tiny apartment, and ate in the nurses' dining room. On the other hand, we all participated in as many activities as we could, such as running for class office, sports, etc. In our third year we received three more women and many more men from the University of Saskatchewan (their program only went to the end of the second year of medicine, and their students then went to the other programs at Manitoba, Alberta, and Ontario). I was fortunate to be voted in as Lady Stick in my last year, which was a valuable experience. After our early graduation, we sought our placements for the required rotating intern year.

Following my intern year, I completed and passed my exams, and stayed on for two years in internal medicine, which also included six months of pediatrics.

In 1947 following my marriage, I moved to Toronto and entered the first year of a three-year training program under the new Dean of Psychiatry at the University of Toronto, Dr. Aldwyn Stokes. This training took place at the Toronto Psychiatric Hospital, later to be called the Clarke Institute. I was fortunate to be able to complete the program, received the Diploma in Psychiatry, and won the University Gold Medal awarded for this program. I applied to write my FRCP(C), but did not get permission because my examiner, a well-known psychiatrist, told me I was pregnant and would not be starting work immediately. This was quite an experience to go through—another example of discrimination against females.

My husband was moved to Winnipeg. We were there for four years where I did part-time work. Then we moved to Vancouver in 1960. I obtained a position in the City of Vancouver Health Department with Dr. H. Gundry, Director of the Mental Health Program. Concurrently, I completed my Certification and Fellowship. At the Health Department, I worked in the various Health units and focussed on children, adolescents, and their families.

I was appointed to succeed Dr. Gundry. The Mental Health Program provided services to the Metropolitan Board of Health, and these experiences really came within the Metropolitan Board of Health, which was then comprised of the City of Vancouver, Richmond, Burnaby, the North Shore, and Simon Fraser Health units. I also held a clinical appointment at the University of British Columbia, Department of Medicine.

Our staff included full and part-time psychiatrists, psychologists, and social workers, all of whom focussed on families, children, and their mental health needs, etc. We worked closely with other agencies. The services were quite comprehensive for a while, but from 1987 on there was a deterioration in services. At the same time there were bed closures at Riverview and the planned closure of Woodlands. I was with the City of Vancouver from 1960 to 1981, latterly as Director of Mental Health Services. In 1981 I came to the North Shore Health Department to work as a sessional child/adolescent psychiatrist where I was a consultant until I retired in June 1993.

My hope has always been to work towards early intervention and, hopefully, the prevention of the mental health problems of children, adolescents, and their families. Such hope seemed to be possible in the seventies and early eighties. However, despite the fact that children are our hope for the future, it has been my experience that the (mental health) needs of children, adolescents, and their families really have never been a primary issue for the public, and especially for politicians at the various levels of government. Today we are witness to the results of this failure because their needs are greater than ever before.

DR. SHIRLEY RUSHTON

My training took place at the University of Newcastle-on-Tyne from 1952 to 1957. Following my training I did a rotating internship at the Orange Memorial Hospital, U.S.A. I then travelled across the U.S.A. by car and fell in love with Vancouver on a beautiful sunny day in July 1959. I worked a year as a Resident in General Practice at the Vancouver General Hospital.

Subsequently, I found an office on West Broadway with a Scotsman, Dr.

Bruce Singleton, and worked with him very happily for several years. When he left I joined Dr. Judy Hornung and her husband Dr. Frank Kalla, and worked with them at MacDonald and Broadway from 1970 to 1993.

It was a great experience for me and was only cut short by my husband getting an interesting job in Brussels, where we have been ever since. My husband is a forester and has always been very supportive of my career. We have raised a daughter and two sons (lawyer, paramedic, and computer wiz), with the aid of a wonderful German housekeeper Oma Wessels and her husband, who have been like grandparents to our kids as both my parents died young. Oma and Opa often moved in as we took holidays around the world.

I remember working hard on several committees for the British Columbia Medical Association, membership and the Sports and Recreation committee, for several years. I was fortunate to be the first woman Chairman of the latter committee. We had a lot of fun pushing Physical Fitness and trying to get one hour daily of PE in the School System. I was also a vice delegate for District No. 3.

My practice was partially geared to Sports Medicine, as I was very active in field hockey, playing on the National Team and acting as the Team Doctor for several years. I played for B.C. and was the Provincial and Local President, as well as being on the National Executive for a while. I was also active in tennis and skiing.

In 1971 I was a member of the Pan American Games Medical Team in South America, Team Doctor for the National Volleyball Team to China, worked at the Montreal Olympics, was a member of The Commonwealth Games Team, and looked after the Elite Tennis Team from the west in the eighties.

Maternity played a large part in my family practice; we all worked long hours but enjoyed it very much. I was also active in the Federation of Medical Women, being the local President for a while.

We all worked very hard balancing family life and work, and it was a struggle, particularly if one of the kids got sick.

Here in Brussels, I have been able to work because of my British licence and have been doing some family practice out of our home. We have been impressed with the standard of Belgian medicine.

Curriculum Vitae

Advanced Education: 1952–57: Medical School: University of Newcastle-on-Tyne, England.

Medical Practice: 1958: Royal Victoria Infirmary, Newcastle, England. Six months of internship. 1958–59: Orange Memorial Hospital, New Jersey, U.S.A. One year internship. 1959–60: Vancouver General Hospital, Canada. One year family practice residency. 1960–92: Family Practice (own private office), Vancouver, Canada. Standard general practice including obstetrics, one-to-one counselling, workshops on relaxation techniques, and hypnotism.

Appointments: 1963–70: Canadian National Field Hockey Team. Team doctor. 1971: Pan American Games. Member of Canadian Medical Team. 1978: Commonwealth Games. Member of Canadian Medical Team. 1980–86: Planned Parenthood British Columbia, Canada. President (two years) and Board Member. 1983–88: Canadian National Tennis Centre, Vancouver, Team Doctor.

Personal: Birth date: February 24, 1934.

Place of birth: Leeds, England.

Nationality: Canadian and British.

Married; one daughter (29), two sons (26 and 25).

My husband is a forester employed by Canadian Pulp and Paper Information Centre- Europe, in Brussels.

1961

DR. BARBARA ALLAN

I was born in Vancouver, British Columbia, grew up in the Dunbar area, and attended Queen Elizabeth Elementary and Lord Byng High Schools. During my school years I belonged to the MacMillan Fine Arts Club (founded by Miss Marjorie Agnew, a counsellor at Vancouver Technical School that was named after Sir Ernest MacMillan). Music played a large part in my school activities during those years, especially piano. I won prizes in the British Columbia Music Festival, Welsh Festival, and in the Royal Conservatory of Toronto exams. At age fifteen, I completed the degree as solo performer from the Association of Royal Conservatory of Toronto (ARCT). I taught piano and theory to neighbourhood children.

A musical career was suggested by teachers, but I decided to pursue other interests, which led to undergraduate studies at the University of British Columbia majoring in Sciences, with minors in English literature, German, and Art courses (the highlights of those years).

Acceptance into the first year of Medicine at UBC followed in 1954. There were sixty students in the class, including five young women. Two of the women withdrew after their first year. The three of us remaining continued our studies and graduated in 1958. During the medical student days, I was not aware of any specific examples of prejudice of discrimination, although in retrospect I realize that both were present. On the whole, we were accepted and treated well.

He came in to see his patients that morning, dressed in his morning suit, en route to the House of Lords.

After receiving my MD from UBC, I interned at St. Paul's Hospital, with the intention to do General Practice. However, during my next year of training as a Resident in Internal Medicine at Shaughnessy Hospital (at that time a division of Veterans Affairs Hospital), my long-time interest in the brain and nervous system anatomy and physiology was stimulated by my few months of experience in the Neurology Service, headed by Dr. Charles Gould, and also staffed by Drs. David Jones and Norman Auckland, all of whom were superb teachers. The following year I interned as Neurology Resident at Vancouver General Hospital with the same neurologists and two other excellent neurologists Dr. Ludmilla Zeldowicz and Dr. S.W. Turvey. The combination of clinical neurology and access to neuro-anatomy and neurophysiology led me to decide to proceed with training in Neurology, with plans to complete requirements for FRCPC and practise Neurology in Vancouver. The thought of leaving the sea and mountains was not acceptable to me, except for short periods for further training.

Following a few months of General Practice locums, it was clear that General Practice was not what I wanted to do. During these years, I investigated places where I might go for further training in Neurology. I was very much influenced by many of the clinicians who had taught me, who had done their neurologic training in London, England, at the two 'meccas' for Neurology, Queen Square and Maida Vale Hospitals. Despite recommendations by the Vancouver group that I should obtain my Canadian fellowship before going to London, I left Vancouver having completed the two Residency years in Neurology. I had no job and no training position to go to, but after a few weeks as a clinical clerk at Queen Square, I was appointed as Resident Medical Officer (equivalent to our Chief Resident's position) at Maida Vale Hospital, the sister hospital of Queen Square. The Chief at that time was Sir Russell Brain who was known and respected for his writing of the textbook *Diseases of the Nervous System.*

The job was exciting and the consultants were outstanding. The hours were long and there was little time off, but nevertheless, I was able to indulge my musical and artistic interests at superb performances at Covent Garden Opera House, the Festival Hall, Wigmore Hall, and many small concert venues.

During my first few months in Maida Vale Hospital, Sir Russell Brain was named a Baron in the Queen's New Year's Honour List. He came in to see his patients that morning, dressed in his morning suit, en route to the House of Lords. I was uncertain how to address him, but he quickly advised that I should now address him as Lord Brain.

Shortly after my appointment at Maida Vale Hospital in London, I managed to get a ticket to the opera at Covent Garden. The performance was Beethoven's *Fidelio*, conducted by Klemperer, with the outstanding Belgian soprano Rita Gorr in the lead role. It was a thrilling performance. I was alone, not knowing anyone who would go with me then, because the long work hours allowed for little socializing. When the performance ended, I could not stand the thought of getting on a bus or going into the underground to get back to the hospital. It was late and very dark and foggy. Having come from Vancouver, I was used to fog and thought little of it. I decided to walk home, with *Fidelio* very much in my mind. Outside the opera house, I passed the people setting up their fruit and vegetables for the Covent Garden Market which would open in the early morning. I kept on walking with this incredibly beautiful music playing in my mind and soon was frightened by footsteps following behind me. When the footsteps picked up their pace, so did I. Then there was a voice—"I'm a London bobby, miss, may I help you? Do you know where you are?" By this time, the bobby was right beside me, which was just as well because I was in a state of near collapse! He asked what I was doing in this district, which did not look very desirable to me as I plodded on. He said this was no place for a young lady to be, and I told him I had just been to the opera and was so overwhelmed by the performance that I did not want to ruin it by being squashed by the throngs on a bus or an underground train. A sermon about such unwise behaviour was then gently delivered. He asked if he could show me the correct way home, and I of course delightfully accepted his offer. By this time, it was very late and the fog was pure pea soup. As we approached the hospital, he slowed his pace and said, "I'll leave you here, miss, but I'll watch that you get to the entrance of the hospital safely. You'll not want anyone to see you arriving home by a police escort!" I thanked him profusely and his parting words were, "Please don't go walking alone at night in London, no matter how marvelous the performance is!"

Another marvelous experience was attending the annual family dinner of the Apothecaries' Guild, held in a hall in Fleet Street where Shakespeare's *Cymbeline* was first staged. I was invited by one of the senior consultants, a delightful gentleman who happened to be a Wagner fan. He had attended many Wagnerian performances in Bayreuth, which to me was fascinating, as one of my ambitions, then and now, was and is to go to Bayreuth where Wagner built a theatre specifically for the performance of his operas. A musical bond developed in short order after my appointment to the hospital, and this led to the invitation to the guild dinner. Shortly after receiving the very beautiful engraved invitation by mail, I got a telephone call from his secretary, who said she just wanted to be sure the invitation had come and, "By the way, it is customary for ladies to wear above-elbow gloves." This was a very formal affair, and I was in big trouble, as my entire wardrobe was sitting in a trunk on

a dock in Quebec, where a strike was going on at the time. All I had to wear was what I could bring in my suitcase, and that did not include anything resembling a formal dress or gloves of this type. Furthermore, I had very little money, having not yet received my first paycheque.

The cheque came a few days later. Its arrival coincided with a trip, via ambulance, to Queen Square, to the National Hospital for Nervous Diseases, where I had to look after a young man with respiratory distress due to Guillain-Barre Syndrome. Once the patient was settled in the other hospital, the ambulance drivers asked if they could take me back to Maida Vale Hospital. I said that I was hoping to go to the Bank of Canada at Trafalgar Square to cash my cheque (so that I could buy my gloves) and then take the underground to the hospital. They kindly offered to drive me to Trafalgar

I instituted in British Columbia the use of Methadone, a powerful narcotic analgesic, as an alternative to morphine and its congeners with success.

Square and back to the Maida Vale Hospital. After I withdrew the cash I ran back to the ambulance and they drove me to Maida Vale at high speed with siren blasting. They delivered me in time to meet my chief Sir Russell Brain, who was just arriving to do his afternoon rounds. I, as Resident Medical Officer, was expected always to meet him for tea. Upon meeting me in the courtyard, he said, "And who comes to meet *you* when you arrive at the hospital?"

The guild dinner was an exciting experience. I hoped that I had been an acceptable dinner guest, having practised proper use of my above-elbow gloves when eating.

Approximately two years after my training in London, I returned to Vancouver to complete training for the fellowship requirements. In 1964, I obtained the FRCPC (Neurology) qualification and began private practice in January 1965. During the ensuing years I was appointed Clinical Professor of the Department of Medicine, Division of Neurology at the University of British Columbia; Consultant in Neurology for the B.C. Cancer Agency; and Active Staff to G.F. Strong Rehabilitation Centre. In the past fifteen years, I was in charge of the Pain Clinic at the B.C. Cancer Agency (Vancouver Clinic), with appointment to Active Staff in the Division of

Medical Oncology. All of these appointments involved much teaching and many lectures on pain diagnosis and management.

Because of injuries sustained in a boating accident in 1996, I closed my clinical practice and resigned my appointments at the Cancer Agency. However, I have continued a certain amount of committee work and medical-legal work, which I find fascinating. My work at the Cancer Agency was extremely demanding and very challenging. During those years, success in cancer pain management was limited, to some extent, by the few treatment options available and also by attitudes of some physicians and patients about the use and abuse of narcotics. Much of my time was spent not only in the diagnosis and treatment of pain, but in education. I instituted in British Columbia the use of Methadone, a powerful narcotic analgesic, as an alternative to morphine and its congeners with success. Methadone was particularly useful in patients with severe cancer-related pain, who were either allergic to morphine and its congeners, or those who suffered prolonged and intolerable side effects of the morphine group of drugs. A very satisfying aspect of Methadone is that it is not equianalgesic to the morphine group of drugs. It can be used in a much lower dose than the apparent equivalent dose of morphine, thus eliminating many of the very troublesome side effects of morphine and its congeners, when high doses are required to control pain.

On the personal side, I am married to a surgeon who retired early to study philosophy. He and I share musical and artistic interests—he having served on the Board of Directors of the Friends of Chamber Music, and I of the Vancouver Recital Society. I was Board President of the latter Society for a number of years. We have one son who is trained and actively involved in computer work. For the past twenty-five years, we have enjoyed our time at the small island paradise Hernando Island, situated about 100 miles north of Vancouver. For over thirty years we have cherished the companionship of Harlequin Great Danes, and have bred two female dogs with success, allowing us to continue the line and keep a pup or two from each litter, on each occasion.

I have thoroughly enjoyed my years in training and in practice, and would not hesitate to do it again, were it not for the abysmal state of affairs in our health system at present.

DR. JANET HALLEY

I always wanted to practise medicine as far back as I can remember. When I was about nine or ten, I had a friend from France who called himself "Froggy." He often addressed me in his cards as "The Future Doctor." When I left school I had an altercation with the headmistress, so she did not give me a reference for medical school. For a back-up, I did a three-year stint as a laboratory technician and wrote the exams required for my applications.

Both Aberdeen and Liverpool Universities accepted my applications. My uncles and cousins had gone to Aberdeen, but I chose Liverpool as I could reduce my expenses by living at home. So I joined the gang in 1953. There were a hundred medical students in our year, twenty-five being female. A few of both sexes dropped out at the difficult exam of 2nd MB.

It was a good time: we worked hard and played hard. I was on the Fencing team for the university. I remember two incidents that made me wonder how I had passed. The first was when in our *viva voce* on Anatomy, I had the misfortune of having the Professor of Anatomy as my inquisitor. He asked me what I had identified in the spermatic cord. I replied, "Well, you have the vas deferens, you have etc, etc." After a few minutes he turned his baby blue eyes on me and said, "Well, Miss Halley, I hope I have." The second incident was in the Pathology final when I identified the large muscle contained in a pot as the gastronemius. When I was asked if it wasn't a bit too large, I said, "You haven't seen mine, Sir."

On qualifying, I didn't want to wait for people to die off before I could climb the ladder. I investigated the career possibilities for women doctors in Canada as my aunt lived in White Rock, B.C. I found that the Vancouver General Hospital had medical reciprocity with the United Kingdom, and if I did a rotating internship I would be accepted in both countries; whereas if I did my house job in England, I would have to do extra training in Canada. I came straight out to Canada, taking the required exam at the end of the year.

I soon experienced cultural shock when I noticed the greater gender inequalities in Canada, the different names for common drugs, and the accent. There was one such occasion when I told a consultant in a gynecological seminar that I could not understand his accent after he had asked me a question four times. A stunned pause followed before he announced that he did not have an accent, whereas I did.

Differences in attitudes between Canada, the U.K., and U.S.A. regarding women in medicine amused me. In the U.K. women doctors were treated with respect and formality; in Canada, less respect and less formality. Once I attended a convention in Miami. I was virtually ignored at the introductory cocktail party because I had arrived late on a Friday night and did not receive an ID tag. When I received my tag the next day, the reception I got was like night and day. It had been thought I was a nurse anaesthetist.

I had promised my parents that I would return to England after a year, so I took a position as a Junior House Medical Officer at my local hospital, but I couldn't stay away from Vancouver. After nine months I returned to VGH to start the course in anaesthesia, then went back to England for eighteen months to continue my training in anaesthesia. In England, we used the Liverpool Method, a technique to administer anaesthetic by giving large doses of curare and hyperventilating by hand with nitrous oxide and oxygen. It worked very well and no patient ever woke up. The United States tried to emulate the technique, but the anaesthetist did not sit at the end of the table squeezing the bag furiously for six months of training, so some of their patients did wake intra-operatively. Also, the British surgeons were extremely quick. Only in very major operations did we put an IV in, usually just a Mitchell needle to have a line available. I stayed in England long enough to take my Diploma in Anaesthesia before emigrating for the third time. It was difficult leaving family and friends, but I knew I wanted Vancouver as my permanent home.

Life was good, sailing in the summer and skiing in the winter while honing my anaesthetic skills. At VGH I hypnotised a small boy with a fractured arm as the surgeon was late. I gave him a very light anaesthetic, much less than the usual dosage. Then at Mount St. Joseph I had an opportunity to try my skills on a mentally-challenged woman who could not have a general anaesthetic. However, I had to give up because of the impatience of the surgeons; and it was not practical to start a pre-op clinic.

I did not have the problem of bringing up children as I had only a little Chihuahua to care for, and when I married, I was already ensconced at Mount St. Joseph Hospital. I did miss the excitement and challenge offered at VGH as I got involved with some of the administrative aspects and lecturing, giving the CPR course, and doing committee work. I had taken a course in hypnosis, and was thinking of going abroad for further training, but I preferred to marry.

When we started cataract surgery at the hospital, most of the ophthalmologists allowed the anaesthetists to give the blocks. The patients were usually older, and the nurses would tell me how good I was with them, and how the patients had found me very gentle—a good boost for the old ego. Technically I was good with the needle. One paramedic said, "Gosh, she can even get a vein in a dead person." Over the years I received many accolades from patients, which was interesting to me since they just saw me pre- and post-op, not knowing what went on in-between.

There are always interesting incidents in a hospital setting. Once I was called out at 3 a.m. for an abdominal emergency. The surgeon asked me to put down a Levine tube and when I went to do so, there was one already in his throat and it wiggled in the forceps; it was quickly noted to be a very long live worm, mistaken as spaghetti from lunch!

I enjoyed the new technology when computerization came in, but did emphasize to the younger generation that machines could fail, and that the eye, the hand, and the art were basically more important. It is said the practice of anaesthesia is ninety-five percent boredom and five percent panic: do not believe it. My career in anaesthesia has certainly proven the opposite!

DR. VIOLET LARSEN

Dr. Violet Larsen graduated in Medicine from the University of Alberta in 1940 and practised in Saskatoon. She enrolled in the post-graduate course in Anesthesia at UBC in 1954, and completed training in Regina. She practised both in Saskatchewan and British Columbia for many years.

Dr. Larsen died in 1970.

DR. MAGDALENE SARA SCHMIDT LASZLO

Magdalene Schmidt was born in Nagykanizsa, in southwest Hungary in 1925. At the Gymnasium (high school) she studied several languages including Italian, Latin, and German, but no English. Her mother was a teacher. The only school in Magda's home town that taught English was one run by the Catholic nuns. The war was part of Magda's girlhood when the Germans invaded Hungary in 1944.

From the Gymnasium school she went directly into medical school in Budapest, graduating in 1950. There were 100 in her class, half of them women students. She interned for a year and was assigned by the government (who controlled the placement of medical graduates) to work in a sanatorium for tuberculosis patients. Magna was married and had a daughter, Shari. Life was difficult with the Russians now occupying Hungary. She divorced in 1954, then married George Laszlo, a structural engineer, who had recovered from tuberculosis. The revolution in Hungary in 1956 was terrible, and although the Russians won and things were better after the revolution, many people decided to leave Hungary, escaping to Austria. Magda and George decided to join those leaving and try to get permission to go to the United States or Canada. Since neither spoke English they decided to leave Magda's daughter, whom George had adopted, with Magda's mother until they became financially able to look after her. They were accepted as immigrants to Canada in 1957.

Magda and George were landed immigrants for five years, struggling to learn English and working at menial jobs in Vancouver, British Columbia. Then George got a job with the railway in Nelson, B.C. in charge of constructing warehouses. Magda was hired in nearby Castlegar as a radiology technician, and continued her studies for the LMCC exams. People were kind to them.

They returned to Vancouver when George decided to study at the University of British Columbia, where he received a Master's degree, while Magda worked in a nursing home. Finally Magda was accepted to intern at Shaughnessy Hospital 1959–1960, and at the Royal Columbian Hospital for the obstetrics requirements. After getting her license, she registered with the College of Physicians and Surgeons of British Columbia in 1961.

Magda and George were now able to have their daughter, Shari, come to Canada from Hungary. In no time she learned English and became a typical Canadian schoolgirl. Over the years Magda had returned three times to Hungary and had brought her mother to Canada for a year. Her mother decided to return to Hungary as she found it too difficult to learn another language at her age.

Magda first began practising by doing a locum for Dr. Rosarina D'Amico for a year, making use of the Italian she learned in school in Hungary. Next she started her own general practice in Burnaby and joined the staff of the Burnaby General Hospital. She worked in her busy practice full time until 1998. She continued in the practice of medicine by doing locums for doctors in the Burnaby area, in New Westminster, and in the Commercial Drive area. With few doctors available for locums she was in great demand. Her husband had died in 1985 of COPD (Chronic Obstructive Pulmonary Disease).

Magda was a tennis player and routinely played at least once a week. She is an expert photographer and has made videos of her travels, including one to the Galapagos Islands when several women MDs and some spouses from British Columbia travelled there after a Pan-American Women Doctors' meeting in Ecuador. She is active in the B.C. Branch of the Federation of Medical Women of Canada.

Magda has survived another difficult time and has shown her wonderful spirit to enjoy life again. She suffered a stroke affecting her right side in December, 2002. With great medical care and attention she is walking with a cane in her penthouse apartment in Burnaby and is able to drive her motorized wheelchair to Metrotown to shop! She can now spend more time with her daughter and three grandchildren.

DR. JOY C. LONGLEY

I entered medicine at the University of British Columbia in 1956 following a B.A. degree with majors in chemistry and zoology. At that time, the class quota was sixty students of which six were women. I married Dr. Donald Longley, a second-year resident in radiology at the Vancouver General Hospital, at the end of my first-year of medicine (1957). We had met over a cadaver in my first year when he was demonstrating in anatomy. This fact led to a myriad of family jokes, as you can imagine. We lived in an apartment on West 10th Avenue, right opposite the Venereal Disease Clinic and the Tuberculosis Wing. Although our parents were appalled, we were delighted, as it meant that we were close enough to the hospital that we did not have to sleep in residence and were able to see one another once in awhile.

At this time—at least in the west—women students in medicine were still very much of a novelty. Nurses, generally, were particularly welcoming, whereas the male response ranged through barely concealed hostility (residents so desperately overworked that their only view was that a woman could not possibly hold her end up), condescension (from general surgeons and orthopods who, with vast quantities of testosterone, delighted in trying to shock us and demonstrate that we could not possibly do their job), and gallantry (mainly the older doctors who did not know what to make of us but were polite and paternal). In fairness though, I would have to mention that there were many excellent doctors who accepted us for our own merits and went out of their way to teach and help us in any way they could.

I graduated in 1960 and began my internship at the Vancouver General Hospital in June of that year. I shall never forget those twelve months of internship. The quota of interns for the hospital was sixty, if I remember correctly, and there were only twenty-four of us. We had to cover the general wards, plus the infectious disease hospital, health centre for children, maternity, emergency, and the relatively new 500-bed Centennial Pavilion. I think Emergency was everyone's favourite rotation because the shift was twelve hours on and twelve hours off. You actually could sleep!

All the other rotations required alternate nights, that was, you worked from 8 a.m. to 5 p.m., then all night, and again from 8 a.m. to 5 p.m., and if you were lucky you had that night off. It was beyond exhausting. We were divided to four in a group. I was the only woman in my group and the only member who did not require hospitalization during the year. When I was on the 8 p.m. to 8 a.m. emergency shift, there were times when no male orderlies or doctors were available, and so on Saturday nights, if we had trouble with rambunctious patients, a policeman would be suited and masked and designated to sit in the operating room to maintain order if he had to. There was one time I stayed in the operating room with a very gallant policeman all night sewing up lacerations after a major brawl with broken beer bottles outside the liquor store at Carrall and Hastings Streets.

The stipend at this time for an intern was about $98 per month, from which some $60 to $80 was subtracted for room, board, and uniforms. In those years, as now, interns were constantly subject to tests of physical endurance brought on by work overload and sleep deprivation. On top of this the emotional rollercoaster that we experienced through coping with the first death of a child, the continual fear of making a mistake, to the triumph of saving a life gradually developed in us a recipe for dealing with disaster. I remember well that towards the end of our year two interns in Montreal went on strike and were dismissed without accreditation—a punishment we could not bear, especially when we were so nearly finished! The following year saw the formation of a medical residents and interns' union, which, I understand, still struggles with these same issues. The hours required are still atrocious and would never be tolerated in any other field where people's lives are at stake. Perhaps by 2050, they will automatically treat interns for post-traumatic stress disorder.

Memories of my internship still remain vivid in my mind, but the one which I recall most often is when I assisted in drilling burr holes into the skull of a young university student who suffered from an acute subdural haemorrhage after a car accident. In the end, we had to drill ten holes in order to find the bleeder. Thankfully, today, because of the CT Scan, this scenario is gone forever.

My greatest achievement as an intern, apart from getting qualified, was finishing the year four months pregnant with twins. Ironically my last rotation was obstetrics and no one besides my family, the obstetrician, and my intern

Bill was wonderful at covering up for me at early morning rounds where I always stood at the back of the bunch if we had been up all night in order to 'nip to the loo' with morning sickness. Thankfully I was never tempted to take the thalidomide samples showered upon us by others at that time.

partner Bill, knew about my condition. Bill, who was a gem, had to be let in on the secret as we 'roomed together' during nights on call, since there was no separate accommodation for women. (This was true throughout the hospital at this time. Women did not walk into 'doctors' changing rooms without announcing themselves as some startling scenes as well as considerable annoyance might be encountered.) Bill was wonderful at covering up for me at early morning rounds where I always stood at the back of the bunch if we had been up all night in order to 'nip to the loo' with morning sickness. Thankfully I was never tempted to take the thalidomide samples showered upon us by others at that time. June 1961 saw the end of my internship year. I remember walking home from the hospital just after 8 a.m. in brilliant sunshine and marvelling that I had made it and a whole new life was beginning.

With twins expected in five months, full-time work in general practice did not seem feasible, and part-time positions were extremely rare. However, the Municipality of Burnaby was looking for a woman physician to do their Well Baby Clinics as well as some school readiness screening. They considered my pregnancy an asset, as my credibility with mothers would be greatly enhanced by my firsthand experience. This work was sessional, meaning that you did sessions of three-and-one-half hours mornings and afternoons, and were paid by the session with virtually no on-call work. There were no additional benefits, but it allowed me to use my medical training while still enjoying a family life. Thus began a career of some thirty years in public health.

Burnaby Municipality, in 1961, was a vast, underdeveloped tract of land which lay between New Westminster in the east and Vancouver in the west—a real transition zone between the two cities. Public transportation was poor with only a few routes available and doctors were scarce, with most families travelling to either city for medical advice. The baby clinics were a great boon to mothers. Most families did not have a second car and these clinics were set up in church basements and schools right within the area.

All mothers with new-borns were visited by a public health nurse within a week of discharge from the hospital and invited to come to the baby clinic nearest to their home for weighing and immunization. (Immunization included vaccines for diphtheria, pertussus, and tetanus as well as smallpox, and what a joy it was to have a vaccine for polio. While in medical school and during the internship, we had visited polio patients from the 1957 epidemic who were still in iron lungs. Each of us was also placed in the lung for a few minutes for the experience! At that time we had never imagined that this dreadful disease would soon become a rarity world-wide. At first we gave the injectable Salk vaccine, and then this was replaced in a few years by the oral Sabin vaccine given on a sugar lump. Another product which was just becoming available was the MMR vaccine for measles, mumps, and German measles.) Babies were routinely booked for a physical examination on their second visit to the clinic unless some problems or worries had surfaced earlier, in which case they would be seen sooner and an assessment would be made, which either ended in reassurance or immediate referral to their own family doctor. Occasionally I would make a home visit where the nurse had concerns and the mother, for whatever reason, was unable to attend a clinic.

The baby clinic work was very satisfying. The mothers were very appreciative of a woman practitioner who seemed to have time to listen, and the more I listened the more problems we were able to discover and bring about early intervention. In 1961 there were nowhere near the screening programs in place in the hospitals that we now more or less take for granted. As well, Burnaby seemed to be a transitional area for immigrant and migrant families passing through with children who had never been seen by any doctor following birth. As a result, almost any condition could and did turn up in clinics—failure to thrive, developmental delay, congenital hearts and hips, and neurological abnormalities were just a few of the conditions that came our way as yet undiagnosed. I like to think that our clinics spurred the area hospitals on to routinely screening for congenital hip disease, a condition which required early diagnosis in order to be treated. At times considerable diplomacy was necessary in referring patients to their family doctors. There was a tendency for parents to think that their doctor had missed something and for family doctors to feel that we were critical of their care. Over time, though, a really positive rapport was developed in the community, as parents realized that so many of these conditions were not present at birth, and family doctors realized that all cases were immediately referred to them for further evaluation and care if required. Not being able to treat the conditions found was one of the great frustrations of this work. However, I had to learn to take great satisfaction from having identified them and knowing that a goodly number of children were helped by my vigilance. This was the price of regular hours and the luxury of a family life.

At this time as well, I became involved with Dr. Henry Dunns' premature infant survey. All premature babies born at the Vancouver General Hospital, if their parents gave permission, were ultimately followed from birth through the early school years. Dr. Dunn was primarily interested in neurological dysfunction, but of course this work really honed my screening skills and helped to develop school readiness examinations. I think school readiness can be historically divided as "Before Sesame Street and After." The difference that the program made to pre-school children was astounding. Prior to "Sesame Street" we were very satisfied if a five- or six-year-old child could count to ten, repeat the alphabet, and identify a few colours. After "Sesame Street" it was not at all unusual to have a two-year old performing these tasks! I suppose the next huge step in the progression of learning will be before and after computers!

The school work done by the doctor was not nearly as simple as the screening done in the baby clinics. We did 'catch-up' immunization clinics, checked on injuries that might not be healing satisfactorily, saw children with physical complaints such as headache, fatigue, limp, etc; we were constantly on the alert for any illness which could be contagious, from lice and scabies to streptococcus and staphylococcal infections. Educational programs in general hygiene, dental hygiene, and nutrition were taught in the schools by the public health nurses. Sexual education was still the preserve of parents and religious teachers. Dental, hearing, speech, and visual services were available through the public health unit. We screened children for these problems routinely and referred to these services. However, a large part of the school doctors' role, particularly in the secondary schools, was one of trying to unravel economic, emotional, and family problems which were leading to school failure, early drop-out, and unsatisfactory behaviour. Child abuse was just beginning to be recognized. Although we had psychological testing available, we were very sadly lacking in counselling services and in residential psychiatric care for young persons.

Over the years the nature of our work gradually changed. Hospitals did more and more of the screening which had been done in the clinics, and as Burnaby grew in residential population, doctors became plentiful through-out the area to do immunization and the follow-up examinations which were so important in paediatric care. Our focus increasingly centered on the social issues of child abuse, parenting, sex education, dysfunctional families, and earlier intervention in recognized emotional difficulties.

The past thirty-some years have been a wonderful journey for me. I feel very fortunate to have been a part of the educational process and to have seen the amazing technological advances which have empowered us greatly in our fight against physical disease, rendering a large part of my work obsolete and enabling us to move on to other issues. I can only hope that these social issues would be resolved as rapidly as have been the more physical disease issues of my time.

DR. ANNE (PATTY) VOGEL

I was born on June 6, 1934, in Inverness, Cape Breton Island, and given the name Anne MacRae MacLeod. My older brother called me Patty for most of my life, so everyone else did too. My father was a GP surgeon and loved by his patients. I attended the local school (where students from Grades One to Three were taught in the same classroom) until I was thirteen when I was sent to a boarding school called Edgehill. I enjoyed my years there and learned some very good study habits. After finishing school I enrolled at Dalhousie University in Halifax intending to take a Bachelor of Science in Nursing. This was a new program that year which didn't materialize, so I just continued in a general science program. I did not consider medicine because in those days it was not something women did unless they really had unusual ambition, and I was just a good-time girl having fun. I loved boys, parties, and sports. After my third year in science I was engaged to a nice young man. He died suddenly that summer from bulbar polio. I was distraught, I felt my life was over, and I needed to throw myself into something that would consume my energy and give meaning to my life, something that would also make my father happy. My marks were good so I was accepted into the medical school at Dalhousie.

There were two other women in my class. This was considered a large number as most years there were none. After the first year, I recovered my spunk and began to enjoy life again and had a good time in medical school. I worked hard, but enjoyed extra curricular activities as well. After finishing my internship and graduating, in 1958 I married a young lawyer from B.C. During my final years, I was encouraged by the Head of Psychiatry, Dr. R.O. Jones, to study psychiatry. He arranged a place for me at the Maudsley Hospital in London. My husband also wanted to study in London, so we made plans to begin a new adventure.

Before leaving, we went to visit my parents and say goodbye. While we were there my father died suddenly. My husband left for England and I stayed with my mother for a few months and then joined him and started my studies at the Maudsley.

London was still recovering from the war and there was still a lot of bomb damage. Housing was scarce, luxuries were few, it was cold everywhere, and everything was covered in coal dust and soot. But the people were wonderful and, remembering the war, they wanted to be nice to young Canadians.

The exception was the Maudsley Hospital. They did not care for 'colonials' and I was not enjoying it at all, so when I was offered a job with the RCAF in Germany, I accepted it without any hesitation. For the next eighteen months, I worked in Germany and my husband studied in London, and we met on weekends in Calais or Dover. We had inexpensive holidays all over Europe. This was before the big influx of young travelling students and we were a novelty and very well-treated.

In late 1960, we returned by ship from Liverpool to Halifax, bringing with us our little Volkswagen convertible which we had bought for $1500. We spent a few days in Halifax and then set off in our little car to drive across Canada to B.C. It was now late November. We left Calgary and ran into a snow storm in the mountains but managed to make it to Cranbrook for the night. My husband had a friend who was a lawyer in Cranbrook. We arranged to meet him at a bar where the town's lawyers met after work and had a jolly evening. They all said, "Don't go to Vancouver, stay in Cranbrook, it's a great place to live!" We carried on to Vancouver, but after looking around for a few weeks we decided to go back to Cranbrook.

In those days, every small town in B.C. had only one clinic with a group of doctors who controlled things. A few towns had competing clinics and there was a lot of nastiness. The Green Clinic in Cranbrook accepted me; I cannot remember what the terms were. The other doctors were all old men, and I don't think they knew what to make of me. One thing they wanted me to do was to look after the two old people's homes, so I dutifully visited them regularly, but did not find that very exciting. I was very young and soon became pregnant. I did not want to go to one of the doctors I worked with every day for my maternity care (girls were still a bit shy in those days), so I picked a doctor from the clinic in another town. I was not aware that there was great rivalry between the two clinics. So here I was, young, pregnant and naïve, working as a GP in a small town in B.C., definitely an oddity. On the Friday before Labour Day of 1961, I said goodbye to my colleagues. They asked me when I would be back, and I said, "Oh, two weeks after the baby is born." I expected to have a month to get ready for this baby. Instead, my son decided to come early and was born on Monday, September 4th, Labour Day, after an easy labour. He weighed just less than six pounds. The day after he was born I received a letter from the Green Clinic saying, "Since you didn't consider any of us good enough to deliver your baby, we no longer wish to be associated with you." I was very angry. The Kimberley doctors who had delivered me said, "Come and join us." In the meantime, there was a growing discontent in Cranbrook with the Green Clinic, and I think that their treatment of me was the spark for developing a new and competing facility. All of this was chaotic as I had a new baby. A lawyer in Creston wanted my husband to go to work with him, so we left Cranbroook and moved to the farming community of Creston. We bought a farm, and I had two more babies. I worked part-time with a congenial group of male doctors and was still the only female physician in the Kootenays.

We stayed and worked in Creston for twelve years. I loved being a family doctor there. You grew to know your patients well; you knew their families and the fabric of their lives. You knew them when they were well, so it was easier to diagnose them when they were sick; you helped them to get well again and comforted them if they did not. As a woman, I brought a different perspective to things. I was the first person to prescribe birth control pills, I introduced sex education in the schools, organized the first Pap screening program, and got the local hospital to change the by-laws so that women could have tubal legations without their husbands' permission. I persuaded the older and well-respected surgeons to perform the first abortions in the

Kootenays, and I helped organize daycares and preschools. Those twelve years were a very happy and fulfilling time for me, and I was very sad to leave when my husband decided to move to Vancouver. I knew it was best to move as our son was now twelve and it was difficult for him growing up in a small town with parents who were a doctor and a lawyer.

When I first came to Vancouver, I was quite depressed for awhile, as I did not know anyone, and I missed my patients. I was not working and felt worthless. It was a good experience as I had never been in this situation before, and it made me a more understanding and compassionate person. After a short time, I began to enjoy my freedom, doing activities with my children and learning things I had not previously had time to do. After a few months, I decided I'd better get back to work. I remembered comments from my classmates in medical school: "You shouldn't be in medical school, you will just get married and have babies, and all the training will be wasted." My reply then was, "It's good I'm here or there would just be another dumb boy at the bottom of the class." Anyway, I was determined to not waste my training.

First, I started doing locums. It was quite interesting seeing different practices, some good and some not so good. It was very different from small town practice, and I did not have the same enjoyment from my work. My last locum was to cover for a lady who was on maternity leave for six months at CP Airlines. After I finished my term, my boss said I should talk to his wife who was a medical health officer in Vancouver and was looking for an assistant. I applied and got the job. I have been involved in the Public Health system ever since and I attended UBC and received a Master's Degree in Health Services. I spent thirty years in various positions within the Vancouver Health Department where I worked with a very collegial group of physicians and I enjoyed the variety. I was never bored as there was always a new challenge, a new program to develop to help people live happier, healthier lives. I retired in June 2004, just after my seventieth birthday. When I think back, it's been a very long life, but it has passed quickly. Time has never been heavy on my hands. I have had a wonderful life. I have cared about people, and they have cared about me.

1962

DR. NELLY AUERSPERG

Dr. Nelly Auersperg received an MD degree from the University of Washington and a PhD in cell biology from the University of British Columbia. She joined the faculty of Zoology Department at UBC in 1968 and became professor of Anatomy in 1974. Professor Emeritus of the Anatomy Department and Honorary Professor of the Department of Obstetrics and Gynecology at UBC, she is a cancer cell biologist who studies ovarian cancer, hoping to make discoveries that will lead to earlier detection of the disease.

A Research Associate of the National Cancer Institute of Canada since 1974, Dr. Auersperg was awarded the most prestigious award for cancer research in Canada in 1985, a Terry Fox Cancer Centre Research Scientist. In September, 1998, she received a three-year grant from the Terry Fox Foundation providing about $80,000 each year for her research. She and her colleagues were the first researchers to isolate ovarian surface epithelial cells, the specific group of ovarian cells that give rise to cancer.

Dr. Auersperg served in executive positions in learned societies, as President of the Canadian Society for Cell Biology, and Vice-president of the U.S. Tissue Culture Association. An Associate Editor of the *Journal of Biochemistry and Cell Biology and of Differentiation*, she has organized many symposia and conferences. She received a Lifetime Achievement Award from the Society of In Vitro Biology, the first scientific society that she joined when she started her independent research. The Society's former name, the Tissue Culture Association, had led to some amusing misunderstandings— at one time Dr. Auersperg was asked by a hotel clerk, while she was registering in a hotel to attend one of the annual Tissue Culture Association meetings, whether or not the organization sold bathroom tissues!

Many of the Society's members encouraged her in her work, including George Martin, George Gey, the creator of the HeLa cell line, Sergy Fedoroff, and Charity Waymouth. Dr. Auersperg has taught courses in tissue culture, and in 1993 she taught tissue culture methods to a group of reproductive endocrinology scientists and students in Beijing, China.

Dr. Auersperg was appointed ISD (International Society for Differentiation) Secretary-Treasurer in 1993. In that capacity she serves as the Chief Operating Officer of the Society. Her service to ISD includes organizing the sixth International Conference of ISD in 1990 in Vancouver and serving on the Board of Directors since 1991.

Dr. Auersperg's research centres on the cell biology of cancer. Her main contributions in this field are in three main areas:

The development of specialized human cervical cancer cell lines has contributed greatly to the understanding of the growth and invasiveness of this cancer. Currently, two of her cell lines are used commercially in test kits, one to detect papillomavirus in cervical cytology specimens, and the other to measure CA 125, a serum marker for ovarian cancer. Her work on cytogenetics of cervical carcinomas contributed significantly to the understanding of chromosome changes in early preneoplastic lesions.

The transformation of highly specialized cells with ras oncogene-carrying retroviruses and vectors. One of the most significant contributions of this work is the demonstration of the pattern by which changes in signal transduction and differentiation of ras oncogene-transformed cells reflect their developmental history.

The establishment of the first experimental system for the study of the normal precursor cells (ovarian surface epithelium) that give rise to epithelial ovarian carcinomas. This development made it possible for the first time to compare ovarian cancer cells to their normal counterparts, and to investigate early changes in ovarian carcinogenesis.

Dr. Auersperg is married with two children, a daughter and a son (who is a medical doctor), and three grandchildren.

DR. YANG-SHU HSIEH

Yang-Shu Hsieh was born on 17 July 1927 in Hangchow, China, a city well-known for its beautiful scenery and women. Yang-Shu was the youngest of the family, with one older sister and three older brothers. In her early years, she studied ancient Chinese literature and traditions, and later attended a Catholic school. She demonstrated herself to be ethical, intelligent, and physically fit since she was young. She enjoyed school, and in fact did so well she skipped grades, and at the young age of seventeen, entered Shanghai Tung-Nan Medical College. That year, 1944, she met her future husband Shou-Hsin, who was also attending the Medical College.

In early 1949, Yang-Shu and Shou-Hsin (with the permission of both of their families) joined a number of other university students in moving to Guangzhou to attend the National Sun Yat-Sen University Medical School. Later that year, they went to Taiwan. In that initial period, all communication with her family was cut off and it was a very difficult time. She completed her medical internship in Taiwan, and did specialist training at Taiwan Provincial Women's Hospital. She married Shou-Hsin in 1952, and had a son David in 1953.

In 1956, she came to Canada and worked at the Ottawa Civic Hospital, starting again as an intern, then completing her specialty training in obstetrics and gynecology and becoming a Fellow of the Royal College of Physicians and Surgeons of Canada. In 1958, she began a Research Fellowship at the Royal Victoria Hospital in Montreal.

Yang-Shu, Shou-Hsin, and David moved to Vancouver in 1962. Yang-Shu began a specialty practice in obstetrics and gynecology; Shou-Hsin worked as a specialist in anaesthesia. In 1965, she had a daughter, Dorothy Jeannette. In spite of being a wife and mother to two children, Yang-Shu continued her full-time medical practice. Over the next three decades, she remained in Vancouver, working at most of the hospitals in the city, but later, mainly at Grace Hospital and Shaughnessy. She worked at Mount St. Joseph's Hospital towards the end of her career. Over these many years, she had thousands of patients, and delivered over 10,000 babies. In fact, many of the mothers of these babies had also been delivered by Yang-Shu.

As well as attending to her busy practice, she was on the Clinical Faculty of the UBC Medical School, teaching medical students and residents in obstetrics and gynecology. She was given the Excellence in Teaching Award.

Yang-Shu began her practice at a time when it was not common for women to become physicians, and she was active in promoting and encouraging other women in medical practice. She served as President of the B.C.

Branch of the Federation of Medical Women of Canada. She very much enjoyed teaching, and felt that education was of great importance. To further that end, she and Shou-Hsin established the Hsu & Hsieh Foundation to assist overseas students to attend Canadian universities, and were planning to establish a scholarship in Yang-Shu's name for medical students.

Sadly, Dr. Yang-Shu Hsieh died of cancer on 7 September 1996, aged sixty-nine.

DR. PATRICIA KIRKWOOD JOHNSTON

Curriculum Vitae

Born: July 30, 1932.
Marital Status: Single.
Education: St. Margaret's School, 1943–1950.
Degrees: BA (Honours Bacteriology) UBC, 1954; MD UBC, 1960; CCFP, 1975.
Work Experience: Research Assistant, Department of Pharmacology UBC, 1954–1955; Research Assistant USC Medical School, Los Angeles, 1956.
Professional Experience: Internship, Victoria General Hospital, London, Ontario, 1960–1961; Family Practice, Victoria, B.C., 1962–1986.
Licensure: Ontario, 1961; British Columbia, 1962–present.
Positions Held: Chief of Department of Family Practice, St. Joseph's Hospital, 1973–74; President of the Victoria Medical Society, 1978–79; Medical Advisor, Pearkes Centre for Children, 1963–1985; Acting Medical Director, Queen Alexandra Centre for Children's Health, 1944–1995.
Professional Memberships: BCMA; B.C. Chapter of General Practitioners; College of Family Practice.
Hospital Affiliation: Active Staff, Capital Health Region.
Honours: Honorary Member of Victoria Medical Society; Honorary Member of Pearkes Foundation for Children; Listerian Memorial Orator, 1990.
Community Activities: University of Victoria Senate, 1984–1988; Member North and South Saanich Agricultural Society.

Hobbies: Gardening, photography, horse breeding.

Dr. Johnston was awarded Senior Membership by the Canadian Medical Association in 2001.

Dr. Pat Johnston writes: "The only thing I can think of to add is that I was the first female president of the Victoria Medical Society, which was remarked on numerous times by my male associates. I don't know if they felt that it was an unusual achievement for a woman or if they felt it was to their credit for voting for me!"

DR. BETTY WOOD
(1930–2002)

After completing Medical School at the University of Manitoba and an internship at St. Boniface Hospital in 1954, I began a Pediatric Residency at the Winnipeg Children's Hospital. From there I went to the Children's Hospital in Buffalo, New York, where I spent a year in Pediatric Pathology. Subsequently, I did a year at the Hospital for Sick Children in Toronto, and then a year at the Children's Hospital in Pittsburgh, Pennsylvania. By this time I had realized that Pediatric Radiology was the way I wanted to go, so I tailored the Pittsburgh year to six months in Cardiology and six months in Radiology. I then returned to Winnipeg to complete Radiology training and passed my specialty exams in both Pediatrics and Radiology.

Having obtained my exams in 1960, I accepted a position at the University of Alberta Hospital in Edmonton. This was to have been mainly Pediatric Radiology, but turned out to be mostly adult work, which was interesting but not what I had hoped. An opening came up in Vancouver at the Health Centre for Children, which was part of the Vancouver General Hospital, with 212 Pediatric beds. I accepted this position in December 1962. The X-ray Department consisted of one room which contained a very antiquated fluoro unit (a Roentgen original). There was no image intensifier. When one wanted to take a picture at fluoro, one had to pull the cassette over by hand causing the machine to shake, and s/he wouldn't be able to see what picture s/he was taking (I hate to think of the radiation it emitted.) Eventually, we had to transport the patients through the old tunnel over to the main X-ray Department in the Heather Pavilion where there was an image intensifier. It was several years before we got a new fluoro unit and a 2nd X-ray room. My office was set up in the doctor's cloak room, and I got many funny glances for a while as Pediatricians came in to leave their coats or to use the adjacent washroom. They soon realized who I was and why I was there, then kept dropping in to see the X-rays and to discuss their cases. When we got the 2nd X-ray room it went into my office, and I moved into a small area down the hill which was a converted bathroom. About this time Dr. Don Newman joined the Radiology Department, spending mornings at the old Children's Hospital on 59th Avenue and afternoons with me in Pediatric Radiology. Plans for the new Children's Hospital were advancing, and as the building started to take shape, we recruited Dr. Gordon Culham and later Dr. Olof Flodmark as our new Radiology staff. We moved into the new facility in June 1982. Dr. Helen Nadel later joined the group. It was then possible to have all plain films, ultrasound, CT, and nuclear medicine in the one area which facilitated better care and total assessment for patients. Growth of the Department continued and magnetic resonance imaging became a valuable tool. Working with the pediatricians, surgeons, and orthopods was a very satisfying experience. They appreciated our help and were keen to share the details of their patients with us, which made diagnoses a lot easier and more accurate. It was a great time in Radiology, and I am grateful to have been a part of it.

(Sadly, Betty died in 2002 from cancer. Her story was written in 2000.)

Curriculum Vitae

Born: May 20, 1930, Winnipeg, Manitoba.
Marital Status: Single.
Rank Obtained UBC: Associate Professor.
Undergraduate Education: University of Manitoba. Obtained MD 1954.
Special Professional Education: Internship: St. Boniface General Hospital, 1953–54; Pediatric Residencies: Winnipeg Children's Hospital, 1954–55; Buffalo Children's Hospital, Buffalo, NY, 1955–56; Sick Children's Hospital, Pittsburgh, Pa., 1957–58; Radiology Residency, Winnipeg General Hospital 1958–60.

Professional Employment Record: Radiologist University of Alberta Hospital, Edmonton, Jan 1961–Dec 1962; Radiologist Vancouver General Hospital—Health Centre for Children, Dec 1962–June 1982; Consultant Radiology Health Sciences Hospital, 1971–1979; Visiting Staff, Radiology, Children's Hospital, Vancouver, 1972–1982; 1st appointment at UBC 1963 as Instructor. Subsequently Clinical Assistant; Professor, Dept. of Paeds. 1965, then Associate Member Dept. of Paeds.; Assistant Professor Dept. of Diagnostic Radiology, 1972; Associate Professor Dept. of Diagnostic Radiology, 1980.

Professional Activities: B.C. Radiological Society, Past Program Chairperson; Pacific Northwest Radiological Society, past Secretary-Treasurer; Pacific Coast Paediatric Radiologists Association, past President; Canadian Radiological Association; Society for Paediatric Radiology; Radiological Society of North America, past counsellor; North Pacific Paediatric Society, founding member and past President; American Journal of Radiology past abstractor; Past Member Medical Board Vancouver General Hospital; Elected Member, Faculty Executive, UBC, 1979-1982; Chairperson, Radiation Control Committee, B.C. Children's Hospital; Secretary Medical Advisory Committee, B.C. Children's Hospital.

Publications:

Robinson G., Wood B.J., Miller J., Baillie. "Hereditary Brachydactyly and Hip Disease." *J. Ped.* 72:539, 1968

Lowry B., Wood B.J., Birkbeck J., Padwick P. "Cartilage Hair Hypoplasia: A rare and recessive form of dwarfism." *Clin Ped* 9:44, 1970

Mullinger M., Wood B.J., Kliman M., Robinson G. "Intramural Hematoma of the Duodenum: An unusual complication of small bowel biopsy." *J. Ped.* 78:323, 1971

Lowry B., Wood B.J. "Syndrome of Epiphyseal Dysplasia, Short Stature, Microcephaly and Nystagmus." *Clin Genetics 8:269, 1975*

Lwin T.O., Wood B.J. "Nitrofurantoin Lung." *B.C. Med J.* Vol 16, No. 8: p. 234, Aug 1974

Wood B.J., Robinson G.C. "Drug Induced Bone Changes in Myositis Ossificans Progressiva." *Ped. Radiol* 5:40, 1976

Lowry B., Wood B.J. "Multiple Epiphyseal Dysplasia & Turner Syndrome Variant Associated with Advanced Maternal Age." *Birth Defects.* Original Article series XIII:24, 1977

Wood B.J. "The Aspirated Foreign Body." *B.C.'s Children* 1:1, 1977

Rogers P.C., Wood B.J., Smith D.F., Teasdale J.M. "Slow Growth of an Untreated Wilms Tumor in the Adolescent." *Arch Dis Childhood 53:82,* 1978

Rowen M., Thompson J.R., Williamson R.A., Wood B.J. "Diffuse Pulmonary Hemangiomatosis." *Radiology 127:445, 1978*

Smith D.F., Sandor G., McLeod P.M., Tredwell S.J., Wood B.J., Newman D.R. "Intrinsic Defects in the Fetal Alcohol Syndrome: Studies on 76 cases from B.C. and the Yukon Territory." *Neurobehav Toxicol Terat* 3:145, 1981

Wood B.J., Newman D.E. "Fetal Alcohol Syndrome: Radiological findings." *BC Med. J.* 23:324, 1981

Tredwell S.J., Smith D.S., McLeod P.J., Wood B.J. "Cervical Spine Anomalies in Fetal Alcohol Syndrome." *Spine 7:331, 1982*

Newman D.E., Wood B.J. Chapter on Pediatric Radiology in *Focus on Clinical Diagnosis*, Eds. Burhenne & Li, 1985

Machan L., Pon M., Wood B.J., Wong A. "The Coffee Bean Sign in Periappendiceal and Peridiverticular Abscess." *J. Ultrasound Med.* 6: 487, 1987

Blumhagen J.D., Wood B.J., Rosenhaum D.M. "Sonographic Evaluation of Abdominal Lymphangiomas in Children." *J. Ultrasound Med.* 6:487, 1987

Southwood T.R., Degado E.A., Wood B.J., Petty R.E., Hunt D.W.C., Malleson P.N. "Psoriatic Arthritis (PsA) in Children." *Arthritis Rheum* 31: (suppl): 119, 1988

Chan K.W., Wood B.J., Johnson H.W. "Testicular Adhesion: A Potential Complication from Wedge Testicular Biopsy in Childhood Leukemia." *Medical & Pediatric Oncology* 16:366, 1988

Nadel H., Kirby L., Ed. Wood B.J. "Radiation Protection" Manual—Nuclear Medicine', *BCCH*

Silverthorn K.G., Houston C.S., Newman D.E., Wood B.J. "Radiographic Findings in Liveborn Triploidy." *Pediatric Radiology.*

MacLean J.R., Lowry R.B., Wood B.J. "The Grant Syndrome." *Clin Genetics* 29:523, 1986

Southwood T., Petty R., Malleson P., Delgado E., Hunt D., Wood B.J., Schroeder M. "Psoriatic Arthritis in Children." *Arthritis and Rheumatism* 32:1007, 1989

Albersheim S.G., Solimani A.J., Sharma A.K., Smyth J.A., Rothschild A., Wood B.J., Sheps S. "A Randomized Double-Blind Controlled Trial of Long-Term Diuretic Therapy in Bronchopulmonary Dysplasia." *J. Pediatrics* 115:615, 1989

Lowry R.B., Wood B.J., Cox T.A., Hayden M.R. "Epiphyseal Dysplasia, Microcephaly, Nystagmus, and Retinitis Pigmentosa." *Am J. Med Genet.* 33:341, 1989

Pike M., Applegarth D., Dunn H., Bamforth S., Tingle A., Wood B.J., Dimmick J., Harris H., Chantter J., Hall J. "Congenital Rubella Infection Associated with Calcific Epiphyseal Stippling and Peroxisomal Dysfunction." *J. Pediatrics 116:89, 1990*

Sparling M., Malleson P., Wood B.J., Petty R. "Radiographic Follow-Up of Joints with Triamcinolone Hexacetonide in the Management of Childhood Arthritis." *Arthr & Rheum* 33:821, 1990

Dimmick J., Wood B.J. Chapter in "Skeletal Disorders of the Fetus" in book *Developmental Pathology of the Embryo and Fetus*, Lippincott, 1992

1963

DR. DANICA MARIA BEGGS

I was the first child born to my twenty-year-old immigrant mother, in Schumacher, Ontario in 1937. She had just arrived in Canada from Montenegro with a husband fifteen years her senior only to become a widow when I was one year old. While she grieved and held me very close she was setting the groundwork for me becoming a doctor. I reasoned that doctors fixed people who were hurting, and as early as age three I decided that this was what I was going to do when I grew up.

When I was three my mother married a wonderful man who was kind and gentle. He assured her that he would love me as his own child and he did that well. I adored him. We moved west, first to the Yukon, then when I was seven to Vancouver. I grew up and lived in the same house with three sisters and two brothers until I was married. My mother respected medicine above all professions and was a driving positive force in our family. She awoke early every morning to be sure we all got up and were not late for school. Our parents valued university education so highly that all six of us have university degrees from UBC.

The Downtown Eastside was a place where I learned about the plight of people who lived in extreme poverty and the street lives of addicts and the mentally ill.

In 1958 after three years pre-med in Arts and Science, I was accepted to UBC Medical School. Receiving that notification letter is a high point in my memory. The feelings of elation and relief were explosive and are still vivid. I remember hugging my mother, lifting her and twirling her around in the kitchen, both of us squealing with joy.

In 1962 when I turned twenty-five I married a classmate, William (Bill) H.C. Holt, and we both interned at VGH. There were no co-ed residences at the hospital, so we lived across the street from each other, sometimes sneaking onto forbidden territory to be together. Bill went on to specialize in psychiatry, but after thinking about the various specialties I decided to stay in general practice with Dr. L.A. Patterson. Then in 1969, after seven years of marriage, Bill and I decided to change our lives and we amicably separated, then divorced without telling anyone for some time. It was the least stressful way we could do it because we both dreaded giving the news to our families. I was thirty-two and on my own for the first time in my life. The day I moved into my own apartment I felt as giddy and ecstatic as the day when I learned that I was accepted to Medical School. This was definitely the right move.

Marriage may not have been what I had hoped it would be, but neither was general practice. In a very large downtown clinic, I found that the few minutes I had with each patient were insufficient. The charts were often large and I had no time to review the patient's past history. This way of seeing patients was too stressful, very dissatisfying, and I wondered if there was a way to practice that would give me more time to think about each case.

I had been doing sessional work for the Richmond Health Department as a 'school doctor' performing hundreds of preschool medical and psychological examinations on basically healthy children about to enter the school system. I found that kind of work a challenge and totally delightful. My ideal wish was to learn how to help people prevent disease, and at that time in Vancouver, 1969, the only option I could see was to work within the Public Health system.

Once I had made my decision I was amazed at how easily I found a job. I was hired as Medical Health Officer II by Dr. G.H. Bonham with the Vancouver Health Department and spent the next thirteen years there, first in South Health Unit, then in the challenging North Health Unit which included the Downtown Eastside and Chinatown.

Being young, I wanted to 'change the system,' and to be in a position where I could influence changes in outdated bureaucratic policies and practices was interesting to me. One influence I did not initiate consciously was as a dress code trend-setter. I remember being the first woman to wear slacks to work and creating some interest to do the same amongst the nurses who were required to always wear skirts at that time. The school system would not let doctors or nurses address classrooms of children because we did not have teaching certificates. I was determined to change that and in the early 1970s introduced some of the first classes on such topics as normal anatomy, sexual education to prevent unwanted pregnancies and STD, and the dangers of smoking and illicit drug use. I convinced the Health Department to equip each community health nurse with her own otoscope, because calling a doctor out to look at the ear drum of every child who presented at the school nurse's office complaining of an earache was an inefficient use of physician time. I remember that many members of the nursing staff were pleased to expand their clinical examination skills, and that I enjoyed teaching them how to visualize the eardrum and what required a referral to the family physician.

The Downtown Eastside was a place where I learned about the plight of people who lived in extreme poverty and the street lives of addicts and the mentally ill. In 1979 after many exhaustive meetings with Human Resources, Health and community workers in an attempt to solve the 're-volving door' misuse of emergency services by 'hard-to-house' clients in the downtown core, I chaired a Task Force and authored the cost-analysis report to the B.C. government. This report was used to obtain $500,000 in Development Funds for the Triage Centre which accepts the extremely difficult to house clients. It has continued over the years and is still func-tioning today in 2003.

What I remember most about that time was that I had married Hagan Beggs the summer before and was now second mother to Morgan and Noah, age ten and eight, who lived with us. This was prior to computers, and our living room was covered with piles of paper as I sorted out the data on 174 cli-ents we were following over a three-month period. Our aim was to prove that not having a special facility to house and process these cases cost more than if one existed. For reasons of confidentiality all the data was coded with num-bers instead of client's names, and the data I needed was forwarded to me by one person, Margaret Davies of the Ministry of Human Resources. We were like-minded and decided that the two of us could make the government understand what was needed if we worked together, and we were right. The report was effective, and it further assured me that I was right to take the pro-ject in hand and just do it, instead of talking endlessly in meetings about what needed to be done while doing nothing. This task was not considered part of my job as Medical Health Officer, which meant that I had to spend hundreds of hours of my own time completing the report. My new husband was amaz-ingly supportive and gave me the space and time I needed to continue the work at home. He took all this in his stride, as did the boys.

To step back for a moment, in early 1970 I discovered Chinese medicine through Dr. Kok Yuen Leung. I was particularly fascinated by the practice of acupuncture. What in the world were they attempting to accomplish by stick-ing little needles in people? I invited Dr. Leung to staff rounds and had him demonstrate using a volunteer, a nurse who happened to be a major sceptic of "this nonsense." When her wrist pain was gone in fifteen minutes after one needle insertion in her forearm and stayed away so she could play golf, we were all interested. I remember asking, "What did that needle do?" I suspected that

he had numbed her sprained wrist by touching the median nerve, but he said that that specific point was called 'Pericardium 6' and by needling it he was tak-ing the pain away and stimulating the kidneys to remove the swelling in the sprained area. This was beyond my comprehension, but because it worked so dramatically I was hooked. I had to find out how he did it. I first studied with him, then with the Acupuncture Foundation of Canada Institute where I met chief lecturer Joseph Wong MD, FRCPC, PhD, who taught the neurological approach to acupuncture and continues to be the physician who has impressed me more than any other with his medical acumen. He has not only his degree in Chinese medicine, but also is exten-sively trained in Western medicine. I learned enough to assist at seminars instructing colleagues about acupunc-ture technique and theory, and met other physicians who were looking for ways to expand their treatment skills, which I found encouraging. A group of Vancouver physicians expressed interest in meeting on a regular basis to have acupuncture rounds, but there was con-cern by some in the group that our

The afternoon classes became very popular and the spectacle of as many as forty to fifty people practising the 'laying on of the hands' with each other created a stir amongst some of the more conservative members working in that building.

licensing body, the College of Physicians and Surgeons, might disapprove of us using this new modality. Not believing that this would be an obstacle, I met with the Registrar of the College to discuss our concerns and asked if we could use the College boardroom for our meetings on weekends. He agreed that it was a good idea and about time someone did something about acupuncture because the College had so many calls from the public. We could not have the boardroom because he thought his chambers, where we would have audiovisual equipment available for our presentations, would be a better place for the meetings.

As I learned about acupuncture myself, I started free community self-help classes at the North Health Unit every Friday afternoon teaching 'acupressure massage for stress relief.' The afternoon classes became very popular and the spectacle of as many as forty to fifty people practising the 'laying on of the hands' with each other created a stir amongst some of the more conservative members working in that building. Anne Ironsides from the Continuing Education Department at UBC invited me to start teaching these classes at UBC, and I did weekend workshops there several times a year for seventeen years, from 1979 to 1996. These classes were open to both lay and professionals alike, and because the concepts of acupuncture and oriental medicine were new to most of us, the mixed classes worked. I remember a scene in one of my classes when a dear friend who assisted me and was a professional actress from Los Angeles very confidently gave excellent psychological advice to one of my students. She was completely unaware that he was a prominent psychiatrist in town, so I listened with some degree of amusement and decided not to intercede.

The idea of treating the body as a complex whole including the physical, emotional, mental, and spiritual levels of functioning fascinated me.

Throughout each year I was invited to give seminars or weekend workshops to lay community groups or professional groups in B.C. on Preventive Medicine and 'self-help' approaches. The groups varied and included lectures to the general public, school counsellors, police departments, Mental Health Services workers, Ministry of Human Resources social workers, physiotherapy and massage therapy associations, and the UBC School of Nursing, to name a few. The curiosity people had about acupuncture was often used as the drawing card, which opened the door to discussing other issues regarding health.

I realized that I enjoyed teaching and dealing with such a wide cross section of the public.

As I dealt with groups of people, at times I wished I had a place to see certain people individually as patients. They were usually cases that I thought I could help if I had a private clinic set-up.

In 1982 I visited hospitals in a number of different cities in mainland China on the invitation of the Chinese Medical Association. This was the time when few North Americans had been allowed to visit China as yet, but Canadian physicians were very welcome because of the respect the Chinese had for Dr. Norman Bethune. Giant murals of his face could be seen in many hospitals across China. On the streets I remember the sea of blue and grey Mao jackets and bicycles everywhere. Had I not been married with a commitment to return to Vancouver, I would have loved to stay in China and work there for a while.

In 1983, after thirteen years as a community doctor, I wanted to try out my acupuncture skills in private practice. I decided to quit the Health Department, but was offered a leave of absence in case I wanted to return to my job. Moved by the gesture, I took the offer; however, once out on my own I found I could not go back. I started a solo practice and used only acupuncture and related techniques to treat musculoskeletal and neurological pain and dysfunction. My challenge was to use my western training to diagnose, then to work with German electro-acupuncture, and traditional Chinese acupuncture, soft or 'cold' laser therapy, and other related modalities to treat pain without using pharmaceuticals. It was extremely important to me to conduct this new practice appropriately and not to replace western medicine if it had a better treatment to offer patients. I would only see patients who were referred by their family doctors because I did not wish to do general practice, but wished to run a pain clinic.

My dear friend Dr. Frank McCaffrey offered me room in his pain clinic in Surrey, but I chose to stay in Vancouver. He had specialized in anaesthesia and after many years working in operating room settings, had started treating patients with pain symptoms, and using some of these alternative modalities in his clinic. Frank and I remained close friends until his death in February, 2003. As I write this I realize that I miss him more than I could have ever imagined. He was my friend and mentor and I could talk to him about any topic; healing, medicine, pain, life, mortality, death, and in his last days, our final goodbye.

Since I turned sixty I have slowly let go of my active practice, though I still do stick a few pins in my friends if they need a treatment. I always marvelled at how acupuncture motivated me to relearn my anatomy and neuroanatomy and to study 'functional' anatomy, which was not taught well in medical school. I integrated a great deal of knowledge about how human emotions relate to the physical body and how the mental attitudes and spiritual aspects of being influence health. The idea of treating the body as a complex whole including the physical, emotional, mental, and spiritual levels of functioning fascinated me, and I learned to use these new methods to give patients energy 'tune-ups' by balancing their meridians after having treated their specific complaints. It was a complicated and time-consuming procedure, but very effective in creating a sense of complete relaxation and well-being in the patient.

Looking back, I realize that my life always gave me what I needed to fill the gaps, the areas that seemed empty and dissatisfying. When I could not find a comfortable place in medicine after internship in 1963, there was Dr. Pat, as we affectionately referred to him, who did not discriminate against female doctors. When I needed to find a way to learn about preventive medicine, there was Dr. Bonham. When I needed to move out on my own to explore pain, degenerative disorders, and bioenergetic medicine, there was Dr. Frank, my mentor. When I wanted children but felt it was too late to have them 'from scratch,' along came a darling man with children and I fell in love with all three of them. In 1978 I had not met nor heard of many single fathers who were living with their children. I am now a grandmother; though I did not bear my sons I am grateful to their birth mother Anna for moving on so I could take over for a while. Now our grandchildren have two loving paternal grandmothers and we are all the richer for it. Our son Morgan has brought us a beautiful daughter-in-law Colleen and so far since 1997, Holden, the twins Lachlan and Bridget, and Ciaran. Our younger son Noah went on to complete his Master's degree in philosophy with honours and is still single.

I have a number of mother-daughter type relationships with younger women that I value greatly and that are extremely rewarding. Their daughters, all under age four, call me Gramma-D, and they are the ones for whom I sew designer costumes for dress-up. I have been told I should start a business designing Las Vegas type outfits for little princesses, but I suspect that will not happen. In order as they came are Anna, Bridget, Imajyn, Clara, and Indica, my little girls who speak the truth as they see it, threatening to keep me feeling young and in tune with life.

Retirement is a welcome but slow adjustment period in some ways. All the time that I used to spend working has somehow been magically filled up and I am still very busy. I have to plan carefully if I want to have periods of uninterrupted solitude. Happy and satisfied with my life, I am ready for what is next on the slate. I sense that I am not completely finished with medicine, and what shape it will take next intrigues me.

DR. BEVERLEY TAMBOLINE

Beverley Tamboline was born and raised in Vancouver, British Columbia. She attended the University of British Columbia, graduating with a BA (Chemistry) in 1953. Although at age five she had told her parents she was going to be a doctor, she did not go directly to medical school after receiving a BA but first spent three years working in UBC's Department of Biochemistry. Her choice of profession was somewhat of a surprise to her parents, as no one in either of the families was involved in health care. She graduated with an MD from UBC in 1960 at a time when the number of women in each class at UBC usually did not exceed ten percent, and often was less.

After her internship in Toronto followed by two years in Medicine at Shaughnessy Hospital, Vancouver, Beverley joined the small group of women then practising in the province. A brief time in general practice was followed by six years with the Provincial Mental Health Service before going to the Workers' Compensation Board of B.C., where she remained until retirement in 1997.

Between 1955 and 1975, she served in the Naval Reserve at HMCS *Discovery* in Vancouver, and was Principal Medical Officer from 1968–1975.

Outside practice, Beverley held several offices with the Federation of Medical Women of Canada, including Vancouver Branch President in the 1970s and National President from 1980–81. She also served as FMWC's representative to CMA General Council for three years prior to being FMWC president. She now chairs the Archives and Bylaws Committee, a position held since 1994, and also has served as an advisor to some of the National Presidents in the 1990s.

Beverley was the first Canadian to be elected President of the Medical Women's International Association from 1984 to 1987, having previously served as Vice President for the North America region for two terms before becoming president elect.

Her long association with the B.C. Medical Association has included being on the Board of Directors and serving on Committees. She also chaired the Section of Salaried Physician and participated in negotiations for that group. Currently, she chairs the Archives and Museum Committee.

Following retirement from HMCS *Discovery*, Beverley joined the Defence Medical Association of Canada, serving for a number of years as President of the Vancouver Branch. She was the first woman elected as President of DMA from 1981–82. In 1982, she was the second woman to hold the top office in the Vancouver Medical Association. She also was a member of the Medical Advisory Council of St. John Ambulance for many years.

A recipient of the Vancouver Medical Association's "Primus Inter Pares" award in 1987, Beverley was also named an officer of the Order of St. John in 1995.

A music lover, particularly opera, from an early age, she has served on the Board of Directors of the Vancouver Opera Association and now is a member of one of VOA's committees.

Since retirement, Beverley has been a volunteer at the Museum of Anthropology, UBC, and was president of the Volunteer Associates from 2000–01. She was the UBC Medical Alumni Association's President from 2000–03, and since then has been a *Newsletter* Editor. She also serves on a church committee.

Dr. Carole Guzman of Ottawa, President of the Canadian Medical Association in 1990–91, has described leadership qualities as: "vision, ideas, goals, passion, the capacity to inspire followers, and willingness to seize opportunities." Dr. Beverley Tamboline possesses all these qualities and rightfully deserved the honour of becoming a Senior Member of the Canadian Medical Association in 2000.

1964

DR. PATRICIA A. BAIRD

Dr. Patricia Baird was born in the United Kingdom and received her medical degree from McGill University in 1963. She did residency training in Pediatrics, becoming a Fellow of the Royal College of Physicians of Canada in Pediatrics in 1968 and going on to specialize in Genetics. She joined the Faculty of Medicine at the University of British Columbia and became a Professor and was Head of the Department of Medical Genetics at UBC for over a decade until 1989. Dr. Baird was the first female Department Head at UBC Medical School. During her tenure as Head, the department grew to have an outstanding reputation for combining activities in research and clinical care in an exemplary way. She was extensively involved both in developing services for patients and children with genetic diseases, as well as developing research in genetics.

Dr. Baird is the author of more than 350 papers and abstracts, and her research work has been in two phases. The first was a focus in the field of genetic epidemiology, and her contributions in this field are widely recognized. She has elucidated the distribution, natural history, life expectancy, and prognosis for several birth defects, and genetic diseases. Successful in obtaining grant support and extremely productive, she has made major contributions to the knowledge about the incidence, prevalence, life expectancy, and clinical course of Down Syndrome, neural tube defects, and congenital limb reduction defects, among other conditions. The information produced using the British Columbia population-based registry was published in prestigious journals and continues to be used widely throughout Europe and North America in counselling families and planning programs. The studies are widely known and cited; for example, her findings on genetic load in a population of more than a million consecutive live births has been widely quoted and is a landmark paper on the topic. The regard in which her academic research is held is evidenced by her invitation to be a charter member in the Canadian Institute of Academic Medicine—a category limited to fifty individuals in Canada who have made outstanding academic as well as clinical contributions.

Dr. Baird's second phase of work has been at the interface of the application of genetic and reproductive technology, and its societal and policy implications. She headed the Royal Commission on New Reproductive Technologies, during the course of which there were 300 researchers at some fifty institutions engaged in studies for the research program of the Commission. The Final Report of that Commission in 1993 has been very highly regarded internationally and is viewed by many in the interested international community as a landmark contribution to the field.

She has been a member of several national bodies, among them the National Advisory Board on Science and Technology, chaired by the Prime Minister; the Medical Research Council of Canada; the Standing Committee on Ethics in Experimentation of that Council; the Research Council of the Canadian Institute for Advanced Research; and the Ethics Panel of the International Pediatric Association, as well as being a member of the influential Ethics Committee of the International Federation of Obstetricians and Gynecologists Societies, which recommends the policy to its more than 100 national organizations.

Dr. Baird has been honoured as the Distinguished Faculty Lecturer, Faculty of Medicine, University of British Columbia (1989); has received the YWCA Woman of Distinction Award for outstanding contributions to health and education (1988); and was the Osler Lecturer for the Vancouver Medical Association in 1991. She received the Commemorative Medal (125th Anniversary of Canadian Confederation) for significant contribution to Canada and the community. She has received a DSc (*hon causa*) from McMaster University and D Univ (*hon causa*) from the University of Ottawa. She was awarded the Order of British Columbia in 1992. In July 1994, Dr. Baird became the sixth person and first woman to be given the position of University Killam Distinguished Professor at the University of British Columbia.

At the University of British Columbia, she has served on committees at every level, including being elected for the maximum of two terms (six years) to the Board of Governors, and being on the Search Committee for the new President. She has served in various capacities in the professional bodies of her specialty (Canadian College of Medical Geneticists, and the American Society of Human Genetics), in particular chairing for its first six years the committee that set standards for the evaluation of Centres of accreditation for service and training across this country. Dr. Baird chaired the Medical Research Council working group that developed guidelines for Gene Therapy in Canada, and was founding member of the Alumnae and Friends of MRC. She chaired the MRC Grants Committee on Genetics from 1982–87 and following this, was a member of the Council for several years.

Dr. Baird has been an invited visitor at many universities, both in Canada and abroad. At the Genetics 2000 Conference at the University of British Columbia, she warned the geneticists that "the aggressive commercialization of scientific research and the public's false expectation that genetic research will provide 'silver bullets' for complex diseases are the two biggest perils facing scientists in the coming years." She advised her colleagues "not to allow their ethics to be corrupted by biotechnology companies offering to use their work."

Patricia Baird, MD, CM, FRCPC, FCCMG, was awarded the Order of Canada in 2001.

DR. MARGARET ELIZABETH (LOVE) PATRIARCHE

Dr. Elizabeth Patriarche was born in Winnipeg in 1912 and graduated from Manitoba Medical College in 1936. She was one of three female interns at the Winnipeg General Hospital from 1935–1936. Although her ambition was to become a medical missionary in India, she was diverted by one of her teachers, Dr. William Boyd, into radiology, a field he predicted would require little night work and allow time for a family. After doing radiology at the Winnipeg General, the Children's Memorial Hospital in Montreal, and the Montreal Neurological Institute, she found that Dr. Boyd's assumption was far from accurate. She recalled with affection working part-time with Dr. Bruce Chown in Winnipeg and meeting Dr. Wilder Pennfield in Montreal during those years. She worked as a general practitioner and a part-time radiologist in Winnipeg before the Second World War.

In 1936 she married Valance H. Patriarche, a bush pilot, who joined the Royal Canadian Air Force and became an Air Commodore. Dr. Betty Patriarche and her growing family accompanied him to various bases, where Betty gave courses in family life, marriage counselling, and sex education in the RCAF Women's Division. After the war, her husband's duties in the permanent force took them to London and Washington. Although unable to practise abroad, Betty maintained her interest in medical affairs.

During the 1950s she gave a series of broadcasts for the CBC explaining medical matters to a wide audience. It was an experience that taught her, she said, to put medical terminology into lay language. When her husband retired she found herself again in practice, in Victoria now; and she has made outstanding contributions in preventive medicine, health education, and family therapy. Dr. Patriarche was probably best known as director and teacher of the Family Life Education Program for the Greater Victoria School Board from 1965 to 1972. She was also a sessional staff physician for the Greater Victoria Metropolitan Board of Health from 1964 to 1971, and in 1976 she published her book, *Family Life Education.*

Dr. Patriarche has been an active member of the Federation of Medical Women of Canada. She has been national secretary, editor of the newsletter and president of the Victoria branch FMWC, and was made an honorary life member of the Federation and the Victoria Medical Society. A Fellow of the Royal Society of Medicine in London, England, she was also a member of the Medical Women's International Association and became a Senior Member of the Canadian Medical Association in 1984. Dr. Patriarche was a Listerian Orator of the Victoria Medical Society, and was especially proud of her Silver Medal of Service awarded by the British Columbia Medical Association.

Dr. Patriarche and her husband had four children (one daughter and three sons) and several grandchildren.

Dr. Elizabeth Patriarche died on November 16, 1994. Her husband, Air Commodore Valance Heath Patriarche, predeceased her.

(Information was extracted from "In Memorium," section of the B.C. Medical Journal *of February, 1995, written by Dr. Frances Forrest-Richards, MD, who has given permission for this to be included.)*

DR. BETTY POLAND

Dr. Betty Poland was born in England in 1919, and was a graduate of the Royal Free Hospital in 1943 at the University of London. On completion of post-graduate training in Britain, Betty came to Canada and practised obstetrics and gynecology in Toronto from 1955 to 1964.

Following the family's move to Vancouver in 1964, she chose to pursue her specialty interest in prenatal development through research and teaching. Betty played an important role in the B.C. Planned Parenthood Association. She served on the special advisory committee, appointed by the Minister of National Health and Welfare, to advise on oral contraception and menopause-related issues. Her pioneering work, which was based on close collaboration with colleagues in Medical Genetics and Embryo-Pathology, helped to establish the place of prenatal diagnostic methods and genetic counselling in modern reproductive care.

From 1984–85, she was elected President of the Society of Obstetrics and Gynecology of Canada. She shared with her husband, Dr. Stefan Grzybowski, an interest in the international health field and service in developing countries, to which she brought her wealth of experience in family planning and organisation.

With great and apparently effortless skill, she maintained the delicate balance of a productive academic career with a full and active family life. She had three sons and a daughter.

She died in 1992, aged seventy-three.

(Written by Dr. Fred E Bryans, published in B.C.M.J. *Vol. 34, number 9, September 1992.)*

1965

DR. PAMELA ALDIS

Being a Woman in a Man's World
I have been asked to put into words my life as a female physician. When I started my medical career in 1959, there were still many hurdles for women to get over in order to survive and practise medicine with dignity. But let's go back to the beginning—when and why did I decide to do medicine?

After sailing to England from Australia at the end of World War II, I had a very happy childhood on a farm in Norfolk, where my father had a Jersey herd and several orchards varying from black currants to apples to pear trees. He also had quite a large greenhouse business that catered to Covent

Garden (a flower market in London) and Christmas markets, with wonderful large single bloom chrysanthemums. Starting from a very young age I earned pocket money by de-budding them.

I should have been a boy. I had an older brother, and of course we roamed across the farm. It was my duty, before the age of eleven, to shoot at pigeons that came to pillage the crop of kale that was grown for the cattle. My brother and I would be sent out to get a rabbit for dinner because England was still in the depths of food rationing at that time. Fortunately, we had lots of milk, and our parents also had chickens for eggs and meat. I used to love hiking around the fields and sneaking around corners, looking for unsuspecting rabbits and hares. On my eleventh birthday my parents allowed me to buy my first shotgun, a 410, which I still have to this day and use for grouse hunting.

Our herd was Jersey cows, and when the heifers were in labour, I would get called out to help my father, since my hands and arms were smaller than both my father's and the cowman's. It was not unusual to hear a rock hit on my window and cowman yelling, "Are you there?" Both my father and I would at once rise out of bed and race up to the calving shed. It was during the calving sessions that I realized what I wanted to do when I grew up. Once, having delivered a particularly difficult calf, I turned and looked at the mother as she lay licking her young one. I was stunned to see her sad, big brown eyes looking at me. She could not tell me how much we had hurt her. I could only see the relief she felt as she tried to get her calf to breathe and nudge it into standing. It was at that stage that I started to notice the importance of communicating clearly with whoever I was helping. I was somewhere between ten and twelve at that time, but I kept my mouth shut because there were very few women in medicine then. Furthermore, all the money we had was poured into my brother's education since he was to be the breadwinner in the family. I would, of course, just be expected to become someone's wife.

Perhaps that last statement is a little unfair, for my parents never discouraged me from pursuing higher education, though my brother did go to the boarding school and I the public school. My uncle, who was the owner of the farm running a seed breeding business, had made it quite clear that I, as a woman, was not welcome to go into his firm, even though my brother's scholastic abilities shone brightest in literature and history rather than agriculture. Even at that early age, I was upset and mystified by male beliefs that women really should stay at home, and I also realized early on that very few men could accept the idea of women having a career outside the domestic realm.

We left the farm when I was about fourteen. It was, indeed, a very sad day for me. I understood that my father had saved enough money to buy a small acreage for our family where he could build a bungalow. At the time of purchase, the property had two very derelict greenhouses, which he put back into order and subsequently built one-quarter acre of glass buildings on a two-acre property. He grew everything and anything that rooted in eleven days, which he sold as rooted cuttings, cash with order. I missed the farm, however, especially the opportunity to walk miles in the countryside, the solitude, the smells, and the animals. But I did not tell my family how much I missed the farm, and when asked what I was going to do when I grew up, I always stated that I would follow my father's footsteps and do horticulture.

In England, the system of education was such that at sixteen, one took

"Both your mother and I will back you fully, and we feel that we will hold the ladder firmly at the bottom, but don't be thinking that you can climb up and fall, climb up and fall. It's straight up to the top for you, or nothing. So go for it, kiddo!"

what was called the "O Level" exams, which were general examinations in as many different subjects as one was able to take. After that, one had to specialize in languages or science, with a view to entry into university. I knew that the Science program at our high school was pretty terrible. In fact, our Physics mistress could not even do the simplest physics experiment without obviously faking an end to prove it, which was why the experiment always failed with this particular instructor. Because of these shortcomings, I felt it might be difficult for me to take the advanced subjects necessary for entry into medical school. I also wondered what the principal of the school would think about my long-term desire to study medicine.

I was taking English, French, Latin, History, Geography, Mathematics,

Science, and my play one, Art, and it was just before "O Levels" when I decided to tell my father that I wanted to study medicine and did not want to do horticulture. He replied, "Well, you simply can't do that, because we can't afford two children going to University at the same time, and since your brother has to do National Service (i.e., enforced enlistment), that will put him two years back, and you would both be entering University at the same stage." He said he could probably manage if I studied a regular program at University, but he simply could not afford to keep paying if I went into medicine, which was a much longer program. I was completely shattered, of course. In fact, I think I probably had one of the worst temper tantrums in my life then, slamming the door out of the dining room, into the hall and my bedroom, whereupon I was hauled back and asked to close the door quietly. I certainly would never have dreamt of disobeying my parents, but I simply could not control myself at that time.

The next day after school, while I was doing my homework, my father knocked on my bedroom door. "Come in," I said, and to my horror he walked in and closed the door. This usually meant that I was in deep trouble, so I was quite frightened by whatever I was going to be told. His face burst into wreaths of smiles, to my surprise, and he said, "Well, if you wish to do medicine, I found out that with both my children having eight ordinary level subjects, you both should be able to get county major scholarships, and there is absolutely no reason why you shouldn't go to medical school—if you can get in. Both your mother and I will back you fully, and we feel that we will hold the ladder firmly at the bottom, but don't be thinking that you can climb up and fall, climb up and fall. It's straight up to the top for you, or nothing. So go for it, kiddo!" And off he went. I cried.

The next day at breakfast, there was this huge discussion about taking my "A Levels," which would have to be in Physics, Chemistry, Botany, and Zoology. I kept the Botany because if I could not get into a medical school, I could still do horticulture. It was a subject I gradually became fascinated with, having helped my father and mother, who both worked very hard in our nursery. My father, of course, phoned the head mistress and informed her that I wanted to take the four sciences at the advanced level, which were necessary for getting the admission into the second year of medicine. The head mistress stated that one of the very bright sixth formers was verging on

a nervous breakdown trying to do four "A Levels," and that I was not half as bright as she was. In fact, she really did not know whether I was going to pass my "O Levels"; I, on the other hand, knew I was going to pass them as I had studied very hard.

My father rose to my defence and pointed out that at the City College in Norwich, England, students taking four sciences at the advanced level was the norm, and that the college's well-developed Science program had attracted many bright foreign students. At this point, my head mistress stated that I need not ask her for a reference because she would not give me one. My father then hit the roof and said we would not ask for one then. Two days later she came back and said I could take four "A levels," but by that time I knew I would never pass Biochemistry and Physics with our terrible Physics instructor. So, off I went to Norwich City College, where we had excellent instructors and laboratories that were properly set up. We had some extracurricular time and I played a lot of tennis, both female doubles and mixed doubles, as well as lacrosse in the winter for the Norwich team. During my last year at Norwich, I sailed through all of my four "A levels," one of them at scholarship level.

But I digress. First of all, I had to get a place in medical school. How did a woman go about getting into medical school? I had made many inquiries about various universities, and I learned that each school had about one thousand applicants for one hundred places. Therefore, my chances were pretty slim. But then I did some mathematics and realized that if I applied to at least ten different medical schools, surely I would get into one of them. If each medical school accepted one hundred students every year, there would be one thousand students getting admitted into ten medical schools. So I figured my chances were good. I set about writing to ten different universities, including all the London Teaching Hospitals. I waited for the application forms to come in and filled out every single one.

Fortunately I got an interview at St. Bartholomew's Hospital, the oldest teaching hospital in London, established in 1123 A.D. The medical school was approximately one block away from the main hospital. It was separated by the Smithfield Meat Market, which was frequented by medical students, not to buy meat, but to stitch countless lacerations there. On the other side of St. Bart's was the Old Bailey, where we constantly went to skip classes and sit in the gallery if there was a particularly newsworthy case going on, such as the Christine Keeler, Mandy Rice-Davis (Profumo) affair back in the early '60s. We also watched several murder trials, and it was amazing how people told diametrically opposite stories after swearing on a bible. I never could understand how the jury ever sorted out those murder cases. Each time after hearing a trial, we would come away aghast and discuss the case with horror and fascination.

I want to mention what had happened at my interview for acceptance to St. Bart's. I was asked what I would do if I failed to get into medical school, and I replied that if this should happen, I could always fall back on horticulture since I was studying Botany. I said, however, that I had always wanted to do medicine since a very young age. To my extreme delight, I was accepted to St. Bart's. After I wrote my exams with great trepidation and passed them, I made arrangements to move to London. This was a very difficult move for a country bumpkin—I can assure you. My clothes made me stand out in a crowd, and I was not sophisticated. I liked to sit in the ditch to shoot pigeons and get my hands dirty in the soil. But I also liked people and wanted to help them, so I had to knuckle under and head for a life in the grimy city.

Life at St. Bart's
Life at St. Bart's was very intimidating. When I arrived, I went into a Catholic Hostel in Kensington because I thought it would be a safe place to live. I had to commute on the "Circle Line" (underground) for at least twenty-five minutes to get to St. Bart's every morning. On the first day of my arrival, I was horrified to discover that we were only the second intake of women into St. Bart's. The first intake of students was from Oxford and Cambridge, and had taken place six months earlier. Out of one hundred students in my group, there were only ten women. This was formidable for us as our Anatomy professor, in particular, absolutely hated women. He wore a winged collar with an extremely old bow tie, and he liked to make pointed jokes to put down all the women students. One had to learn to hold one's head up and laugh with the crowd so as not to appear a prude.

After two weeks of classes I was approached by a girl who introduced herself as Deanna. "Say, buddy," she said, "I've been reading a book on how women should get through medicine and I understand that one has to pick a pal, and I've been looking around for the last two weeks. You're the only person I think I could possibly pick to become a pal." The idea of having a "pal" was that one should have someone to work together with, studying the books and the bones, throwing questions and making up cue cards to ask each other about various topics when riding on the train or at odd times when there were no lectures. "I saw that you were riding on the Circle Line and I'm on that line, so we could co-ordinate trains in the morning and do quite a bit of work during the train ride. Also, the idea is that both should study hard all week and then spend one evening together and throw the books and bones or whatever at each other so that we could study and make sure that we pass the tests. If you've noticed, they really have it in for us women, so we have to work very hard to make sure that we don't fail anything all the way through school." Wow, I thought, this woman has really got it together. It sounds like a great idea. So I said, "Certainly, I'd love to give it a try, but I live in a hostel so I wouldn't be able to invite you to my place." She said this was no problem, and that I could go to her house once a week and we would have our brush-up sessions there.

The consultants in our hospital were like gods to us. When they came into the room, the routine went like this: we all stood up and followed them like a flock of sheep around the ward.

Well, I tell you. On my first visit to her home, we took the tube to Putney then a bus up Putney Hill, and hiked into a posh area with huge mansions on either side of the road. We walked down a driveway, and I said, "Oh my goodness, you live in quite a big house." She said, "Oh, well, I guess so." When we got to the door it was swung open by two of the little people. My goodness, I thought, these people have maids! Not only that, while the husband took our coats, the wife offered us a silver tray with a couple of gin and tonics on it. Oh dear, I knew I was really out of my depth. But, I was made to feel 100% welcome, and was taken in to be introduced to my pal's parents, who turned out to be Lord and Lady Layton.

Well, you could have knocked me over with a feather. They received me into their home as though I was a long-time friend. I was welcomed with open arms, and on several occasions they even entertained my parents, making them feel extremely welcome. Deanna and I hit it off very well and found that we could study together with lots of laughs. After that first visit, I think I spent at least one night a week at her house all the way through medical school.

Just to give you an idea as to how calculating we were in our studying—we had pulled out every single examination dating back to 1928, and had cue cards for the answers for every single question on each paper. It was surprising how often similar questions were posed over the years, and we discovered that there was only one new topic every year, which tended to be about new medical treatment. For example, when radiotherapy first came in it was the top question of that year. As chemotherapy and various other medical and surgical techniques kept advancing each year, Deanna and I simply focussed on studying these new techniques and knew them by heart. Therefore, to say that Deanna and I were prepared for exams was an understatement.

Now, thinking to myself, I'm not the brightest in the world. Which prize could I win? Well, I think I can win the Skins Prize (dermatology, to you and me).

As time went by, we became more accepted in our class and began to have a lot of fun. We certainly were good tennis players, heavily involved with representing the hospital against other clubs and playing both girls' doubles and mixed doubles for the hospital. I played lacrosse for London University and obtained a half-purple since lacrosse was only rated a 'half colour,' not a full colour as with rowing, rugby, etc. We also had fun starting a fencing school and a squash team for the hospital.

At Christmas, we always entertained the wards by putting on a skit. We rotated around each ward and our skit was expected to last somewhere between twenty minutes to half an hour. A barrel of beer was supplied by the hospital and travelled with us from ward to ward. At the beginning, our performances were slightly stilted and at the end, we thought our skit was very funny. I am not sure how funny it was, but everyone seemed to enjoy it and had a good time. Could it have been the beer? We gave up our Christmases in order to entertain the patients, and of course, the brunt of all the jokes pointed mainly towards the Sisters, the Pinks (who were the half-sisters or second-in-command), and the various consultants.

Of course the consultants in our hospital were like gods to us (we had to walk the wards for three years of our four-and-a-half years of training). When they came into the room, the routine went like this: we all stood up and followed them like a flock of sheep around the ward. The consultant would come in, say good morning to the sister, then to the crowd. The sister would then walk him around the ward. He would stop at the foot of a bed, turn to the medical student who had supposedly worked up the case, and say, "Tell me about this patient." The medical student would stammer out a few things, and the consultant would stroke his face and say, "Well really, really, what about this and what about that," leaving the medical student stammering.

Before going on, I should point out that the first year and a half of our training was strictly academic in the form of Anatomy, Physiology, Pharmacology, and Biochemistry. At the end of that time, we took an exam called Second MB, having been granted the first MB with our advanced levels exams from school. It was after these sets of exams that we graduated to 'walking the wards,' which was a three-year program. During those three years we did rotations in all of the departments—Pediatrics, Obstetrics, Surgery, Medicine, and the sub-specialties of Urology, Orthopaedics, Dermatology, ENT, and Gynecology. Our work usually ran from 8 a.m. until approximately 3:30 p.m., and there was one lecture everyday from 3:30–4:30 p.m. which was open to all the medical students who were walking the wards. These lectures were run on an annual basis and covered every topic that we needed to know in order to pass our exams.

If we attended every lecture for three years, we would have done the same lecture three times; but during the course of our education we were farmed out to various other hospitals to do extra medical and surgical training, and particularly, obstetrics and gyne training. For the first half of my obstetrics training I was lucky enough to be sent to Peterborough, a small Italian community just north of London. During this time my friend who came with me became ill, and I had to deliver one hundred babies in a month, alone. What a feat. I was exhausted.

The practice in Peterborough was divided between a proper hospital and a cottage hospital (housed in a converted Elizabethan manor), where all the 'normal' deliveries were supposed to take place. The former was for complications, twins, C-sections, gynecological surgery, etc. We lived in the cottage hospital, and had to ride a bike down to the other hospital to assist at surgery, attend rounds, and go to any emergency. Occasionally patients would be transferred from one hospital to the other at breakneck speed. The obstetrics was run mainly by midwives who had so much experience that they would merely look at the women's eyes, and say, "Call the Registrar," and we would know there was trouble. And they were always right.

As we were coming up to our finals, it became apparent to us, watching the girls who were a half-year ahead of us, that women did not get house jobs at their own teaching hospitals. There were very few house jobs available; only ten to fifteen students achieved a house job each year. The rest had to find house jobs at other hospitals. If one wished to get on in medicine and pursue a certain career, one virtually had to have a house job at one's teaching hospital.

By this time, I had become very interested in Ear, Nose and Throat work and wondered how I could get a job at St. Bart's. "Well," I said, "I better win a prize." Now, thinking to myself, I'm not the brightest in the world. Which prize could I win? Well, I think I can win the Skins Prize (dermatology, to you and me). And so, instead of putting my efforts into writing six or seven scholarship prize exams, I read and learned the Skins book backwards. Naturally, I won the Skins prize. I could not *not* win it! This accomplishment gave me a house job, and I was, in fact, offered the Ear, Nose and Throat house job. I loved the work. I got to do many sets of tonsils and assisted at some very interesting operations, like stapes replacement.

Indeed, when I started my work in ENT, my hand was so steady, I would often be the one who dropped the bone into place or repaired the drum using the operating microscope. Halfway through the six-month job, however, I began to develop intention tremor, and this was a nightmare for me, because my mother's intention tremor (and her brother's) was so bad that she could not pass a cup of tea across a table without nearly shaking it off the saucer. I had to do a lot of soul-searching, and realized that I might be chasing a moonbeam. I really didn't know where my intention tremor was going, but should it develop into one as severe as my mother's, I certainly could not do Ear, Nose and Throat surgery.

So, I decided I should head for general practice, and make sure I was at least of some use to society, having achieved my goal and become a physician. For this reason, I left the teaching hospital at the end of my house job and went down to the Royal Devon and Exeter Hospital to do a medical rotation (this being the custom in England in order to register). Exeter was an absolutely wonderful place to work, although extremely busy. We had very little time left to think about ourselves. We got into gear and we worked. I was lucky enough to be there in the spring, and I did get down to Steps Bridges, where the British poet William Wordsworth wrote his poem about the daffodils. As I sat there and watched these little wild daffodils "dancing and fluttering in the breeze," I felt very much like crying. The beauty that Wordsworth had written about years before was still truly present in England at that time.

It was about half-way through my rotation at Exeter that I decided I was going to 'save the world' and I would head to India first to do my 'saving.' Of course my father was horrified. Being very practical, and having been in Malaya as a rubber planter and caught in the fall of Singapore from which we fled as children, he said, "Don't be ridiculous, child, you can't save the world. At least start in a country where the climate is a little better and the people speak the same language, and see if you can get over the loneliness of being away from home and then travel on from there." I thought, "What does he know about it?" but as I thought harder I realized that my father was right, and I better take his advice.

So I picked Canada, which of course was his suggestion. He suggested western Canada, specifically Victoria or Vancouver, where he had visited and worked during his youth prior to going to Malaya to become a rubber planter. I applied to the hospitals in Victoria and the Vancouver General, and was accepted by the Vancouver General. I was told that I could go into a residency program if I did six weeks of pediatrics and six weeks of obstetrics. I later discovered that an intern at the Vancouver General had to have delivered five babies, and since I had already delivered a hundred in a month, I failed to understand the rationale! But I was in no position to argue, and I chose to re-do the internship year because the drug names and the style of medicine were totally different. Moving to Canada was a very big step in my life, and I was quite intimidated by the whole deal, especially when I came closer and closer to leaving England. I began to wonder why on earth I had chosen to make this move.

But wait—I forgot to tell the story about how I did my first 'stitch-up' while I was still a medical student in the Emergency Department. It went like this: I was on duty when a big, burly meat porter came in with a huge slash down his forearm. I was dutifully sent to stitch him up, since I had, by then, watched my sixth suture job, and arrived with the nurse who was in charge of the operation. Well, the man lay down on the table, and I withdrew some local anesthetic, having cleansed his laceration. After I had explained to him what I was going to do, I stuck the needle in to begin the freezing, then he suddenly let out a whole pile of expletives and whipped his arm away, whereupon I promptly passed out! This was humiliating, to say the least, as the patient leaned over the side of the table, and asked, "Where's the doctor gone?" Grey and green around the gills, I crawled off the floor and said to him, "Well you know, I don't like hurting people, and when I thought I was hurting you it made me feel really ill and I guess I just passed out." "Oh luv," he said, "that didn't really hurt that much! I'll be good this time!" Well, he was a honey. He sat there gritting his teeth, saying, "Oh luv, it don't hurt half! It don't hurt a bit! You ain't hurtin me nothin!" I got him stitched up, and was so happy when he gave me a great big hug and told me to come by for a leg-o'-lamb, anytime. Of course I never did go and get my leg of lamb, nor did I see the stitches come out, but the nurse in charge went back to Emergency in gales of laughter to recount the story of the green Dr. Pam lying on the floor.

"Oh, Pam, I've got bad news for you. The 'Old Boys' voted against having a female practitioner join in any of the groups, and that should you insist on working, they would not refer patients to your husband."

Canada

I flew to Vancouver and started to work at the Vancouver General the next day. My, Canada was prudish! We were segregated into a 'women's building' for lodgings, with a 'men's building' across the road. The men were only allowed into the living room and had to be out of the building by 11 p.m. It certainly seemed different to me as we, a group of graduated physicians, were treated like high school kids.

The next thing I realized was that I was way ahead of the rotating interns as far as history taking, physicals, and decision-making. In England, I had walked the wards for eleven years, and had done an additional year as a houseman. In our training we had had so much more experience with patients than what the North American training could offer. I was pretty bored, but was lucky enough to be on some rotations with various specialists. They soon noticed my boredom, and assigned me some more challenging tasks to perform.

In the winter I took up skiing and, as fate would have it, after my second time up Mt. Seymour, I got taken out by some avid idiot who knocked me off my skis. Unfortunately, I had actually torn my ligaments, and with no one in sight, I crawled up to the top of the hill and sat in the snow, hoping my buddies would come to search for me at the end of the day.

Driving down the mountain was certainly a nightmare. I spent a terrible night with my right knee swelling to the size of a football and the left the size of a baseball. Eventually, the orthopaedic registrar came to visit, and told me that I had indeed wrecked my knees. He arranged for me to meet with an orthopaedic specialist in the morning. I had an EUA and woke up with a huge cast from groin to ankle, having had my medial collateral ligament repaired. I was lucky that I had not got the meniscus or cruciate ligaments; however, the specialist suggested that I needed to be put on 1,000-calorie diet.

With my huge leg cast, I soon returned to work in order to get through my internship. After spending six weeks in the Outpatient Department, I finished my rotating internship and began applying for jobs. In the meantime, we each received a wonderful certificate presented to us by Dr. Lawrence E. Ranta, who was the CEO of the Vancouver General. I was shocked to find that all women interns were addressed as men in our certificates. And when I asked for a female version of the certificate, Dr. Ranta simply replied, "Well, nobody else has complained. What's your problem? You've got the certificate, you've got the year."

"Yes," I replied, "but I am not a him."

"Well," he said, "you'll just have to like it or lump it."

I told him that this certificate would never go up on my wall, and suggested that he should order some female versions for oncoming groups. It was a bit sad, however, that I could never put this certificate on the wall. It was a huge insult, but only one of many more to come.

Towards the end of my rotating internship year, I had decided that I would work for a year or so in Canada before proceeding on to 'save the world.' My parents were not remotely surprised, but they were a little sad that I was not going home to England. I applied to many advertisements, and it was extremely interesting to notice how, when I applied to practices that were run by men, nine times out of ten I would not even get an answer, not even a refusal, from the male doctors. If I had the gall to phone them up, they would say, "Well, we didn't think you would fit in with our practice. We're men, you know." When I pointed out that I could perhaps enhance their practice, I was simply told, "I don't think so." I do not think this had anything to do with me as a doctor, but with the fact that I was *female*, since most of these people had never even heard of me at that time, let alone met me.

I was offered a job in Kamloops and another in Kelowna, but I was also offered a job at the Seymour Clinic in Vancouver. Since I was quite enjoying Vancouver, the entertainment and sports, I decided to work in the Seymour Clinic. At that time, the clinic was kitty-corner to The Bay on the corner of Georgia and Seymour Street. I was the first female physician in the clinic, and I have to give everybody top marks for welcoming me into this group. I quickly became extremely busy, and was paid a straight salary, $750 a month! I soon realized I was lining the pockets of the partners. I expected to line their pockets to a degree, but felt that there should be some sort of incentive program. In the end, I did manage to get a somewhat inadequate incentive program started.

I worked a lot longer hours than most of the partners, and made them a lot of money. And my hard work was finally recognized by a practitioner in Emergency who offered me his practice (much to my surprise) during one holiday weekend. He must have thought that I was hard-working and capable enough to take good care of his patients. After I looked at his books and his office, I decided to buy his practice, including the equipment, and kept his nurse.

Throughout my ten years in Vancouver I worked very hard. I delivered up to 120 babies each year, became a member of the teaching staff for the family practice unit, and co-lectured on sexology to medical students as a joint team with my husband. As you can gather, I got married and had two

children during this period. My husband was an obstetrician and the itinerant surgeon for Courtenay, Comox, and Campbell River. After barely seeing my husband for several years and the children had gone from babies to Grade 1, my husband finally came to suggest that we should move to the Comox Valley where both of us could certainly make a good living, and our children would have more relaxed and happy lives.

So we packed and moved to Vancouver Island, and I was immediately approached by an ex-student of mine who asked me to fill his position in Comox for a year while he was on sabbatical. This was an absolute Godsend for me at the time, as my husband was planning to do consulting work in Courtenay, Comox, and Campbell River. When we arrived on the Island and got the children into school, this poor young man arrived on our doorstep one day and said, "Oh, Pam, I've got bad news for you. You could do my job for the year, but there was a meeting of the Medical staff last night and the 'Old Boys' voted against having a female practitioner join in any of the groups, and that should you insist on working, they would not refer patients to your husband."

This intervention was, of course, akin to blackmail, but we could not take it to the Medical Association because they would have said, "Oh, nonsense," and still not referred patients to my husband. One time, when I went to the hospital and asked for an application form to obtain hospital privileges, I was sent to see Sister Christine, who looked at me and said, "Well, how do I know you are Dr. Aldis?"

"Sister Christine," I said, "I have my references with me and I wonder, do you ask the male doctors this same question?" She did have the grace to blush and admit that she did not. It was a very cold reception, nevertheless, and slightly surprising, since this was a Catholic hospital and I thought they were supposed to be charitable and Christian.

But I have to tell you the physicians in Campbell River opened their arms and welcomed a female physician. I finally got work in Campbell River and could have worked there forever, but the commute from where we lived in Royston to Campbell River was rather onerous. After working in Campbell River for six months non-stop, I was offered two days a week at the Cumberland Clinic and three days a week out at the air base as a civilian doctor. This was a wonderful job, and I was extremely lucky to be able to get on some of the mercy flights with 442 squadron (Search and Rescue), even though the physicians working at the base found the flights somewhat *passé*.

I, on the other hand, was very excited about going in helicopters and being dropped down into God-forsaken places. I can remember one flight to the end of Bute Inlet where we went to pick up a crushed logger. As we were hovering over the dock and I was waiting to get strapped and dropped, one of the pilots said, "Don't hover right over the dock. You have to hover over the ocean, because should you lose power you would squish this doc on that dock!" To my horror, I realized that "this doc" was me! Of course, I also realized that if he had been hovering over the ocean and lost his power, I probably would have been decapitated by the blades, but I did not have much time to think about it at that moment.

Sometimes during our mercy flights, we would find that the Snowbirds had beaten us into town. Thus, we could not get into the base and had to do practice drops somewhere while they were flying. One day the pilot asked, "Would you like to be dropped onto the Glacier?" Well, it would take a lot to beat that experience. Another time, just as the kids were coming out of school, they decided to drop me into the field after circling around our house and taking some aerial pictures for me. This caused much merriment among the kids, of course, as they saw this wild woman whistling down the wire and dropping from forty feet, sixty feet, 100 feet and so on, practising.

I had a lot of fun working in the services, and became the Lt. Commander at the cadet camp for three summers doing sick parades. There were some hilarious stories from kids trying to get out of a day's doubling, an overnight sail, or hiking a mountain. It was amazing how they *all* had sick grandmothers whose kidneys were being taken out, or mothers who had just come down with pneumonia, or some such thing, and were terrified lest they would miss a phone call. I later found that what they really needed was a cup of hot chocolate, a night in bed, and they would be back on their feet the next day.

Around this time, I was approached by another physician who was taking a sabbatical. Since my arrival in the area, there had been three or four other women doctors entering the work force in the Comox Valley. Somehow the 'Old Boys' team could no longer veto my working. I was offered the job for a year and thoroughly enjoyed working in the group. Eventually I took

over, as the doctor did not return. Two of the original 'Old Boys' owned the building, however, and again told me that I was not welcome there. I really began to get a thing about 'Old Boys,' and wondered what my problem was, only to find that the nurses supported me 100%, as did the other two young doctors in the group. We were all told, however, that if they liked me so much, they could all move out with me. The nurses had no choice, of course, and neither did the other young doctors.

I decided not to be intimidated. I bought a house half a block down the road and set up my practice which I had purchased from a doctor whose charts were now officially mine. My patients would run up to the old office, pick up their chart, and run back with it. I have to tell you that I had fantastic co-operation from the nurses in the group, and have remained friends with them to this day. I also became good friends with the young physicians in that group with whom I often shared weekend calls.

It was of great interest to me that when the two 'Old Boys' retired, the young physicians refused to buy their building because the asking price was much too high, and the much-needed repairs would have cost far too much. In the end, the two old physicians were left with an empty office, which they had to sell some four or five years later at a tremendous loss. This turn of events gave me some small pleasure.

I am happy to say that I am now in a converted house working with a delightful young couple, who have recently purchased the house from me. Now, I am "the old renter." These days, I work three days one week and four days the next, and am completely enjoying my life. About ten years ago, at the age of fifty, I gave up Obstetrics and Emergency work. So life has become extremely easy for me. I have my office and hospital practices, and I also assist at surgery. I enjoy my work completely as I am turning sixty-one. I smile at the thought of probably working until I am sixty-five and accepting that everybody needs to retire, some sooner, some later. Who knows? Maybe I might retire sooner. This year is the start of my thirty-eighth year in practice.

Not everything turns out well in medicine, of course, and I remember the sad times too. There are the pacts you make with dying people in Palliative Care when they say, "Doctor, it's time now for you to let me go." There are the discussions and family consultations, when heroic measures have to be stopped and adequate pain relief given. This is a very sad part of our practice, even sadder when children die. As you get older, it is hard to see your patients whom you have known and looked after for twenty to twenty-five years dying.

There are also the times when bad diagnoses come in. After numerous sleepless nights and thrashing around, we often wonder if we could have caught it earlier or done something different. But I know this is all part of the process of ageing. All we can hope for is to grow old gracefully, and to have a wonderful retirement.

I think by now women in medicine are no longer discriminated against as much by other physicians since there are a huge number of us in practice now. However, I do find that I can be discriminated against by the public. For some reason, the public seems to think that we, women physicians, are unapproachable. I find this very sad because I believe we are like everybody else who needs just as many friends as one would want in all walks of life. We are doctors simply because we love this profession. We need to be accepted as friends for who we are, not for what we are.

I love my job, my life, my children, home, and pets. I would never consider a change of occupation. For me, life as a medical doctor has always brought tears of sadness and joy, but I regret nothing. It was a struggle, but women are totally accepted now and rightly so, for we have a different slant to offer people, and not everyone wants a male doctor.

DR. VIVIEN ELISABETH BASCO

Dr. Basco writes about her interesting career as follows:
The professional highlights that seem of most importance to me include of course the fact that we immigrated to Canada in 1964 and Dr. Max Evans—the Director of what was the B.C. Cancer Institute at that time—gave me the opportunity to work there. There was no vacancy as such, so I obtained what was called a Special Interim Certificate from the College of Physicians and Surgeons of British Columbia and worked without pay for a bit (I think not possible today)! After he cast a somewhat beady eye over me, he nominated me for the Shane Fellowship—$6,000 per annum—which I held until an additional position was created in 1966. This brought the establishment of full-time Oncologists to seven, together with two part-time Medical Oncologists and, I think, two non-specialist Clinic Physicians.

My initial clinical responsibilities were for children with malignancies, with Dr. Mavis Teasdale, as well as being responsible for patients when their Oncologists were away on up-country clinics. Around 1971 we recruited a Radiologist Oncologist who was a Pediatrician, and I changed my main area of interest to Malignant Lymphomas. I became Chair of the Lymphoma Group after Dr. Mac Whitelaw retired in 1974, and this group of diseases remained my focus until 1980.

In 1980 I joined Dr. Glen Crawford in the Breast Tumour Group and became the Chair in 1982, which I held until I retired in 1991.

My major research interest included the following:
Lymphography, which I introduced to British Columbia when I arrived, was mainly useful in the localization of the para-aortic lymph nodes in men with seminomas, staging in lymphomas and gynecological malignancies, and in some patients with melanomas of the lower limb. This procedure has been largely superceded by CT scanning and now I presume by MRIs, if the waiting list is not impossible.

I was involved in Clinical Trials with the NCIC in Hodgkin's disease and chaired the Canadian Stage 4 Study.

In the Breast Cancer area, I (along with Dr. Pat Rebbick and Dr. Urve Kuusk) did a historically controlled study looking at the comparability of local excision and radiation therapy with Modified Radical Mastectomy in British Columbia. Other studies we did looked at the place of radiation therapy following Modified Radical Mastectomy, management of chest wall recurrence following mastectomy, and management of lymphoedema.

In 1983 we joined the NCIC Breast Screening study for women forty to forty-nine and fifty to fifty-nine years.

When this was completed in 1988 we started the Screening Mammography Program of B.C., which was not only the first in Canada, but the first population-based program in North America. When we started, this program was unique, since with the blessing of the B.C. Medical Association, among others, women did not need a referral providing they gave the name of a Family Doctor to whom reports could be sent. (Some physicians were surprised to find that they were considered by a woman to be her GP even though they last saw her thirty years earlier when they had delivered her last child!) Another new aspect of the reporting was that the reports were also sent directly to the patients as well, which was much appreciated.

Administrative responsibilities included a spell on the Board of Directors of the CCABC in 1975–1976 as the Medical Staff representative, Vice-Chair and then Chair of the Medical Advisory Committee of the CABC from 1980–1983, which meant a second term on the Board. After I retired I became a Ministry of Health appointee to the Board from 1993–1998. Nationally I was on the Board of the NCIC from 1978–1984.

The four professional awards of which I am most proud are the Primus Inter-Pares of the Vancouver Medical Association in 1990, the Canadian Breast Cancer Association Award in 1991, the Order of British Columbia in 1991, and the award of the Terry Fox Lectureship and Medal by the BCMA in 1993. I have to state the obvious—none, or at least very little of this, would have been possible without the more than whole-hearted support of my husband. He was aeons ahead of his time in shouldering at least half of the work, problems, and responsibilities (as well as the joy!) involved in raising our two children. This despite being a Chemistry Professor at UBC all these years; in fact it was his job that brought us to Vancouver in the first place.

Our daughter, Debbie, is now a rural Family Doctor who seems to spend her time at the moment between Iqaluit and Sioux Lookout. Our son, Mark, works in Computer Science doing things I don't understand at all!

I could embellish with the sorts of experiences women of my generation had. One I liked perhaps least at the time, and became funnier and funnier as the years went by, was in England at the dinner they used to give to honour successful candidates at the Royal College of Surgeons following the Fellowship in Radiology. We were assigned seats and I found myself next to Sir E.S. from a Scottish Medical School who opened the usual small talk at this type of function by saying, "I suppose I should congratulate you, but I may as well tell you now that I have never appointed a woman to my department, and never will!"

Curriculum Vitae

Present Rank: Clinical Professor Emerita, University of British Columbia Faculty of Medicine / Department of Surgery (the Department of Surgery at UBC is the academic 'home' of Radiation Oncology).

Place and Date of Birth: Shrewsbury, England; July 23, 1935.

Marital Status: Married; two children.

Undergraduate Education: Birmingham University, England, MB, ChB, 1953–1958.

Special Professional (Internships, Residencies, Specialty Board Qualifications): Jul. 1958–Jan. 1959, House Physician, Newmarket General Hospital, England; Jan. 1959–Jul. 1959, House Surgeon, Newmarket General Hospital, England; Jul. 1959–Jan. 1960, Senior House Officer, Department of Radiotherapeutics, University of Cambridge; Jan. 1960–Aug. 1961, Registrar, Sheffield National Centre for Radiotherapy; Sept. 1961–Aug. 1964, Senior Pegistrar, Sheffield National Centre for Radiotherapy.

Specialty Board Qualifications: 1961, DMRT, London; 1963, FRCR, London; 1965, LMCC, Canada; 1965, CRCP, Canada; 1972, FRCP, Canada.

Academic awards and distinctions (prior to final degree): State Scholarship, England and Wales, 1953–1958.

Teaching, professional or research positions held prior to UBC appointment: Oct. 1964–May 1965, B.C. Cancer Institute Radiotherapy Fellowship; May 1965–Aug. 1966, Shane Fellowship, UBC.

Date of first appointment at University of British Columbia: 1969.

Rank at which first appointed: Clinical Instructor.

Subsequent ranks including dates of promotion: Clinical Assistant Professor, 1974; Clinical Associate Professor, 1981; Clinical Professor, July 1, 1988; Clinical Professor Emerita, Oct. 1, 1991. Principal University and UBC Department of Surgery teaching and service responsibilities over the last five years (including all university administrative positions; research/teaching administrative committees, honorary/associate appointment; lectures—undergraduate/postgraduate, continuing medical education).

Teaching—Undergraduate: 1979–1980, Breast Cancer, Anatomical, Clinical Correlation lecture to first-year medical students; 1977–1988, General Cancer lecture to second-year medical students; 1978–Apr. 1988, MSI. Co-ordinator, MSI Programme Radiation Oncology; Feb. 1981–1988, Director, Undergraduate Teaching in Radiation Oncology; 1977–Aug. 1991, third-year medical student teaching; 1985–1991, Systems Breast Examination, second-year students; 1985–1991, Lecturer, second-year radiotherapy technician students.

Teaching—Postgraduate: Aug. 6, 1987, Breast Cancer Seminar, Department of Surgery Residents; Dec. 10, 1987, UBC Department of Surgery, General Surgery Seminar Series; June 6, 1989, Victoria Cancer Clinic—Inservice, Review of Radiotherapy, Techniques in Breast Cancer; 1980-Aug. 1991, Family Practice Resident—lectures and clinic teaching; 1968–1991, involved in teaching of Residents at BCCA (clinical oncology).

Committees: 1981–Mar. 1988, Member, Department of Surgical Curriculum Committee.

Continuing Medical Education Lectures: Fall 1978, BCCA Continuing Education Meeting, Qualicum, B.C.; Apr. 1980, Cancer Course, Powell River, B.C.; Sept. 1980, Cancer Course, Nanaimo, B.C.; Feb. 9, 1991, Topics in Internal Medicine—Update on Breast Malignancy for Primary Physicians, Whistler, B.C.

Membership in professional and learned societies: B.C. College of Physicians and Surgeons—Honorary Member, 1992-present; B.C. Medical Association, 1965-present; Canadian Medical Association, 1965-present; Founding Member, Canadian Oncology Society, 1975-present; Canadian Society of Clinical Hypnosis, 1984-present; Faculty of Radiologists, London, England, 1963-present; Royal College of Physicians and Surgeons of Canada, 1965-present; Founding Member, Canadian Association of Radiation Oncologists, 1986-present; Canadian Association of Medical Education, 1987-1989.

Offices Held: Royal College of Physicians and Surgeons of Canada: Specialty Committee in Radiation Oncology—Nucleus Member, 1986-1990; Surgical Oncology Specialty Committee—Nucleus Member, 1989-1990.

Academic or professional awards and distinctions: Shane Fellowship, University of British Columbia, 1965–1966; Primus Inter Pares, Vancouver Medical Association, Mar. 15, 1990; Canadian Breast Cancer Foundation Award, 1991; Order of British Columbia, 1991.

Professional service and experience: Alberta Cancer Research Centre: Member, Advisory Committee, 1979–1984; Maxwell Evans Clinic: President, Medical Staff Advisory Association, 1979–1980; Executive, Medical Staff Advisory Association, 1989–1991; B.C. Cancer Foundation: Member, Research Committee, 1982–1988; B.C. Cancer Agency: Acting Head, Radiation Oncology, Sept. 1976–Mar. 1977; Radiation Oncologist, Sept. 1966–1991; Board of Trustees, 1993–present; B.C. Cancer Agency/Committees/Groups: Medical Staff Representative, Board of Directors, 1975–1976; Chair, Lymphoma Tumour Group, 1974–1980; Vice-Chair, Professional Advisory Committee, 1980–1982; Chair, Professional Advisory Committee, 1982–1983; Member, Medical Records Committee, 1985; Member, Clinical Investigations Committee, Nov. 1987–Jan. 1989; Vice-Chair, Investigations Committee, Nov. 1987–Jan. 1989; Member, Joint Conference Committee, 1984–1991; Chair, Breast Tumour Group, 1982–1990; Chair, Breast Screening Subcommittee, Breast Tumour Group, May 1987–1991; Development of Pilot Project and formation of SMP of B.C.; Member, Co-operative Osteoporosis Project Committee, May 1988–1991; Chair, Task Force on Education, 1988–1989; Canadian Breast Cancer Foundation; Board of Directors—B.C. Division, 1992–present; Canadian Breast Cancer Funds; Chair, Management Committee (MRC/NCIC/DHW), 1993–present; National Cancer Institute of Canada; Director, June 1978–1984; National Cancer Institute of Canada/Committees; Chair, Hodgkin's Disease Committee, 1971–1975; Member, Working Party on Haematological Malignancies of Cancer Research Co-ordinating Committee, 1974–1979; Chair, Advanced Hodgkin's Disease Group, Clinical Trials Section, 1976–1980; Member, Clinical Trials Committee, 1976–1980; Search Committee, Clinical Trials Director, 1980; Member, Terry Fox Liaison Committee, 1984; National Cancer Institute / Canadian Cancer Society; Member, Joint Professional

Affairs Committee, 1981–1984; National Cancer Institute / Health and Welfare Canada; Chair, Advisory Committee for Breast Screening, 1979-1991; Invited Lecturer / Discussant / Chair at many meetings across British Columbia and Canada, as well as U.S.A., France, and China; forty-nine are listed in her CV.

Research grants received as principal investigator include those from: B.C. Cancer Foundation (1984–85), for "Breast Tumour Studies"; B.C. Cancer Foundation (1985–86), "Breast Tumour Studies" continued; ICI Pharma Clinical Trial for Node Positive Post-Menopausal Breast Cancer Patients (NCIC) 1985–86, a grant given for two years.

Dr. Basco's CV lists dozens of publications, including chapters and abstracts for journals, as well as videotapes she has produced. She has co-authored with many doctors, including women colleagues—Dr. Gwen Ballantyne, Dr. Pat Rebbeck, Dr. Mavis Teasdale, Dr. Urve Ruusk, Dr. Linda Warren-Burhenne, and Dr. Ann Worth.

DR. VICTORIA BERNSTEIN

Curriculum Vitae

Education: University of Witwatersand, Undergraduate, 1962; University of Liverpool, LRCP (London), 1965; University of Liverpool, MRCS (England), 1965; Sefton General Hospital, England, Intern, 1965–1966; Shaughnessy Hospital, Vancouver, Resident, 1966–1968; Shaughnessy Hospital, Vancouver, Cardiac Fellow, 1968–1969; St. Paul's Hospital, Vancouver, Cardiac Fellow, 1969–1970; St. Paul's Hospital, Vancouver, Chief Resident, 1970–1971; St. Paul's Hospital, Vancouver, FRCP Internal Medicine, Nov. 1971; St. Paul's Hospital, Vancouver, Asst. Dir. ICU, 1971–1972.

University or Organization Employment: University of British Columbia: Teaching Fellow, 1971; Clinical Instructor, 1972–1976; Clinical Assistant Prof., June 1976–1981; Site, Director—ICU, University Hospitals, July 1981-June 1994, Clinical Assoc. Prof., 1984–1987; Clinical Prof., June 1987.; VGH & UBC Hospitals: Consultant Cardiologist, July 1994– ____.

Areas of special interest and accomplishments: Lipids; Heart Disease in Women; Hypertension; Ischemic Heart Disease; Cardiac Congestive Failure.

Courses taught at UBC: 1999, 2nd year Cardiology; 1998, 1st year Cardiology; 1998, 3rd year Cardiology; 1998, 2nd year Cardiology; 1999, 2nd year Cardiology.

Continuing Education activities include Grand Rounds in towns of British Columbia and in Departments of VGH, speaking at Seminars, Continuing Medical Education lectures, Post-Graduate Symposiums, as well as chairing a Canadian Congress in Cardiology in Vancouver and being a Visiting Lecturer at Dalhousie University Cardiology Course. Dr. Bernstein was the principal investigator for many research projects receiving grants from 1994 to the present. As Guest Speaker she has travelled all over British Columbia, the United States, Argentina, Czechoslovakia, the Canary Islands, England, and Italy; she has been the Guest Speaker on the Art Hister Show, CKNW many times.

Dr. Bernstein's awards include a Finalist Certificate at the New York Film Festival, a Gold Medal at the Houston Film Festival, and a teaching video on congestive heart failure won a Globe Award which represents the best in Health Care Communications worldwide. She was elected Prince of Good Fellow, Vancouver Medical Association, 1998, has published over forty journal articles and Conference Proceedings from 1966 to the present.

DR. MARGARET SHIRLEY NEAVE
(1910–1997)

Dr. Margaret Neave was born in Winnipeg on 3 December, 1910. She graduated from the Manitoba Medical College in 1934, a rare achievement for a woman at that time, and later studied pediatrics in England, graduating with honours in 1936. That same year, she achieved another goal that she had set for herself: climbing the 14,000-foot Jungfrau in Switzerland. She loved mountaineering and hiking, and met her husband Hugh on a climb in England; after their marriage in 1939, they enjoyed a lifetime of mountaineering together.

Throughout the Second World War, Dr. Neave lived in a cottage in rural Yorkshire and practised medicine there while Hugh fought in Italy and North Africa. Their daughter Felicity was born during the years of the British Blackout. In 1946 the family immigrated to Canada, and in 1949 they settled in Victoria.

Dr. Neave returned to medicine in 1959, when she accepted a position at the Manitoba School for the handicapped in Portage la Prairie. But she found the prairies too flat, and when, in 1985, she was appointed superintendent of the Tranquille residential school, the family moved to Kamloops. She stayed only five years, preferring work among the residents to administration, and believing that small group homes provided a better life for the handicapped than larger institutions. She devoted the rest of her life to caring for and assisting mentally handicapped people and children with learning disabilities, first in private practice and, following her retirement in 1980, as a volunteer and advisor for group homes. Dr. Neave was also a founding member of the Kamloops Child Development Society (1973), where she continued to make a positive contribution until her death.

Children gravitated to Dr. Neave, and she offered solid, caring support to hundreds of anxious parents, who responded well to her informed and realistic guidance. Years after her retirement, she was always well-informed and up-to-date in her medical knowledge.

Dr. Neave had a long-time dream of owning a Jaguar, and she finally acquired an XJ-6 in 1987. Even in her eighties, she loved to beat everyone else away from the stoplight. There was never a speck of dust on her car.

During her last few years, she struggled with Parkinson's disease, but despite her increasing incapacities, she was determined to remain in her home, and she never lost her concern for others.

Dr. Neave was predeceased by her husband in 1988. She died in her sleep on 27 June, 1997. On her final day, two of her grandchildren visited her and read her their report cards for Grade 2 and kindergarten. She is remembered as a well-known, respected, and much-loved physician in Kamloops, B.C. She leaves her daughter Felicity Ross and her husband David; Roland and his wife Anne; six grandchildren, and three brothers and two sisters. She will be sadly missed by many.

(This obituary was written for the BCMA Journal *by Margaret Horne, MD, and Roland Neave, of Kamloops.)*

DR. IRENE PUETZ

During internship in 1963 at the Vancouver General Hospital, Dr. Irene Puetz was interviewed by Nikki Moir of *The Province* newspaper. Dr. Puetz gave me a copy to print as the first part of her story. Dr. Puetz later became a very busy General Practitioner for many years in Richmond, B.C.

"There were fourteen children in grain farmer Puetz's family when daughter Irene left school at the end of Grade Eight to take a business course in nearby Humboldt, Saskatchewan.

"On June 15, 1963 Irene turned up at Vancouver General Hospital, having been accepted for internship there. Young Irene, who left school at the end of Grade Eight, is now Dr. Irene, a fully qualified medical doctor doing an internship at one of the continent's finest teaching hospitals.

"There was little help from home, naturally, so she worked in an office, took Grade Nine and 10 by correspondence, finally getting into Regina College for Grade 12. There, a kindly dean encouraged her to go to the University of Saskatchewan. Loans, good friends, working summers and Christmas holidays, and six years later Irene Puetz changed the Miss before her name to Dr. She chose one of the three most expensive forms of education in Canada. Ranking with medicine are dentistry and the law. Annual cost per student, according to Dominion Bureau of Statistics is between $2,050 and $3,465 (in 1963). Dr. Irene says of her struggle, 'I just carried on,' as though it was that simple. Her desire to 'help people' and a love for children steered her into medicine.

"Her years in college were fraught with penny-pinching. Every time it looked impossible a scholarship would come along. 'Don't stop,' friends and associates encouraged her. There was a summertime job as a medical secretary with the Grey Nuns in Regina; another stop-gap with a stockbrokerage firm.

"When she graduated from the University of Saskatchewan, there were four girls in a class of thirty-one students. In the last year, as the Medicare battle waxed hot and heavy in Saskatchewan, it looked for a time that students might have to pick up the balance of their education elsewhere. But the school went on, without any undue disturbance.

"With three other women doctors and a complement of thirty-one interns in all, Dr. Irene Puetz began internship on June 15, 1963 at Vancouver General Hospital. She has a room in the residence for women doctors on Heather. An intern gets $226 a month, less income tax, living allowance. As an intern she works from 8 a.m. to 5 p.m. and when on call can work an eighteen-hour day."

—excerpted from *The Province*, November 2, 1963

Dr. Puetz continues with her story:
During my year of internship I could not decide what field of medicine I wanted to pursue. That led to my decision to take a year of Residency at Shaughnessy Military Hospital. I registered for six months medicine and six months surgery.

Many people suggested, because I was a woman, that Obstetrics and Gynecology would be a good choice. I was not convinced. I liked surgery, but because that field was so dominated by men I did not stay with the thought of a surgical specialty. Many years later I thought that if I had to do it over I would choose Plastic Surgery.

While at Shaughnessy I met the man who would become my husband, Dr. Gwilym Evans. He had come over from Wales where he had worked in a number of fields of medicine and spent time at Shaughnessy while studying for his Canadian exams. We married and decided to go into General Practice in Richmond where we worked together for twenty-five years. Most of my practice was women and children, but I did have a few husbands of my female patients.

I recall that when interning, during my Residency, and during my first five to eight years of practice, the topic of 'women doctors' came up. A number of people did not feel truly confident to see a female doctor. It is interesting that as time went by we, as women doctors, became more and more sought after.

I enjoyed my busy General Practice. Seeing the children grow up, following the health and happiness of families, and being intimately involved in their lives was rewarding. I took numerous counselling courses throughout the years and used some hypnosis in my work. Interested in Palliative Care, I began to hold meetings of doctors and nurses in the early stages of planning for a Palliative Care ward in Richmond Hospital. After retirement I spent many years with the Richmond Hospice Association wearing many hats as fund-raiser, office manager, volunteer co-ordinator, and filling in where necessary. I had a special interest in bereavement counselling and spent many hours with bereaved clients.

I meet some of my former patients from time to time. It is nice to hear that I am missed and to get brought up to date on the grandchildren, marriages, travels, etc.

I feel very fortunate to have served the years I did as a doctor. When my husband, who had already worked for a number of years in Wales, suggested retirement I did not hesitate to retire with him. I miss my patient contact and often say that on my own I would probably have worked in some capacity till I was eighty years old.

1966

DR. MARGARET CARLSON

I first thought of medicine as a career when I was fifteen. My family was very surprised because no one had ever gone to university except cousins on my mother's side.

My father wanted me to go to university not so much to further my education, but because he thought that I might learn to meet people confidently and easily. He felt he did not have that capacity even though he did very well in his profession. At the age of fourteen, he ran away to sea. He moved up through the ranks of seamanship and eventually obtained his master's ticket and sailed Imperial Oil tankers on the east and west coasts of North and South America and on the Great Lakes. My mother was a nurse.

She was married before her final year of nursing school but was allowed to complete her course, which was an unusual occurrence in the mid-1920s. She did not practise after graduation. I had no siblings.

Time went by. I enrolled in the Faculty of Arts at the University of British Columbia, and in my final year I met Glen Carlson, a second year medical student. We fell in love and agreed that we would marry whenever we could find the time. I graduated with a B.Sc. in 1958, the first year this degree had been conferred by UBC. I was still thinking about medical school but made no move to apply for admission. I worked as a research assistant with Dr. Gordon Dower in the Department of Pharmacology, Faculty of Medicine.

During the year following graduation, I made up my mind to apply. Not only was my family surprised, but so was Glen. At first he was not happy about it at all, but after a few days of thinking, he told me that the decision was entirely mine and that he had no right to interfere. My parents were not particularly encouraging, but neither were they discouraging. I think they were really rather pleased.

I entered UBC medical school in September 1959 and did well academically in my first two years. At the end of my second year, when Glen was finishing junior internship at St. Paul's Hospital, we were married on May 27, 1961. Glen went into general practice with older colleagues in Burnaby, and I went to my summer job with Dr. Dower and then into third year. Having had atopic dermatitis, eczema, and neurodermatitis all my life, I began to feel the stress of medical studies and its effects on my skin and had to give up my year. I am sure most people thought I would never go back, but I finished my studies with the help of Glen and my parents. My marks suffered, but I struggled through to the end and graduated in May 1964.

Glen had not been happy practising in Burnaby, and during 1963 he began looking for an opportunity to do general practice in a rural setting. He decided to move to Merritt, a small community eighty kilometres south of Kamloops, between Christmas and New Year of 1963. I went with him, but returned to Vancouver to live with my parents until graduation. After graduation, I moved to Merritt but could not practise because I had not yet interned. In December 1964, in the depths of a very cold and snowy winter, we moved to Kingston, Ontario where I did my junior rotating internship and Glen did fifteen months as an anesthesia resident. When our terms were finished at Kingston General Hospital, we were asked to come back to Merritt. And we have remained here ever since.

I never felt strongly that there was prejudice against me as a female medical student and physician. There was one occasion during a clinical session when I was picked on because I was a woman. I did not let it worry me and was backed up by my male colleagues who thought the whole episode was rather silly. During internship, while on the one-month orthopedic rotation, I was suddenly relieved of my responsibilities and placed back on the pediatric service. I never questioned this change. Perhaps I was being discriminated against as it was probably thought that I would never do any orthopedics.

During my twenty-six-and-a-half years of practising in Merritt, there was only one other female physician.

In April 1966, we returned to Merritt, a community located in the Nicola Valley with 5,000 to 6,000 population. There were four physicians in the community with offices for five. Glen became the fifth doctor and I was asked to be a more-or-less permanent locum. My first night on-call was interesting. All of our colleagues turned up at our apartment unannounced. I think the reason they all appeared was to see who exactly was going to take calls. I don't know whether they were surprised or not, but I always took my own calls.

Being a permanent locum meant that I worked steadily all summer and only once in a while during the winter. I did not find this arrangement very satisfactory and soon began to work almost full-time. There were now six physicians and five offices, so I used the one that happened to be vacant. I had a little private cubby-hole where I could do my paper work undisturbed.

There were comings and goings amongst the medical staff over the next twelve years until 1978 when our clinic finally stabilized, and remained so for the next seventeen years. By this time there were only five physicians in our group and another clinic of two. In our clinic there were two surgeons, both of whom had their fellowships, and two GP-anesthetists. I was none of those, but did almost all the surgical assisting.

Our 'new' hospital had opened in April 1964. It had forty-nine beds. We saw medical, surgical, pediatric, and obstetric patients. Our main referral centre was Royal Inland Hospital in Kamloops. With the expertise available we were able to handle almost all our complicated obstetrics, as well as cholecystectomies, hysterectomies, hernias, varicose veins, some orthopedics, and other surgical procedures. As well, one surgeon was doing highly selective vagotomies and fundoplications which were the surgical treatments of choice at that time for peptic ulcer and symptomatic hiatus hernia respectively.

We all took turns on-call. I did not take weekend calls, but always took one night on during the week. The men shared weekends until we were able to acquire an emergency room physician for the weekends. My colleagues were very understanding about the call rota. Only once did anyone try to make me do weekend calls.

During holiday time, everyone usually just closed ranks, but it was more difficult for the others when Glen and I were away together. At times, particularly during the summer, we were able to get locums for a long time, and the same semi-retired physician returned to Merritt every year to help us out.

During my twenty-six-and-a-half years of practising in Merritt, there was only one other female physician. She was with the other clinic and stayed only about a year or so. Occasionally our locums were women doctors.

The women of Merritt seemed to appreciate having a woman physician in their community. Most of my practice consisted of women and children, although there were a couple of instances when the husband came to me while his wife saw Glen. Naturally, I saw many obstetrical cases, but never had the pleasure of delivering a baby whose mother (or father) I had delivered.

Merritt is surrounded by five Indian reserves which makes for a large Native population. When we first arrived in the Nicola Valley, many of the older First Nations people did not speak English and were accompanied to the doctor's office by an interpreter, usually a younger member of the family. Unfortunately, it seems that the languages are being lost despite the efforts of some elders to preserve them. Many babies were brought in swaddled in gaily-decorated papoose boards even up to the present time. The babies seemed very contented.

My medical activities outside of the practice included occasionally giving talks to groups organized by the public health nurses. One nurse and I made two videos on medical topics for our local TV station . I was on the inaugural board of directors for the long-term care facility built here in the early 1980s. Because of a deemed conflict of interest, I had to leave the board at the time the facility was to be opened. Later, I was medical director for several years.

I have been the accompanist for the Merritt Community Choir since the early seventies. Efforts to get away from the job for any length of time have been unsuccessful, but eventually they are going to have to find someone else. I enjoy accompanying and occasionally working with others besides the choir. During the late 1980s and early 1990s, I chaired a committee in its various incarnations that was eventually responsible for the building of a community aquatic centre. I was on the first board of directors for Shimyim House, a safe home for battered women and their children on the Coldwater Indian Reserve. Since retirement, I have become active in the Arts Council, and am on the Recreation Commission for the City of Merritt and on the board of directors of the Nicola Valley Health Care Society Endowment Foundation. We are very interested in the out-of-doors and belong to many naturalist groups. We record common loon activity at our summer home at Lac Le Jeune for Bird Studies Canada and monitor a bluebird trail near Merritt for the Southern Interior Bluebird Trail Society.

In 1992, the long run of stability in our clinic came to an end. The youngest member in our group decided that it would be best for his family to move to a larger community. Later that year a physician couple indicated an interest in coming to Merritt at a time when I was looking for an opportunity to retire. At the end of October 1992, I hung up my stethoscope and took down my shingle. I remained medical director of the long-term care facility for about another year. In March 1995, Glen retired and shortly after that the last of the five joined us in retirement. The medical community in Merritt is very different now.

I am glad I went into medicine. It provided many interesting and challenging experiences. I cannot say that I miss it a lot, though I sometimes think of my loss of that unique place we physicians have in the lives of our patients. As a child living in Vancouver, I always wanted to live in a rural area. I was wise enough even at that time to know that it might be wishful thinking, but when the time came to move to a small community, I came readily. Both of us have never regretted it and are now enjoying the community from a different point of view.

DR. ANNE DERKS

I started my studies at the Free University of Amsterdam in 1957 and received my medical degree in 1965. Over the years I developed this dream of coming to Canada and wrote many applications for internship. To my surprise, I was accepted at the Royal Jubilee Hospital in Victoria, British Columbia, where I started my internship in December, 1965.

My knowledge of the English language was pitiful textbook English—not as efficiently taught at school as it is nowadays with all the audio equipment. Somehow I muddled through the first few weeks, then started to understand and speak better. While in Victoria I met some wonderful women doctors: Dr. Patricia Johnston, Dr. Ilse Destrube, Dr. Joyce Clearihue, and Dr. Mary Leith. Their teaching and friendship meant a lot to me.

At the end of the year, I decided to share an apartment for a while with Dr. Barbara Wilson, an intern from St. Joseph at the time. Meanwhile, I began to apply for a position in general practice in Vancouver. The opportunity to start my own practice in Vancouver came in August, 1967, when I took over some patients from Dr. Mary McMurray, who moved to Boston, and later from Dr. Mary Garner, who moved to Texada Island.

Vancouver in the 1960s was a big city in the making, a much larger community than Victoria. Personal interactions between doctors and patients were less frequent because doctors in Vancouver did not just practise at one hospital. Most doctors had privileges at several hospitals and would visit their patients in all these different locations. There were only a few women physicians, and we knew almost everyone as we were also members of the Federation of Medical Women of Canada.

I married Dr. Michael Roburn in 1968, and we have two boys and two girls. For each baby I took two months of maternity leave. Pregnancy and childbirth did not seem such a big issue in those days, at least male colleagues hardly noticed or paid attention.

The children were a lot of fun to be with, yet the days were never long enough for us to get things done. I left the Federation of Medical Women and stopped doing obstetrics after our youngest child arrived.

In some ways, practising medicine in the 1960s was easier. We did not have ultrasound, CT scanners, or MRIs. Internal medicine was a specialty back then, now subdivided into nephrology, cardiology, gastroenterology, rheumatology, and so on. Patients were less demanding, less inclined to see themselves as victims, and more capable of accepting misfortunes as part of the human condition. There were fewer forms to be filled out and fewer medical legal letters. Whiplash injury hardly existed. Balancing home and work was just as hard as it is for young people today.

Looking back, I can hardly believe we have arrived in the 21st century. Life has been busy, the years have gone fast. Medicine has shown incredible progress, with the emergence of new diagnostic techniques, new treatment, and new drugs.

I hope to continue to be part of this great profession!

DR. KATHLEEN A. ELLIOTT
(1918–1986)

Kaye Elliott was born in 1918 in Northumberland, England, where her family had deep roots. She received a classical private school education in Wycombe Abbey School and then entered the Medical School of the University of Durham. She qualified at age twenty-four in 1942 with the MBBS. During the remainder of the Second World War she worked as a medical officer at various British armaments companies. Post war she obtained the MRCS, England, and LRCP, London.

In 1945 she married Dr. George B. Elliott, and in 1947, they emigrated to Canada. Eight years later when their first two daughters were aged six and four, she returned with them to London, England, to complete her training as a radiologist at Middlesex Hospital. She received the DMRD, England, and later the FRCPC in Canada. In 1960, their third daughter was born, and five years later the family moved from Calgary to Vancouver. Dr. Elliott initially worked in the Department of Radiology at St. Paul's

Hospital and subsequently in private practice in Vancouver. After the tragic death (because of a drunk driver) of her second daughter, Alison, a law student, in 1972, the family moved to Victoria where Dr. Elliott continued her private practice with Dr. Bill Lewes.

Aside from her dedication to the medical world, Dr. Elliott had diverse interests. Her garden and house were always full of exotic and beautiful blooms she had grown from seed. In addition to being an accomplished cellist, horsewoman, skier, and chef, she started learning German at age fifty, and at age sixty-six took up scuba diving.

She is survived in Canada by her husband Dr. G.B. Elliot, Professor Emeritus of Pathology, University of British Columbia, her daughter Dr. Jean Carruthers, a pediatric ophthalmologist and her husband Alastair and their three sons, and her daughter Christine Elliott, a lawyer. She will be remembered by her family, friends, and staff as a person of great gentleness, equanimity, and kindness who was able to wed consistently and successfully her family and career life.

Dr. Kathleen A. Elliott, consultant radiologist, Victoria, British Columbia, died suddenly while scuba diving on June 28, 1986, aged sixty-eight.
(Written by Jean Carruthers, MD, FRCSC for the BCMJ, *October, 1986.)*

DR. LOUISE JILEK-AALL

I was born in Oslo, Norway, on April 21, 1931, the middle of three children. My one-year-older brother Cato Aall became a physician and worked for many years in developing countries for the United Nations agency FAO; he now has a family medical practice in Norway. My sister Ingrid Aall, two years younger, is Professor of Asian Arts at the California State University, Long Beach. My father Anathon Aall was Professor of Philosophy and Psychology at the University of Oslo, Norway. My mother Lily Weiser-Aall was an ethnologist and psychologist and one of the organizers and Directors of the Norwegian Folk Museum in Oslo.

We three siblings spent our early childhood in Oslo, but our family retreated to the countryside during the German occupation of Norway in World War II. We were a closely knit family; both my parents have had a profound influence on my life and choice of profession. After graduation from high school I at first took a degree in philosophy at the University of Oslo. Since I always had planned to become a physician, I followed the European tradition of seeking out the best teachers in academic disciplines and moved on to study medicine at the Universities of Tubingen and Saarland in Germany, then at the University of Zurich in Switzerland from where I graduated in 1958. While attending medical school I also heard lectures in philosophy of religion and in anthropology, and became increasingly fascinated with Africa. As a consequence I took a diploma course in tropical diseases at the Swiss Tropical Institute in Basel. Upon graduating I obtained a small grant to do research on tropical diseases in the then British Trust Territory of Tanganyika, East Africa.

There in Africa as a young doctor in the interior of what is now Tanzania, I assumed responsibility for the medical service of outpost mission stations throughout the Ulanga District, riding on trucks, biking, and walking through the bush many days' journeys from one place to another. In these mission stations hundreds of sick people were cared for at the field hospitals and dispensaries by nuns trained as nurses and by auxiliary nurses' helpers, together with whom I treated the patients. I have described some of the hardships and adventures I experienced in this service in my book *Call Mama Doctor* (Hancock House Publishers, 1979) which has also been published in translation in Japan, China, and Hungary. It was in the interior of Tanzania that I founded and maintained the Mahenge Epilepsy Clinic.

When the first Congo civil war broke out in 1960 and the Belgian physicians fled this former Belgian colony, I responded to calls from the International Red Cross Society and the United Nations, who had sent a peacekeeping force to the Congo. I had to provide medical service in the general hospital of Matadi on the Congo River which was overcrowded with the hitherto unattended, severely ill patients. I worked in the hazardous civil war situation of the Congo for three months, together with Scandinavian colleagues, protected by Canadian UN soldiers. I was later awarded a citation and medal by the International Red Cross.

After that exhausting experience I decided to make a sea voyage around the southern half of Africa. But the Dutch freighter I was to board in the

Congolese port of Pointe Noire was delayed for at least a week. Standing there in the hot little travel office looking at a map of West Africa, my eyes caught the place name "Lambarene" in Gabon, only a couple hours' flight from Pointe Noire. Remembering that old Dr. Albert Schweitzer, whom we had welcomed as students in the 1950s when he received the Nobel Prize in Oslo, was still active at his hospital in Lambarene, I decided to pay him a visit while I waited for my ship.

When I arrived in Lambarene, Dr. Schweitzer told me that he was in desperate need of another physician due to an outbreak of a measles epidemic, which sent scores of severely sick children to his hospital. He asked me to help out and instead of a few days, I stayed for months on end, working at his jungle hospital. My unforgettable time in Lambarene turned out to be decisive in my eventually choosing Psychiatry as my medical specialty. Many years later I used my diaries to capture this experience in my book *Working with Dr. Schweitzer—Sharing his Reverance for Life* (Hancock House Publishers, 1990) which has been translated into Japanese and German.

Returning to East Africa, I organized the epilepsy clinic at Mahenge in the interior of Tanzania with the help of a Swiss mission nurse, as it had become evident that very simple medical treatment could in most cases control the seizures suffered by the many epileptic patients of the area. Effective seizure control would free them not only from physical but also from social and emotional suffering inflicted upon them due to the people's superstitious beliefs about epilepsy, held to be a demonic and contagious affliction called 'kifafa,' 'dying a little.' Because anti-epileptic medication has to be taken regularly, with my knowledge of their culture and of the Swahili language, I started treatment by getting the family members of the epilepsy sufferers together and explaining to them the treatment procedures, soliciting their co-operation. Working with the epileptics and their families had to be done after my daily medical duties; I often worked until late at night, and sometimes I was too tired to eat. As the Mahenge Epilepsy Clinic became known throughout the region, new epileptic patients arrived at the clinic every day with their relatives. As there was no prospect of another colleague joining me in Mahenge and I was running out of financial resources, I realized that I would have to leave or the mission station would be inundated with epilepsy sufferers coming from near and far. I

therefore returned to Europe in late 1961, hoping to find financial support to build up the Mahenge Epilepsy Clinic, and to start a research project investigating the apparently unusually high prevalence of seizure disorder in the region.

Little did I know that it would take me thirty years of presentations at international congresses, writing in scientific and popular publications, and soliciting at public and private agencies and pharmaceutical companies before achieving a substantial response. For all those years I maintained close consultative contact with the African nurse who had been trained to be in charge of the clinic which I tried to support and supply with the help of a few friends and colleagues.

I continued my psychiatric and neurologic training in Switzerland at the Psychiatric University Clinic Zurich under Professor M. Bleuler and at the Swiss Institute for Epilepsy under Professor H. Landolt. There I

Effective seizure control would free them not only from physical but also from social and emotional suffering inflicted upon them due to the people's superstitious beliefs about epilepsy, held to be a demonic and contagious affliction called 'kifafa,' 'dying a little.'

met my husband-to-be, Dr. Wolfgang Jilek from Austria. He accompanied me to East Africa to assist in a one-month follow-up of the epilepsy patients at the Mahenge Clinic whose number had grown to over 200.

We had both independently been planning to continue our specialization by taking the Diploma Course in Psychiatry at McGill University, Montreal, to which we were attracted by the pioneering research in transcultural psychiatry and epidemiology undertaken by Professors E. Wittkower and H.B.M. Murphy, with whom we later became closely associated. After a double wedding in Oslo and Vienna, we sailed by Cunard Line to Canada in 1963, on immigrant visas which the interviewing Canadian consul offered us instead of the student visas we had applied for, and thus we eventually became Canadians.

We completed our rather lengthy professional education by 1965. We had to repeat our previous European examinations in general medicine for the Medical Council of Canada and obtained the McGill Diploma in

Psychiatry, then the Specialist Certification, and later the Fellowship of the Royal College of Physicians and Surgeons of Canada.

On a cross-country vacation trip through Canada by Volkswagen we discovered the unique scenic beauty of British Columbia and decided that this was where we wanted to settle. In 1966 we received our licences to practise medicine in British Columbia and from then to 1975 we were the only psychiatrists in the Fraser Valley. We opened our office in Chilliwack.

We built our first Canadian home near Harrison Lake. Besides my office practice I worked at the Mental Health Centre, newly organized by my husband, and at the psychiatric unit of Chilliwack Hospital which we had helped to design, providing psychiatric consultation and running travelling mental health clinics from Hope to Langley.

We were especially interested in the First Nation peoples, and many of our publications derived from experiences in assisting Native patients with psychosocial problems associated with rapid culture change. Even after moving to Delta in 1975 where we built our second home in Tsawassen, I maintained my special interest in the psychosocial problems of the indigenous peoples of British Columbia and other minority groups, providing outreach consultation service to the Pacific Northwest coast and gathering experience in "intercultural psychotherapy." I also became actively involved in the Canadian Psychiatric Association's Section on Native Peoples' Mental Health, and the World Psychiatric Association's Transcultural Section. We joined the faculty of the Department of Psychiatry of UBC, of which I became Clinical Assistant Professor in 1975, Clinical Associate Professor in 1982, and Clinical Professor of Psychiatry in 1986, teaching students and residents and working at UBC, Vancouver General, Shaughnessy, and Children's Hospitals from 1975 to 1995, and also at the Greater Vancouver Mental Health Service and in recent years at the Delta Mental Health Centre and our local office.

When my husband was WHO consultant in Papua, New Guinea and later UNHCR Refugee Mental Health Co-ordinator in Thailand, I took on volunteer psychiatric consultations, especially in refugee camps in Thailand during the year 1988.

Throughout all my years in Canada I continued my efforts to keep the Mahenge Epilepsy Clinic in Tanzania going, mainly through regular consultative contacts with the nurse in charge of the clinic, and through securing an ongoing supply of anti-epileptic medication. In many guest lectures at universities in Canada and abroad, and in numerous congress presentations and publications, I described and illustrated the plight of African epilepsy sufferers and tried to attract international scientific interest for research on the causes of the high prevalence of seizure disorders in the Mahenge region and in other regions of Africa, where this problem had meanwhile also been reported. In 1991 I returned to Tanzania at my own expense, to do further research on epilepsy among rural populations together with Dr. H. Rwiza, Neurologist-in-Chief at the Dar-es-Salaam University Hospital, and to upgrade operations at the Mahenge Clinic for Epilepsy. Finally in 1992 I succeeded in obtaining a substantial research grant from the International Development Research Council of Canada so that I was able to organize a team of specialists from UBC and from the University of Dar-es-Salaam, Tanzania, and procure the necessary equipment in order to investigate the causes of seizure disorder in Mahenge region, and explore this problem's most appropriate therapeutic management and possible ways of prevention. We conducted a well-prepared research project of three years duration. The data confirmed the high prevalence and familiar incidence of epilepsy with the neurological and psychiatric complications in the population.

In 1994 I made my last field research trip to Tanzania, this time accompanied only by my daughter Martica Jilek, now an RN, who as a student nurse volunteer assisted me throughout the project. On one occasion my daughter saved my life when I was stabbed by robbers in Dar-es-Salaam; she provided first aid and took me to a safe hospital for emergency treatment.

The research results and my clinical observations led me to suspect that a regionally endemic filaria parasite is the significant factor causing seizure disorder through interference with brain function. Unfortunately I have not been able to pursue this investigation because of the drastic cuts in Canadian funding of medical research in developing countries. The Mahenge Epilepsy Clinic which I founded forty years ago and assisted ever since, is currently treating close to 900 patients and continues a health education program I inaugurated in 1994 in co-operation with the Tanzania Epilepsy Association.

DR. PATRICIA REBBECK

Dr. Patricia Rebbeck, general surgeon, is indeed a "woman for all seasons." She can safely be lauded as one of the outstanding female physicians in British Columbia. The above praise was written in the *Newsletter of the Federation of Medical Women of Canada* in 1979. Pat has continued to be outstanding during the decades of the eighties and nineties. She became even more famous on May 24, 1979 when she was the first woman to receive the President's chain of office in the history of the eighty-one-year-old Vancouver Medical Association. In the '70s she was the second woman to be elected as a member of the Board of Directors of the British Columbia Medical Association. She was also chairman of the BCMA Health Care Delivery Committee and member of the Editorial Board of the *BCMA Journal* and for several years was a delegate from the FMWC to the Canadian Medical Association's General Council. She was chairman of the National Services to Patients Committee of the Canadian Cancer Society, Consultant in general surgery to the Cancer Control Agency of British Columbia, and Director of the Section of General Surgery for the Surgical Society.

Her main surgical practice was treating cancer of the breast. One colleague, Dr. Urve Kuusk, who practised with her for ten years, praised her for breaking ground for other B.C. surgeons by saving as much of cancer patients' breasts as possible. She was doing partial mastectomies ten years before her male colleagues and she pioneered this surgical treatment for breast cancer and developed innovative alternatives to radical mastectomy.

Her advice to women who wish to become surgeons is, "If you want to do something then go ahead and do it . . . it also helps if you are fairly 'bloody-minded.'" In her days of training as the only woman surgical resident, she received no encouragement whatsoever.

Dr. Rebbeck was associate professor in the Faculty of Medicine at the University of British Columbia. She was the Osler Lecturer in 1986 and began her oration on "Communication: Things Osler Never Taught Me," with some humour stating, "It was a shock [to be so honored], as I had thought that the Osler lectureship, like honorary membership in medical societies, was for the elderly physicians on the point of retiring, one foot in the grave and the other on a banana skin. Perhaps the Vancouver Medical Association know something I do not—or perhaps it is my white hair that misled them."

In 1991 she became President of the College of Physicians and Surgeons. In 1993 she was chosen as one of the eight recipients to receive the YWCA Women of Distinction Award in the Health, Science, and Technology category.

Pat's interests were many; she was volunteer medical officer, Canadian Air Cadets, Westwood Race Track; she taught post-mastectomy volunteers; she was on the GVRD committee on Ambulatory Care; and lectured on health to lay groups.

Patricia Rebbeck was born in 1934 in Ipswich, Suffolk, England. She spent most of her young life in as many countries of the world as her engineer father's job led his family, and attended nine different schools during her elementary and high schooling. She did her undergraduate training first at the University of Western Australia, later at the University of South Australia. She attended medical school at the University of Edinburgh, Scotland, and graduated with MB, ChB in 1959. Internship followed at the Montreal General Hospital 1959–1960 and she wrote the LMCC exams in 1960. She began a surgical residency in Vancouver on the advice of Dr. Rocke Robertson, formerly of Vancouver and Head of Surgery at McGill while Pat was at McGill. (She had left her decision to do surgery too late to be part of McGill's residency program.) There was no precedent of a woman surgical resident and she had no mentor. After two years, at the insistence of her mother in England who was missing her only daughter, she left the residency course and did two years of general practice in Swansea, Wales, the first woman doctor in that area. That experience only confirmed her stubborn wish to do surgery and she completed her residency in Vancouver at Vancouver General Hospital, St. Paul's, and Riverview Hospitals; and then a year of Pathology at Shaughnessy Hospital. When she was at the General Hospital she lived in the Female Residence which is now the Family Practice Unit. At the residence the interns and residents used to get together and play strip poker. There were some games when the males lost and left with most of their clothing "stripped"! While on the surgery rotation at St. Paul's her room was on the top floor with the nuns. The residency was very demanding.

Pat became a Fellow of the Royal College of Surgeons of Canada in 1967. She was the first woman general surgeon in British Columbia.

After twenty-eight years in surgical practice she had to quit surgery because of arthritis in her hands. She took a position as Deputy Registrar of the College of Physicians and Surgeons of B.C. where she was responsible for impaired physicians, sexual misconduct cases, ethics, and publishing. She was the first woman ever elected to the College. As President of the College in 1991, she was appointed Head of a special committee struck to review the problem of sexual offences committed by physicians against their patients. Dr. Rebbeck and Dr. Mary Donlevy, an elected member of the College council, spent time teaching respect for the boundaries between doctors and patients. As a result, Dr. Donlevy with lawyer Barbara Fisher wrote the 1992 report on physician sexual misconduct, which has been a guide for other medical institutions.

Dr. Patricia Rebbeck was made clinical associate professor emerita University of British Columbia. She retired from the College of Physicians and Surgeons in 1999 and received a further honour when the College Council awarded her honorary membership. She is also a Senior member of the Canadian Medical Association.

Pat continues to be busy with the College of Physicians and Surgeons of British Columbia, working part-time inspecting private medical and surgical facilities, and publishing the *Quarterly Bulletin* of the College.

DR. MARY ALICE SUTTER

I was the only child in the family, born in the midst of the depression in Edmonton, Alberta. We moved to Victoria when I was one and lived at Cordova Bay, just footsteps from the beach, next to an abandoned daffodil farm. It was idyllic as I spent most of my childhood exploring the seashore and tide pools or playing with garter snakes. I even met Emily Carr.

A church group had started a craft class for small children, but I was soon expelled because as soon as I got a needle in my hands, I proceeded to "vaccinate" my fellow three- and four-year-olds who didn't admit to having had that procedure done. My father rejoined the army with the onset of WW II,

so my mother and I moved to Victoria. I started school at St. Ann's Academy because it was the only school that would take me at age five. I remember playing in the sandbox with the other child in the class who was not preparing for first Communion, so as a result when we moved east to join my father at Pembroke, Ontario, in December, my education was quite deficient and I passed Grade 1 'On Condition.' I had had the adventure of travelling from Victoria to Vancouver by boat and from Vancouver to Edmonton by train all by myself after I turned six. I stayed with my aunt while my mother was packing up. This was right after Pearl Harbor and a Japanese sub had been caught at Victoria Harbour. My Grade 2 was better except for a brief suspension for being inappropriately clothed. My mother made clothes from whatever material she could get, but some people considered the blouse I was wearing under my pinafore 'too sheer'! It was during this time I developed my interest in becoming a doctor. My mother was a nurse and would answer any of my medical questions she didn't know with "a doctor would have the answer to that." (Medical school later taught me that doctors did not know everything!)

Because of the nursing shortage, when I developed pneumonia the hospital had me admitted so my mother didn't have to stay home to care for me. I thought it was a fascinating place, especially when the doctors would show me things, like a drop of blood, under the microscope. I also had to have my tonsils out and my father's military friends slipped me into the base hospital for this. They let me see all the preparations in the operating room. I went to sleep with the promise that my tonsils would be in a jar beside my bed. They were!

I also had stepped on broken glass, and my foot became seriously infected with lovely red streaks spreading on my leg. Again the military friends came through with a new medicine they had just received—Penicillin—with miraculous results. My father was then posted to Brockville where there was an Office Training Centre. Because I had always been interested in the insides of fish and chicken, it was my chore to clean them, and my mother volunteered my services to teach the new brides of the young officers who had never had to deal with this before—a simple introduction to anatomy and surgery of which our children miss out today.

My family finally decided to settle in Vancouver. I attended John Norquay

Elementary School, and was tossed out of Sunday School at age eleven when I asked what circumcision meant in the Bible reading. I went home and looked it up in the dictionary. It became obvious to me that I wanted to become a doctor as I grew older. But I was always discouraged whenever I told people about my aspiration. My guidance teacher from John Oliver High School told me to be more realistic, that girls didn't become doctors.

Fortunately, my family had no problem with it (except financially), but my father had really hoped I would become an engineer as he had had to abandon his studies when he had joined up for World War I. He had a cousin who had graduated in medicine, but she had married and moved east so he had no contact with her. My maternal grandfather didn't really think women needed much education (my mother had had to run away to go into nursing), but when I was instrumental in getting him medical care when he was ill and was with him in a surgery, he told me he had changed his attitude and offered to pay my school fees.

Even though I really appreciated my grandfather's respect, I was able to say in my fourth year that I didn't need his financial support after having worked at Woodwards since the age of fifteen, a couple of summers at a Uranium Mine in the north, research in pharmacology at UBC, and a summer on the nursing payroll at Burnaby General Hospital acting as an intern in the Emergency, OR, and Laser Room.

I graduated from UBC in Medicine in 1960 and did a rotating internship at the Montreal General Hospital, which included a couple of months in North Carolina. I did six months of residency in Medicine and six months in Surgery at Shaughnessy Hospital in Vancouver before returning to the Montreal General Hospital to complete my Obstetrics and Gynecology training. This included one year at the Margaret Hague Maternity Hospital in Jersey City, which at that time did 20,000 deliveries a year.

I returned to Vancouver and joined the Seymour Medical Clinic as an Obstetrician and Gynecologist, working mainly at the Vancouver General and Grace Hospitals, then B.C. Women's and Children's Hospital with UBC Medical School teaching responsibilities. When I started in practice I had privileges at St. Paul's, St. Vincent's, St. Joseph's, Burnaby, and Richmond, but logistics made going to all those hospitals impossible. It is difficult nowadays for a physician to get privileges at one hospital.

I married a Family Physician, Blake Wright, who was also at the Seymour Clinic, and we adopted two children—a boy and a girl. Early in my career I would go to Bella Bella and Bella Coola to see patients and later to the Queen Charlottes, but with two children this was too difficult. I practised until I was sixty-three when I took a medical leave of absence. I was sixty-five by the time I was able to return to work, but would not have been able to keep up my hospital work because of age limits, so I quit. I don't think I could have found time to return to practice as I have become involved with quilting (we give away about 400 quilts a year to various charities) and a grandchild (with another on the way). I was surprised that I hadn't missed doing what I had loved doing for so long, but many of my patients have become friends and I see many of my babies, so I have wonderful memories of those years.

1967

DR. MARLENE E. HUNTER

I decided to become a doctor when I was eleven years old. I remember various members of my family smiling at me in a way that I later realized was fondly patronizing, and saying, "That's nice, dear," or "I'm sure you'll make a wonderful nurse, dear." I had not then, nor have I ever had, anything but the greatest respect for nurses, but I was determined to become a doctor.

A bunch of tear-jerking circumstances got in the way, as circumstances are wont to do. My mother died from metastatic breast cancer at the age of forty-eight. She had been ill for more than two years and there was no Medicare in those days. My father would never have done anything different, but in looking for a wonder cure, a lot of money was spent, money that we did not have. Dad looked at the world through rose-coloured glasses, and Mum kept things going in a way that always astonished me. She could take the wildest of his schemes, siphon off some workable fragment, make it work, and let him think that it was all his idea. Incredible.

When Mum died, Dad was lost. I was just at the end of my first year of university. He married an old friend a year and a half later—poor woman; she did not know about the rose-coloured glasses and could not compete with my mother's talents. Nevertheless, they were fond of each other and the marriage lasted for about fifteen years. They became good friends and got along much better with each other after the divorce.

Despite my family situation and various complications, I worked my way through university, becoming a good employee of the B.C Telephone Company. I was quick and enjoyed the work, usually taking the 4-11 o'clock shift. If the schedule did not work out for me and I was slated for a day shift, there was almost always someone who would change with me, and the supervisors were lenient in allowing this. (Theoretically, we were all supposed to take our turns with day, split, and evening shifts.) The stressful circumstances did take their toll, and I graduated with lower marks than I think I otherwise would have achieved. A big part of the problem was that I was too stubborn to cut back on a lot of my extracurricular activities: I was president or secretary of various societies and a member of the musical society. Consequently, I was mostly in the high-second or low-first-class brackets. There is nothing wrong with marks like that, but they do not get you into medical school, especially if you are a female in the early 1950s. I was very unhappy about not getting into medical school that year. Knowing that I needed to be very busy, I went to talk to my Bishop, asking if he knew of any demanding job that I might do. He suggested that I should contact the Bishop of Caledonia, the northernmost diocese in the province.

I was mostly in the high-second or low-first-class brackets. There is nothing wrong with marks like that, but they do not get you into medical school, especially if you are a female in the early 1950s.

And that is how I came to spend a wonderful, rewarding and restorative year living in a First Nations village along the B.C. coast—the village of Kitkatla on Dolphin Island. It was five hours by fish boat to Prince Rupert. My title was Field Matron—highly unsuitable, as Field Matrons were experienced nurses and I was neither experienced nor a nurse, but there I was.

Two weeks before I was to leave for Kitkatla, I had received a telegram from the Department of Indian Affairs saying that they were short of a teacher and asking if I would be interested in teaching. Although I had never wanted to be a teacher and lacked training, I accepted the DIA's offer and was hired as a teacher for a remote Indian village. (In much later years I was able to boast that Roy Vickers, the artist, was a snotty-nosed kid in Grade 2 when I taught him in Kitkatla.) There was another teacher, older and very experienced, so with my complete ignorance of the whole process we agreed that I would teach Grades 1 and 2, and she would teach three to eight, inclusive. However, she worked herself into burnout and left at Christmas, and I had to take Grade 3 into my room; that gave me forty-eight children in the first three grades.

I learned so much in Kitkatla. I began to understand what exploitation was all about. I discovered the gentle caring of the Tsimpsian people— nothing bad would ever have happened to me in that village. I realized that, on the few days of the year when the tides were really low and everybody went out clamming to augment their incomes and their food supply, I would defy the edict to report the parents for keeping their kids out of school, just as I refused to punish them for speaking their own language. And there were a lot of fun times. I organized a Junior and Senior choir, girls' homemaking course (we did that in those days) and held confirmation classes (I was basically working for the Church afterall!). I had a happy social life, especially with the Vickers family. Also, I learned a little of the Tsimpsian language, enough to get the basic symptoms if someone was sick. It was really a learning experience.

Aside from my communication with the Department of Indian Affairs, another important event happened just before I left for Kitkatla. I had had an on-again-off-again romance with a boyfriend since we were in Grade 9. We had been 'off-again' for a year or so, but I wanted him to know I was going away, so I sneakily sent a birthday card to his mother, telling her about my posting and when I was to depart. I thought he was away for the summer working, but it turned out he was home. He phoned and invited me for dinner at his house with the family. On the bus as he was seeing me home, I wanted him to say he was sorry for whatever quarrels we had that led to a breakup. Much to my surprise, he asked me to marry him. Wordless, I nodded my head as hard as I could. So John Hunter and I were married just after I got home from Kitkatla in the following August.

And a week later, I got pregnant. John was doing his articling, having graduated in law. We were still two kids, really, with very little money, and we were going to have a baby. I had a happy pregnancy, working right up to eight-and-a-half months; our first son was born nine months and a week after our wedding. I used to watch people as they mentally calculated the dates, and wished that the baby would come early so that they would *really* have something to gossip about. John got a raise to $60 a month after the baby was born. I had enough Unemployment Insurance to last us for almost a year, so we made out quite well. The following summer he was called to the Bar, and our financial situation improved considerably. I went back to work, and the lady living downstairs offered to babysit for me during the day. However, there was not enough money to even consider going to medical school, and besides, the baby was too young for me to want to leave him.

I was happy enough. I started to do some writing, selling enough to pay for stamps and stationery and keeping me encouraged to continue. In time, we had another baby, four years after our first son was born. It seemed as if my long-held dream had been put on the shelf permanently. Then one day, when our younger son was about a year old, John asked me if I wanted to go on to medical school, I was stunned. "Oh, I couldn't," I said. Then, "Could I?"

I went to the University of British Columbia to have a chat with the screening committee. They were distinctly unenthusiastic about my aspiration of wanting to go back to school, especially medical school. I was female, and married with two children! Besides, having applied at the end of both my third and fourth years, I already had two refusals.

Eventually, I convinced them that we had thought about it very carefully, and I wished to apply. With a collective sigh, they told me that I would have to do a post-graduate year (to prove that I was not senile? After all, I was almost twenty-nine years old!). Furthermore, I would have to get a first-class average to even be considered, and that would be no guarantee of acceptance. To their chagrin, I accepted, saying as long as I knew the condi-

tions, I would abide by them. They told me to fill out an application form, even though I was not going into medicine until the following year. However, that was what they wanted me to do, so I did. Of course, I received my third rejection letter.

Accordingly, I started the year in September, taking the courses they had prescribed for me. For some of the demands, I was lucky—bacteriology, for instance, because I had been working as a bacteriologist (learning on the job, with one undergraduate course to fall back on) for two-and-a-half years. On the other hand, they suggested calculus. As I had always loved math, I thought "sure!" Little did I realize I had had no math for twelve years. Furthermore, everyone else in the class had had eight weeks of calculus in their previous year. I got a tutor. Everybody told me that I should stop worrying and that one day the light would just come on. It never did. Eventually, I wrote and colour-coded every example problem that I could think of: red for the question; blue for the formula; green for the working out; black for the solu-

All communication between me and the Faculty of Medicine went through my husband. They even called him to tell him that they were going to accept me—to give him a chance to rethink the whole thing and back out, I presume.

tion. Then I sat down and memorized them, praying that I would recognize enough to get me through. I made a bare second class in the course.

In the middle of the year, I came back to the car to find John sitting there. It turned out that he had intercepted a letter to me from the screening committee—a refusal. I was keeping my part of the bargain, but they had just broken theirs. Angry on my behalf, he had arranged an appointment with the Dean. When he went to the Dean's office, my folder was on the desk—inches thick by now, with four refusals! The Dean spoke quietly, "That wasn't fair, was it?" John replied, "I didn't think so." The Dean said, "She'll be reconsidered when her final marks come out." So John had come to the car to tell me all this, full of contrition for having opened my mail—as if I cared!

An interesting side effect of this was that all communication between me and the Faculty of Medicine went through my husband. They even called him to tell him that they were going to accept me—to give him a chance to rethink the whole thing and back out, I presume. And so I entered medical school at the University of British Columbia at the advanced age of twenty-nine years and nine months.

Two days after I began my second year, John had a subarachnoid haemorrhage from a ruptured berry aneurysm. He died six hours later. He had turned thirty-two the day before his death.

I thought I was managing quite well, and I was, but I failed my year. The faculty had done their best to help me, allowing me to write three supplemental exams (the limit was supposed to be two), but I just could not manage it. Although my pride took a beating, repeating the year was the best thing I could have done, and I was home free from then on. This second time around was a cinch, and then came the clinical years which, for me, were my natural métier.

Through medical school, I became more and more interested in doing an overseas tour of duty. I had never given it much thought before, because John certainly would not have been interested. I had a good friend who had graduated from medical school three years before who was, by that time, in India. He and his wife (a nurse) were planning to stay there for few more years. The idea began to grow. I also investigated other possibilities, such as working for CUSO and the Department of External Affairs. My friends had gone over with the United Church and were certainly happy with their arrangements. In the long run, it was clear that the United Church offered the best options, considering the fact that I had two kids to think about. People might take risks for themselves, but when it comes to any risk for their children, no matter how unlikely, that is a different situation. I applied and was accepted. It was agreed that I would take over the little hospital where my friend worked (the only doctor), which would give us a few months to overlap. I liked that idea; I could learn a little of the language and the local customs, and be introduced to the village of 60,000 people by someone they knew and trusted. The boys liked the idea, especially when they realized that it was uncommon for children at their age to be going to India—it gave them a special stature in the classroom.

I graduated very comfortably in the top three of the class, and had been accepted for my internship at St. Paul's Hospital in Vancouver. The administration at St. Paul's was very good to me, allowing me to live at home except for my on-call nights when had to stay in the nuns' sleeping quarters. They also allowed me to start my internship one month later than usual, in August, so that I could spend one of the summer holiday months with my sons. Accordingly, I finished my internship at the end of the following July. We were due to leave on August 7th, as I was to have interviews in Toronto with the United Church Board of World Mission before leaving for India on August 9th. It was a busy week, having had to pack up the house. I had been able to find suitable tenants and a real estate firm to keep their eyes on things, as I was renting it furnished.

There was one little hitch. Before that year (1967), all requests for visas had gone through the Indian High Commission in Ottawa. That year, we had been told that all requests would go to New Delhi for processing, so we were to allow two months for our visas to be approved. Accordingly, I had sent off all applications and documentation on Feb. 1st, knowing that we would be leaving at the beginning of August. I thought six months would allow sufficient time for our applications to be processed. But I was wrong. So here we were with no job, our home leased, and our car sold. I believe there are times in life when one just has to take the next step, not knowing what the following step will be or where it might lead. This seemed to be one of those times. On August 7th, therefore, according to plan, we set off for Toronto. Fortunately, we had friends who had invited us to stay with them for the few days while we were planning to head for Toronto.

At the Board of World Mission, I found that we were one of seven families in the same situation. That was the year when the first EXPO took place in Montreal. We also had friends, that is, parents of our friends there. I am not much of an exposition person, but this promised to be special, so it seemed like a good idea to spend a week in Montreal. Surely our visas would be waiting when we got back to Toronto. It *was* a good idea, and EXPO was wonderful. When we got back to Toronto, however, there was no sign of any visas for any of the families awaiting them. We went back to stay with the friends who had first invited us. Two weeks went by, and two situations arose: the boys had to start school, and it was definitely time to stop imposing on our friends. I found a minimal bed-sitting suite on Avenue Road. The Board of World Mission agreed to pay the rent, as all their accommodation facilities were in use. There was one bedroom; to open the chest of drawers, one had to close the bedroom door. There was also a pull-down sofa in the sitting room. I put the boys in the bedroom and took the couch, and on many nights I perched precariously on a V-shaped piece of furniture, not knowing whether I would be folded up in it like a sandwich or flung unceremoniously to the floor if it decided to extend to its full position. There was also a closet kitchen: if I stood in the middle and extended my arms, I could touch all four walls.

As soon as school started, I went to the Ontario Medical Association. I knew that I could not bear to be in the cramped little apartment all day, and I badly needed something to do. I told them that they would not have to pay me (I was on salary with the United Church by then) but please, please could they find me a temporary job. It would have to be one which I could leave on very short notice. The next day I was taken on as a temporary junior resident in surgery at Women's College Hospital. What a life-saver that turned out to be. The medical staff was wonderful to me, knowing where I was headed, and I got to do all kinds of procedures (being supervised very carefully, I hasten to add) which I had never had a chance to do as an intern. Besides that, I worked straight day shifts, had no weekend work, and was never on-call. I did, however, stay after my usual chores were finished so that I could do an admission or two for the other hardworking residents who did not have my generous working conditions.

By the end of November, it was clear that our visas were unlikely to be approved, so when refusal came on November 26th, I was prepared. I had been offered Nepal, Hong Kong, or Kenya. I chose Kenya, as did one other family with whom we had become good friends. Six of the eleven families were refused, with the sole exception of this family who had a personal association with someone in a southern Indian city. After four years of looking forward to India, it seemed strange to reorganize our thoughts toward Kenya. Our friends, Menai and Alun Hughes and their two sons, left Toronto to spend the Christmas season with their families in Wales. We met up again in London at the end of December and travelled together to Kenya, arriving on December 30th.

The Hughes were to be stationed in Nairobi, so we said goodbye at the airport, where we had been met by someone from the hospital. I was to be the 'second doctor' at the hospital in Tumu Tumu, near the town of Nyeri. (Nyeri is the capital of Central province, and near the famous Treetops Hotel.) We were welcomed at Tumu Tumu. The hospital was run by the Presbyterian Church of East Africa. So there I was, an Anglican, working for the United Church of Canada which was second to the Presbyterian Church of East Africa. Ecumenism in action!

Besides the hospital, there was (and still is) a girls' secondary school, and of course, the Church. The hospital also had a nursing school, graduating what we would call Licensed Practical Nurses. They are called Enrolled Nurses in Kenya. It was a 120-bed hospital, and there were supposed to be doctors. Luckily, when I arrived there was a very experienced physician who had been there for several years. He came from Scotland, as were several other members of the expatriate staff—matron, administrator, and another nurse; as well, there were two VSO nurses (equivalent to our CUSO), a Canadian nurse, and a German lab technician. Other than those, the rest of the staff were Kenyan, including of course the student nurses. The hospital was extremely well run and the staff sufficiently large. There was an X-ray, run by the person without whom the hospital would have collapsed. Kimunyu was a registered nurse who had taken an extra year of training to become a physician's assistant. He did everything from finding out why my bread had not been delivered to giving the anaesthetics. The lab was small but adequate, and we could get most of the usual tests done there without sending them into Nairobi. There was a fairly large pharmacy, presided over by Kimunyu. Although we did not have all the newest miracle drugs, we certainly had all the important basic medications and could get some of the 'hifalutin' ones from Nairobi if necessary.

We saw a wide variety of problems and I soon realized that I would have to turn my differential diagnoses upside down. Tuberculosis and every variety of intestinalailment were rampant; hypertension and coronary heart disease were almost never seen. We were too high for malaria (5,400 feet) although we did see the occasional cases when someone who had been on the coast contracted it. There was a leper colony attached to the hospital with about two dozen dear souls who had lived there for years and would spend the rest of their lives there. They worked around the hospital grounds, happy to have a secure home. They were no longer infectious (leprosy is not very infectious anyway), but did have problems with their limbs from time to time as some of them might have lost their fingers or toes because of this disease.

There were strange benign tumours, elephantiasis, and neurofibromatosis, but rarely did we see malignancies. There was, however, Kaposi's sarcoma. And, looking back on it now, I can remember cases where, no matter how hard we tried, the patients who often were too young withered away and died. I now believe they probably had AIDS.

Trauma, especially severe burns and ghastly panga slashes, were very common. Co-wives would come in with their noses badly bitten. Male circumcision occurred after puberty, and was seldom done in hospital; and female circumcision, although theoretically outlawed, was still practised. (When I arrived home, I had to adjust my impressions of what normal female genitalia looks like.) Female circumcision often predicted whether the woman needed an episiotomy or not, as there were major perineal tears when the circumcision had been more like a vulvectomy. And then there were the common problems: various dermatitides, bronchial infections, stomach and digestive complaints, painful joints, and sore ears.

There was a leper colony attached to the hospital with about two dozen dear souls who had lived there for years and would spend the rest of their lives there. They worked around the hospital grounds, happy to have a secure home.

It has always been difficult for me to write or even talk about Tumu Tumu. Many people have told me I should write a book. However, I have a keen memory of one woman in the community who said that, "Some [white] people just come to Kenya so that they can go home and write a book about us." Obviously, she felt that such books were derogatory and disrespectful, and I was determined that I would never become one of those "white" people. It is difficult to write about living in a different culture, because those aspects of life are so different from our own. And it does sound demeaning and patronizing, even though one may not intend to give such a portrayal.

Ten weeks after I arrived in Tumu Tumu, the other doctor had to go to the PCEA sister hospital in Chogoria, as the only doctor there had been flown out with a bowel obstruction. So I was all by my lonely self to be in charge of a 120-bed hospital in rural Kenya. Lucky for me that the other staff was so knowledgeable and experienced. They led me carefully through various diagnostic minefields and made disingenuous suggestions when they obviously knew much more about some situations than I did. Nowhere was this more apparent than in the obstetrical ward: "Did you say that you would like us to start a pit drip, doctor?" or, "I can check the foetal heart again for you, if you'd like." In the two days prior to his leaving for Chogoria, my senior partner called me three times for a C-section: "You'd better do it," he said, "never know when I'm going to be back." And so I diligently learned and learned.

Never did I say, or think, that I was sorry to have gone to Kenya—not even on the worst days when things were challenging to the point of total frustration. But there were also many times when I was looking forward to going home. This was especially true during the last six months of our time there. We had been there more than three years, without a home furlough. I could hardly wait to leave. Not the case for my sons, though, who loved Kenya unreservedly and would have been happy to stay much longer. We left on April 1, 1971. I had accrued three months furlough pay, which took us through East Africa and large parts of Europe on the way home. We finally arrived back in Vancouver on August 18, the day before my father's birthday. We turned up at his birthday party unexpectedly. It was a wonderful reunion for us all.

Back in West Vancouver, our home was waiting for us. Not selling our house was the best decision I had ever made. It was a security blanket for all three of us, knowing that we had a house to fall back on. I bought a little family practice from a colleague who had been away for two years anyhow, and his locum did not want to buy it. There had been some attrition, which almost always happens if the doctor is gone for a long time, so the cost was not terribly high. It was only five minutes away by car, or an easy twenty-minute walk. I settled in happily, and was invited to join an on-call group, which made life seem incredibly easier after Tumu Tumu. As it turned out, for about two of the three-and-a-half years I was in Tumu

Tumu, I had been the only doctor in the area. Thus, being on call for weeks at a time seemed normal. The senior nurses there, who were also referred to as "Sisters" (as it was a British-run hospital), always took the first call and only contacted me when absolutely necessary. Most problems were dealt with by the night staff, including deliveries. It often caused me wry amusement that I was called for the very things I knew nothing about. When I got home, it again caused wry amusement when I was not supposed to do those procedures with which I was then competent such as doing a prolapsed cord, vacuum extraction, or even Caesarean sections. I joined the medical staff at Lions Gate Hospital in North Vancouver and to me, it quickly became the epitome of what a good community hospital should be. My practice grew quickly (as did all practices of women physicians) and I was feeling very satisfied with life in general.

One day, a friend who was my medical school classmate as well as on staff at Lions Gate, asked if I would like to come to dinner with him and his wife (who was my jogging friend). His friend's wife had died a couple of years before, he said, and he thought that the friend and I would get along well together. My classmate's name was John. I can remember my light-hearted response as clearly as if it was yesterday, "Sure, John, what have I got to lose?" The arrangement was that we would all have dinner at their home. Two days before the dinner, the friend whose name was Redner Jones phoned me. "How about us meeting before we go to this dinner?" he suggested. It seemed like a good idea to me, and we arranged that he could come over to my house the next evening. That was November 2, 1971. We were married on July 31, 1972.

Redner had three daughters from his first marriage. All were adopted and multiracial. My classmate had described them as "pretty well grown up." In fact, when I met them they were four, ten, and fourteen years of age; whereas my sons were twelve and sixteen. Challenges were all around. I was used to sons, and got a package deal with three young girls. Redner was used to girls, and he got a package which included sons—teenage sons who were used to having their mother all to themselves. There have been some very rocky times, but somehow we all survived and become a real family. We now have six grandchildren.

During the first months after my return to West Vancouver, while my practice was growing I worked one night a week in the emergency room at Lions Gate. I became very distressed at how we used to treat children when they came into the emergency room. We had to take them away from their parents, "bundled" them so they could not move, took them down the hall where there were people in strange clothes and masks, and bright lights and funny smells, and they were made to lie down on a hard table with us telling them not to cry. Of course, they howled their heads off, and I thought this was cruel, and surely we could find a better way. Just at that time came my serendipity (which I always say follows me around): a brochure came across my desk from the American Society of Clinical Hypnosis. They were coming to give a weekend workshop in Vancouver, and on the agenda was hypnosis with children. So I went to this workshop. It was in the autumn of 1972. I found it absolutely fascinating,

I loved Cuba immediately, and in time became associated with the Cuban Ministry of Public Health, and some years later, also with the Ministry of the Interior. I now teach throughout Cuba.

and it did seem as if this would be a useful tool for many things besides calming children in the emergency room. We were advised to start using the techniques, within our competence, as soon as possible; so when a youngster with terrible warts all over his hands turned up in my office on the following Monday, I took a deep breath and thought, "Well, here goes!" I saw him twice, and the results were unbelievably successful. He and his mother were ecstatic, but no more than I.

I cautiously began using hypnosis within my practice to relax a woman for a vaginal exam, or to soothe children who had a few stitches, or to allay anxiety and relieve pain. After about two years, the word had spread, and my colleagues began to refer their patients for problems of pain, anxiety, and insomnia, etc. I continued to go to workshops and take courses. I joined the Canadian Society of Clinical Hypnosis (B.C. Division); I had joined the American Society at that first workshop. Those who know me already know the long-term results. The clinical use of hypnosis in medicine and psychology became a major part of my professional life, and brought with it wonderful experiences in the international community, and the most delightful acquaintances with colleagues around the world. In time, I found myself as President of both the B.C. Division and the American Society of Clinical Hypnosis, and a lecturer and workshop leader in seventeen countries. What wonderful gifts that first tentative workshop had brought to me!

In 1974, I entered a writing contest of a leisure magazine for physicians, *Canadian Doctor*. The first prize was a trip for two for a week in Barbados; second and third prizes were money; and then there were nine additional prizes, including having one's submission printed in the magazine. I was aiming for one of the nine prizes, yet I won the first prize! There was one little hitch. Redner did not want to go to Barbados, it being (in his opinion) elitist, colonialist, and all other 'ists' which he deplores. At that time I had encouraged him to go back to university to pursue his teaching degree. (It was fascinating to see the transformation of his features with the emotions flashing across his face as they had once flashed across mine when John encouraged me to go back to medical school.) His courses included one on the political sociology of revolutionary countries. So where did he want to go? Cuba! "Cuba?" I yelped. Afterall, this was 1974. Nobody in their right mind went to Cuba, did they? He generously told me I could take somebody else to Barbados if I wanted to. We had been married a little over two years. I agreed to go to Cuba, which proved to be somewhat of a challenge as the flight was offered by Air Canada and they did not fly to Cuba, and there was no reciprocity of hotels, no such thing as credit cards, and various other little glitches. "Couldn't you choose any other Caribbean Island?" The editor of *Canadian Doctor* moaned to me at one point. In the end, they flew us to Miami and gave us money to fly on through Mexico, and covered our expenses for a week (they hoped). In fact, the trip lasted for two weeks in May 1975.

The night before we left from Toronto, we were staying with Redner's younger brother and family. I was so nervous about going that I began weeping. My sister-in-law embraced me and told me that I could stay there if I wanted, and Redner could go by himself. "N-no," I quivered, "I'll g-g-go." I always did enjoy a little theatre. So we went to Cuba. And from the moment we entered Havana Airport, I understood more about propaganda than I had ever realized before. I had been fearful because of what I had heard and read, not because of what I knew. I loved Cuba immediately, and in time became associated with the Cuban Ministry of Public Health, and some years later, also with the Ministry of the Interior. I now teach throughout Cuba. I often teach clinical hypnosis and the treatment of trauma survivors. Soon I will be going back for my eighteenth Cuban experience.

In 1977, I had another experience which dramatically changed the direction of my medical career. A colleague was leaving town. She phoned and said, "Marlene, I know you're not taking new patients [the first warning signal], but I wonder if you'll take this woman [louder warning signals]. She needs you." (Deafening warning signals!) She was twenty-eight years old, intelligent and pleasant. She held a responsible job with government, which she did well. She was estranged from her family and had a documented history of early childhood abuse. She also had a plethora of somatic complaints, which defied solution. We could just get one under control and another would surface like Ogopogo. Among these problems were terrible headaches, digestive problems, and various unexplainable aches and pains. I had absolutely no reason to think she was malingering, but I could figure out neither her nor her conditions. I would give her the newest pharmaceutical miracle for her headache, and she would phone from work and say, "That stuff is wonderful! Why didn't you give it to me before?" Then, a few hours later, she would be sitting in my waiting room, and when I went out to get her, would growl at me, "Why did you give me that crap? It isn't worth the paper it's written on!" Help. I knew that my colleague, who did hypnosis, had at the patient's request done a hypnotic back-to-birth experience with her. During that experience the patient said that, when she was born, her mother had said, "Take the little bitch away." Now, whether or not that really happened is not the issue; if one believes that that is what happened when s/he was born, it does not augur well for that person's emotional comfort throughout life. In fact, the mother abandoned the family when the little girl was three weeks old. Her father was a labourer, poorly educated, and in no way able to take care of this small babe. She was passed from one household to another among his cronies, and at thirteen months old she was found on the beach at Ambleside in West Vancouver, wrapped in newspaper and left for dead. She had been hit on the head by a beer bottle. She was apprehended and in the ensuing years had been in four foster homes. At age five, she was adopted by a family who were pillars of the community on the outside, but it was (as she perceived it) a very emotionally harsh environment. I was bewailing my inability to figure this woman out at an ASCH meeting where one could discuss problem cases with older, experienced clinicians. Luckily (serendipity again) I spoke with a wise psychiatrist from California who listened carefully, asked all the right questions, and finally said to me, "Have you ever thought of Multiple Personality Disorder?" "No," I croaked. Nor did I want to! I could go on at length, but I will not. Eventually, I did something that I would not do now: I asked a direct question, when we were again doing hypnosis for her headaches. "Is there any other person who would like to come to speak with me?" And this entirely different voice said, "Of course! What took you so long?"

As it turned out, she was highly dissociative with more than twenty identifiable ego states. I learned that the family physician when she was young had told her adoptive parents bluntly that she had a "split personality" and they had better accept her condition. He made it clear that he did not mean schizophrenia. In time, I recognized similar behaviour patterns in two other patients in my own practice, and I realized that this disorder was not nearly as rare as people were saying it was.

And so my medical career took another sharp turn. It was very difficult, working with MPD, as it was called in those days. There was little support and recognition, and much opprobrium from my colleagues. (In fairness, however, because I felt so alone, I began to see dissociation behind every bush, and was in grave danger of believing that I was God's gift to Multiples. In that mode, I did not allow myself to recognize offers of help, as I felt that those who were offering were on the wrong track.) In 1984, another brochure came across my desk; hypnosis colleagues in the U.S. were planning the "First Annual Conference of the International Society for the Study of Multiple Personality and Dissociation." Wow! Help was at hand! So I went to this conference. Initially they had hoped for 150 registrants so that they could cover the hotel costs. Eventually, 452 registrants turned up. What bliss—all of a sudden, there were 451 people who understood what I was talking about. For the first two years, we spent a lot of time patting each other on the back saying, "There, there, I understand." Then we gathered ourselves together, and the research started.

I have never understood the antipathy toward dissociative disorders. To me, it makes so much sense: a small child, or someone being traumatized, somehow has to get themselves away. To do so, they dissociate. When trauma or abuse is chronic, it becomes the modus operandi of dealing with painful, abusive, frightening, and confusing situations. In doing so, the personality structure becomes compartmentalized. What's hard to understand about that? Further recognition about attachment process offers another aspect towards clarification. What is fascinating is the elegant, sophisticated research that has been going on in many parts of the world for two decades now, which involves neurophysiological, epidemiological, biochemical, brain waves studies, endocrinological investigations and comparisons, CT scans and PET scans, and SPECT studies. Yet, there seems to be so much resistance to even looking at this data. Why? Can't they read?

I have never understood the antipathy toward dissociative disorders. To me, it makes so much sense: a small child, or someone being traumatized, somehow has to get themselves away. To do so, they dissociate.

In time, the name was changed, thank goodness, to Dissociative Identity Disorder and the association became the International Society for the Study of Dissociation (ISSD). There is a Canadian Branch, now called the Canadian Society for Studies in Trauma and Dissociation. I was with the ISSD from the beginning, and in time became the President; I was also a past National Co-Chair of the Canadian Society. If hypnosis changed my professional life, that is nothing compared to understanding about dissociative phenomena. I have learned more about the art of medicine from my dissociative patients than I could have dreamt possible. Their creativity, resilience in the face of devastating trauma, determination never to give in, as well as head-shaking evidence of how mind and body communicate (for better or for worse) have all helped to shape my education. And so I have had the opportunity to add Dissociative Disorders to my lectures and workshops around the world.

Early in the 1980s, the B.C. College of Family Physicians was looking for an outreach program at the same time that a small community up north was looking for medical services. This resulted in an establishment of a small family medical centre in Dease Lake, in northwestern B.C., which is about 150 miles from the Yukon border. I became one of the rota of physicians and went up regularly throughout the latter half of the 1980s and the first half of the 1990s.

By 1994, the community had opened its own Stikine Health Centre. By then, I was the identified Medical Director of the little clinic (read: trouble shooter) and so I went up for the opening, a sort of a semi-official handing-over. I felt quite nostalgic, thinking that that was the last time I would be going because the new centre had two full-time doctors. I loved going up north. The clinic also took care of Telegraph Creek and Iskut (both are First Nations communities) and the scenery was so beautiful. Within about a year and a half, one of the doctors quit and I got a call asking if I could come up for a while to give the remaining doctor some time off. Happily, I went up for a month and I have been going regularly ever since. Now, however, because I have been out of family practice for so long, I go to do psychotherapy and counselling instead. This is part of the world where Residential School Syndrome, alcoholism, family violence, and sexual abuse are all rampant. It's a prescription for dissociative disorders, and almost no one has known anything about them. Hard to believe.

I have also done three locums at Mills Memorial Hospital, in Terrace, as Clinical Director of the Psychiatry Unit. These have been thoroughly enjoyable, due entirely to a wonderful nursing staff and the pleasant working and living conditions provided. (Besides, it pays well!) While there I have taught the nurses about dissociative disorders. They have understood immediately, and I could see them whispering to each other, "So-and-so! She's talking about so-and-so. . . ." (So why do medical colleagues have such a hard time with it? C'est la vie, I guess.)

Along this idiosyncratic career journey of mine, I have developed a penchant for collecting presidencies. Besides those to which I have already referred, I have been President of the B.C. College of Family Physicians (Ha! Again to that old selection committee!); and for years I was an Associate Clinical Professor in the Department of Family Medicine at UBC.

In 1989, I sold my practice. It was a difficult decision which had taken me a year and a half to make, because I loved being a family doctor. However, there were many good family physicians on the North Shore, but very few people who could treat patients with dissociative disorders; thus I opened a little office in West Vancouver. I worked in this office on a strictly referral basis, happy as a clam and busy as a bee until I decided to retire at the end of 1996, on my sixty-fifth birthday. That left me free to write, and do my lecture/workshop tours.

In 1999, we moved to Victoria, where I had grown up and still have family and friends. We bought a little heritage house which had been kept up but never been fixed, and so this has become our current project. Our plans have been approved by the Heritage Committee; we will do it in small steps, as finances allow.

And, in my 'retirement,' I have fulfilled a dream and opened a centre for the treatment of trauma and dissociative disorders. It is called Labyrinth Victoria Centre for Dissociation Inc. Besides myself, I have two part-time workers—a PhD psychologist who is a Registered Social Worker, and a Clinical Counsellor. It is the only centre in British Columbia devoted to psychotherapy of this deserving, hard-working, yet under-serviced population. My staff is dedicated and knowledgeable, and the centre will grow. In another two or three years, I will probably sell it. Then what? I will find something!

Curriculum Vitae

Education and Professional Records: BA (Zoology and Psychology), University of British Columbia, 1953; MD University of British Columbia, 1966; Medical Officer, PCEA Hospital, Tumu Tumu, Kenya, 1967–71; Certification in Family Medicine, College of Family Physicians of Canada, 1977; Awarded Fellowship, College of Family Physicians of Canada, 1987; President, B.C. College of Family Physicians, 1986–87; Associate Clinical Professor, Dept. of Family Practice, UBC, 1992–98; Active Staff, Lions Gate Hospital, 1971-89; Courtesy Staff 1989–1996; Chief, Dept. of General Practice, Lions Gate Hospital, 1975–1979; Deputy Chief, Dept. of Medicine, Lions Gate Hospital, 1980; Private Practice in Family Medicine, 1971–89; Consulting Practice in Psychomatic Medicine, Clinical Hypnosis, and Dissociative Disorders, 1989–96; Director, Labyrinth Victoria Centre for Dissociation, 2001–present; Fellow, American Society of Clinical Hyponosis; President, American Society of Clinical Hyposis, 1991–1992; President, Canadian Society of Clinical Hypnosis (B.C. Div.) 1978–83; Member: Cuban Society of Hypnosis, Swedish Society of Clinical and Experimental Hypnosis, International Society of Hypnosis; Teaching Faculty: ASCH, CSCH (B.C.) since 1975; ISH since 1985. Papers presented at the Annual Conferences of the International Society for Studies in Dissociation (previously called the Int. Soc. for the Study of Multiple Personality and Dissociation) since the establishment of the Society in 1983, until 1992; teaching faculty since 1989; Awarded Fellowship by ISSD, 1993; International Member-at-Large, Executive Council ISSD, 1991–1994; National Co-Chair, Canadian Society for Studies in Dissociation (previously called CSSMP&D) 1987–89; actively involved in the treatment of dissociative disorders since 1977; Scientific Co-Chair, International Society of Hypnosis triennial Meeting, San Diego June 1997; Member, Clinical Advisory Committee, Tzu Chi Institute for Complementary Alternative Medicine, 1995–1999; Scientific Co-Chair, Joint Meeting, Tzu Chi Institute and B.C. College of Family Physicians, 1998; Alternate Representative, College of Family Physicians of Canada, to the Health Protection Branch ad hoc Committee on Herbal Remedies, 1997–98; Locum Clinical Director, Psychiatric Unit, Mills Memorial Hospital, Terrace, B.C., Nov.-Dec. 1998, July 2000, Dec. 2000; Rotating Locum Service (Family Medicine), Dease Lake Medical Clinic / Stikine Health Centre, B.C., 1984–2000; Psychotherapy Service, Stikine Health Centre, Sept. 2000–present; international lecturer and workshop leader on Dissociative Disorders in Canada, United States, England, Scotland, Sweden, Germany, Austria, the Netherlands, Australia, New Zealand, Japan, and Cuba.

Memberships: Associate Member, Canadian Psychiatric Association (requirements include the recommendation of two psychiatrists); Member, Lions Gate Institute of Psychotherapy (membership limited to psychiatrists and physicians approved by them for membership): Institute no longer active; Member, Dept. of Psychiatry, Lions Gate Hospital, Category B, (i.e. no mandatory Psychiatric consultation required when admitting and treating patients), 1972–89; maintenance of department membership, Category B, required attendance at Rounds and Dept. meetings, presentation of cases, literature reviews, etc., on a regular basis.

Publications:

Psych Yourself In! Hypnosis and Health (Sea Walk Press), 1985

Daydreams for Discovery: A Manual for Hypnotherapists (Sea Walk Press), 1988

Creative Scripts for Hypnotherapy (Brunner/Mazel), 1994.

Making Peace with Chronic Pain: A Whole-Life Strategy (Brunner/Mazel), 1996

Numerous papers in international journals on clinical hypnosis and on the phenomena and treatment of dissociative disorders

DR. MARA LOVE

I am a family physician. I graduated in Medicine from the University of Western Ontario, London, Ontario in 1966 at the age of twenty-three, and interned at the Montreal General Hospital. In July, 1967, I married my classmate, Robert, and we headed 'out west' to practise medicine.

Why did I choose to be a doctor? I was born in 1943 in Riga, Latvia, during the Second World War. I fled with my family to Germany in 1945, where we stayed in a Displaced Persons' Camp until I was six years old. We then moved to London, Ontario, where my father had a job as a geology professor at the University of Western Ontario. My grandfather was a history teacher and theologian, my mother, a librarian, and my grandmother cooked and kept house. My sister and I were free to pursue any academic studies we desired. My passion was for art and the piano. I finished my Associate of Music degree while in Grade 12, but realized I was not meant to be a concert pianist. At this time I read a book about Dr. Albert Schweitzer, and my dream changed to that of a medical missionary in Africa. I already played the organ for the Latvian Church, so I figured I had a good start.

I started pre-med (a two-year university course) after finishing Grade 13. There I met my husband-to-be, Robert Love, the tall funny guy with glasses who helped me boil water in chemistry lab. I was a romantic in other ways, too. I loved English, philosophy, psychology, and dancing.

After pre-med, we moved to London, south to the old, dark Medical School, which stood across the street from Victoria Hospital. In my class there were sixty students, six of whom were girls. I have to admit that we girls were all serious and had little fun, compared to the men and the nurses. I always felt left out when the guys told dirty jokes (I could not 'get' them) or went to the pub or to fraternity parties. I still lived at home with my parents and grandparents and had to be home by 1 a.m. Robert and his two roommates lived in a house and could do what they wanted.

At Medical School, the biggest challenge for me was anatomy: we were put into groups of four and assigned a cadaver each. I will never forget the formaldehyde smell and grease that got all over our books, and the trials of dissecting tissue that all looked the same grey-green to me. I preferred pathology with all the colourful slides and the hint of detective work. I worked hard and became a member of the honours society, *Alpha Omega Alpha*. We wrote essays and presented them to our faculty advisor, a well-known heart surgeon, on whom we girls had a crush. I did well until the fourth year. At that time, my boyfriend and I broke up, so my clinical year was a blur of lonely hospital beds and disorganized teachings, some of which were held at the new Medical School on campus. I did graduate and went to intern in Montreal while Robert went to Detroit.

My internship in Montreal was my most memorable year. I was finally on my own, in interns' and residents' quarters at the Montreal General Hospital, which bordered on the beautiful Park Royal in the middle of Montreal. We got to do exciting things like riding the ambulance to deliveries and murders, delivering babies on our own (one of us gave nitrous oxide while the other intern delivered the baby), and being in charge of Emergency. Besides, Expo '67 was on in Montreal and we got to visit often. Robert and I got back together after he proposed to me, and we spent memorable weekends in Vermont and Mont Tremblant. At the end of the year, we got married in London, Ontario, and immediately set off in Robert's blue Plymouth convertible for the west. We were to start practice in a clinic in Squamish, British Columbia, in one week. Our honeymoon became four days travelling across the country. We have been trying to make up for that since then and have had some wonderful exotic holidays.

Squamish was a mixture of heaven and hell. We drove into heavy dust from road construction and a dense cloud of wood fibre smell and smoke, with white ash remaining on our car. Above us stretched the magnificent white glaciers and rising mists. We stayed in the comfortable house of the doctor we were working for. In ten days time both Robert and I came down with infectious hepatitis! No one had told us there was an epidemic in Squamish. Robert became very ill and was transferred to St. Paul's Hospital for two weeks. Eventually we had our own apartment. Robert worked full-time and I did part-time. We both enjoyed the Native people, and Robert travelled to Pemberton once a week to hold clinics there and sometimes I accompanied him.

The Squamish hospital had twenty-two beds, two operating rooms, and an X-ray department. There was a surgeon, and we took turns attending a six-week course in anaesthesia at Vancouver General Hospital. We got to know the Squamish highway very well indeed, as we drove back and forth so we could see each other at least once a week in a little damp trailer under the Lion's Gate Bridge.

I enjoyed the medical practice in Squamish. It was exciting, with great variety. We were on-call every second weekend and got out of town when off duty, because patients would come to the house. I got to ride the ambulance again with emergencies to be transferred to Vancouver. We presented a course on Sex Education to Grades 10 and 11.

We took a Search and Rescue Course, and learned how to rappel from a hydro pole down a cliff. We'd spent two years in Squamish when an opportunity came from the Irving Clinic in Kamloops, asking us to join their

Squamish was a mixture of heaven and hell. We drove into heavy dust from road construction and a dense cloud of wood fibre smell and smoke. Above us stretched the magnificent white glaciers and rising mists.

clinic. We planned to work for another two years and then take a year off to travel before children arrived. The Irving Clinic agreed.

In Kamloops there were specialists, so weekend call was only one out of seven, and we took turns being on-call once a week. We both worked full-time for the two years as agreed.

Then, in 1971, Robert and I boarded a Quantas flight to the South Seas. We visited Fiji, New Zealand, Australia, New Guinea, then South East Asia, India, Nepal, Africa, and finally Europe—indeed we had a wonderful travelling year.

We arrived back in Kamloops in the fall of 1972. I was five months pregnant and played housewife until Maria was born in March, 1973. I nursed Maria for six months and went back to the Irving Clinic as Laboratory Supervisor (the Government had decided that all private labs needed a doctor to supervise them). It was an easy job which kept me in touch with medicine. In September, 1974, I delivered our son, Toby. I found life with two babies very stressful and decided to go back into general practice part-time at the Irving Clinic.

On my first day back I was so slow that I got locked in by the janitor, and had to phone Robert to come get me. I often felt guilty, as I was the last Mom to pick up the children from the baby-sitter. Robert often did the picking-up, but it took him quite a while to figure out that he could make dinner as well and keep the children happy. I have to admit that I love chatting with my patients and have never learned to speed up my practice. I also enjoyed being on-call as then I got to do emergency and more complicated medicine, and I loved delivering babies.

In 1979 I left the Irving Clinic to share a private practice with another woman doctor, Audrey. We both had young children and we practised medicine in a similar way. On the days when one of us was out of the office, each could relax, knowing that everything was taken care of and our patients were happy. We had an added benefit as another woman doctor with small children moved into town and offered to work occasional days when both of us had to attend school trips or workshops. This ideal setup continued until 1992. Audrey's husband had to do a year-long course in Edmonton, so we decided to get a locum for a year. He was a young man

who did work out well for us, but we lost a few patients! I took a sketching course and continued piano lessons after a ten-year lapse. Audrey returned and we practised together for one more year, but she retired because of illness. I decided to join my husband and his partner in their office part-time. This worked well for six years, as Robert covered my hospital patients and emergencies on the days I did not work.

As far as holidays go I was lucky in having a good locum, Roberta, who moved into our house for the summer, and I had all summer to spend with the children. A terrible tragedy struck our family in 1983 when our nine-year old son was killed in a car accident. We had a lot of grief-work to do and were blessed to have a supportive church family and community, and a life-changing workshop with Elizabeth Kubler Ross. I went back to work in three weeks and my patients gave me such loving support.

As a doctor I have felt privileged to be involved in so many people's lives and hopes. In 1984 we received the gift of our adopted son, Matthew, at the age of three days. I took time off from work until a wonderful lady asked to be Matthew's Nana. She even made meals for us. Robert and I have made family and our marriage a priority. We spent most of the summer at our cabin at Shuswap Lake. Once we took time off for two months to take the children to Fiji and Hawaii. We hiked Lake O'Hara every summer. Every winter Robert and I took two weeks to travel, and we skied together.

I retired from medical practice in May, 1999, at the age of fifty-six. The final two years had been quite stressful. I took my turn as Chief of General Practice during the time of turmoil at our hospital. Then I developed dizziness and was happy when I could hand over my practice to an eager young woman doctor.

I am looking forward to a gentler life-style, with time at home to garden, play the piano, and maybe take art classes. Matthew is still a teenager, and we do schoolwork at night. I am looking forward to my husband's retirement so that we can travel and do more medical mission clinics in the future.

What have I accomplished in my medical work? My goal was to help people, which I feel I have done. In return I have received love, support, fulfillment, and adventure. Our daughter, Maria, who is in her twenties, used to complain bitterly as a teenager about her doctor parents, saying we always talked shop at dinner and psychoanalyzed her. Now she says that she actually found it exciting to share in our conversations about medicine and human psychology.

DR. SUE PENFOLD

I would like to claim that my career, marriages, and family fit together as a harmonious whole and moved from strength to strength. Instead, it tends, in places, to resemble a soap opera or a bad novel. As one of my friends remarked, truth is stranger than fiction. The reader interested in the vicissitudes of my early life and later tribulations can find them in my book, *Sexual Abuse by Health Professionals: A Personal Search for Meaning and Healing* (University of Toronto Press, 1998). Despite, and perhaps even because of this, I have managed to have a very stimulating and successful career. In addition to rewarding clinical work with children, women, and families, I have taught, been a role model and mentor for medical students and residents, taken on administrative and leadership roles, done volunteer work, and produced two books and seventy articles.

As a medical student at St. Mary's Hospital, London, from 1954–60, I remained grateful to be allowed into this male-dominated environment and did not question the right of some elderly consultants who refused to acknowledge female medical students. We were not allowed into the male VD clinic. Was it to avoid corrupting our minds or embarrassing the patients? I never asked. Because of National Health Service regulations, we had ten women in our class of fifty, which provided an excellent support group. We coped with harassment and comments like, "What is a pretty girl like you doing here? You're just looking for a husband, and taking the place some poor man deserves." Attendance for lectures was poorly monitored; fifty signatures on a sign-up sheet might translate into ten bodies in the classroom. We took long weekends on some rotations, including sailing at the United Hospitals Sailing Club at Burnham-on-Crouch. Sailing to various pubs on Sundays complemented inter-hospital races on Saturdays. At St. Mary's, psychiatry was considered laughable and we bet on how many times our analyst lecturer would mention sex. My flat-mate Maggie and I discussed careers and decided that we could not choose psychiatry or anaesthetics, both of which we perceived to be at the bottom of the totem pole. And guess what happened, years later!

Following graduation, I emigrated to Canada in 1960 with my new husband and found that women doctors here were a rare species. As an intern at Victoria Hospital, London, Ontario, I approached an elderly farmer who was slated for surgery. When I announced my purpose, he shouted, "History, yes, physical, no!" He believed that I was a young nurse masquerading as a doctor. Doctors, he insisted, were always men.

In early 1961 I became pregnant during my internship and managed to conceal my expansion in the shapeless uniform. When I fainted after standing for hours holding a retractor and was caught by a fellow intern before I collapsed into the middle of a cardiac operation, I found that my state had unexpected benefits. Henceforth I was assigned only to very short procedures. Caught up in the 'feminine mystique' at the time, I fully expected that I would become a stay-at-home mother for the next many years. Curiously enough, my male obstetrician felt very strongly that I should not shelve my talents and abilities and sent me to see some women physicians who, despite husbands and children, were carving out careers for themselves.

Before my pregnancy I had decided on a career in Internal Medicine; now I found myself trying to decide what I could manage as a wife and mother. In January 1962 I began work at the local mental hospital. I was given a month's 'training' and found myself responsible for a ward full of institutionalised women as well as on a rotation for night call and new admissions. Later, I was assigned to a men's ward where a previous physician had suffered brain damage after having been hit on the head by a large vase. There was a strong resemblance to "One Flew Over the Cuckoo's Nest." Naively, I was determined to get some of these institutionalised patients, who no longer had any active symptoms, out of the hospital. But I met fierce resistance from relatives, patients, community, and even the hospital itself that stood to lose a gardener, cook's assistant, or laundry worker. One of my most frightening duties was giving patients ECT—all by myself. Only once did a patient stop breathing, and he was held up by the heels by a burly attendant and clapped on the back.

In June 1963 we moved to Vancouver, where my husband had obtained a residency in Pediatrics. I had applied to Psychiatry, but heard nothing. When I inquired, they welcomed me with open arms, saying that Dr. Tyhurst had forgotten to reply to the applications that year. As one of five residents at Vancouver General Hospital, I quickly realised that the chief resident was no more experienced than I. Half-way through, one resident resigned, claiming overwork! We were on call frequently for Emergency and the rest of the hospital and I learned to navigate the rabbit warren of tunnels below VGH. In the Emergency there was no psychiatric space and at night we used the head physician's office. Once I asked a brawny man what he wanted. "You," he answered, advancing round the desk. Lacking call buttons or attendants, I had to rely on my quick wit to escape. One other occasion I was called urgently, to find three patients waiting. One was preoccupied with writing messages on toilet paper, another had tried to drown himself in a sink, and a tiny woman had hit several nurses with her handbag. Although it was a brutal year, I struggled on.

We had found a wonderful daycare mother for our son, and my husband and I managed our call schedules so that someone was always home with Paul. My second year at VGH, or third residency year, was somewhat easier although very disorganised. I was the first resident in child psychiatry at VGH, working with Dr. Hamish Nichol. He was always busy, perpetually late, and had little time for teaching. But I found that I loved child psychiatry. Minimal interventions could lead to major changes. It was more complex in that the child, parents, siblings, teachers, and others were all involved. Yet it was also more stimulating and hopeful, I felt, than trying to work with adults who had major mental illnesses.

From July 1963 to June 1965 we lived in Seattle where my husband had a fellowship in Pediatrics and I had a fellowship in Child Psychiatry. Compared to Canada there was more teaching and supervision, and we even had those new-fangled video cameras. People worked at a faster pace and under greater pressure. I thought they were joking, at first, when they decided to compress every hour into fifty minutes so that our day, with patient visits and teaching schedules, went 8–8.50; 8.50–9.40; 9.40–10.30, and so on. But there was not much night call, and Paul attended a daycare for University of Washington staff and faculty. There was time for skiing and sailing. Although

I had initially thought that I would work in a child mental health clinic when I returned to Canada, Dr. Nichol persuaded me to accept a faculty position on my return to Canada. This was part-time for several years, during which I had two more children.

It was in the last few months of my fellowship in Seattle that I had the misfortune to get trapped into an extremely damaging 'therapy' that massively influenced my life, relationships, and career over the subsequent years. A psychiatrist supervisor convinced me that I had "identity problems" and needed therapy with him. As described in my book, I travelled back to see him from Vancouver for the next five years. Claiming that he could restore my trust in men, which had been damaged by my sexual abuse as a child, he sexually exploited me and turned me against my mother, whom he blamed for all my supposed problems. It was my reading of feminist literature in the early seventies that facilitated my escape, letting me begin to see through his pronouncements that I should never challenge men, never be angry, and should rely on "feminine wiles." While this experience propelled me into feminism and a continuing concern about abuse of power in doctor-patient relationships, I also felt deeply ashamed about letting myself be so duped and used, and felt partly responsible. The psychiatric literature of the time tended to blame women patients who were abused, and portrayed them as deeply disturbed, seductive, and manipulative. If I was such a flake, I thought, how could I possibly be an effective psychiatrist?

In the Emergency there was no psychiatric space and at night we used the head physician's office. Once I asked a brawny man what he wanted. "You," he answered, advancing round the desk.

At the same time, however, my career in child and family psychiatry was prospering. As a faculty member I have had various work assignments which are used to teach medical students and residents on the job. My experiences have included working in psychiatric outpatient departments, a child welfare agency, the juvenile court, a child development program, a child inpatient unit with a clinic for women and children with HIV/AIDS, and doing outreach to Nelson, B.C. As well, I have always had a small private practice seeing mainly children, but more recently seeing adults, who were sexually abused as children, at various stages in their lives. I have learned to do eye movement desensitisation and reprocessing, which I find very effective for children and adults with post-traumatic stress disorder.

When my youngest was three, we employed a wonderfully warm and efficient Scottish woman as a live-in housekeeper. Working full-time with Ellen at home was much easier than working part-time and doing most of the childcare, cleaning, and cooking. In 1972 I worked part-time with the Family Law Commission headed by Justice Tom Berger, a very interesting and stimulating assignment. To keep up with the 'publish or perish' dictates of the medical school, I was writing articles, which increasingly included a feminist perspective on psychiatry. In 1975 a colleague and I founded the Task Force on Women's Issues of the Canadian Psychiatric Association and I served as the co-ordinator for the next five years. My children were a continuing joy, and I made new friends, including joining a women's consciousness-raising group, and had a little time for outdoor interests. But the damage caused by my sexual exploitation and long entrapment by "Dr. A" caught up with me. My marriage had been weakened by my withdrawal from my husband during my preoccupation with Dr. A, and my husband left me for a younger woman in 1978. I was devastated and the children were distraught. Caught up in a hedonist cult-like organisation that promoted self-fulfillment, seemingly at the expense of everyone else, their father further traumatised the children.

To keep up with the 'publish or perish' dictates of the medical school, I was writing articles, which increasingly included a feminist perspective on psychiatry.

Struggling as a single parent, my women friends were a great support. At that time, Gillian Walker and I were working on *Women and the Psychiatric Paradox*, which was published in 1983. Ellen had moved out, and her place was taken by an au pair. This was another loss for the family. But we muddled through and gradually things improved. During this difficult time, my work assignment was with the Child Development Program at the Children's Diagnostic Centre on West 10th Avenue. This was a friendly atmosphere in an old house, and proceeded at a fairly leisurely pace by current standards. I was able to get the children to school and start at 9 a.m. and be home again by 5 p.m. My writing was done at home in my 'spare time.' My daughter Mary was by that time approaching her teens; after talking with friends and colleagues, I was convinced that girls that had a horse would be much less likely to get involved in early sexual experimentation. In later years Mary told me that I was quite wrong, that some of the girls regularly invited boys into the hayloft at the barn!

In 1982, I decided to have another go at a relationship and, with the children, moved in with a man friend. As I had such distrust of the institution of matrimony, we lived together for fourteen years until we finally married in 1996. In some ways, this proved harder than single parenting. At times we had as many as five teenagers—two of his, three of mine—living with us. Drawing on my experiences of working with blended families, I tried to provide structure and organization, but it occasionally degenerated into huge arguments, his 'side' versus mine. It was harder for me to write in my (vanishing) spare time and it was not until 1989 that I achieved a full professorship in the Department of Psychiatry. By this time the children were scattered and Keith and I moved out to Tsawwassen.

In 1982, I was one of only two child psychiatrists in the newly-opened B.C.'s Children's Hospital, and the 'acting head' of the fledgling department. With mounting stresses at home and at work, I suddenly began, in 1984, to have panic attacks, anxiety, fatigue, and flashbacks of my abuse by Dr. A. I spent the next two years in therapy with a wonderful woman psychologist, Dr. Naida Hyde. During this time I realised how much I still blamed myself for my abuse by Dr. A, and became more aware of the pervasive power of shame in silencing victims.

Towards the end of this time, a marvelous opportunity opened and I spent a year at Simon Fraser University as the first Chair of the Women's Studies Program. This year away from medicine, dialogue with SFU faculty and students, and presentations to community groups gave me a renewed focus on the possibilities of abuse of power and trust by psychiatry and other branches of medicine. I began to talk openly about my own abuse to women's groups. At the end of the 1980s I joined a group, the Therapist Abuse Action Group, which was dedicated to advocacy for and education about sexual abuse of patients by therapists, psychiatrists, and other health professionals. This group and several friends urged me to make a complaint about Dr. A. In 1976, I had visited Seattle and confronted him in his office, telling him how he had harmed me. At that time I dared not make a formal complaint; victims fared badly, were often dismissed as sick or lying, and I judged that my career and reputation would likely face damages far worse than his. So it was not until 1991 that I got up the courage to write a letter of complaint, which led to some restrictions being put on his licence.

In the 1990s I continued my very rewarding work with our marvelous multidisciplinary team on the Child Psychiatry Inpatient Unit at B.C.'s Children's Hospital. I enjoy working with children and their families, trying to understand the traumas and vicissitudes of their lives, and working with them to find a feasible plan that will help them begin to transcend their difficulties. In the mid-1990s I began to consult with the Oak Tree Clinic, a joint project of BCCH and Women's Hospital for women and children with HIV/AIDS. The terrible sadness, loss, and devastation of their stories surpassed even those of some of the sexual abuse victims.

Sabbaticals are extremely difficult to obtain in the medical field, and I had my first sabbatical from 1995 to 1996. In addition to spending time in England, I managed a first draft of my book on sexual abuse by health professionals. Lingering shame and embarrassment caused me to procrastinate for several months, but finally I got started. My involvement with other survivors, fellow professionals, and the public had convinced me that I could make a helpful contribution to understanding victims of sexual abuse. I decided to disclose my own experiences of abuse, the after-effects and the recovery process, and linked my experiences with those of other victims and with relevant literature.

In the seventies, a major concern with our task force on Women's Issues was the over-medication of women with psychotropic drugs like valium. Women, it seemed, were sometimes medicated to help them cope with difficult husbands and obstreperous children. In the 1990s, I also noticed that children were suffering a similar fate. The rate of medications prescribed to children has grown astronomically in the last decade. Children are admitted to our inpatient unit who are on two, three, even four medications at once. Currently, I am researching and writing about the multidimensional factors involved, such as cutbacks in educational resources, society's focus on a 'quick fix,' the medical system's demands for cost-effective short-term treatments, education and practice in psychiatry that ascribe more psychiatric problems to neurotransmitter abnormalities, and the pervasive growing power and influence of the pharmaceutical industry.

In May of 2000, I was honoured to be chosen as a YWCA Woman of Distinction in the category of Health and Wellness. The Head of the Department of Psychiatry at UBC nominated me for this competition. This was a nice gesture, as sometimes my feminism and outspoken criticism of psychiatry has not endeared me to colleagues. As of writing this in August 2000, I am soon to go to England for the fortieth reunion of my medical class graduation. Next year, I will move into semi-retirement, which will hopefully give me more time to follow my passion for hiking, scrambling, kayaking, sailing, skiing, and snow-shoeing before I become too ancient. My fantasy is to write some novels or short stories as well. I wish I could say that I am destined for a tranquil old age, but crises still tend to dog me. Two of my three children have developed chronic illnesses. Luckily any tendency to feel sorry for myself has usually vanished momentarily when I think about the terrible traumas and losses suffered by some of my unfortunate patients. I recommend a career in psychiatry to keep one humble and understanding of the amazing variations of human nature through treating those who are less fortunate. Speaking from my own experience, I firmly believe that healing can sometimes be achieved with dedication and persistence.

DR. EVE ROTEM

Most of my life I have been an itinerant—as both a consequence of circumstance, and by choice.

When I was just about five years old, my parents decided to emigrate to Palestine (under British Mandatory Government). It was a very hard choice for them and caused a great upheaval in their lives. My father at the time had just shortly before started his practice as a young dental surgeon in

Berlin. But as the Nazis came to power my parents decided that that was not the kind of place they wanted to bring up their daughter, so, being allowed to take only a few possessions, the family left for Palestine. My mother, who had artistic interests but had never had to perform any housework on her own, suddenly found herself not only in a totally new and strange country, but also in altered circumstances. She had to shop and cook and clean all by herself, having never done so before.

At the time, the streets of Tel-Aviv were mostly unpaved, and camels walked through the sand slowly and majestically. Milk and fruit were delivered to the streets by 'merchants' from the bags on the sides of donkeys. My parents had a hard time adjusting to a totally different culture, language, climate, and habits from those of northern Europe. I had very little trouble, quickly picking up Hebrew, which became my language. Gradually, my father built up his practice; many of his patients were British Government officials and some were new immigrants who at the time mingled freely with the richer Arab families. My father's brother (a general surgeon)

They predicted that the three female students would faint on entering the dissection room. However, only two did, and they were males!

also arrived in those days, but all the rest (of an extensive family) stayed behind only to end up in various concentration camps.

By the age of five, I was already quite determined to become a doctor, despite my uncle's and my father's protestations that that was really not a suitable occupation for a woman!

It did not take me very long to learn to read, and once learned, I was free to roam the world through books at will, and I seemed to gravitate to tales about or by doctors, explorers, and scientists. Later, at school, even with peer pressure to become an actress or a nurse (fashionable and acceptable at the time), I persisted in the idea of studying medicine despite being told this was considered to be bad or ill-considered behaviour. I soon skipped some classes at school. The years between 1936–1939 were quite traumatic as the 'troubles' between Jews and Arabs had started and were violent.

In 1939, after the agonizing negotiations between Britain and Germany, WW II began. My father and uncle had already joined the British Army as surgeons. My uncle was stationed all over the Middle East (Egypt, Iraq, North Africa) while my father remained in Palestine. By 1940, it became evident that he was ill and was diagnosed a year later with TB. Of course, there were no antibiotics. Despite a pneumothorax, his condition worsened and in the winter of 1941, he developed a lobar pneumonia—again no antibiotics. He died in 1942 at the age of forty-two. This was very devastating to myself and my mother, and laid a whole new burden on her. During my father's illness, he had to borrow money from his life insurance for our living, and when he died, hardly any money was left. My poor mother quickly learned how to design, cut, and sew dresses.

We moved into a small apartment, and as there was no money to pay for my school, I started to give tutorials to other students to pay for my school and books. The war was a bitter experience for all—food was rationed and there were queues for everything. Then the bombardments started, mostly by the Italians, often not only getting us up at night to spend hours in the shelter, but also during day-time in the school shelter. I saw quite a few casualties—people who were innocent pedestrians—that constantly reinforced my determination to become a doctor and be of help.

At that time I took on another job, taking care of young kids after school. I completed my high school by the time I was seventeen, and as I had rejected my uncle's idea of applying to the University of Cairo or Beirut, I tried to get into a university in Britain. However, I was not accepted (even though I had passed the required Entrance Examinations) because having been too young to serve during the War, they rejected my application; at the time, they were only taking veterans. I then tried to register in France: not only did I not know enough French, but they also insisted on a French "baccalaureat." My parents had taught me some German when I was ten, so I tried to enroll in a Swiss German University, but they insisted on an entrance exam in Latin, which was another thing I had not had at school. Finally, out of desperation and with cheekiness, I applied to the University of Geneva (with the help of a family friend who could write a decent letter in French) and was accepted.

At the time one had to deposit a sum of money in the bank to prove to the Swiss authorities that one was well provided for and would not require any assistance. By working several months as a kindergarten teacher, I managed to deposit that sum. My mother thought that it was a harebrained idea since there was no chance of completing my medical studies as there was no money in the family to help me, and she thought I should keep it as my 'dowry' since I already had a serious boyfriend.

After enquiring about cheap transportation, I booked on a 400-ton Greek freighter, and left for Genoa. Before leaving, my uncle had given me a tin with DDT powder. While the ship was still in port I saw my quarters—a cabin shared by six people, with multiple storey bunks right next to the kitchen and the goats tethered next to it. Lifting the straw mattress, the whole bunk was crawling with bedbugs, the first but not the last time I encountered these critters. I put the DDT powder there liberally, but never had occasion to test its efficacy as I became violently sea-sick as soon as the ship left port. I lay in an upper deck passageway all the way to Genoa, neither eating nor drinking. Arriving in Genoa I realized that 'our' war in Palestine had not been nearly as bad as that of Italy. It was 1946, but there was still no glass in the trams, no heating, no milk for the ersatz coffee, and people wore sandals made of straw or wood! I eventually made it to Geneva, which was a Garden of Eden for me. Yes, they had rations, but one got everything permitted, and still being on a child's rations, I got extra milk, bread, and chocolate—real chocolate, the likes of which I could not even remember.

Then started a whole new chapter: first of all, I discovered that the little French I had from high school was not even sufficient to buy the simplest groceries. I had to pass my first Bachelor of Medicine nine months after arrival, in French, and I also realized that my money was not going to see me through even part of the year. So I had to pick a rented room farther from University which did not have adequate heating, allowing only one bath per week. I found that there were some small cafés in the University quarter where one could sit all day over one cup of coffee in a heated place, and that one could also put newspapers and books on top of the inadequate blanket for extra weight (giving at least the illusion of warmth). I tried to avoid the company of other students speaking Hebrew or English and took my little dictionary with me everywhere.

After nine months I managed to pass the exams in French (not brilliantly, but a pass nevertheless). I then returned to Palestine, and despite everybody's opposition, my boyfriend and I got married. He was studying at the Technion (later Israel Institute of Technology). Since he could not study at Geneva but was accepted at Lausanne Ecole Polytechnique, I enrolled in Lausanne as well. So shortly after the wedding, we left for Switzerland, with very little money and some gifts of old clothes ("suitable for Europe") as well as some old medical textbooks. Since the University and the EPUL are in widely different areas, we each had a good distance to walk twice a day (to save money, we had to have lunch at home). We studied the best we could and put up with a cold room and skimping wherever we could.

The attitude in Switzerland to aspiring women students and doctors was very nonchalant. My fellow students had the idea that women only went into med school "to catch a good husband." When they heard I was already married, I became an oddity. They also predicted that the three female students would faint on entering the dissection room. However, only two did, and they were males! We had not a single female professor or a female physician. The women physicians took great pains to hide their gender, and the only way was to wear strictly male-looking attire: hair in a severe bun, no make-up whatsoever, and of course, flat shoes. We had one specialist in TB who spent all her days in the dark, fluoroscoping patients. Her voice was deep, and she was proud to be addressed as "monsieur."

I ended up in the Medical Service even though I was certainly not yet a doctor nor even a nurse or orderly. I soon picked up what I had to do and willy-nilly learned a lot about medicine, surgery, burns, etc.

By 1948, I had noted a funny rash which would not go away, and marked deterioration in my eyesight. I finally went to the Polyclinique where the examining doctors hemmed and hawed, until finally a post-graduate student from Japan came by and told the shocked audience that he had seen that condition in POW camps and it resulted from malnutrition. His diagnosis shook them all up: What? In wealthy Switzerland? Then they found out that we basically existed on French bread and jam and little else. The only advice I got was to go home and give up Medicine. I was not prepared to do so.

Fortunately, my professor of Bacteriology came by and when he knew about the diagnosis and recommendation, he suggested that since I was a good student, if I could pass a BSc course in Bacteriology, Parasitology, and

Hygiene, he could employ me as an assistant to teach the medical students, and the University would waive my fees (which were pretty hefty as a loan without interest). Meanwhile, I got multivitamin samples and took the courses. After I passed all the requirements, I started my extra career as an assistant. Later, I got half a stipend from the Jewish Community, and in return I taught Hebrew and took care of displaced youngsters in a place close to Lausanne on the weekends.

May 1, 1948, marked the birth of the State of Israel. At the same time, the Arab Nations jointly attacked the new young state which had no army. But prior to the British leaving, the Hagana (the Jewish Self-Defence Organization) had been founded. Both my husband and I belonged to it and had been trained in the use of arms. Word was sent out to all previous members of the Hagana abroad to volunteer. We both volunteered and were sent to a location in southern France where they had camps of displaced persons, survivors of the Nazi camps and the war. These were desperate and devastated people.

As my husband and I had been brought up in a thoroughly democratic society, we shared the tents, food, and all facilities with the inmates of the camp. My husband was trying to teach them some elementary discipline and use of various arms, while I was supposed to see to the hygiene and nutrition of the camp. There was no proper physician. After about six weeks, the long-awaited ship arrived to take about a thousand of them (and us) to Israel. It was an old, derelict transport ship. I was to be the only doctor on board (still not having had any clinical experience), and it was quite a frightening challenge. We were supposed to board quickly and quietly at night, supposedly so we would be undetected. I had the only key to the sparse supply of IV penicillin which at that time came in 10,000 u. vials and was worth more than gold. Hoping to make it easier on myself and all, I said that only healthy people—no woman in the last week of pregnancy and no newborns—were to embark. Before embarkment, my husband and I had placed our few belongings on one of the wooden planks which were to be used as sleeping quarters. After everyone had boarded, I dealt with a woman who had a stabbing wound and went into labour. We returned to 'our' bunk only to discover that it along with all our belongings had been taken over by others. Those poor people had not yet managed to shed their camp personality.

Another edict of mine was disregarded: I had asked everyone not to expose themselves to the burning Mediterranean sun as they were all white from years of internment. They felt, however, that I was just another 'enemy' not wanting them and their children to be nicely tanned like the children in Israel. In a few hours, we had all our tiny sick bay full of badly burned and some badly dehydrated adults and babies. At the time I had never had to put in an IV, and most certainly not in a baby. It was quite a traumatic experience for me. To make matters worse, my sea-sickness returned and it was hard to manage.

Fortunately, the trip took only five days, and when we reached the port of Haifa and had unloaded the people without deaths or major disasters, we immediately joined the Army without even notifying our respective parents of our arrival! My husband was sent right away to an early anti-tank unit, whereas I did a stint at boot camp until they could decide where to put me. I ended up in the Medical Service even though I was certainly not yet a doctor nor even a nurse or orderly. I soon picked up what I had to do and willy-nilly learned a lot about medicine, surgery, burns, etc. I saw cases I would never see later, like diphtheria in adults, tetanus, medical and surgical emergencies.

Six months later the Medical Services decided to take all the volunteer medical students to the newly opened Faculty of Medicine in Jerusalem. At the time the Faculty of Medicine on Mount Scopus was under Jordanian occupation and Jerusalem was under siege. The road between Tel-Aviv and Jerusalem was constantly shelled, so water was only brought up weekly in an armoured convoy. The soldier-students were housed in tents in the yard of a hospital where various professors and physicians taught us some of the courses. Meanwhile, we were also supposed to spend some hours at the hospital helping out.

I was asked to assist at the amputation of a young soldier's leg which had been shattered beyond repair. This was the first surgery I assisted at, and had no idea how heavy a person's leg was when unattached. I felt really faint. Later that day and for several days I received that same leg as an anatomical specimen to dissect. Gradually, while being under military discipline, we passed the equivalent of the second MB.

At that time, the authorities also decided to have a formal opening of the Faculty of Medicine, in defiance of the Arabs, to show that life continued on in Jerusalem. Many dignitaries arrived from Israel, the U.S.A., and Britain, and the soldier-students were paraded.

Finally, in 1949, my husband and I were able to return to Switzerland where fortunately my exams were recognized, and I also got the scholarship back. So we started all over again in another small grim room. In 1951, my husband graduated, but I had another year remaining. Luckily, he found a job at a large factory in Zurich and he moved there. We had a long-distance relationship, but just prior to my final exams I found I was pregnant. The morning sickness did not make studying for exams any easier. As soon as I got my MD, I left for Zurich and joined my husband at the small flat in an outlying blue-collar suburb. As a foreigner, even a graduate of Switzerland, I was not allowed to accept a paid position, so I tried my best to do my 'rotating internship.' I worked in a university for premature infants. There I learned a lot about all the congenital malformations and complications of prematurity. On April 18, 1953, my first daughter was born. Amidst our financial difficulty and little family support, she was quite content in a drawer of our chest of drawers and in an 'inherited' pram which could be placed in the kitchenette at night. I made diapers out of old sheets, but also received fresh ones and clothes as presents from my fellow students.

We then decided that we needed to return to England and to find a place where we could both work. My husband got a job with English Electric Company, and I got an interview at the Leicester Chest and Isolation Unit, which was quite a big hospital. I applied to become a House Surgeon since I dreamed of doing surgery. Much to my surprise while waiting to be interviewed and wearing my black 'exam suit' with my hair in a bun, no make-up, flat shoes—all "comme il faut"—I heard the clicking heels of a woman talking gaily, and then appeared Miss S. the surgeon, second in command, fashionably dressed in a red suit with perfect make-up and well-coiffed hair. Her demeanour was quite a wake-up call! She was a pleasant lady, and I worked with her and Mr. C. well for a long time.

Besides assisting at surgery which was quite back-breaking as we had a lot of thoracoplasties for non-healing cavities, we also did very early cardiac surgery: closure of atrial septal defects, ligation cutting of ductus arteriosus, and of course closed mitral and pulmonic valvotomies, and the earliest replacement of aortic valves for severe aortic regurgitation with the noisy Hufnagel valve. In those days we obviously did not have any heart-lung machines, so the patients had to be cooled. After being given a "lytic cocktail," they were immersed in a bath full of ice cubes and when their temperature had dropped to a level meeting the approval of the anaesthetist, who had no monitoring equipment of any kind, the patient was placed on the operating table on top of a cooling blanket and then opened very quickly. Fortunately, the anaesthetist was very competent and calm: he continued reading his paper, commenting occasionally on what was going on in the world while from time to time he would press the bag a little. The patient was attached to a blood pressure cuff, and blood was on stand-by. Surprisingly, the patients often recovered and did well.

I had my first unpleasant encounter with Jehovah's Witnesses. We had admitted a three-year old girl who resembled my daughter a lot. She had a ductus which was ligated. Since it was very large, it had to be cut, and all went well for a few hours and then things got worse as the ligature seemed to have slipped, and she was bleeding profusely. We knew she had to go back to the OR and needed blood. Her parents adamantly refused. As a young 'houseman' I felt I could not let her die, and made her a "ward of the court." We took her back to the OR to stop the bleeding and she steadily recovered. Then I discovered to my horror that the parents had not only disappeared, but refused to see her or take her back. Finally, she had to be adopted. This haunted me for years. Later, in Vancouver, I had several adults who also emphatically refused any blood for or after surgery, and some died because of their choices. And I could never quite accept their faith.

We also did numerous lobectomies and pneumonectomies for bronchiectasies and for cancer of the lung. It was the time when Hill & Doll's

Working on the wards was a delight; the Sister (head nurse) knew all about each and every patient, their diagnosis, progress, and daily condition. We also had to have a 'sluice room' inspection to look at all the bed pans, urinals, sputum mugs—definitely not a pleasant job.

articles regarding the relationship of smoking to lung cancer first appeared, and my experience in thoracic surgery only demonstrated the truth of their research!

By the time I finished the first six months of this job I found out that in order to go into surgery, I would have to do a lot more general surgery and would have to go to London. Balancing work and family was hard enough. After discussing this issue with my colleagues and family, I decided to switch to a Registrarship in Medicine. Now I had two infectious wards and two wards with fourty TB patients each. Working on the wards was a delight; the Sister (head nurse) knew all about each and every patient, their diagnosis, progress, and daily condition. We also had to have a 'sluice room' inspection to look at all the bed pans, urinals, sputum mugs—definitely not a pleasant job. But this was most helpful for diagnosis and treatment, and I was very sorry that in the U.S.A. and Canada we did not have anything like it. In those days the registrars were also supposed to do the dimple checks on blood: haemoglobin, urinalysis, and plating of sputa. We learned once and for all the unforgettable appearance and smell of melena, the appearance of sputum of TB, bronchiectasis, and the various stages of bacterial pneumonia. In those years in England, TB meningitis was common along with all other meningitides, and it became routine for us to give daily lumbar punctures for those poor patients who needed intrathecal streptomycin. I also visited Dr. Honey in Oxford and witnessed her pioneering work on intrathecal PPD.

I had not even heard of Vancouver. I felt Canada was a country of eternal snow, igloos, and Mounties. My husband reassured me that it was quite a civilized country, and brought me some pamphlets which showed houses and buses and the beautiful weather.

In the late 1950s, we had an outbreak of poliomyelitis. Since ours was the only Isolation Hospital in Leicestershire, we got all the acute patients, including all the paralytic cases. We had several iron lungs (and later, alligator respirators) but no way of knowing how well the respiration was controlled. We had no oximeters and no blood gases. By that time some early articles about blood gases had appeared in the medical literature, but there was only one hospital in the city which undertook this test. Nobody was used to taking arterial blood samples, so it was a big deal to obtain a sample, call a taxi, and the sample dispatched to the Leicester Royal Infirmary. If one was lucky one got a phone message by late afternoon. Meanwhile, we had to continue the age-old clinically based judgment: if the patient was pink, calm, and fell asleep, the blood gases were functioning well. It was during that epidemic that I also delivered the last baby to a woman in a respirator. Fortunately, both survived, and years later, on a return visit to Leicester, I met her and her teenaged son. To make it more interesting we had several cases of viral meningitides, including ECHO virus, measles, and mumps, as well as cases due to Listeria Monocytogenes. In addition to the common meningitides such as meningococcal, H. Influenza, and S. Pneumoniae, there were always cases of TB.

We had to be on call every second night and second weekend, and this work schedule was very hard on my family and me. When I approached my boss, he said patronizingly, "My dear girl, if you cannot manage the schedule the way it is, then look for another job. I did not ask you to come!" and that was the end of it—I never approached him again. Since we had only mercurial diuretics for patients who often developed pulmonary oedema at night, the only thing one could do was a therapeutic bronchoscopy and suction of the oedema. For severe peripheral oedema, we used the nasty Suthey's tubes: little bronze tubes inserted into the distended legs and then with the patient's legs in a basin, the fluid drained—of course we had no idea about electrolytes, nor were we able to measure them.

A colleague of mine on the medical service was the cardiologist for the hospital. He was the only one who could and did read ECG's, which in those days were considered absolutely diagnostic. It was also a lengthy procedure to obtain them; they were recorded on light sensitive strips and had to be developed. He talked me into developing an interest in Cardiology and said that ECGs, despite their appearance, were not so enigmatic after all. He taught me patiently and took me on rounds with him. At the same time I continued my work on the general medical wards and paid a lot more attention to the cardiac status of all patients. Gradually, I even managed to hear more and more different murmurs, finally believing they were not some invention of the professor, and they were not 'built in into some specialists' stethoscopes.' There were actually quite a lot of cardiac patients: acute and chronic rheumatic fever were common conditions and with it the murmurs of valvular stenosis and regurgitation, and acute as well as sub-acute bacterial endocarditis. In addition, we got a fair number of congenital heart disease, found mostly in babies and small children. We had a visiting Cardiologist who ran the Congenital Heart Disease Program. He only had his ears, ECG's, and X-rays at his disposal, as ultrasound and CT scans had not been developed yet. He did his best at this guessing game, and I often wondered at the responsibility of subjecting patients to risky surgery on that basis.

In 1957, it became obvious that doing only the clinical assessment of cardiac conditions was no longer enough. The first tentative cardiac catheterizations were done. Only the right side of the heart was accessible via a cut-down on the right median vein, a procedure which at the time was not yet done at Leicester, and as a result I went several times a week to Sheffield. My guru was a young cardiologist who had sustained a traumatic hemiplegia due to a MVA. His left hand was useless, but he was fiercely independent and resisted all assistance. He used the paralyzed left hand as a weight to hold the patient's arm and swab down. When the vein was isolated, a catheter was passed through the vein under fluoroscopy and into the right side of the heart. Other than measuring the arterial pressure (at first indirectly with a blood pressure cuff and then through a needle into the brachial artery), the left side of the heart was not accessible. Even so, I quickly learned that even our regional specialist in congenital heart disease was prone to make mistakes in diagnosis.

Gradually, I knew enough to start the cardiac catheterizations at Leicester, using the X-ray room for it. After a while, it became all too obvious that other techniques were required to gain access to the left side of the heart. More publications regarding such a technique appeared, and I learned to pass a long needle through the bronchoscope, directly into the left atrium. That was, of course, very useful in the many cases of suspected mitral stenosis: if the blood spurted right up the bronchoscope, the pressure was elevated (but we could not measure the height). The anxiety then was to remove the bronchoscope without any means of stopping the bleeding or applying pressure to the punctured atrium. Later yet, we started to insert a long needle (initially a lumbar puncture needle) through the chest wall and into the left ventricle. Again, if the pressure was very elevated, the blood spurted right across the room. To get a gradient, we measured the pressure in the brachial artery as well, although mostly not simultaneously. We were lucky because we knew virtually nothing about the anatomy of the coronary arterial system, or I would have never dared to do that blindly. Because of the high incidence of pulmonary diseases, I got good exposure to pulmonary pathology and treatment.

In early 1958, my colleague in medicine/cardiology persuaded me to try for the Membership. Obtaining the Membership from the Royal College of Physicians of Edinburgh, and preferably, from London, was a "must" to obtain a higher position. The failure rate for these examinations (and particularly the London Membership of the RCP) was so high that people took out a 'subscription' twice a year. I had watched other Registrars try time and time again, and doubted if I would be able to pass either. The London Membership was known to be particularly difficult, coupled with the disadvantage that I am a woman. I hesitated, studied, and finally decided to go for both. Each consisted of several parts. First was a written examination and if one passed, one had to present oneself for the clinical part, followed by the last two "vivas." Much to my surprise and delight, I passed all these examinations. I proceeded on to obtaining London Membership, although the mere idea of it was too intimidating. After I finished all the examinations, I waited for the results, which would be posted in front of the Secretaries' office. I had passed that as well. As luck would have it, before I left Leicester for Edinburgh, I discovered I was pregnant. Studying and working thus became much more difficult with all my symptoms coming along.

During the previous year my husband, who had always wanted to get his PhD, had started his studies at the University of Nottingham. With autumn came the fog and endless drizzle, and he began to find the commuting between London and Nottingham increasingly difficult. He therefore corresponded with the authorities at the Israel Institute of Technology and was accepted. Having passed my Membership exams, and even though obviously pregnant, I obtained the position of Senior Registrar at the same hospital. So I continued as usual and my husband left for Israel. As it became too difficult to manage the work, my daughter, and the house, I decided to take the opportunity and apply to buy a house right across from the hospital. I continued to work until two weeks prior to the expected date of delivery, and painted all the walls and ceilings in the house. My second daughter was born on Labour Day, 1959. In those ten days at the hospital, my surgical colleague and his wife kindly took care of our first daughter (as my husband did not return until six months later). Four weeks after the birth, having dealt with a newborn and hordes of visitors, I returned to work. In those days we were fortunate to have a doctors' maid who not only brought us a cup of tea early in the morning when on duty, but also kept an eye on the baby for me while I was on the wards shuttling between breast-feeding and the patients.

Eventually, my husband returned for a short time, but again found it too hard to commute to Nottingham, and he decided to return to Israel. I stayed behind with the children. After I completed my stint as a Senior Registrar, I could not get a post as consultant. After several months of hopeful waiting, I sold the house, packed up all our belongings, and went to Israel with my kids.

Fortunately, all my degrees were recognized, but I had great difficulty trying to find a paying job. Since my husband was working on his PhD, he only had a symbolic salary which hardly sustained the expenses of the whole family. I finally got a job with the Edinburgh Medical Missionary Hospital at Nazareth. This meant a two-hour long trip twice daily, including a long strenuous walk in the heat. I enjoyed the work and the camaraderie there. It only lasted for about three months as I then came down very ill with infectious hepatitis.

After my discharge from hospital, I got temporary jobs, first with a team of doctors employed by the National Institute of Health of the U.S.A. to do a survey of the prevalence of high blood pressure amongst people of different descent and origins in Israel. The research was held at a large hospital in Haifa. Later, I worked for a short time at a municipal hospital; the problem in Israel was (and is) that there were too many doctors, many of whom were underpaid, and oftentimes there was more than one doctor for a patient. After a year of this unsatisfactory situation and having wasted my specialty

training, we decided to leave. We applied for a scholarship each to Stanford University (U.S.A.) and were fortunate to be accepted—my husband in chemical engineering and I at the Medical Centre.

In 1962, we went to Stanford and experienced a great cultural shock. Besides finding people and attitudes to be totally different, we experienced a language barrier, as we both had not spoken English for a long time. Other doctors and I were thinking in different terms. I found it most frustrating that the head nurse was unable to tell me anything much about the problem and condition of a patient other than knowing how many aspirins s/he had had or how many bandages, etc.

I was finally accepted in surgery while the first experiments in auto-transplantation of the heart in dogs were in progress. I also learned a lot from the later experiments in dogs' hetero-transplantation. Meanwhile, I worked at the hospital and learned newer techniques for left heart catheterization (transseptal catheterization using the Brockenbrough technique, whereas I had only used the Ross needle and technique in England). I later did some other work in cardiology using the "hydrogen electrode" and studying "corrected congenital transposition of the great vessels." I even got a couple of papers published based on this work.

In 1964, my husband had the brilliant idea of coming to Vancouver for a year. I had not even heard of Vancouver, only of Montreal and Toronto. I felt Canada was a country of eternal snow, igloos, and Mounties. My husband reassured me that it was quite a civilized country, and brought me some pamphlets which showed houses and buses and the beautiful weather. He got a position as visiting professor at UBC and asked me to clarify my position as a doctor. I utterly refused to do so, telling him that as I possessed the highest qualifications in the Empire, and Canada was part of the Empire, I should not hide my qualifications. We rented a U-Haul, loaded kids, guinea pigs, and our few belongings, and drove due north. We briefly stopped on the way at Crater Lake, Mount Lassen, drove Highway 99, and finally on one beautiful late-summer day we arrived to see Vancouver at its best. We promptly fell in love with it.

My husband's job was confirmed at UBC, and he started work as soon as we found a rental house. I later learned that however much my MRCP (Edinburgh and London) were appreciated, I still had to get my Canadian

FRCP. By then I was working at Shaughnessy Hospital with Dr. W. at Cardiac Catheterization. For years, in the U.K., at Stanford, and in Vancouver, each cardiologist adapted the catheter at the time of the procedure to suit the curve of the patient's thoracic veins, or aorta (by shaping it with the aid of a wire and a bowl of boiling water). The shaping procedure of the catheter was not only cumbersome, but slow and often painful. After discussing these issues with one of the catheter salesmen, the pre-shaped catheters were introduced. In 1967, Dr. W., the Chief of Medicine at Shaughnessy, put pressure on me to get the Canadian FRCP as soon as possible. I started studying, but my mother came to visit, and the whole family drove across Canada in celebration of the Centenary Project. Not too much time was left for studying, and I managed only to get the Certificate (there were two levels of the FRCP in those days). The Chief was not happy and said I had to go back the following year. I had no choice; this time I got it without any trouble. This was not the end of the problems, however; after having had my finals from Switzerland and the U.K., I had to pass them in Canada. It was harder to study for FRCP, mainly because I had not had any contact with gynecology, obstetrics, and forensic medicine or public health in over ten years! I passed these finals, even though I wasn't aware of the most up-to-date techniques in gynecology. After proposing a D&C several times, I was told by the examiner that I was "bloody-minded."

Over the years at Shaughnessy I had numerous residents and stayed in touch with many of them for years. When I joined Shaughnessy, it was active and large with 1,200 beds, chronic wards, and a ward for seamen. In all those early years we had three administrators: one director who was an ex-army physician and two ex-army nurses who ran the hospital most pleasantly and efficiently. They managed to make complete rounds, stopping daily in all wards, talking to patients, residents, heads of services, and listening to complaints or suggestions. One could also phone them directly with whatever problem came up and they would see to it.

Later, the hospital was sold to the Province as the aging veterans required more and more chronic care. I believe it was sold for all of one dollar. Gradually, from that time onwards, there was a marked change in the hospital. No longer was it primarily a hospital caring for a large population of patients (and their relatives), giving the physicians a chance to practise the best medical care possible with good teaching facilities for students and residents, the hospital also aimed to deliver medical care humanely. At Christmas, for example, the staff administration as well as all senior consultants were expected to be there to serve Christmas dinner to all patients and their families, cheerfully and quite lavishly (Army style: officers serving men). Before the sale we had a doctors' dining room where one could not only get a cup of coffee and buy one's lunch, but one could also discuss one's problem case in a congenial atmosphere with an attentive colleague. In the name of 'democratization,' this was abolished soon after the sale of the hospital: the dining room became a place for one and all so families of patients, patients themselves, and physicians were allowed to queue up together and to share tables with everybody. Thus, we lost all informal colleaguial contact and the chance to discuss problems in a discreet atmosphere, for we now only met at councils and formal rounds.

With these changes and the advent of more administrators being hired, more ward space was lost to patients and more reams of paper were spewed forth from all the administrators. The specially developed "office-speak" consequently became a time-consuming chore and frustration. Basically little was done to benefit patients and the running of the hospital, and any requests we submitted needed endless meetings, discussions, submissions, and re-submissions. Physicians became more and more frustrated and disillusioned. To make matter worse, under the guise of needing to cut down on expenses, the merging of the Shaughnessy Hospital with another became a forefront issue.

I wasn't aware of the most up-to-date techniques in gynecology. After proposing a D&C several times, I was told by the examiner that I was "bloody-minded."

Shaughnessy occupied a large area in a centrally located site with ample parking (which the patients appreciated); on the same site the Children's Hospital and the Women's Hospital (formerly Grace) were established. We had good co-operation, and often consultants from various departments were asked for a consultation or help in management of particular patients. For us the most logical and most economical solution would have been to merge laboratory services and kitchens and dining rooms of the three sites (preferably with decreased administration). What was proposed, discussed, and basically rejected by the staff was to merge with the University Hospital at UBC.

But this was done nevertheless. The lack of logic in this decision was incredible, for there is a distance of several miles between the two hospitals. In any case, long before a decision had been reached by the staff, the final decision was handed down by the administration and for a while, many doctors would commute at all hours between the UBC and Shaughnessy sites, resulting in a loss of time to care for patients, inability to supervise them properly, and loss of revenue. I am sure the Province never saved a penny on this arrangement.

Finally, Shaughnessy was closed altogether, and in one fell swoop, the patients and physicians lost a great hospital at a prime location. The main building was said to be too old, requiring demolition. I had worked at Hotel Dieu in Paris which dates back to the Middle Ages, and in ancient Hospitals at Edinburgh and London which with some renovations and moderniza-tion, served patients and physicians very well for many more than the fifty-odd years of Shaughnessy.

I had been teaching in Leicester, Stanford, and Shaughnessy for many years, and gradually progressed from lecturer to a full clinical professor of medicine. Yet when the hospital closed and many physicians were left to fend for themselves and find another hospital association, UBC literally wrote us off with a few written lines: "Thank you for the many years of teaching."

My colleagues in Cardiology and I decided to go to Richmond as we were not offered positions at any of the University Hospitals. We had numerous meetings and were promised that we would have a Cardiac Catheterization Laboratory to lighten the load of cardiac patients in the Vancouver Hospital ("bringing the hospitals to the community" was the slogan of the Government). After waiting for quite a while, the cardiolo-gists decided that as there was no money we would raise it, and after solicit-ing our patients, we managed to raise enough money for the equipment required, but the Government did not come up with the funds to operate it. And after a year or so this expensive equipment had to be donated to a third world country. Meanwhile, Shaughnessy patients for years had longer and longer waiting lists, to be seen by one or another of the very busy cardiolo-gists in town (again costing a consultation fee) and then had to wait again for a place in the cardiac laboratory and then similarly for surgery. And after having waited for so long, they often became urgent in-patients!

After thirty-five years of doing on-call, I was dissatisfied with all the bureaucracy and the hardship imposed on my patients and decided to quit. Thus ended a long career in a specialty I enjoyed practising through which I believe I did some good.

1968

DR. ERICA PIA CRICHTON
(1924–2005)

I spent my early childhood in Vienna with my parents and three brothers. I was a fairly good student with an aptitude for mathematics. My mother was a musi-cian, an accomplished pianist, and my father was a lawyer. I did not think par-ticularly about a career when I was at school. In 1938, I was separated from my family and was moved to England with my younger brother. We went to a boarding school in Kent. I thought that I should take my higher school certifi-cate in arts, as science, I thought, was just a matter of memorizing facts. After I had accomplished that I happened to read a book, *Mathematics for the Million* by Lancelot Hogben, and it opened my eyes to the fascination of science and the wonders of the world. I then ruminated about which science subject and what profession I wanted to choose. It came to me that medicine would be the most difficult and the most challenging discipline that would provide the broadest base to branch out into another career if I should so choose later. By that time I already had a job as Girl Friday at Cadbury's in Birmingham. I asked for and obtained a part-time educational leave to take the higher school certificate in science in order to get into a medical school. I succeeded and was accepted by the University of Glasgow as a medical student in 1943. It was a five-year course with the first year for chemistry, physics, botany, and zool-ogy, the second-year physiology and anatomy.

The medical class was big: 180 students of whom forty-two were female. A roll call was held every morning. After a few sessions a student representative asked the class to stay behind (I do not remember the pretext) and the girls were asked to parade in front and to show their knees. Another female student and I bolted from the room. I guess the others liked to show their knees.

After the first term I was called to the president's office. Sir Hector Hetherington asked me how I was seeing myself through the university. At that time I earned some pay as a teller at the dogtracks, so I replied, "I am going to the dogs." He smiled and gave me a scholarship for the rest of my medical training, and also asked me to help out in the bacteriology department during my vacation. There was a great need to test for penicillin susceptibility for Staphylococcus aureus. After that I spent my vacations of the first two years in the laboratory under the direction of Dr. Iwo Lominski, a brilliant scientist who became my mentor and supporter in my own investigations which resulted in my first publication as a second-year medical student. I was slogging and plain-sailing until the finals in 1948, when for the oral examination I was presented with patients whom I happened to have looked after in the Professorial unit. That was fun. When they finally found a patient whom I had not seen before, a patient with myasthenia gravis, she told me her diagnosis. That also was fun.

I did my first medical internship in Burnley, Lancashire, in an old rambling municipal hospital with about 300 acute beds and 300 chronic beds where patients had lingered for many months. There were only one medical resident and one medical intern (myself), and two staff physicians. At a small initiation ceremony party I was given a bottle of whisky to taste. I opened it, poured a little for myself, and found it horrible. I reached for an open window just in time to spit it out, as it was varnish and not whisky. The very same night I was on duty and had my first case of tubal pregnancy which I diagnosed, suffering agonies about having to call out a consultant in the middle of the night. When I became used to the place and settled in, I managed to diagnose two of the chronic patients as operable and sent them to Manchester for surgery with very gratifying results. It was a marvelous experience to be exposed to so many patients and to have had the responsibility and authority to deal with problems. I remember a situation in which a patient in an acute ward had a blood pressure of 240/125. I promptly set up an IV with hypertonic mannitol and was delighted when the BP came down promptly. Years later when I

proudly recounted the experience, the comment was, "a phaeochromocytoma, presumably." This had never occurred to me.

The internships were followed by six months in general practice. I was a locum in a husband and wife general practice in three small towns in the environs of Glasgow, while the wife took time off for her first baby. The practice was very busy. In the office we saw about twenty to thirty patients per hour. There was no social talk, just straight to the point about the illness, and a quick but thorough clinical examination. The patients felt well served and I felt useful. We did a lot of house calls which we arranged ourselves by street map, so that we could see many patients in minimum time, from one house to the other. The patients were ready, with their wounds or problems exposed for rapid and thorough inspection. I never had to worry about a patient because I could always see them whenever I wanted.

At that time we had an outbreak of smallpox, when one of the professors in the infectious disease hospital had misdiagnosed a patient from India as a case of chickenpox and demonstrated him to a group of eight medical students. One student died. I had to vaccinate 6,000 people against smallpox; I had my first car accident at that time while rushing from one village to the other. I was prompted back to driving without delay. I thought that I would never hear of that professor again, but he resurfaced and completed a distinguished career.

We gathered our meager possessions and the few pounds we were allowed to bring into Canada and sailed to a new world, to arrive in Calgary on April 9th, 1951, to a temperature of 23° Celsius and clear blue skies. We shed our coats and started a new life.

In December 1950, I married John U. Crichton, who had been the registrar at the Hospital for Sick Children when I was an intern there. The National Health Service had just come in and we felt that we had no control over our future. My brother was already established as an internist in Calgary and he wrote glowing reports to us. So we gathered our meager possessions and the few pounds we were allowed to bring into Canada and sailed to a new world, from Southampton to Montreal and west by train, to arrive in Calgary on April 9th, 1951, at a temperature of twenty-three degrees Celsius and with clear blue skies. We shed our coats and started a new life.

We had to look for jobs. My experience was in Bacteriology and no jobs were available in the hospitals. After being at home for two weeks, I was so bored that I went back to the Provincial Laboratory where the director Dr. Denis Shute had told me that he had been trying to get a position for another medical doctor. I suggested that I would like to work in the laboratory without pay in the hope that this position might materialize. Dr. Shute was happy to take me up on the offer. I would look after the bacteriology section and I could sit in on the histology and read the slides with him. This suited me well. It was interesting and I had the opportunity to learn something new. We did a lot of diagnostic bacteriology for physicians and small hospitals, serology, and of course public health bacteriology. The Provincial Laboratory of Public Health was under the general direction of the Professor of Bacteriology in Edmonton, Dr. Stuart, who had developed the transplant medium for swabs to ensure survival of the organisms when there was delay in delivery. After about six weeks of this arrangement I told Dr. Shute that, regretfully, I would have to look for another position unless something definite became available. He sympathized, and might have written some urgent letters to Edmonton, because I was then appointed as bacteriologist to the Laboratory and assistant professor to the University of Alberta. I learned a lot of histology with Dr. Shute and enjoyed working as a consultant bacteriologist and giving sessions to physicians at outlying hospitals.

I was treading in unknown territory in infection control, and was pleased with the great opportunities at the hospital to visit the wards and see the patients so that I could assess the usefulness and validity of the reports coming from my laboratory.

I had my first child in February 1954, taking four weeks off before delivery and four weeks after. We employed an Italian lady to look after the baby while I was at work, but I did breastfeed her, coming home at lunch time to do so. When her sibling was expected in October 1956, we decided that we needed live-in help and opted to take a small family, with the idea that the mother had her own family interests in the evenings and on weekends, which would give us privacy. To accommodate this arrangement we built a suite in the basement of our small house in Parkdale. After Andrew's arrival and Heather's astounded exclamation upon seeing him: "It is a baby," we employed an Austrian couple whose baby was the same age as Andrew. We arranged for the couple to live downstairs, with Luise looking after the children and preparing meals. Luise cooked separate meals for her family in the kitchen, so we really had separate households.

One and a half years later we moved to a bigger house, built a bigger suite downstairs, and made a similar arrangement with an Italian family who was highly recommended by our first Italian housekeeper. Mida had two children—Luciano who was Andrew's age, and Alfredo who was eight. Her husband Ernesto was a carpenter and had a job as an aide in one of the hospitals. This was a blissful household. Mida was happy looking after the children and the house, cooking for us and separately for her family (the kitchen was located with easy access from downstairs). I was very happy because the children were well taken care of and loved by both sets of parents, and the household chores were handled. And somebody was always there on the occasions when John and I had to go away. The children were perfectly bilingual, called Mida and Ernesto "mama" and "papa" and us "mummy" and "daddy." This lasted until Luciano reached the age of six when he had to go to a Catholic school and the family needed to move. They bought a house and I secured a job for Mida in my laboratory.

In the meantime, though, I realized that it would be good for me to get a specialist certificate to widen my horizon and opportunities. I considered either bacteriology or pathology and found out that I would require additional training for either of these specialties. So I chose pathology because it might possibly open more doors. John also wanted to specialize in neurology. We took six months sabbatical from our respective positions—John to do neurology in London and myself biochemistry in London and haematology in Cardiff. John's sister lived in Cardiff and we stayed there for three months. I also needed more training and experience in doing autopsies. Fortunately, the University of Alberta was very helpful and supportive, as was Dr. D. Shute. We arranged that I should keep my position in Calgary and work in the lab on Mondays and half a day on Saturdays, and do autopsies in the Department of Pathology in Edmonton from Tuesday to Fridays for six to eight months. I rented a room close to the University in Edmonton, and traipsed up there weekly either by night train or driving early in the morning. I never considered such work situations as tough, hard, and stressful. I simply did my work and my training, and the family was happy and managed with the help of Mida and her family. We both passed our specialty examinations. John had to do his oral examination in Vancouver and he was subsequently offered a position at UBC as neurologist in the Department of Paediatrics. We both then had to write our final qualifying medical examination to enable us to work in B.C., which at that time did not recognize our medical degrees from Edinburgh and Glasgow Universities. We did this without a murmur, although we did badly in paediatrics because there was an extremely obtuse question on little-known parasites. I had to repeat paediatrics, but they passed John because they felt that they could not possibly fail a person with his experience and accomplishments in pediatrics.

The University of Calgary was opening a Faculty of Medicine and John was offered the position of Head of Paediatrics. He agonized about the conflict between gown and town and how he would handle it. John was also offered a position in Vancouver associated with UBC in pediatric neurology. We took a holiday in the Caribbean to clear our brains and decided to give Vancouver a try, but we wanted to be sure that at least one of us would like it here. So I kept my job in Calgary and the home and the children, and John took an apartment in Vancouver.

We visited each other every second weekend, alternatively in Calgary and Vancouver, and looked for a house in Vancouver when it became clear that we could get established, though I did not have a job. We bought a house at what seemed to be an exorbitant price at the time, and I moved with the children in July 1967. It was hard on the children, especially my daughter (aged thirteen) who had to adjust to a new school and find new friends. I tried for a position in the Provincial Laboratory and met Dr. E. Bowmer who really wanted to add me to his staff, but he could not create a position. He was probably instrumental in securing me a job at St. Paul's Hospital, where, incidentally, I had performed very well in my oral specialty examination. My knowledge in Bacteriology was much needed and appreciated, as there was nobody in the department of laboratories with special interest or training in this subject.

For me the new job held great challenges, because my experience in bacteri-ology had been at the bench and exclusively in the laboratory. I was treading in unknown territory in infection control, and was pleased with the great opportunities at the hospital to visit the wards and see the patients so that I could assess the usefulness and validity of the reports coming from my laboratory. I used the laboratory as my stethoscope. The clinical application and rapid diagnosis for the benefit of the patient was of major concern for me. Unfortunately, I immediately encountered difficulties with my head technician who had been accustomed to running the laboratory according to standard procedures for the isolation and identification of bacteria, regardless of how long it took to send out a report. It was not easy to get co-operation.

So in desperation to understand and resolve the problems I took a course in sensitivity training and quickly realized that he was painting himself a victim to the other technicians who sympathized with him. I felt isolated. I arranged a meeting with all the pathologists where he stated that he should be running the laboratory, whereas I made it clear that I had to be in charge of methodology and procedures as I carried the ultimate responsibility for the quality of the work. As a result, he resigned and we could move forward. The clinicians welcomed me as an advisor on antibiotics and diagnostition of infectious disease, and the nurses were delighted to have a resourceful person.

In the laboratory we worked as a team, and I think that every one of the technologists was proud to be a part of the process.

There was a great need for accurate information on many issues and it was a wonderful time for investigation and collaboration. We had several minor triumphs with being able to initiate investigations which would result in practical solutions for infection control and procedures. For example, we were the first to establish hibitane as an effective antibacterial agent, demonstrated the ability of various fluids such as water and saline to support the growth of nosocomial bacteria, demonstrated to the clinicians colonization on the hands by Staph aureus and the punctures in surgical gloves, and demonstrated Legionella in direct smears of sputum with concentrated carbol fuchsin. I investigated antimicrobial susceptibility testing and after a visit to Australia introduced the plate dilution method, participated in clinical trails of antimicrobial agents, and many, many other initiatives which were executed promptly and gave great satisfaction to the technical staff, the nurses, and the clinicians.

A nurse was appointed exclusively for infection control and, together with the nursing staff, we developed the infection control program. I was in charge of the laboratory-designated medical microbiologist, acted as infection control officer, and was consultant to clinicians on diagnosis and antibiotic use. I was always on-call for emergencies, but did not mind this as I got great satisfaction in being able to make immediate diagnoses from the Gram smear, for spinal fluids, wounds, and sputa. I would phone the clinician and participate in the selection of the appropriate antibiotic with dramatic results. I was not called out often, but remember my diagnosis of gas gangrene from the stained smear which resulted in the patient being sent to the hyperbaric chamber and the saving of his leg.

Direct diagnosis from the Gram smear was my special interest, especially for the diagnosis of respiratory infection, because it was more accurate and certainly much speedier than the culture, allowing me to phone the clinician immediately with the recommendation for the appropriate antibiotic. The technologists learned the interpretation and reading, and this was incorporated in the bacteriological report and often sent out as a preliminary report from my laboratory. I wanted to publish this work, but the collection of data was very time-consuming, as the diagnosis depended on the presence of bacteria microscopically in the context of respiratory epithelia cells and inflammatory cells. This is where my knowledge of pathology and histology was so useful. It was not part of the standard training for technologists, but it became standard procedure in my laboratory.

In the laboratory we worked as a team, and I think that every one of the technologists was proud to be a part of the process. The infection control nurse was also a member of the team and our moderate rational approach in infection control was much appreciated by the clinicians and the hospital.

Domestic arrangements were also satisfactory. The children were within walking distance from school. After school they would let themselves into the house, do homework, or go to a friend's house. I was usually at home shortly after 5 p.m. They were not neglected; we always had dinner together as a family. I was usually the one who cooked, but later my daughter and my husband helped to take turns with cooking. We had adequate domestic help with cleaning, and spent much time together out walking, or on small excursions and weekend trips. John was absorbed in his work as pediatric neurologist and I supported him in this. Andrew was a social creature and had many friends, so much so that we had to send him to a private school (Brentwood) when they made the University Hill School into an experimental school. Heather continued at University Hill School. Both children graduated from UBC—Andrew in medicine; Heather in architecture.

For me the picture changed somewhat with the appointment of an infectious disease clinician who took over the clinical management of infectious diseases on patients for whom he was consulted by clinicians. I continued to go to the wards, especially the ICU where sputum bacteriology plays a very important role. The infectious disease specialist and I worked as a team. I was welcomed on the wards and often alerted the clinician promptly and directly whenever a laboratory finding indicated the need for urgent clinical attention.

It became evident even to the administration that there was a need for an additional medical microbiologist. The position was advertised and a very suitable candidate was found in the person of Dr. Alison Clarke who was then the medical microbiologist at Lion's Gate Hospital. She agreed to take the position provided that she would be appointed as the director of medical microbiology. She was adamant about this, and I agreed, with some reluctance, in the interests of the laboratory and the hospital. The arrangement worked well for the remaining two years of my appointment, which terminated in March 1989 after twenty-one years.

A few years later I was nominated to the board of the Greater Vancouver Regional District (GVRD) as director for Electoral Area A, which included the University Endowment Lands and UBC. This opportunity was intriguing, as politics had never been part of my occupation, and also because I could see that I would be fed a lot of selected material and information without having to search for it myself. Little did I realize the vast amount of information I would receive. I noted that there was a big gulf in communication and understanding between UBC and the GVRD, and I made it one of my objectives to bridge this gulf. I think that I succeeded somewhat.

Looking back on my professional life, I think that I have been very fortunate in having had the freedom to act according to my best judgment, and the opportunities and the temperament to seize them regardless of possible difficulties. I was also fortunate in having chosen a specialty which allowed me to organize my time so that I could attend to my family responsibilities as well as to my professional obligations.

(Dr. Crichton wrote her story during the winter of 2005. She died May 10, 2005 after a long battle with cancer.)

DR. ELSPETH DAVIES
(C. 1935–1974)

Dr. Elspeth Davies was born in England and graduated in medicine from Durham University in 1959. She enrolled in the post-graduate course at the University of British Columbia and its affiliated hospitals. On completion of training she received Certification from the Royal College of Physicians and Surgeons of Canada in 1968 and Fellowship in 1969. Dr. Davies was a member of the active staff of the Department of Anesthesia of St. Paul's Hospital in Vancouver. Prior to joining the staff of St. Paul's Hospital, she was a member of the staff at the Children's Hospital of Vancouver. She was an active member of the Canadian Anesthetists Society and the B.C. Medical Association. Dr. Elspeth Davies died at thirty-nine years of age in North Burnaby, B.C., a great loss to the Department of Anesthesia.

DR. IRMGARD ELISABETH HERMESH

After being in medicine for most of my life I am now retired. I graduated from the University of Hamburg, Germany in 1948, after having attended universities in Hamburg and in Strasbourg (now France).

I worked in hospitals in Hamburg and also did a locum there. Since times were very bad after the war, my husband, a physician, and I decided to leave Germany. My husband preceded me and settled in Saskatoon, Saskatchewan, Canada. In the summer of 1952, I, with two children aged one year and five years, sailed across the Atlantic to join my husband in Saskatoon.

My husband had done his internship in Canada as required of foreign graduates and had passed the LMCC examination, and we accepted a position in an Outpost hospital in northern Saskatchewan. My youngest son was born there. Since there was no laboratory in the hospital and I had worked in one in Germany, I opened a small laboratory and worked as technician in this small hospital to help my husband.

Finally in 1959 we moved to a bigger town, called Wilkie in Saskatchewan, where my husband opened a family practice. I finally was able to write the LMCC exams in 1959. In those days we had to write the exam in Winnipeg. I then joined my husband in the family practice in Wilkie. Then my husband died in a car accident, which was a horrible shock. I carried on with the practice in Wilkie, until I decided that I did not want to end my days in a small prairie town.

In 1968 I found office space in the Medical Arts Building in Penticton, British Columbia where I moved with my two youngest children. The oldest boy stayed in Saskatchewan where he went to university. It was a fortunate move, but also a demanding time, with two children and a very busy practice. There were five other general practitioners in the building, each with their own private practice, but alternating calls on week nights and weekends. Of course there were always the duties in the Emergency Department of the Penticton Hospital. There were only two female physicians at the hospital at the time I started there, and I was the third. I enjoyed my work, assisted with surgeries, and did small procedures myself. Since the neighbouring town of Keremeos had no local physician, one doctor from our medical building had office hours there once a week; he asked me if I wanted to take another day for office hours there. For seven years I travelled to Keremeos once a week and had office hours. These were usually long days and I arrived home quite late. Finally the municipality of Keremeos built a medical clinic and a local doctor settled there, so my services were no longer required. I was lucky to have a good relationship with the specialists at the Penticton Hospital and with my colleagues at the Medical Arts Building.

At age sixty-eight in 1990, I felt it was time to retire and therefore turned my practice over to a young medical couple. I was sorry to leave my patients, some of whom trusted me for all the twenty-two years I was in Penticton. There are sad and bright moments in every practice, but I am happy to say that I got along well with everyone, both colleagues and patients.

Now I enjoy my retirement.

DR. PATRICIA (PADDY) MARK

I was born in Donegal, Ireland's most northwesterly county, into a family of doctors. My father, uncles, and cousins were physicians. The other alternative was the Presbyterian ministry. Not an option.

Ireland's greatest export is doctors. In a small country with a population of about four million, there are six medical schools, three in Dublin alone. My home was in Northern Ireland, but I chose Trinity College, an ancient university, walled and self-contained, in the heart of Dublin. Once graduated, I moved to Belfast to do my house year in the days before sectarian conflict exploded. Anxious, as are all new doctors, to earn extra money, I became a "night call" physician, quartering the city in my car, armed with a radio telephone and stethoscope, doing house calls wherever I was sent. Three years later, most of these areas were declared "no go" by the British Army. I roamed the streets of Andersontown, the Falls, and Shankill alone, and never once did I feel unsafe. Ulster people are kindly gentle folk. They have paid a terrible price in blood for their betrayal by bigots and fanatics.

Jobs are scarce in a land with so many medical graduates. England beckoned, for junior hospital positions were plentiful. I chose pediatrics, and became a registrar before it came time, once more, to move on.

On January 1st 1967, I landed at Toronto airport, another medical immigrant in search of a future. I had a job—Fellow in Chest Diseases at Toronto's Hospital for Sick Children.

For the last year I had worked as pediatric registrar at a hospital in the south of England. I loved the job, and was, by this time, adept at all the technical aspects of pediatric care, one of my claims to fame being that I could get a needle into any vein no matter how small!

Thursday morning's clinic was for leukemia patients, for medical assessment and drug review, decisions and blood transfusions, and of course, for chemotherapy. It was here I met Simon—Simon who was nine when he developed leukemia. He celebrated his tenth birthday being transfused on the kids' ward, and was my constant Thursday morning companion until I left.

He decided, after a very few weeks, that I was the only person he would trust to do his chemotherapy—a cocktail of the best available drugs. His faith in my ability to get into his vein at the first attempt was complete, and with every passing Thursday, became more difficult to achieve. I used every trick I had been taught by every pediatric resident, consultant, and nurse I had known, so that I would not break faith. It took me longer and longer each week. And in the end, my tricks ran out. I began to take several attempts to get that vein. But Simon was my coach and comforter, never waivering in his confidence. There are few things more humbling than a child's unlimited faith in your limited expertise.

When it became time to tell him of my job in Canada, I was riven with guilt. It felt like a betrayal of the worst kind, and not just medical. After all, there was another registrar who would do my job. No, it was more personal, a gut feeling of abandonment, for I knew that his young life was nearly over. His mother helped us both through the awful moment when I broke my news. Simon, she told me, had never been to London Airport. How would it be if he came to see me off? It was a wonderful idea, a pre-emptive strike for absolution, my absolution, or so I felt it to be. Simon could talk of nothing else during our remaining Thursdays.

And so, on a blustery wet New Year's Day over thirty years ago, I stood with Simon in London Airport, looking at him for the last time. He was puffy from medication, his pale skin stained with tell-tale, smudgy bruises. We heard the last boarding call and he smiled up at me, holding out a parcel wrapped in bright paper and tied with ribbon. It was a necklace of sparkling blue stones with matching earrings, chosen by himself. I have them still.

I struggled onto the plane, blurred with tears, tormented by doubts about a personal decision which seemed, at that moment, to mean leaving behind everything I valued.

Simon died ten days later, at a time when I was in the throes of learning my new job. His mother wrote a long letter describing his last bout of illness. But there had been no more chemotherapy, and they had decided against further heroic blood transfusions. He had talked every day of his trip to see me off. There seemed to have been a certain element of fulfillment. It nearly broke my heart.

When I walked onto the taxi ramp at Toronto Airport that icy evening, I knew what Simon's future held, even if the timing was uncertain. I was thousands of miles away. My world seemed bereft of anything that made it good. But as the taxi crawled through snowy streets, I began to notice a part of Canadian culture which was quite different from anything I had seen in Britain. It was dark, and reflected in the snow were coloured lights, Christmas lights, patterning the outlines of each house, sparkling around windows and garlanded through trees. It seemed magical, that first drive through a Canadian city, and by the time I collapsed in bed, hope for the future had begun to nudge against my grief.

Simon would be forty now if he hadn't had leukemia.

I am still in Canada, a land with which I quickly fell in love. And every New Year, I remember the night I came to Toronto in such despair, grieving for Simon, and being comforted by the beauty of coloured Christmas lights glowing against the crisp fresh snow.

After six months in Toronto, I had had enough. There was a world of difference between my registrar jobs in England and the spider's web of resident politics at Sick Kids. I turned down the preferred residency program and with a friend and my soon-to-be husband, headed west, all our worldly possessions crammed into a battered Volkswagon Beetle.

We spent Canada's 100th birthday in Sudbury, Ontario, got mixed up in time zones in Nipigon, feasted on wild strawberries by the roadside in Manitoba, and marvelled at the soaring splendour of the Rockies. And when we drew to a standstill at the West Coast, we knew that this was where we could make our home.

But first, I had to get a job! Pediatrics was not an option, so I looked for a locum in General Practice. There is, I swear, a guardian angel whose only interest is to save young physicians from the perils of their own ineptitude on first starting General Practice! I had, luckily, some minimal experience in this field. Between hospital appointments in Belfast, I had with all the confidence of youth, hired myself out as a locum in various practices. It was a shambles. Dreary down-at-heel premises, no medical records worth the name, and a first-come-first-served arrangement for patients. Waiting rooms were furnished with benches, along which patients slid until they reached the front of the line. Inside the examining rooms, there was, if you were lucky, a table and a couple of chairs. Examining tables had not yet found their niche as an aid in diagnosis, and patients stood to be examined, the greatest expanse of exposed skin being

"O'Reilly's diamond-shaped space," the product of pulling gently on either side of a single open blouse or shirt button. In one practice, the patient's chair had the front legs cut down by a couple of inches to discourage prolonged consultation. In another, the incumbent left his woolly gloves for me to wear during the colder weather, there being no form of heat provided. All in all, I was under the impression that General Practice was pretty untidy business!

Thirty years in the trenches later, I have regrouped. I know that General Practice is probably the most demanding field of medicine. I also know that, as a General Practitioner, I have the best job in the world.

The best job in the world? In this new millenium, are there many who would agree with me? Hard to say, for there is much dissatisfaction and discontent roiling round medical communities everywhere. And yet, every day in my office, most individual patient encounters are good. Is it easy? No, of course not. Was it ever? No. Never.

We are all the complex result of many parts—genetics, family history, emotional, and intellectual experience. I had the great good fortune to be born at a time when families, communities, and nations were engaged in terrible conflict between good and evil. These were not just local philosophical differences, but overwhelming forces of evil whose aim was total world domination. Every child born during World War II was influenced

There is, I swear, a guardian angel whose only interest is to save young physicians from the perils of their own ineptitude on first starting General Practice!

by the experience even if the personal experience was benign, as mine was. My parents' war was more difficult, and the emotional legacy profound. I was seven months old when my father was captured by the Japanese during the battle for Malaya.

In 1939, my father was twenty-five. He had qualified as a doctor the year before, and within weeks of the outbreak of war, he was a Captain in the Royal Army Medical Corps. On a few days leave at Christmas, he rushed back to Northern Ireland and got married.

I was born at home, a difficult forceps delivery. A letter from my grandmother describes the family's fear that neither mother nor baby would survive. Childbirth, then, was an uncertain business. Three months later, my father's unit left to join the British forces in the Middle East. But on December 7th, 1941, the Japanese bombed Pearl Harbor, changing the course of both history and my father's life.

His unit was diverted to Singapore and arrived in mid-January. Ten days later, after a short desperate battle on the west coast of Malaya, the British troops destroyed their guns and transport and retreated to Singapore on foot, leaving behind their severely wounded. My father and the rest of the Ambulance unit volunteered to stay with these men and surrender, in the full knowledge that the Japanese don't readily take prisoners. They were lucky. Their surrender was accepted and they became prisoners of war. For the next three and a half years my father and his colleagues from several nations worked to treat and protect brutalised and malnourished prisoners on the Burma-Siam railway under conditions far beyond their worst imaginings.

But he survived. He came home when I was four. It was probably thirty years before I began to understand how much cold courage he had shown when he volunteered, that night, to wait in the jungle with the wounded men in his care. While he was missing, my mother demonstrated a different strength. We lived with relatives, always housed and cared for, but we had no home of our own. For three-and-a-half years, she never knew if her husband was alive or dead.

There was little for our family to do but hope and pray. After the war, my father told us POW stories which made us laugh. How he and three friends shared a smuggled bottle of Queen Anne whisky in the darkness of their cell in Kuala Lumpur jail. How one night, the Japanese turned out all fit men to hold up their guard house during a storm, but the men, in great glee, managed to push it over. He never talked about the bad times. But he had nightmares. During my childhood and adolescence, I was regularly wakened by terrified screams which would jolt me upright in bed, heart hammering. His nightmares diminished slowly over the years, but never stopped until he died just before his eightieth birthday. When I became interested in my father's past, I asked more questions, and heard some of the details of his captivity. One day in London, I went to the Imperial War Museum. There, in the circular reading room high under the central dome, I discovered the first of many diaries kept by my father's contemporaries, day-to-day accounts of their work, their play, their hopes, and their fears. I read and marvelled and wept. Those lost years came to life, and I began to understand my past and present. This was my heritage. As with the human animal everywhere, my family's life experiences shaped my way of doing and being, both personal and professional.

When we arrived on the West Coast of Canada, I became a General Practioner, first in Deep Cove in North Vancouver. My husband, Mark Nixon (yes, really! We share a name, his first name is my surname! Great for confusing everyone from banks to Revenue Canada!) is an anaesthetist, and worked at St. Vincent's Hospital in Vancouver until we got the chance to move to Vancouver Island. Nanaimo was a small town then, with a cheerful hospital and a medical staff of about fifty. Both our daughters were born there and grew up in our home in Nanoose Bay where Mark and I still live. We were joined in a few years by Mark's sons by a previous marriage, and our home was as frenetic with work and play as only a household of six can be. I always managed to work school hours so that I was home by mid-afternoon. I was deluded enough to think that when the kids moved on, I would have plenty of spare time to indulge in my passions—historical research, writing, and gardening. But of course, like others before me, I discovered new challenges in the world of medicine and couldn't resist, so that over the last eight or nine years, I moved in some different and complementary directions. I became involved in Quality Assurance and learned that there are great gaps in this field. I became President of the Medical Staff at Nanaimo Regional General Hospital, a fascinating job! With my perpetual interest in history, I started interviewing retired and retiring physicians, capturing their memories on tape. I burrowed through old hospital records and managed to tabulate the dates during which all physicians had had active privileges. There was no memorial for deceased physicians, but with my research and donated medical staff money, an In Memoriam board is now mounted in the hospital lobby.

During these years, the political aspects of medical care became increasingly troublesome. Change has been escalating, and change is not always welcome. As a profession, we are not good adapters. I began to realize, perhaps five years ago, that unless we embraced some new ideas, new ways of doing and being, we would be stuck on tramlines grinding towards professional destruction. The adversarial nature of our relationships with government, with governing bodies such as regional health boards, with administrators, and with each other has not served anyone well. There are, I believe, many lessons to be learned.

For two years, I was Chief of Staff at the Nanaimo Regional General Hospital. My family and personal experience has led me to condense much of my philosophy thus. I believe there is an eternal triangle: good communications lead to solid relationships which build trust, in turn leading to improved communication and so on. Engineers tell us that the triangle has great structural strength. I learned that if this particular triangle remains intact, things work. If any part of it is shattered, nothing works. I discovered that in today's health care climate, there is lousy communication, terrible relationships, and no trust. Here and there, in isolated pockets, my triangle held together, and the people involved reaped the rewards of personal satisfaction, good physical and emotional health, and great patient outcomes. But for the most part, struggles for turf, power, and control overwhelmed valiant efforts to create an infrastructure conducive to clear communication, strong relationships, and mutual trust. In the end, I chose, as many others do, to walk away from such disturbing and destructive environments. Things in hospitals are now so bad that some sort of climactic event will be necessary before a phoenix arises from the ashes.

This year, I turned sixty. I have lived through the years of medicine's greatest achievements, through years when attitudes and expectations have made tectonic shifts. We have had children, now grown, and a wonderful, rewarding life on Vancouver Island's east coast. We are, in my family, a small melting pot: I am Irish, my husband is English, and our children and grandchildren are Canadians. Our friends come from backgrounds all over the world. And as a child of World War II with some understanding of just how difficult life was in the '40s and '50s, I am more content with my lot than many of my younger colleagues. No one is shooting at us. There are no bombs. Our children will not be sent to suffer and die in foreign fields.

Perhaps, amongst the many causes of present medical professional dissatisfaction, is the sense that most of us now have no idea how far we can go, what strength we might display in the face of true adversity. Physicians today challenge themselves on mountain bikes and skis. Physicians of my father's generation had their strengths and weaknesses hammered out in the crucible of death, disease, and damnation the like of which we have not seen in our time. Subsequent generations of doctors might consider counting their blessings rather than cursing their present difficulties.

Canada and British Columbia have been gracious to me and my family. We live well and laugh a lot. I thrive on my General Practice, my colleagues, and my staff. I have ambitions to make my rock and alpine garden the best in B.C., keeping up with my husband's wonderful rhododendron collection, part of which he has grown from wild seeds. We revel in the company of good friends together with great music, food, and wine. By way of giving thanks, we host a garden party every May and invite a couple hundred colleagues, friends, and neighbours to walk round our acres, and enjoy some wine and feast on fresh buns stuffed with hot roasted ham and turkey.

And my fascination with history continues. As a volunteer for the Imperial War Museum in London, I transcribe diaries kept by prisoners of war, many of them medical, so that they are readily available in disk format to researchers.

New challenges? Oh yes! Addictions medicine and methadone programs are taking up more of my time. I am getting back to writing. Our family continues to expand. My life is good.

1969

DR. BETTY HUGGETT CHAN

As Ulysses said, "I am part of all that I have met." I went to high school in the 1950s when the country was booming and University was possible for so many of us. The women in my family live into their eighties or nineties. I wanted to challenge myself and to find a field that would allow a productive and interesting life. By the age of ten, I was fairly sure that housekeeping was not my area of expertise.

The University of British Columbia Medical School was ten years old when I was admitted. I was one of six women (we would have said girls) in a class of sixty. Our classmates managed to ignore us and be good to us at the same time. Medical school was hard, but fun. By graduation I wanted to see other sights, so I applied to University Hospital, Saskatoon, for internship.

During my first weekend on calI, a woman bled from her esophageal varices, and I learned quickly about Sengstaken Tubes from this experience. Pediatrics was the second rotation. A ten-year-old boy had high blood pressure and his pulse went slower and slower. Cardiac resuscitation was fairly new then, and I knew what to do if his heart stopped. Finally, I called a Code. The bed was very soft, so I asked the boy to lie on the floor. I compressed his chest, and asked him to take deep breaths. About this time the anesthesiology first call (a junior intern) arrived. He knew he was supposed to intubate the patient, so he asked the patient to open his mouth. On further reflection, he just asked him to take more deep breaths. Shortly afterwards, a resident and the cardiac fellow arrived on the run. We all helped the patient back to bed and the cardiac fellow patted me on the head.

I occasionally turned up at the hospital with assorted children who played in the doctors' lounge until someone could come and get them.

In my senior year, I did six months Medicine and six months Anesthesiology, and married the cardiac fellow, Fai Chan. Then we went east, he to Hamilton, Ontario for General Medicine, and I to Toronto for Anesthesiology. We stayed for two and a half years, and then went back to Saskatchewan. Fai worked for a cancer clinic in Regina, and I finished my last six months of Medicine in Saskatoon.

Port Alberni, British Columbia was looking for an internist and an anesthetist, so we were invited to go there. We had our first baby, took our specialty exams, visited Fai's family in Hong Kong, and then moved to Port Alberni. We worked as a team. Fai taught the Lab Tech to do ECGs, and set up the pulmonary testing lab. I introduced anesthesia standards and procedures into the operation room. We both began cardiac arrest procedures at the hospital.

In the beginning we looked after very ill patients on the general ward, but this was very wearing for everyone. An Intensive Care Unit was opened, and Fai gave classes to the nurses and doctors on cardiac and respiratory disease, and I handled the respirators. In the evenings we went to meet the bus that delivered all the tracheotomy tubes.

Monitoring patients' oxygen level became a very important procedure. I remember talking myself into tolerating the high-pitched beeps of the first ECG monitors in the OR. When oxygen monitors became available, I ordered two, which was seen as highly extravagant in those days. An 'expert' in Vancouver did not really think this was necessary in the rural setting (read "the boonies") and my reply was that I wanted not only oxygen monitors, but also carbon dioxide monitors as soon as they were reliable. Later these became standard devices in every operating room.

The actual hours of anesthesia were less than full-time, but there were twenty-four hours of call to cover. Some of the general practitioners helped me with call, and in return I was back-up for cases they didn't want to do. Since this could happen at any time, I occasionally turned up at the hospital with assorted children who played in the doctors' lounge until someone could come and get them.

Balancing work, marriage, and family proved a challenge for both of us. We found a full-time housekeeper and indexed her raises to ours. We had invited Fai's nieces and nephews to live with us and finish high school in Canada, thus unwittingly solving the problem of child care when we were both called out at night. Later, the housekeeper and then the neighbours took call for child care. The community definitely wanted a full-time internist, so I took more responsibility in the home area.

Continuing Education was another challenge. I would go to Vancouver for a short course and lurk in the OR to find out what was new. After ten years I went to Toronto for a refresher course and saw another set of friendly faces. I always came back renewed. In later years, some of the anesthetists came up from Victoria to give me a break.

After twenty–some years of practising, I felt I had given what I could and opted for early retirement. I happened to mention my plan in Victoria, and was invited to do locums. This led to other anesthesia locums on the Island. I also did family practice locums in Port Alberni. These were interesting years, with very steep learning curves, and a chance to work on a broader palette.

It seems to me that women usually have to decide between working too little or too much. The deciding factors are usually home–related, and may be abstract. They are often not understood or deemed important by the general public. This should not deter women from finding their own solutions to their own set of circumstances. The devil may be in the details, but so are the angels and the ordinary decent folk who make life and the practice of medicine worthwhile.

DR. BARBARA ROBINSON

I was born in Edmonton, Alberta, in June, 1941. My parents were both forty-three at the time and since they had married late in life they did not expect to become parents. However, they accepted their only child with great humour and affection. As a teenager I did some acting and won a scholarship to the Banff School of Fine Arts to study drama during the summer. I enjoyed this very much and seriously considered a career associated with the dramatic arts, but decided on science instead.

In 1959, I entered the University of Alberta and spent the first four months wondering what the professors were talking about! The English course was the only one I understood. After Christmas, however, things became clear and I managed to pass the year with some good marks. During the summer I spent some time with an old friend who was a medical student and found what he and his friends talked about was very interesting. I investigated the possibility of entering medical school and discovered that I had already taken most of the prerequisites. At that time, you could enter medical school after two years of university if your marks were high enough. I worked very hard in my second year and managed to get accepted.

My parents were totally shocked! They had assumed I would become a teacher like the rest of the family. There were seventy-five students in our class of whom ten were women. Several of the men went to the Dean complaining about the number of women because they would never practice and were taking places from fellows who would work hard all their lives, etc. Fortunately, our Dean was very ahead of his time and told them to grow up in a very nice way. We were also very aware that in the final two clinical years the school could only handle sixty students, which meant fifteen of us would be eliminated. The competition was fierce and sometimes unpleasant, but we also had a lot of fun and many of us remained close.

The big cut in our class came after the first year. We started the second year with five women and fifty men, four of whom we picked up from the class ahead of us. Our numbers remained the same thereafter and we graduated in 1965. As for the idea of women getting married and not practising, of the five girls, one is an anesthetist at St. John's Hospital in Santa Monica, one is a pediatrician in Nanaimo, one is an internist in Grand Prairie, and I am a microbiologist. Unfortunately, the brightest of us died tragically shortly after we graduated. Both the internist and I worked for many years with the Royal College of Physicians and Surgeons of Canada.

Because I was still living at home I (and my long-suffering parents) felt I should go elsewhere to intern, hence I came to the Vancouver General Hospital. The work at VGH in those years was long and hard, with too much responsibility left to the interns and residents, some of whom (such as myself) were ill-prepared to cope with what we had to face. I remember some highlights, however. Particularly enjoyable was my time spent on the ENT unit. Dr. Ken Cambon and the other ENT surgeons there were kind and generous in helping me to learn some skills. We had to work in that terrible old OR which was hot and humid, and the women doctors had to change in the nurses' room. The male surgeons did not seem to mind me barging into their change room to ask questions about the next case or what to do about the problem on the ward.

After my stint with ENT, I seriously considered specializing in surgery, but exhausting the general surgery rotation ended that prospect. The only highlight in general surgery was the day when Pat Rebbeck, the senior resident, and I went in to do a case together. The anesthetist was also a woman resident. The only man in the room was the patient! The senior surgeon came in to see how we were doing and quickly left. Little did he or we know this was the way of the future.

During my internship I met Dr. Bill Cockcroft and became very interested in what he did at the hospital. I had never met a microbiologist who involved himself so much with the clinical side of the field. I was surprised to learn that there was a Royal College training program in the field, a four-year program that I could do in Vancouver. But they had never had a candidate who completed the entire program in microbiology. Dr. Fred Roberts, who was first a General Pathologist, just received his microbiology fellowship. Fred was also very encouraging, so I decided that microbiology was to be my field.

By the time I made up my mind, it was too late for that year and they could not accommodate me. Fortunately, I was able to get a Fellowship in Pulmonary Medicine with Dr. Stephen Grzybowski. It was a very useful year for me because Stephen was doing a lot of work in TB and in particular mycobacteria other than M. TB. I learned more about pulmonary infections and the various manifestations of mycobacterial disease with his unit than I could have anywhere else. Stephen was a great character and a wonderful teacher. We did a research project that demonstrated that M.avium infections were more common in Richmond and found the organisms were present in the soil, a fact which has since been confirmed many times. It is interesting that tuberculosis of all kinds is still a serious public health problem around the world, perhaps even more serious now than thirty and forty years ago when we thought the problem could be solved.

It is interesting that tuberculosis of all kinds is still a serious public health problem around the world, perhaps even more serious now than thirty and forty years ago when we thought the problem could be solved.

To complete my residency I did two years with Dr. Cockcroft at VGH and one year in London, England, at the Royal Post-graduate Hammersmith Hospital. My year in England only served to increase my respect for Bill Cockcroft, who had figured out how to do things properly by himself and knew just as much about microbiology as the big names in the field.

I completed my residency with a year of research at UBC in the Department of Medical microbiology under Dr. Donald McLean. I received my fellowship in 1972 and spent another year as Assistant Professor in Medical Microbiology. When the position of Microbiologist became available at Shaughnessy Hospital I was lucky to be asked to fill it, but I still maintained my ties to UBC and continued as a Clinical Assistant and later Clinical Associate Professor. I taught microbiology to every medical class from 1969 until my retirement in 1996. I loved teaching, especially in the later years when we changed from didactic lectures to small group seminars. I think I learned as much from the students as they learned from me! My biggest thrill was the day I entered the hall to give a lecture to the second-year students, and realized that half were women. These women were different. They were confident of their future success, sure of themselves, and well-rounded in their activities. They did not feel they had to study all the time as we did in our class. They knew they had equal chances as the men.

One morning at the beginning of term I arrived to give a lecture to the medical class on surgical infections. Unfortunately, there was a mistake in the schedule and an undergraduate math class was also booked in the same room. As we had been using the room for a month already, I was able to persuade the poor math professor that he must go elsewhere, and off they went. I started my talk with a small film clip of an abdominal surgery where a huge abscess was discovered and lanced, releasing pus under pressure. All of a sudden a student jumped up, grabbed his books, and ran out shouting, "Oh, no, I'm in the wrong room!" After that I had trouble getting the class to stop laughing and be serious about infection.

There were also times in my career when I experienced the prejudice that women doctors were not as capable as men doctors. One time, Eve Rotem and I were examining a foreign mariner with two female students and a nurse. The nurse was translating for the patient and he gave her a long tirade, which she did not translate for us. Eve said to her that she bet he said he had been in this hospital for a week now and all he had seen was a bunch of women and was wondering when the real doctors were coming. The nurse laughed and admitted that was exactly what he had said.

During my Shaughnessy years I became involved with the Royal College, first on the specialty committee, then as an examiner in General Pathology and Medical Microbiology. In those years, we gathered in Hamilton, Ontario, for a week and put all the candidates through orals and practicals at the same time. McMaster was the only university with enough microscopes and vacant laboratories to accommodate us.

Altogether, I did eight years as an examiner, the last two as Chief Examiner in Medical Microbiology. I really enjoyed the work, and I think we were able to reform the examination process in Pathology and make it more attuned to every-day practice. My own exam had been very academic and somewhat tricky. We tried to remove the tricks and give the process some sense. After my stint as an examiner I finished Dr. Cam Cody's term on the Council of the Royal College. He had become ill shortly after being elected. I considered my appointment an honour, but did not enjoy it very much; it was too stuffy and definitely male-dominated. My term ended in 1989, and I did not seek re-election.

During the Shaughnessy era, I tried to encourage women to enter the field as well, because microbiology is one of the few specialties in medicine that adjusts easily to home and family. A woman in this field can have an interesting career and a normal married life. I am very proud of the residents who trained with us, all of whom have done very well. Alison Clarke, Ann Skidmore, and Judy lsaac-Renton were some of the best.

In 1987 after much thought, I left Shaughnessy for Lions Gate Hospital. I had a funny feeling about the future at Shaughnessy, which proved to be true a few years later. Several of my friends had difficulty finding jobs when the hospital closed. My years at Lions Gate, first as Microbiologist and then as Department Head, were the best for me. I really felt wanted and needed in the community setting. I did seven or eight years as Head and retired in 1996.

About my personal life: my first husband was John L. Williams, the youngest son of Dr. Seriol Williams, a surgeon at St. Paul's. His older brother is Dr. Kibben Williams, a GP in Vancouver. John was in the real estate business. I met him at the Royal Vancouver Yacht Club, which I joined in 1974, having bought a small twenty-four-foot sailboat. John and I raced sailboats for many years, and our adventures took us to Hong Kong, Egypt, England, Lahina, and much of the seven seas. Usually I was the crew, but I was not a particularly good racing helm, whereas John was excellent. However, I did manage to win the first Emily Carr Regatta with a team of six women from the Royal Vancouver Yacht Club. I was also the first woman on the executive of the RVYC and served for two years.

Breaking into that charmed circle of the yachting establishment was much harder than being a woman in medicine. When I joined the club they still had a lounge reserved for men only, although women had been members for years. When I showed up for a skippers' meeting booked in that room, the members were shocked to their eyeballs!

In January 1993 my husband died of cancer at the age of fifty-three. I was fortunate in being able to carry on working, which aided me in recovering from that difficult time. John's best friend, who had been on his own for many years, helped me a great deal and soon we became a couple. We married in 1994. Peter had been a very successful yacht broker for many years, but retired before we were married. I worked until I was fifty-five and could receive my pension from my Shaughnessy days. I retired in June of 1996, and we spent the summer sailing around the Gulf Islands and points north. In the fall we bought a fifth-wheel trailer and a truck to pull it and headed off south with the snowbirds. We ended up in Mesa, Arizona, and liked it so much we decided to establish a permanent winter home there. We have a small house, and travel back and forth in the trailer. We have spent some time in Mexico as well. Last year we travelled about 13,000 kilometres in our trailer. At the moment I am writing this story from our boat. This fall we will leave again for Mesa, returning for my mother's 102nd birthday in December.

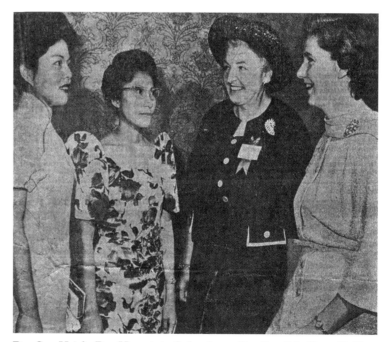

Dr. Sue Hsieh, Dr. Herminia Salvadores, Dr. Eva MacDonald, Dr. Bernice Russell Wylie at the FMWC meeting, June, 1964

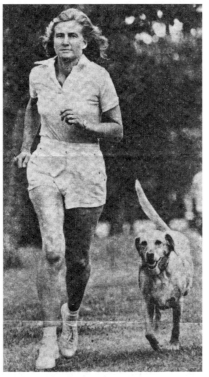

Dr. Shirley Rushton, 1960

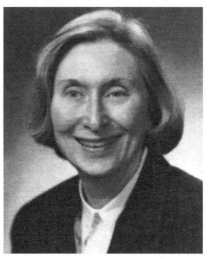

Dr. Beverley Tamboline, 1960

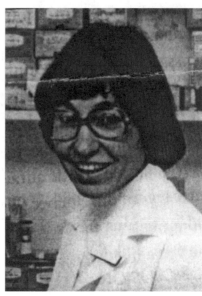

Dr. Molly Towell, 1962

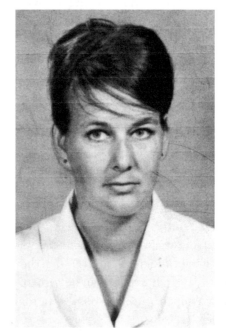

Dr. Pam Aldis, 1963

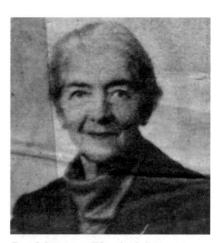

*Dr. Margaret Elizabeth Love
Petriarche, 1964*

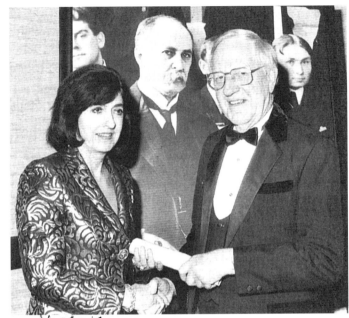

Dr. *Victoria* Bernstein, 1965

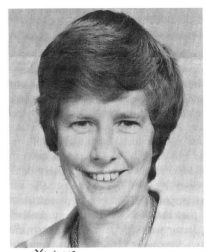

Dr. *Vivien* Basco, 1965

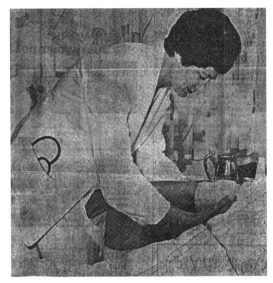

Dr. Irene Puetz, 1965

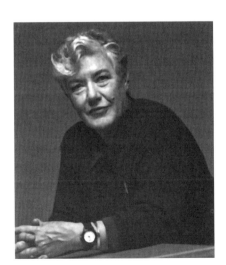

Dr. Patricia Rebbeck, 1966

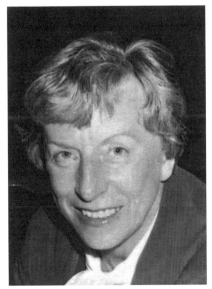

Dr. Erica Chrichton, 1968

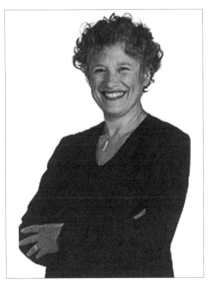

Dr. Jerilynn Prior, 1969

Notes from BC MEDICAL JOURNAL 1961—1969

January, 1961 Of the total 179 admissions to Woodlands School for the first year in 1959–60, 78 were classified as morons, 75 as idiots and imbeciles, while mongols and other low intelligence groups constituted the remainder. Over eighty percent of the idiots and imbeciles admitted were under 10 years of age, while only thirty-one percent of morons were in the same group.

Dr. Jean McLennan of Vancouver will head a special clinic set up by the Health Minister, Eric Martin, to assess the individual needs of retarded children. She and associates will determine if these children should be admitted to such schools as Woodlands or Tranquille or whether they can be satisfactorily treated in their own communities and homes.

February, 1961 Dr. Margaret Kennard, well known to Vancouver doctors and now Director of Mental Health Research for the State of Washington, is doing research in schizophrenia.

Dr. Evelyn Fox of Kitimat, B.C. where she has practised since 1953, is retiring after 16 years of practice in that centre, but is retaining her position of Medical Health Officer for Kitimat. She has a wide circle of friends, including patients, and will be much missed by the latter.

Dr. John McCreary in his address to the Vancouver Institute gave statistics on population per active physicians from 1901 to 1959: 1901: 972; 1911: 970; 1921: 1,008; 1931: 1,034; 1941: 968; 1951: 977; 1959: 918.

April, 1961 Included in the list of B.C. authors is: Dr. Ludmila Zeldowicz, "Paroxysmal motor episode as early manifestation of Multiple Sclerosis," *CMAJ* 84: 937–941, April 29, 1961.

There were double the number of cases of food poisoning in 1960 in B.C., to 714. Polio increased from 132 in 1959 to 165 in 1960, with 12 deaths, mostly in rural areas.

August, 1961 B.C. authors: Dr. Doreen McConnell and Dr. G.C. Robinson, "Simultaneous onset of diabetes, and the nephrotic syndrome," *CMAJ* 85: 81–82, July 8, 1961.

Drs. J.W. Thomas, Ann Worth, and R.C. Hasselbach, "Blood Bank: Organization and Personnel," *CMAJ* 84: 1431–1434, June 24, 1961.

September, 1961 BCMA Annual Reports 1960–61 include: Nutrition report by Chairman, Dr. Margaret Mullinger; Committee on Physical Fitness report by Chairman, Dr. Reba Willits, who also serves on the Child Care Committee.

October, 1961 University of British Columbia opened its Physical Medicine School in September, 1961. Dr. Brock Fahrni is Director, assisted by Dr. Margaret Hood as Supervisor of Occupational Therapy, and Miss Jane Hudson as Supervisor of Physiotherapy Training.

November, 1961 The former Vancouver Preventorium will now be known as the Sunny Hill Hospital for Children. It is situated on 21st Avenue between Slocan and Kaslo Streets on the grounds of Princess Margaret Children's Village. It has 70 beds for long-term illness.

In the November *Journal* there were many B.C. authors, including the following four women with their co-authors: Doris Kavanagh-Gray, Edward Musgrove, and David Stanwood, "Congenital Pericardial Defects," *New England J. Med.* 265: 92–94, Oct. 5, 1961; G.C. Robinson and Jean M. MacLennan, "The Vancouver Health Centre for Children: Evolution of the Outpatient Department during a ten-year period," *CMAJ* 85: 1944–99, July 22, 1961; J. Mavis Teasdale and D.M. Whitelaw, "Vincaleukoblastine in treatment of malignant disease," *CMAJ* 85: 584–91, Sept. 2, 1961; Anna Farewell MD, Kettyls Chilliwack DM, MD, F.E. McNair MD, "Mental Health Services at the Community Level. Project in Chilliwack."

December, 1961 There are 900 physicians in the Vancouver area.

January, 1962 In Toronto Medic-Alert opens a Canadian Office. During five years, 1955–1959, an average of 220 British doctors each year settled in Canada.

April, 1962 Articles: Ludmila Zeldowicz, "Chlorophenoxamine hydrochloride in the treatment of Parkinsonism," *Appl. Ther.* 3: 613–6, Aug., 1961.

June, 1962 University of British Columbia Medical School graduates 50 doctors.

July, 1962 BCMA Annual Meeting will take place in September, 1962. The speakers include Dr. Doris Kavanagh-Gray whose topic will be "The Diagnostic Use of Angio-cardiography."

Doctors were instructed to dispose of all tablets of Thalidomide (Kevadon) (Talimal).

September, 1962 Dr. Joan Ford of Burnaby, who is the B.C. representative of the members of the College of General Practice, was selected (one from each province) to receive the Schering Bursary Award for 1962. These physicians receive a grant which provides for a two-week Refresher Course at a centre to be chosen by themselves for post-graduate study of the newest techniques and therapies which can be applied to General Practice.

The first advertisement to appear in the *BCMJ* on oral contraception Enovid appeared in the September *Journal*, 1962.

Dr. Margaret MacCrostie lectured on Anesthesia at the September Refresher Course. Dr. Margaret Mullinger continues as Chairman of the Nutrition Committee. Dr. Reba Willits continues as Chaiman of the Physical Fitness Committee and as a member of the Child Care Committee.

November, 1962 Those receiving Specialist recognition from the Royal College include: Dr. Nancy Katherine Ironside, Anesthesia; Dr. Doris Kavanagh-Gray, Internal Medicine; Dr. Ruth Kennedy, Psychiatry; Dr. Geraldine Kent, Anesthesia; Dr. Roberta McQueen, Psychiatry; Dr. Molly Towell, Obstetrics and Gynecology.

December, 1962 The December issue of the *BCMA Journal* (*BCMJ*) will be the last issue published under the control of the Editorial Board of the Vancouver Medical Association which has for 38 years made a great contribution to the medical profession of British Columbia. The BCMA as a body that represents the whole profession, rather than one association, will undertake its publication as a truly provincial journal.

Among the B.C. authors: Doris Kavanagh-Gray, "Spontaneous closure of a ventricular septal defect," *CMAJ* 87: 868–870, Oct. 20, 1962.

Thalidomide: As of November, 1962, nine babies have been born with congenital deformities associated with the use of thalidomide by the mother during the early months of pregnancy.

January, 1963 Doctors have been notified that treatment with Tetracycline in the child will cause tooth pigmentation.

In 1958 the average income for practising physicians was $15,264.

Of 250 or more students applying to UBC Medical School, only 60 are selected; of these at least two-thirds progress to graduation. It costs the Provincial Government $16,000 for the four years to graduate a student in medicine. Student fees constitute one-eighth of the total cost. UBC has graduated 466 physicians up to 1962 with the first class graduated in 1954. Of the 466 graduates, 241 are licensed to practise in British Columbia.

February, 1963 Dr. Anna Farewell is doing post-graduate studies at the Child Health Centre.

Admitted to Fellowship of the Royal College: Dr. Doris Kavanagh-Gray, Internal Medicine, and Dr. Molly Towell, Obstetrics and Gynecology.

March, 1963 B.C. authors: Clarissa Dolman, "The morbid anatomy of diabetic neuropathy," *Neurology* 13: 135–142, Feb. 1963; M. Viola Rae, "Bronchogenic carcinoma," *Med. Serv. J. Can.* 18: 651–655, Oct. 1962; Bluma Tischler and Edith McGeer, "Effects of folic acid on the phenylalanine tolerance test in phenylketonurea," *CMAJ* 87: 1331–1332, Dec. 22, 1962.

Diphtheria occurred in B.C. in 1961; one case in Vancouver; and in July, 1962 a diphtheria case died. A second case had an eye infection and the results of a swab examination proved to be diphtheria. A third case in Victoria died.

April, 1963 There was a sharp rise in the incidence of syphilis in 1962, with over one hundred and eighty percent increase between 1961 and 1962.

Infant mortality was at record low in 1962, 22.3 per 1,000, compared to 24.5 in 1961. Relocation of Children's Hospital to the UBC campus has been recommended to the Provincial Government.

May, 1963 Canadian Research Council has awarded research fellowships to four UBC graduates. Of these, Dr. Patricia Emmonds is to receive a grant of $4,000 plus expenses for a year's research in neuro-physiology at Oxford, England.

British Columbia's new Virus Laboratory will be operating by August, 1963. It will be under the Provincial Public Health Department and will be situated in Vancouver at 828 West 10th Avenue.

June, 1963 B.C. authors: Joel B. Chodos and Hedwige Habegger-Chodos, "An epidemiologic study of 100 cases of toxoplasmosis uveitis: implications for diagnosis and prevention," *CMAJ* 88: 505–511, Mar. 9, 1963; Honor M. Kidd, C.E. Gould, and J.W. Thomas, "Free and total vitamin B-12 in cerebrospinal fluid," *CMAJ* 88: 876–881, April 27, 1963; Maria Mate and F.W. McCaffrey, "Methoxyflurane (Penuhrane): A report of 1200 cases," *Can. Anaesthesia Soc. J.* 10: 103–113, March, 1963.

September, 1963 There was an increased incidence of venereal disease in B.C. in 1963.

October, 1963 Dr. Margaret Johnston is President of the BCMA Section of Dermatology and her report was included in the BCMA Annual Reports.

November, 1963 Dr. Marie C.M. Chiasson has recently joined Dr. Jack Matvenko at Burns Lake, B.C. and will assist him for two months. She has previously worked in Kitimat. She is a very ardent big-game hunter.

January, 1964 BCMA President is Dr. N.J. Blair.

High School Career Kits are available for doctors speaking on "Career in Medicine" at High School Career Days, produced jointly by the UBC Faculty of Medicine and B.C. Medical Association.

Virology Laboratory has been established by the Health Branch, and is located in the Provincial Health Building, 828 West 10th Avenue, Vancouver.

February, 1964 At the Clinical Refresher Course at St. Vincent's Hospital, Dr. Bernice Wylie spoke on "Current Concepts of Rehabilitation."

In February, 1964, the BCMA learned of the death of Dr. Myron McDonald Weaver, the first Dean of Medicine at UBC from 1949 to 1956. He died on Christmas Day, 1963.

March, 1964 B.C. authors: P.L. McGeer and Ludmila Zeldowicz, "Administration of Dihydrophenylalanine to Parkinsonian patients," *CMAJ* 90: 463–466, 1964.

The cornerstone of UBC's new Woodward Biomedical Library was laid on February 28, 1964. Chancellor Phyllis Ross, CBC, presided, and the ceremony was performed by Mr. P.A. Woodward. The building cost $950,000; half the cost has been paid by Mr. Woodward in honour of his father, Charles Woodward. In addition, the Woodward Foundation gave a gift of three and a half million dollars to the Health Sciences Centre at UBC.

June, 1964 B.C. authors: Margaret Stuckey, David Osaba, and J.W. Thomas, "Hemolytic transfusion reactions," *CMAJ* 90: 739–741, March 21, 1964.

July, 1964 Increase continues in Venereal Diseases in British Columbia, especially syphilis.

Dr. Bernice Wylie is the President of the Federation of Medical Women of Canada for 1964.

October, 1964 B.C. authors: Doris Kavanagh-Gray, "Comparison of central aortic and peripheral artery pressure curves," *CMAJ* 90: 1468–1471, June 27, 1964; G.C. Robinson, J.R. Miller, F.J. Dill, and Tonka Kamburoff, "Kleinfelter's Syndrome with XXYY sex chromosome complex, with particular reference to prepuberty diagnosis," *J. Paediatrics* 65: 226–232, August, 1964.

Dr. Reba Willits continues as Chairman of the Physical Fitness Committee and Dr. Margaret Mullinger as Chairman of the Nutrition Committee.

December, 1964 Statistics: Expectation of life in 1964 was 66–68 years for men and 72 years for women.

Members of the B.C. Cancer Institute Research Program include Dr. Ann Worth and Dr. Honor Kidd.

January, 1965 Dr. Peter Banks is BCMA President.

B.C. authors: Doris Kavanagh-Gray and A. Gerein, "The preoperative assessment of multiple valve disease," *CMAJ* 91: 887–892, Oct. 24, 1964; Thomas L. Perry and Bluma Tischler, "5-Hydroxytriptophan administration in Phenylketonuri," *Am. J. Diseases of Children* 107: 596–589, June, 1964.

February, 1965 Dr. Patricia Radcliffe of Nanaimo, B.C. has been elected a Fellow of the American College of Obstetrics and Gynecology.

Dr. Barbara Allan Garrow was admitted as Fellow of the Royal College as Specialist in Neurology in January, 1965.

May, 1965 The Canada Pension Plan was approved by the Senate on April 2nd, 1965.

A recent addition to the staff of the B.C. Cancer Institute is Dr. Vivien Basco, a graduate of Birmingham Medical School in the United Kingdom. She has taken extensive training in Radiotherapy and in research especially as regards cancer. She is engaged at present particularly in lymphangio-graphy and its relation to early diagnosis of cancer. Her work is financed by the B.C. Cancer Foundation and she has received an Order of Eastern Star Shane Scholarship.

June, 1965 B.C. authors: D.L. Collins, J.H. Black, and Margaret Mullinger, "Gastrectomy in early childhood," *Am. J. Dis. of Children* 109: 149–155, Feb., 1965; Honor M. Kidd, "Vitamin B12 content of circulating leukocytes as an aid in the differentiation of acute leukemias," *CMAJ* 92: 261–263, Feb. 6, 1965.

UBC 1965 medical graduate, Dr. Virginia Wright, was the winner of the Hamber Medal awarded "to the student graduating in the Faculty of Medicine with the most outstanding record throughout the entire course." She won other medals (the Osler Medal) and awards in her medical years.

Dr. Bluma Tischler, a pediatrician at Woodlands School, and Dr. T.L. Perry, Associate Professor of Pharmacology, have won the Dr. L.A. Kenwood award for mental health research at Woodlands School. They have developed a test which they believe will enable them to detect in advance prospective parents from whom a child could inherit phenyl-ketonuria.

July, 1965 Dr. Kay Belton, formerly of the anaesthesia staff of the Vancouver General Hospital is now practising in Oxnard, California.

Medicare is introduced in Canada.

Faculty of Dentistry: Ground was broken in June, 1965 for construction of accommodation for the Faculty of Dentistry at University of British Columbia.

August, 1965 B.C. authors: J.C. Mitchell and Margaret Hardie, "Treatment of basal cell carcinoma by curettage and electrosurgery," *CMAJ* 93: 349–352, Aug. 21, 1965; Ludmila Zeldowicz and Wm. St. J. Buckley, "Myasthenia gravis: medical aspects," *CMAJ* 93: 189–197, July 31, 1965.

Health Planning Reports: Dr. J. Mavis Teasdale is a member of the Child Care Committee, and Dr. Doris Mackay is a member of the Chronic Care and Rehabilitation Committee.

September, 1965 The B.C. Medical Plan has come into operation, and 95,000 persons are to be covered by September 1. Cost is $5 per person, $10 for two persons, and $12.50 per family.

A project to detect hearing loss in Vancouver School children for Grades 1, 3, 4, and 5 has begun.

October, 1965 Dr. Peter Banks, President of BCMA, gave his Valedictory address in October, 1965.

Membership dues: $30 for the Canadian Medical Association, and $90 for the B.C. Medical Association.

December, 1965 B.C. authors: A.N. Gerein, R.H. Gourley, and Doris Kavanagh-Gray, "Open heart surgery for mitral valve disease," *CMAJ* 93: 643–650, Sept. 18, 1965; J.G. Gills, F.W. Hurlburt, Doris Kavanagh-Gray, R.A. Palmer, B. Shallard, and J.A. Traynor, "Clinical Management of acute myocardial infarction," *CMAJ* 93: 398–403, Aug. 28, 1965; Doris Kavanagh-Gray, "Recommended criteria for cardiac catheterization on patients with aortic valve disease," *CMAJ* 93: 1009–1014, Nov. 6, 1965.

Tuberculosis admissions for B.C. in 1964 were 385; 216 were 50 years or older, with an increase in older female patients. In 1958 there were 734 admissions.

January, 1966 Dr. H.G. Scarrow is President of BCMA.

February, 1966 St. Vincent Hospital's Refresher Course speakers included Dr. Barbara Allan Garrow. She spoke on: "Current Concepts in Management of Cerebral Vascular Disease: Medical Aspects."

March, 1966 An eminent woman physician, a visitor at UBC from March 1 to 26, is Dr. Alice Stewart who is the Nuffield Lecturer for 1966. She is Reader in Social Medicine and Director of the Social Medicine Unit of Oxford University.

B.C. authors: R.B. Lowry, Beverley Tamboline, and A. Bogoch, "Microscopic exams of stools after partial gastrectomy," *CMAJ* 93: 1205–1207, Dec. 4, 1965.

April, 1966 The world population is now three billion and is expected to double by year 2000.

A Canadian Medical Retirement Savings Plan was urged by Dr. E.C. McCoy at the BCMA meeting.

Dr. Barbara Moss, a pediatrician, has begun practice with her husband, Dr. Donald Williston, in Summerland.

May, 1966 B.C. authors: G.C. Robinson, J.R. Miller, E.G. Cook, and Bluma Tischler, "Broad thumbs and toes and mental retardation," *Am. J. of Diseases of Children* 3: 287–290, March, 1966.

Dr. Myrtle Farquharson will become Medical Health Officer in the Fort St. John area of B.C., in July, 1966.

June, 1966 The 1946 Canadian Medical Association President, Dr. Wallace Wilson, died March 12, 1966. His wife is the author, Ethel Wilson.

Dr. Florence Evangeline Perry died April 19, 1966. She was a dedicated doctor for over 30 years.

July, 1966 Biographical profiles are being placed in the Archives of the College of Physicians and Surgeons of B.C.

Influenza and Streptoccal disease occurred during the early months of 1966 with 300 cases of scarlet fever. Virus types A and B in the influenza epidemic caused 50 deaths in Vancouver, 31 in Victoria, and 25 in the remainder of B.C.

Dr. Vivien Basco of the staff of B.C. Cancer Institute has been awarded the $6,000 Shane Fellowship by UBC to enable her to continue her research on body cells. This is the second time she has received this Fellowship, the first having been made in 1965, shortly after her arrival in Vancouver from England.

August, 1966 A Genetic Counselling and Chromosome Service has been established at the University of British Columbia.

Dr. Margaret A. Carlson, UBC MD, 1964, a new member of BCMA in August, practises in Merritt, B.C.

Article by Dr. Eve Rotem and Dr. M.B. Walker on "Six Months' Experience in the Coronary Unit at Shaughnessy Hospital."

September, 1966 Reports of the Health Planning Committee are in the September *Journal*. Dr. J. Mavis Teasdale is a member of the Child Care Committee, Dr. Bernice Wylie and Dr. Doris Mackay are members of the Chronic Care and Rehabilitation Committee, and Dr. Jean Hugill is a member of the Foetus and Newborn Committee.

The Government of British Columbia has set up a Royal Commission on Automobile Insurance.

October, 1966 Dr. Molino Yam and his wife, also a doctor, have decided to practise in Valemont, in the McBride area of B.C. They are from the Philippines and are cordially welcomed by the area concerned.

November, 1966 The "60 and up," a Health Centre for anyone over 60, was inaugerated by the Vancouver Health Department as an extension of its existing health clinic. It is located at Health Unit #5, 2610 Victoria Drive. Dr. Agnes Weston, Assistant Medical Health Officer, will be in charge. A screening counselling service will be offered.

December, 1966 The declining birth rate continues in British Columbia.

Dr. Virginia Josephine Wright is included in the list of new members of BCMA.

January, 1967 Dr. A.M. Johnson is the President of the British Columbia Medical Association.

Between the ages of 15 to 24 the motor vehicle accident death rate among males currently exceeds 60 per 100,000 and is four times that of females.

Dr. Patricia Rebbeck is included in the list of new BCMA members.

February, 1967 There are 79 interns in British Columbia hospitals in 1967, at Vancouver General Hospital, St. Paul's Hospital (Vancouver), and Jubilee Hospital (Victoria).

Dr. Louise M. Jilek-Aall, Chilliwack, B.C., and Dr. Elaine Stephanelli, Trail, B.C. are included in the list of new BCMA members.

March, 1967 Dr. Agnes Weston stated that the response to the "60 and up" clinic was overwhelming. Thirty-three persons were screened and reports sent to their family doctors.

There were 43 new BCMA members, including five women: Dr. Rhoda Ree, Victoria, Dr. Roberta Dalton, Bella Bella, Dr. Gladys Murray, Richmond, Dr. Sheila Rotgan, Sooke, and Dr. Shirley Craddock, Prince George.

Extended Care Hospital Coverage as reported by Dr. Doris Mackay, Consultant to B.C. Hospital Insurance Service, in 1966 amounted to 76.6 million dollars; 1966 daily amount $246,500 compared with 1949 of $50,000 daily. The number of patients treated 329,455 and average stay 9.89 days.

April, 1967 Statistics: Population of British Columbia, 862,000 in 1966, which is 73,000 more than in 1965.

New BCMA members include: Dr. Sylvia Roa, Essondale, Dr. Barbara Ann Wilson, Vancouver, Dr. Frances Horner, Nanaimo, and Dr. Carolyn McGhee, Prince George.

Dr. and Mrs. Charles Gould are travelling around the world on their boat "Astrocyte" and writing their story in the BCMA *Journal* of April and May, 1967.

May, 1967 Neurological Clinic for school children was opened by J.A. Crichton, MB, MRCP.

New BCMA members include Dr. Judith Hornung.

Three doctors in Vancouver have received awards which will help them to devote time to medical research in Canadian medical schools unhampered by teaching duties. The three are Dr. Margaret J. Corey, Dr. Molly Towell, and Dr. John R. Trevithick. Dr. Corey and Dr. Towell will do their research at University of British Columbia and Dr. Trevithick at University of Western Ontario.

July, 1967 Salk Vaccine is to be discontinued. In 1962 Sabin live poliomyelitis vaccine was introduced to augment the protection offered by the Salk killed vaccine.

Dr. Patricia Mullins, Director of the Cariboo Health Unit since 1965, has resigned for family reasons.

August, 1967 There are now 1,683 BCMA members. New members in July and August include Dr. Doreen Bowman, New Westminster, and Dr. Helen Currie, Prince George.

September, 1967 The epidemic of gonorrhea in British Columbia reached a peak in the last quarter of 1964. In 1965, 6,005 cases were reported.

Dr. Ruth Roffmann, a graduate of the University of Breslau, has begun practice at 100 Mile House. She has practised in North Surrey for 12 years and has been a staff member of the Royal Columbian Memorial Hospital.

Dr. J. Mavis Teasdale, Dr. Bernice Wylie, Dr. Doris Mackay, and Dr. Jean Hugill remain active members of the Health Planning Committees of the BCMA.

October, 1967 Dr. Michael Turko is now President of the BCMA.

New members of BCMA include Dr. Mara Love, Squamish, and Dr. Evelyn Englebrecht, Vancouver.

November, 1967 Dr. J.H. "Jack" MacDermot, associated with the *BCMJ* and the *Vancouver Medical Association Bulletin* since its first issue in October, 1924, is retiring after 43 years. The *VMA Bulletin* became the *B.C. Medical Association Journal* in 1959.

Use of gamma-globulin is advised for Rh negative women immediately after the birth of the first child, before the woman has developed antibodies, as she is apt to in later pregnancy.

January, 1968 There is a new Logo for the *BCMJ*. Each issue will contain the list of Officers and contents.

New members for BCMA include Dr. Stephanie Dimoff, Dr. Audrey Mandeville, Dr. Shirley Hazell, and Dr. Eudora Davies.

April, 1968 The new hospital at University of British Columbia is to open in the Fall.

Vancouver General Hospital interns now do not have to do a rotating internship. They can choose specialties they prefer, but must do a three-month period in general medicine.

May and June, 1968 New members of BCMA include Dr. Margaret Hardie, Ladysmith, who for many years was with the B.C. Cancer Institute, Dr. Katherine Vaughan, Victoria, Dr. Anne Duffield, Vancouver, and Dr. Vivien Basco, Vancouver.

Dr. Shirley Rushton became the President of the B.C. Branch, Federation of Medical Women of Canada. Immediate Past President is Dr. Margaret Cox. Other officers: Dr. Doris E. Mackay, Vice President; Dr. Yang-shu Hsieh, Secretary; Dr. Patricia Rebbeck, Treasurer; and Dr. Joan Ford, Social Convener.

Dr. Shirley Rushton is a Vice Delegate for District #3 to BCMA.

August, 1968 In the summer of 1968 there was a Postal Strike.

There was the legal wind-up of affairs of MSI now that the Canadian Health Plan is functioning.

A province-wide Poison Control Centre is being established.

An Arthritis Centre is being built by the Canadian Arthritis and Rheumatism Society at 10th Avenue and Laurel Street, in Vancouver.

Dr. Ethlyn Trapp of West Vancouver has been awarded the Medal of Service of the Order of Canada. During the war years she was acting director of the B.C. Cancer Institute for which she had been a consultant and member of the Board of Directors since its inception in 1937. Dr. Trapp is still an honorary member of the Board. She was the only radiotherapist in Vancouver when Dr. Maxwell Evans, who was the Director of the Institute, joined the armed services. She was President of the B.C. Medical Association in 1946, and served in 1952 as the President of the National Cancer Institute of Canada. Dr. Trapp is a past President of the Federation of Medical Women of Canada. Other honours include a Prince of Good Fellows award from the Vancouver Medical Association.

Hon. Ralph Loffmark is the Minister of Health Services and Hospital Insurance.

September, 1968 The birth rate in Vancouver in 1967 was the lowest since 1936, according to the Annual Report of the Metropolitan Board of Health. The birth rate fell from 15.9 per 1,000 in 1966 to 14.8 per 1,000 in 1967.

Drs. J. Mavis Teasdale, Bernice Wylie, Doris Mackay, and Jean Hugill continue on the Health Planning Committees.

A new committee, the Indian Health Committee, has been formed with Dr. P.E. Termansen as Chairman. The Indian birth rate has declined from 41.4 per 1,000 live births in 1961 to 40 per 1,000 in 1967. Infant mortality dropped from 82.3 per 1,000 live births in 1960 to 61.5 per 1,000 live births in 1965. Overall mortality rate for Indians up to two years of age is eight times the national rate. Recommendation of the Committee to the Provincial and Federal Governments is to develop a comprehensive health plan for the Indians of the province and that this health plan be developed in negotiation with each Band and with local health resources within the area.

Dr. Norma Calder, West Vancouver, had an unusual vacation this year when she acted as "nurse" for the 78 young Musicians of the West Vancouver Band Association's camp at Keats Island. Her husband, Dr. T.L. Calder, is camp director. Dr. Norma Calder is mother of six children, three of whom attended the Band camp. She is a member of the North Shore Medical Advisory Committee on family living and sex programming in the schools.

New members of the BCMA include Dr. Molly Towell, Vancouver.

Referral to Chiropractors: It is illegal under Section 85 of the Medical Act to practise with or in association with an unregistered practitioner. It is also unethical.

October, 1968 Dr. R.M. Lane is the President of the B.C. Medical Association.

The Affiliated Societies of BCMA are first noted in the October, 1968 *Journal*, including the B.C. Branch, Federation of Medical Women of Canada.

In the past 15 months nine cases of diphtheria have occurred with three deaths.

November, 1968 A committee on Payment of Institutions and Special Practice Groups has been set up. Dr. Doris Mackay is a member of the committee.

Dr. J.B. McCaw and his wife, Dr. Pamela McCaw, have arrived from England to practise medicine in Vanderhoof, B.C.

Journal article: "Oral Contraceptives and Their Relationships to Carcinogenesis," by authors: H.K. Fidler MD, D.A. Boyes MD, Ann Worth MD, Central Cytology Laboratory.

December, 1968 Doctors from Czechoslovakia who have arrived in the Vancouver area need a helping hand from local physicians who could "adopt" a Czech family and/or sponsor them. Dr. Libuse Tyhurst is organizing this project.

Over 560 four-year-old children had their hearing assessed, reports the Central Vancouver Health Unit.

The Medical Women's Dinner Party sponsored by the B.C. Branch, Federation of Medical Women of Canada is for all women doctors, for all women residents and interns, with their husbands and escorts, and is to be held on January 11th, 1969 at the home of Dr. Josephine Mallek.

January, 1969 Dr. Donald Patterson, who founded the Health Centre for Children in 1946, has died.

Dr. Shirley Rushton continues as a BCMA vice delegate for District #3. She is also the President of the B.C. Branch, Federation of Medical Women of Canada for 1968–69.

February, 1969 Dr. Pauline Hughes heads Woodlands School in Burnaby. In making the announcement in Victoria, Deputy Minister of Health, Dr. F.J. Tucker, stated that Dr. Hughes is probably the first woman psychiatrist in Canada to head a major psychiatric treatment faculty. She has worked 20 years at Woodlands. The School houses 1,375 patients of all ages. She will encourage a new image for the school and keep the patients as long as necessary, then send them back into society. The more severely retarded are treated at Lady Fatima School in Maillardville, B.C.

New members of BCMA include: Dr. Janet Stewart, Whitehorse, Yukon, Dr. Hilda Stanger, Vancouver, Dr. Vivian Baker, Vancouver, Dr. Nesta Leduc, Whitehorse, Yukon, and Dr. Kathleen Elliott, Vancouver.

March, 1969 Computers are now being used at Government headquarters, for billing purposes.

Free measles (rubeola) vaccine has been added to the Health Branch list in the immunization program. The diseases on this list consist of smallpox, diphtheria, tetanus, pertussis, poliomyelitis, and rubella.

April, 1969 Dr. Mary K. Woods Langston was honoured at Shaughnessy Hospital on her retirement: Dr. Langston originally joined the hospital as a full-time medical officer in anesthesia in 1944. In 1952 she resigned her full-time position to become part-time consultant in anesthesia. She graduated in 1928 from the University of Alberta with her MD and did General Practice in Port Coquitlam, B.C. and Vancouver. She later did her training in anesthesia mostly in England, during the war years.

BCMA membership is now 2,680, an all-time high.

Dr. J.H. MacDermot, the distinguished and beloved former editor of the *BCMJ* and the *VMA Bulletin* for more than four decades, has died. He was the first editor of the *VMA Bulletin* in 1924 and retained the post when in 1959 it became the *B.C. Medical Association Journal*. Dr. Ethlyn Trapp says of him, "To look back over his editorials of more than forty years is an education in itself."

May, 1969 Hepatitis is on the rise since 1953, the year of first reporting. Two thousand cases occurred in 1968; another peak year was 1962–63.

At the North Shore Medical Society Ski Meet on Grouse Mountain the women title-holders were: Dr. Doreen Watson, first; Dr. Mary Anderson, second; and Dr. Roxanne Parson, third. The men title-holders were: Dr. Paul Watson, first; Dr. Dick Anderson, second; and Dr. Gary Morrison, third.

BCMA District #3 is now Vancouver City only.

June, 1969   Dr. Doris Mackay heads the B.C. Branch, Federation of Medical Women of Canada. Other officers: Dr. Yang-shu (Sue) Hsieh, Vice President, Dr. Pat Rebbeck, Secretary, Dr. Joan Ford, Treasurer, Dr. Bev Tamboline, Social Convener, and Dr. Shirley Rushton, Past President.

The Family Practice Unit is to open in September at Vancouver General Hospital in the former Women's Residence on Heather Street.

New members of BCMA include: Dr. Marie Warnock, North Vancouver, Dr. Ruth Arnott, Port Arthur, Ontario, Dr. Pauline Nock, Kamloops, and Dr. Therese Taddeucci, Vancouver.

September, 1969   B.C. Heart Foundation 1969 has awarded 17 grants to faculty members, including Dr. Shirley Hazell of Vancouver.

October, 1969   There was a flurry during the BCMA Meeting over the subject of Doctors' individual incomes listed in the press.

Dr. George Gibson is President of BCMA.

November, 1969   There was a Pediculosis Corpori infestation at Shaughnessy Hospital (Department of Veteran Affairs), according to the Division of Dermatology. All cases were lone men age 45–79. In the city jail there were 86 cases per month from August to November, 1968.

BCMA Reports: Dr. Bernice Wylie and Dr. Doris Mackay continue as members of the Chronic Care and Rehabilitation Committee. Dr. Jean Hugill continues as a member of the Foetus and Newborn Committee. Dr. Joyce Clearihue gave the report of the Section of Dermatology.

Minister of Health, Mr. Ralph Loffmark, has announced that the world's first centre for treatment of autistic children in a home-like setting will soon be established in British Columbia.

New members of BCMA include: Dr. Ruth Lennox, Chetwynd, and Dr. Beverley Barron, Vancouver.

December, 1969   Children's Hospital's Evaluation Centre opened at 901 West 10th Ave. as a Diagnostic Centre for multihandicapped children and adolescents.

The B.C. Branch, FMWC plan to hold four interesting evening meetings and panel discussions for Medical Women in February and March, 1970, in the Academy of Medicine. Dr. Yang-shu (Sue) Hsieh, Vice President, is organizing the meetings.

BCMA has Affiliated Societies in 23 districts in the Province of British Columbia, and also the Yukon Medical Association.

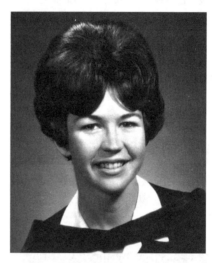

Dr. Mara Love, 1966

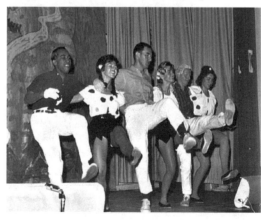

Medical school show featuring Mara Love (second from the left), 1965

Stories from 1970 - 1979

There were 466 new registered women doctors from 1970 to 1979.

1970
Dr. Vera Margarethe Frinton
Dr. Carol Herbert
Dr. Ruth Isaacsen
Dr. D. Ruth (Welch) Lennox
Dr. Teresa Elizabeth Rush
Dr. Linda J. Warren (Mrs. Joachim Burhenne)
Dr. Moira Yeung (Chan-Yeung)

1971
Dr. Mary Marshall Bailey
Dr. Hedy Fry
Dr. Mary Trott

1972
Dr. Roberta C. Ongley
Dr. Alice Caroline Patterson
Dr. Margaret Pendray

1973
Dr. June Estelle Steinson
Dr. Jirina (Strakata) Vavrik
Dr. Elizabeth Whynot

1974
Dr. Kirsten Emmott
Dr. Eleanor Payne
Dr. Lorna Sent
Dr. Emily Sterbak
Dr. Joan R. Stogryn

1975
Dr. Jean Swenerton

1976
Dr. Mary Conley
Dr. Millie Cumming
Dr. Shelley Nan Ross
Dr. Ellen Wiebe

1977
Dr. Wedad Theresa Abraham
Dr. Gillian Arsenault
Dr. Emilia Barton
Dr. Esther Brown
Dr. Diana Ho Yuen
Dr. Betty Kleiman
Dr. Lianne Lacroix
Dr. Wan Ching (Rebecca) Woo

1978
Dr. Lois Blatchford Fuller
Dr. Jerilynn Prior

1979
Dr. Lani Almas
Dr. B. Lynn Beattie
Dr. Suzanne Montemuro
Dr. Holly Stevens

DR. VERA MARGARETHE FRINTON

My father always told the story of how, the night I was born, he dreamed that he took me up the steps of a medical school. Years later, on weekends, I would accompany this small town family doctor on his early morning rounds. The antiseptic smells of Royal Columbian Hospital in the '50s were the stimulants to my love of being in quiet hospital halls.

We travelled as a family in 1957, when I was eleven, to England where my father Ernst started his specialty training. He had always wanted to be an obstetrician, but later had a bad back, which was painful for him when he was doing deliveries. He chose radiology at a colleague's suggestion . . . good hours, great pay. My mother used to work in his office when he was a family doctor in Cloverdale. Later, during summer vacations, I worked in the darkroom of his X-ray office. So, I knew about doctors and medicine . . . a bit. No doubt it played a part in my decision to become a physician.

I always remember what I think of as the 'best year of my life,' which I owe to my late parents, who encouraged travel and exposure to other cultures. After finishing high school in West Van I went to Neuchatel Junior College in Switzerland. Although not the 'finishing school' of the past, it represented something of the completion we require at that age. When I attended in 1962–1963 I took the McGill program which satisfied some of UBC's requirement. Patricia Porte (Blackshaw), now a family doctor in Crescent Beach, was there the same year, and we reconnected in 1971 when she moved west from London, Ontario. The year was spent studying a bit, but mainly learning French and travelling in well-chaperoned buses throughout Europe and North Africa. We had a blast! Since then my daughter Leah has become an alumna, as did Pat's daughters. It gave us the taste to travel and explore.

My dream of becoming a prima ballerina was dashed when I developed the shape I have now! Certainly by the time I was twelve I knew I wished to study medicine. At seventeen, as an undergrad at UBC, I recall buying a book on Operative Gynecology that was on sale at the Bookstore. I hadn't even applied to medical school yet. I later used the book to study for my Fellowship exams. Being accepted into medical school in 1965 was not the challenge it is today, but in any event I was not immediately accepted, as I had an Arts background and only average marks. I had found the science prerequisites very tough, as I had always excelled at languages. I generally memorized what I needed in order to pass the chemistry and physics exams . . . sometimes in the parking lot before running to the examination hall. I was put on the waiting list, and had to have an interview with the Associate Dean prior to my acceptance. (This is making me feel old, as now there are several Associate Deans, and all short-listed applicants have several interviews.) I now enjoy the responsibility of being a member of the Admissions Selection Committee . . . and recognize that the students now are of an extraordinary academic culture, with broad backgrounds and wonderfully varied life experience.

It was during my years at UBC medical school that I really made the important friendships and relationships of my life. We were all so connected, by the new subjects, the incredibly hard work, the pleasure of learning, and, oh, so much fun. The class of '69 (soixante-neuf toujours) still manages to have warm and fairly well-attended reunions.

After graduation it was off to San Francisco with several classmates to experience an American rotating internship. We felt woefully inadequate compared to our new colleagues, with our book learning and little practical experience. We caught up quickly, and soon could actually write orders and start IVs! What a time . . . Haight Ashbury and Jefferson Airplane's home just around the corner.

Despite the nausea of fatigue at 2 a.m. during my Obstetrics and Gynecology rotation, after helping with a frightening forceps delivery, that was still where I wanted to be. But I needed some broader sense of medicine, so decided to do family practice locums for a while. This was a financially driven decision as well . . . work a bit, earn some, travel, and do it again! During a two-month locum in Castlegar in 1970 I learned some important things. Being a young, attractive female doctor with long black hair and a red MG in a small town meant no privacy. I found family practice to be very tough, with the requirement of extensive knowledge in so many areas, that it was not for me. However, I still reflect back on those days and continue to be aware of what it is like in the trenches.

I still maintain that all young doctors should have an exposure to family medicine to understand these stresses, especially in a smaller community. In 1971, I phoned Dr. Fred Bryans, then Professor of Obstetrics and Gynecology, and asked if I could join his program in September. That was it, no interview, no matching program . . . just: "Sure, there is one spot left." The highlight of my years in the residency program was spending six months with Dr. David Boyes at the BCCI, the Cancer Agency. It was from David I learned about respecting and caring for women, our province and country, and our environment.

Early 1973 was an emotional time, what with working with such a mentor and then meeting my best friend Bryan Davis. Although we lived next door to one another, and had had brief encounters on the street in the previous year, it was within weeks of our first lunch together that we decided to get married. Our wedding was in my parents' front yard, under the chupah, on August 5, 1973. We joke: "They said it wouldn't last." Well, it has, and with children. We have two daughters. Leah, born in 1979, has completed her degree in Geography and is hoping to become a teacher. Leah is a beauty with a love of life, endless charm, and wonderful humour. She inherited that from her father. She also got his stubborn streak. Marisa, born in 1984, is our life's challenge. She has been developmentally delayed since birth, a warm sweet child who is significantly mentally handicapped.

I guess I was originally seen to be one of the 'super-moms' who did it all. Not so. I have always had help. We had a series of nannies after Leah's birth and I currently have had my own 'wife' for seventeen years, Sandra. After a telephone interview, Sandra arrived a month before Marisa's birth and has been with our family since. The girls call her their "real mom." In 1980 Bryan switched direction from family lawyer to provincial court judge to be able to help with my career and family obligations.

And I have flourished. I am proud and rather embarrassed to say that I have been a very popular general gynecologist and obstetrician since I opened my doors in February, 1976. There were few females in the field at that time, and we were immediately busy. It seems natural for some women to feel more comfortable with a woman gynecologist. It makes sense. It is why I chose the specialty. Never an academic or one with detailed knowledge, I always tried to have a balanced and commonsense approach to patients and their problems. I enjoy my patients, women of all ages and backgrounds, each one with a person and story behind the face. That is not to say that I don't have days when I am thoroughly fed up with them all! And these seem to be more frequent now, as the health care system fails, and all of us are frustrated.

On staff at St. Paul's Hospital, a UBC teaching hospital, has meant that I have been on the Faculty, and am now designated a Clinical Professor. I thoroughly enjoy teaching, especially keen young medical students and the public. I have done my share of CME lectures to family physicians, particularly on the subject of Menopause. On a daily basis we all teach residents and nurses. I feel I have accomplished something when I teach a student or resident how to perform a beautiful gentle delivery!

The highlight of my years in the residency program was spending six months with Dr. David Boyes at the BCCI, the Cancer Agency. It was from David I learned about respecting and caring for women, our province and country, and our environment

For a change of pace, and a broadening experience, I was elected to the Council of the College of Physicians and Surgeons of British Columbia in 1993. I have worked on virtually all the College Committees and have had a year as President. I am proud to have been elected for my third term in 2000. Working with the profession and the public in this capacity has been very rewarding.

Now at age fifty-five I find it hard to believe that I am able to contemplate retirement, and I must say I often do. We have just returned from two luscious months of freedom in Europe and realize there is much to see and do. I love my work, especially the one-on-one caring of patients, but find it increasingly difficult to tolerate the obstacles to being able to 'do the job.' I often wonder if there is another road to take, a career change of some sort, but realize that is not likely or easy.

(In 2003 Dr. Frinton got her wish of a career change by being appointed Associate Dean of Admissions, UBC Faculty of Medicine.)

Curriculum Vitae

Born: May 19, 1946, Glasgow, Scotland.

Citizenship: Canadian.

Undergraduate Education: West Vancouver Senior Secondary School, graduated 1962; Neuchatel Junior College, Switzerland, 1962–1963; University of British Columbia Faculty of Arts & Science, 1963–1965; Faculty of Medicine, 1965–1969 (MD).

Post-graduate Education: Rotating Internship, St. Mary's Hospital, San Francisco, Ca., 1969–1970; *Residency:* Obestrics & Gynecology, University of B.C., 1971–1975; FRCS(C) O&G, November 1975.

Clinical Practice: Family practice locum tenens in British Columbia 1970–1971; private practice in general obstetrics & gynecology from February 1976 until present.

University Appointments: Clinical Professor (from July 1999), Faculty of Medicine UBC; Assistant Head, Department of Obstetrics & Gynecology, St. Paul's Hospital from April 1991 until January 1966; previous member, Faculty Executive Committee, Faculty of Medicine (1993); previous member, President's Advisory Committee for selection of Dean of Medicine (June 1955–February 1996); also a member of previous selection committee in 1991; member of the ad hoc "Jubilee Committee" for the Faculty of Medicine; member of (Faculty of Medicine) Admissions Selection Committee from 2000.

Hospital Appointments: Active Staff, St. Paul's Hospital; Courtesy Staff, B.C. Women's and Children's Hospital.

Past and Current Committee Involvements: Past Chairman, Quality of Medical Care Committee, St. Paul's Hospital; past Member, Quality Assurance Committee, University Hospital; past Medical Director, Planned Parenthood B.C.; past President, Federation of Medical Women of Canada, B.C. Branch; previous member, COUTH Committee on Women's Health; previous member, COUTH Committee on Obstetrical & Neonatal Program; previous member, Medical Education Committee, St. Paul's Hospital; previous member, Perinatal Committee, St. Paul's Hospital; previous member, Midwifery Committee, St. Paul's Hospital; elected Member of Council of the College of Physicians & Surgeons of B.C. (from 1993, 4-year term). Elected for second term, April 1997 until present; member of Executive Committee intermittently since 1995; Chairman of the Quality of Medical Performance Committee (1995/1996); Chairman of the Ethics Committee (1996/1997); member of other CPSBC committees; president of Council 1997–1998.

Association and Society Memberships: British Columbia Medical Association; Society of Obstetricians and Gynecologists of Canada; David Boyes Society; Planned Parenthood Federation of Canada; Federation of Medical Women of Canada; North American Menopause Society; Pacific Northwest Obstetrical & Gynecological Society.

Publications:

"Contraception in the Older Woman," *Canadian Doctor*, August 1986

"Pap Smear Positive: Next Steps in Investigations," *BCMJ*, November 1984

Other Appointments: Past Member, Board of Governors, Crofton House School; Resource Gynecologist & Obstetrician for the "Fitness Group"; nominee, 1988, Woman of Distinction, YWCA; Co-Chairman, 1984, Medical Women's International Association Congress (in Vancouver); Speakers' List, BCMA, with resultant TV and radio interviews, health education; member of Medical Advisory Panel, Checkpoints Women's Health Fair; SOGC Stress Manager; Advisory Board Member, PT Group personal training; Medical Program Director, Reproductive Health: B.C. Women's Hospital and Health Centre Society (from July 1995 until 1996); Examiner MCQE Part 11.

Awards: Mike Turko Award, presented by the Section of Obstetrics & Gynecology, BCMA 1998; Roberts Award in recognition of work in Reproductive Health, presented by the Federation of Medical Women of Canada, 1999; Teaching Awards, St. Paul's Hospital house staff 1989, 1990.

DR. CAROL HERBERT

Carol Herbert's medical career is indeed outstanding. A Vancouverite, she attended the University of British Columbia where she received a BSc, followed by an MD in 1969. Her internship was at St. Paul's Hospital. After additional pediatric training, she began practice at the REACH Clinic, the storefront clinic which followed a forerunner community information centre which she started in her fourth year of medical school with a nurse and social work student. REACH is a Commercial Drive multidisciplinary health centre caring for a community of people with complex medical and social needs.

After 1982 Carol moved to a full-time position in the Department of Family Practice. Ever an ardent advocate for family medicine, Carol helped put Family Practice on the map. She was Professor of Family Medicine and was Head of the UBC Department of Family Practice from 1988 to 1998. She was an early recipient of CCFP, and later was awarded a fellowship by the College of Family Physicians of Canada.

Her work has often been in poorly explored areas: adolescent health, addiction, poverty, aboriginal health, family violence, and sexual abuse. Carol pioneered services for sexually abused children and was founder and co-director of the Sexual Assault Service for Vancouver. She is an international leader in the area of primary care research, her current interests being clinical health promotion, patient-doctor communication, physician behaviour, and decision-making, especially prescribing. She has been Chair of the National Research Committee of the College of Family Physicians, and President of the North American Primary Care Research Group, the major international primary care research organization. All this she has done while raising three children!

As well as eighty-five peer-reviewed publications, book authorships, and editorial board memberships, Carol received extensive grant funding. She has been a Visiting Professor in New Zealand, Austria, Israel, San Francisco, and Cambridge University in the U.K.

In September 1999 Carol was appointed Dean of Medicine and Dentistry at the University of Western Ontario. To date four UBC medical graduates have been appointed Deans of Medicine, but Carol is the first woman and the first family physician.

Awards are not new to Carol. These include the YWCA Woman of Distinction Award, the UBC Faculty Citation Award, and the Faculty of Medicine's 50th Anniversary Award of Excellence. She was the 2002 recipient of the UBC Medical Alumni's Wallace Wilson Leadership Award.

Carol is a long-time member of the Federation of Medical Women of Canada, and was co-chair of the scientific program for the Medical Women's International Association Congress held in Vancouver in 1984. In an interview for the 1999 summer issue of the *Newsletter* of the Federation of Medical Women of Canada, Carol submitted this summary of her involvement with FMWC: "I joined the Federation as a medical student, where I met role models who demonstrated more than one way to combine identities—woman, wife, mother, and physician. For many years the Federation was the only place where we could talk safely about issues facing women in medicine without feeling defensive or 'wimpy,' and where we focused on women's health issues. As medical women have become more numerous and more politically active, that discourse has entered the agenda of other organizations such as the CMA, but the Federation still acts to bring issues affecting women to the forefront."

DR. RUTH ISAACSEN
(1911–1985)

Dr. Ruth Isaacsen was born in Hamburg, Germany, in 1911. Her father had moved from Denmark to establish an import firm in Germany. It was in a Danish newspaper that he was made aware of the persecution of the Jews. He moved his family to Barcelona, then Portugal. On a ship in the mid-Atlantic, the vessel was boarded by German U-boat crew, who ordered all passengers into lifeboats. They spent twenty-four hours in the lifeboats, and fortunately, the ship did not blow up. The Captain decided the passengers could return to the ship and Ruth's family continued their journey to New York, later going on to Toronto.

Ruth Isaacsen was admitted to University of Toronto Medical School despite the limited quota for women and Jews. She could speak six languages. After her graduation she practised in Edmonton as a family physician, and was on staff at Miseracordia Hospital. At age seventy she moved to British Columbia and did locums for three years, retiring in 1984. She died on June 5, 1985.
(This was written for the BCMA Journal *by a friend, P.E. Simmonds, MD, of Edmonton, Alberta.)*

DR. D. RUTH (WELCH) LENNOX

I was born in Luton just north of London, England. Most of my school years were in the Midlands in England, but my final two years of high school were in Yorkshire. I went to the Medical School of Newcastle University on Tyne, and graduated in 1957 with an MB, BS. This was followed by six months each of internship in surgery, pediatrics, internal medicine, and obstetrics. In 1958 I married Dr. John Lennox, a classmate in medical school. In June 1960, we went to West Africa. We had one baby and I did not work at that time. I became a Midwifery Tutor in 1964 and for five years taught the student midwives. During one leave in 1966 we went back to England and I obtained the Diploma in Obstetrics from the Royal College of Obstetricians and Gynaecologists (D. Obst. RCOG).

We left West Africa in January 1969, and my husband spent some months in general practice in England. My husband had an aunt in Trail, British Columbia, and had a longing to settle in this beautiful province. With three children, then aged nine, six, and three, we flew from London to Vancouver and up to Fort St. John where we were taken to Chetwynd.

We arrived in Chetwynd in September 1969. There was no office space available, so we rented two rooms in the Chetwynd Hotel to start our practice—one as the examining/consulting room and the other as the reception, records keeping, and waiting room. It was scary going back into general practice after ten years away from it, but I always had John to consult with, and the specialists in Dawson Creek were very helpful. John and I passed the LMCC examination in May 1970, which gave me the confidence I needed. The Chetwynd Hospital had a board but no building when we arrived. The hospital board invited our whole family out for supper two days after our arrival. We were all jet-lagged, and our youngest child, who was then only three years old, fell asleep with his head on the table while we ate and were interviewed by the board.

The construction of the hospital was completed two years later, but in the meantime all patients needing hospitalization went to Dawson Creek. On the Big Day—the hospital opening ceremony—W.A.C. Bennett, then premier of B.C., came to open the hospital. He insisted on having his photograph taken with the hospital medical staff (both of us) just to prove that physicians were still friends with him.

Now the pattern of practice changed. John could go back to doing surgery and I could follow obstetric patients through and deliver them. Any patients whom we suspected would have complications were sent to Dawson Creek, but I did low forceps deliveries, vacuum extractions, and manual removal of placenta when necessary. John did Caesarean sections and I assisted. And these sections were also made possible by the arrival of a third doctor who came from Scotland with anaesthetic experience. When we examined our Caesarean rate we found it was higher than would be expected, and we wondered if we were doing too many since I had only attempted low forceps. We asked the obstetrician from Dawson Creek to come and review all our deliveries. He came and commented that we had all the adequate reasons to do operative deliveries.

We decided to ask for inspection and applied for accreditation. We were delighted when the thirty-bed Chetwynd General Hospital was granted accreditation at the first attempt after only two years in existence.

When we first went to Chetwynd there was no pharmacist in town. We kept a small amount of urgent drugs on hand and could dispense these ourselves when necessary. Everything else that we requested by phone was sent out on the next bus by the pharmacist in Dawson Creek. When a local businessman built a professional building, we were happy to leave the local hotel and move into the new building. Then a pharmacist came to town and that improved service a lot. We had no X-ray department, but did take some X-rays in the office and sent them to the radiologist in Dawson to be checked.

Chetwynd never did have veterinary services while we were there. I remember a dog who came to the office to be sutured and dripped blood on the waiting room floor. John even stitched up a horse on one of the local farms.

It was Christmas Day in 1970. The phone rang at ten in the morning: Could Dr. Ruth please come and see Mrs. B. who was expecting her third child in the near future? Her husband thought she might be in labour. They did not want to spoil their Christmas Day by driving sixty-four miles to Dawson Creek only to find that she was not in labour.

I went to the home, taking sterile gloves and fetal stethoscope with me. I examined the wife. She was having fairly regular mild contractions about every five minutes, and the cervix was about three centimetres dilated.

I made my decision. "She is in labour," I confidently announced. "It looks like you may have a Christmas baby. You'd better be on your way to the hospital."

So they altered their plans for Christmas day, found a baby-sitter for the other two small children, and set off for Dawson Creek. When I next saw her in the office she was obviously still pregnant. It had been a false alarm which made me separate a family on Christmas Day. The baby did not come until 1971.

I remember a Métis woman who was a grand multipara. She had previously delivered in Dawson Creek and was not used to having prenatal care available in Chetwynd. We first met in the labour delivery area. On examining her, one small leg was already in the vagina. It was not a difficult breech delivery as the baby was small and the outcome was fine. Although I had done some breech deliveries under supervision in England and I knew that the nearest obstetrician was just sixty miles away, the feel of that leg in the vagina was not an experience I would like to repeat.

When my family decided to move because we wanted different educational opportunities for our children, we thought of living on Vancouver Island. John and I visited with two of the local GPs in the town where we hoped to locate. The discussion was cordial until John explained that we would be one-and-a-half physicians since I was also a doctor and would want to work part-time. The tone changed and one of the doctors said, "We don't want any women doctors here. We've never known a good woman doctor." John was very upset at this—certainly more than I was. We decided not to fight the issue, but to make Abbotsford our new home.

Matsqui-Sumas-Abbotsford Hospital was quite unprepared for a woman doctor on staff. The obstetrical delivery unit had one tiny room for doctors to change in, 'sleep' in if necessary, and do dictation. Sleep was impossible unless there was only one patient in labour, and other physicians were coming and going all the time as the staff washroom in the delivery suite could only be accessed through this room. Later an even smaller room was allocated as a change and sleep room for the women doctors, and the dictation was moved out into the hallway.

We went back to Chetwynd in 1996 for the twenty-fifth anniversary of the hospital. We visited the little museum, and there we found our pictures which had been taken on the day of our arrival as the first doctors in town. When we told our children we were museum pieces, they were quite amused. I also had my picture displayed in the Abbotsford museum as the first woman doctor in town. Being 'exhibited' in two museums surely makes me feel very old!

DR. TERESA ELIZABETH RUSH
(1926-1979)

Dr. Rush was born in Saskatchewan. She qualified in three professions, obtaining her Teacher's diploma from Saskatoon Normal School when she was seventeen years old in 1943, graduating in Nursing from the Vancouver General Hospital in 1952, and qualifying as an MD from the University of Ottawa Medical School in 1962. She registered in British Columbia in 1970. Dr. Rush was married to Mr. B.J. Therice and had three children. She died suddenly at home in Crescent Beach in August 1979, at the age of fifty-three years.

DR. LINDA J. WARREN
(MRS. JOACHIM BURHENNE)

The Early Years
My history began in a small town with a population of 14,000 on Vancouver Island. Port Alberni at that time was a forestry dependent town; my father, as a businessman, was in a small minority of parents who did not work at "The Mill." The eldest of two children, I was always serious about school, always bringing home school work even before it was required.

My parents encouraged my scholarly approach to things, even at a young age; and, as many of my schoolmates were more interested in things other than homework, it was not too difficult to stay at or near the top academically.

Never very good at sports, I concentrated on my studies and my music. As valedictorian at my high school graduation, I was really inspired when quoting from Alfred Lord Tennyson's Ulysses: "I am a part of all that I have met, yet all experience is an arch where through gleams that untravelled world, whose margin fades forever and forever when I move." Grade 13 was available then; and I chose to stay home another year. None of my close friends thought this was a very good idea and went off to UBC.

Pre-med

I arrived at UBC and moved into Phyllis Ross House in September 1962. Very soon I understood what it was like to be the classic small frog in a gigantic pond and found this experience quite overwhelming. I knew then that I was interested in science and found these courses challenging. Joining the UBC chapter of the Kappa Alpha Theta sorority helped to save me from being swallowed up in the enormity of what UBC was even then— there were suddenly many friends which I have to this day; and there was acknowledgement of my musical skills. Difficult as it was to fit these social activities into my schedule, I knew somehow that it was important

After about a year, however, it was clear that I needed to make an important decision. What profession should I choose, and how? All I could think of was to gather together the people I trusted most—my family—and try to make a decision in a scientific way. I made a list in alphabetical order of all careers. After crossing off those which were "not suitable for girls" or which I thought I would not like, medicine and pharmacy were left. My dad's best friend was a pharmacist; and after consulting with him and discovering that pharmacy involved selling cameras and chewing gum as well as dispensing prescriptions, my Mom and Dad advised me against this choice. That left medicine. All I knew about medicine was that I respected my family doctor, a dear friend of the family; I knew that I liked science and I wanted to help people. It was decided that I would apply for medicine; a few months later I was fortunate to receive an early acceptance. The die was cast, and I could not even imagine turning back.

Medical School

The first days of medical school in September of 1964, although on the same campus that I already knew, were different from anything I had imagined.

We had a class of sixty students, four of whom were women, one of whom dropped out after a few months. I will never forget the aura of expectation and requirement for accomplishment which was present on the first day when Dr. Sidney Friedman, Head of Anatomy, first spoke to us.

Those were dramatic, challenging, agonizing, and wonderful days with what seemed to be more emphasis on competition than on what we now know as problem solving. We memorized everything, and in second year those of us who could write fast enough transcribed up to seventeen pages of notes at each pharmacology lecture. We all felt more comfortable in our clinics, as we had always assumed that seeing and caring for patients was what medicine was all about. All of us worked hard, but it was probably more difficult for those of us who believed we could not afford to take any time off, assuming that this would lead to certain failure.

I always took a summer job in my hometown where I could visit with my family and friends. Those were wonderful times, as I was able to spend time with my best friend, my younger brother Rick.

Internship

After an academic career that began in kindergarten and which increased almost exponentially in intensity, I felt somehow that it would not be a good idea for me to stay home or even choose another Canadian city in which to intern. Through the national matching program, I received my first choice posting—the most exotic sounding place on the list—Honolulu. However, the most important reason for choosing the University of Hawaii was that at that time a rotating surgical internship was offered—six months surgery and six months internal medicine.

By then I had decided that I would apply for a residency in ophthalmology at UBC and for that a rotating surgical internship—with so much experience in surgery—was considered quite valuable. The opportunity, in the few off hours, to learn to surf, to tour the Hawaiian Islands, experience the Polynesian lifestyle, and meet fellow interns and residents from all over North America were bonuses.

However, the experience in ophthalmological surgery was important from the standpoint, that, as compared with the other surgical subspecialties, the surgery seemed curiously tedious; and it was at that point that I realized I should return to my first choice— radiology. During a third year externship summer at the West Coast General Hospital in Port Alberni, I had the opportunity to spend a lot of time with Dr. Hans Waldman, a highly skilled and comprehensively trained radiologist. He seemed to know about every specialty and was the resource to whom other physicians, including specialists, turned for advice. At that time, the radiology four-year residency required a "year out," which was typically done in either internal medicine or pathology.

Residency

With my decision to pursue diagnostic radiology firm, I returned to Vancouver to begin my year in the Department of Internal Medicine at the University of B.C. The work made me feel at home; internal medicine had always been one of my great interests. The radiology years of the residency were to commence the following year.

I entered Radiology in January of 1971 after a few months' break. When I arrived in December 1970 to meet with the Department Head and staff, I was surprised to learn that the funds for residencies that year had "run out" and there would be no funding for me to commence my training in January. As I did not wish to delay any further, I chose to begin my radiology training without funding. A couple of months later, after a meeting with the Minister of Health, I was allocated a $200 a month stipend for the remaining four months of the year. The three years in radiology were full and inspiring. The first Professor of Radiology, Dr. J. Scott Dunbar, arrived around the same time I did, and introduced academic radiology to the department. I received my FRCPC in November of 1973.

The Practice

Subspecialty Fellowships were uncommon in those times and radiology was such a general broad field of which I enjoyed every aspect. I did not see a very good reason to pursue one small area of this specialty which I so embraced. I was privileged to join a busy prestigious general radiology practice in the community, conducted by six respected male radiologists.

Mammography was in its infancy, and was not taught in residency programs. In fact, a fellow resident organizing radiology pathology rounds, on finding insufficient general radiology material, apologized to me for giving me a breast case. I had never seen a mammogram before, and literally had to go to the books to come up with a reasonable differential diagnosis. However, my senior colleagues helped me on my way, encouraging me to "take over the breast" segment of the practice and build it. I started out earnestly learning from the texts which were available, taking courses, teaching residents and staff and speaking to the public. In those days we had the time to interview patients directly and do a breast physical examination on all women presenting for mammography. Later on when the volume was too great, I taught our technologists to take on these tasks.

It was during the late 1970s and early 1980s that the first reports of mortality benefit from mammography screening were published, with the landmark report from Sweden in *The Lancet* in 1985. International bodies made recommendations for screening of asymptomatic women which we began to apply in our practice. In 1986 reports were published from the United States on low-cost mammography screening centres and their success. It was in 1986 that my husband and I spent six months in Europe on sabbatical. Our major project was to study the technique of operative cholangiography throughout Europe. My project, to visit five established European mammography screening centres, was quite secondary. The knowledge and experience I derived from these visits contributed to Dr. Vivien Basco's (of B.C. Cancer Agency) and my successful applications at our practices, which subsequently led the Provincial Health Ministry in 1987 to grant us funds for a Pilot Project on Screening Mammography in B.C.

The first patient was examined in July of 1988, and, based upon the early success, the Ministry of Health encouraged us to expand within a year. The

I had never seen a mammogram before, and literally had to go to the books to come up with a reasonable differential diagnosis. My senior colleagues helped me on my way, encouraging me to "take over the breast" segment of the practice and build it.

early years were exciting, as I had taken on the post as Executive Director of the Screening Mammography Program as an after hours job. Since I felt I should know what was happening "on the front," I became a screening radiologist. This work, also of necessity, was conducted away from my private practice. Our data collection and analysis yielded new and unique information which was important to the international medical community. Invitations to speak in Europe, North and South America, and in Asia followed, and in 1979, the Chilean Society of Obstetrics and Gynecology appointed me an honorary member. Subsequently, in 1993, I arrived at work one day to find a little box with a silver medal—the Governor General's Commemorative Medal for Public Service. However, what really made these busy years, the long hours of work and travel a joy, was the opportunity to share everything with my beloved husband. The story of my marriage follows.

We travelled to continents and countries together where we helped organize and participate in radiology meetings, lecture and train other physicians, and meet old and new friends.

The Marriage

It was on a dull rainy January 10th afternoon in 1977 when one of my senior colleagues encouraged me to attend a farewell tea party which was being held at the Radiology Department in the General Hospital for four fellow residents who were leaving for other posts. Although reluctant to leave my colleague with the busy office afternoon, I finally accepted the invitation.

Arriving at the Radiology library, I had barely greeted my departing colleagues when a senior resident invited me to meet the visiting Professor. He was H. Joachim Burhenne, of San Francisco, an international authority in gastrointestinal radiology and one of the two founders of interventional radiology. He was spending a month as visiting professor at the Vancouver General Hospital and was fitting in as much skiing as possible on the weekends. Though the idea of a "date" never occurred to me, it turned out that he had been invited for a ski weekend at Whistler and wondered if I had planned to go skiing that weekend. Joachim, it turned out, was an expert skier, a former member of the Junior Team for West Germany. This was the first of uncountable ski weekends which were to come, following a whirlwind long-distance courtship after his return to San Francisco. He took up the post of Professor and Head of the Department of Radiology in the Faculty of Medicine at UBC in April 1978. We were married in October 1978, nearly two years after our first meeting. The nearly eighteen years which followed were a dream marriage. We travelled to continents and countries together where we helped organize and participate in radiology meetings, lecture and train other physicians, and meet old and new friends. On sabbatical in Europe in 1986 we visited twenty-two different medical schools in nine different countries, and put 25,000 kilometres on our Subaru four-wheel station wagon. We went riding in the foothills of the Andes, hiked the Rockies, cruised to Alaska and through the Mediterranean, and spent our summers swimming, water-skiing, windsurfing, rowing, and blackberry picking at the lake.

Abruptly in 1995, Joachim's health failed, and he was diagnosed with amyotrophic lateral sclerosis. Despite progressive weakness, we determined to carry on with our lifestyle as best we could. We were able to pursue our love of travelling and completed fourteen trips during 1995 and early 1996. I had the unique privilege as a wife to be his in-house physician, nurse, and friend, and to essentially administer a mini-hospital in our home. During the last six months of his life, he enjoyed to the fullest his music, excursions to Stanley Park, and our unobstructed view of the mountains. As he very much wanted to see San Francisco one final time, we undertook a risky weekend trip there two weeks before he died, on June 1st of 1996.

Years as a Widow

Fortunate to have a challenging career, I returned to work two weeks after my husband's death. Immediately there were manuscripts to write, invitations to participate on international committees, lectures, and refresher courses to prepare for. The opportunity to edit the biography, together with Professor Brian Lentle, Joachim's successor, gave me an enormous satisfaction: *Hans Joachim Burhenne, A Pioneer in Radiology*, was thus published in November 1999.

Opportunities to be creative, to return to ballroom dancing, the piano, to subscribe to Bard on the Beach and Ballet B.C. are important as the challenges involved in conducting a private practice in radiology grow. At a more global level, physicians everywhere now understand that there is no universal ideal or quick solution to the provision of high quality health care. The future of medicine stays bright with the promise of modern technology and the innovative ideas of our younger colleagues. However, it is individuals, not only the new bright young minds, but also those with the wisdom of experience, who are responsible for these prospects.

Indeed, in *The Idea of a University*, John Henry Cardinal Newman observed: "One of the best companions is a man who to the accuracy and research of a profession has joined a free excursive of acquaintance with various learning and caught from it the spirit of general observation."

It is probably because so much good has come out of it all that I hardly remember, at this point, the fateful day, when after anatomy lab, one of my male colleagues saw fit to put my head underneath the water in the dissection wash-up room—as I recall for no apparent reason. Everyone in that class has gone on to have a full and productive career. I cherish all of these memories from the "good old days."

I see my medical education and career as my most important accomplishment. The opportunity to serve, particularly in the realm of breast health, to build, to teach, and to create visions for the future are treasures that relate directly to this medical education. Had I not become a radiologist, I would not have had the opportunity to meet my husband and live the incomparable life we shared. His approach to life and now mine is again symbolized by Tennyson's Ulysses, who encourages us "to strive, to seek, to find and not to yield."

DR. MOIRA YEUNG (CHAN-YEUNG)

Curriculum Vitae

UBC Department of Medicine: Present Rank: Professor since July, 1982.

Post-Secondary Education: Hong Kong University, MBBS, Medicine, 1962; Queen Mary Hospital, Department of Medicine, Hong Kong, Intern/Resident, 1962–66.

Special Professional Qualifications: Royal College of Physicians, MRCP, 1967; Royal College of Physicians, Edinburgh, MRCPE, 1967; Royal College of Physicians & Surgeons, Canada, CRCPC, 1969; Royal College of Physicians & Surgeons, Canada, FRCPC; American College of Physicians, FACP, 1972; American College of Chest Physicians, FCCP, 1972; Royal College of Physicians, Edinburgh, FRCP, 1976; Fellow of Hong Kong College of Physicians, 1996; Fellow of Hong Kong Academy of Medicine, 1996.

Employment Record: University of Hong Kong, Department of Medicine, Assistant Lecturer, 1963–65; University of Hong Kong, Department of Medicine, Lecturer, 1965–66; Institute of Diseases of the Chest, Clinical Research, 1966–67; Brompton Hospital, London, England, Assistant Research Fellow, 1967–68; University of Edinburgh, Edinburgh, Scotland, Clinical Endocrinology, Research Unit; UBC Teaching Fellow, 1968–70; UBC Research Associate, 1970–72; UBC Clinical Assistant, 1972–73; UBC Assistant Professor, 1973–76; UBC Associate Professor, 1976–82; granted tenure: July, 1978.

Scholarly and Professional Activities:

Occupational Asthma: Over the years I have conducted research in occupational asthma and in particular occupational asthma due to western red cedar exposure. I have accomplished the following:

- Identified a low molecular weight compound (M.W. 400 Daltons) plicated acid, present uniquely in red cedar, to be the agent responsible for red cedar asthma.
- Demonstrated the presence of specific IgE antibodies in a proportion of patients with red cedar asthma to indicate that it is partly immunologically mediated.
- Showed that other nonimmunologic mechanisms such as nonspecific bronchial reactivity and activation of the complement pathway may be important in the pathogenesis of occupational asthma.
- Documented that about half of the patients with red cedar asthma failed to recover after removal from exposure and that early diagnosis and early removal predict recovery.
- Demonstrated that occupational asthma is the most common form of occupational lung disease in developed countries.

My work has contributed to the recognition by the Workers' Compensation Board of British Columbia and across Canada that occupational asthma is a compensatory disease. Because of this, guidelines have been established for impairment/disability evaluation specifically for patients with asthma by working experts in this area within the American Thoracic Society. These guidelines are being used in North America. Guidelines have also been established for the diagnosis and management of occupational asthma through a consensus statement organized by the American College of Chest Physicians. The scientific community now recognizes that asthma can be caused by low molecular weight compounds and that occupational asthma is an excellent model to study the natural history of asthma.

Occupational Lung Diseases: The Occupational Lung Diseases Research Unit has conducted many epidemiological health studies of workers in different industries in British Columbia to assess the effects of exposure to various air contaminants on the respiratory and other systems. Health surveys were carried out in most of the major industries in British Columbia: sawmills, grain elevators, pulp and paper mills, aluminum smelter, foundry, bakeries, together with a number of control populations. Altogether 15,000 workers in British Columbia have been examined over the years, and many of them were studied on several occasions in a longitudinal manner.

As a result of the monitoring program on grain elevator workers in this province, the level of dust in the elevators has been reduced considerably over the years. Our work has shown that the permissible concentration of grain dust should be below 10 mg/m. The Association of American Governmental Hygienists has recommended that the permissible concentration of grain dust be 4 mg/m based on the result of our studies.

We described acute decline in lung function over the course of a work shift in grain workers and demonstrated that this acute airway response is predictive of longitudinal decline in lung function. This has been demonstrated with workers exposed to cotton dust as well. This acute airway response may prove to be the biologic marker of future respiratory impairment/disability with continuous exposure. This is important as longitudinal studies are expensive and difficult to conduct.

Research in Asthma and Hypersensitivity Lung Diseases: Studies of environmental risk factors in asthma were conducted, particularly the indoor aeroallergens in two cities, Vancouver and Winnipeg. Our results showed that in children, the level of house dust mites is an important determinant of asthma severity, indicating that house dust mite avoidance is important in the management of asthma in children.

University committees: Director, Occupational Lung Disease Research Unit, Respiratory Division, Department of Medicine, Vancouver General Hospital, 1979–present; Acting Head, Respiratory Division, Vancouver General Hospital, December 1982 to June 1983; Head, Tuberculosis Inpatient Service, Vancouver General Hospital, 1983–1990; Head, Respiratory Division, Vancouver General Hospital, 1983–1990; Member of the Science Council, Vancouver Hospital, 1983–1986; Acting Head, University of British Columbia Respiratory Division, 1993–1994.

Dr. Yeung is a member of eighteen scholarly societies and has been on numerous committees and chairperson of several. She is a regular reviewer of thirteen journals and has held the position of Editor of three: *Clinical and Experimental Allergy*, 1990–1992, the *American Journal of Industrial Medicine*, 1991–1999, and the *Canadian Respiratory Journal*, 1994–1999.

Her awards include the Killam Fellowship Award for senior investigator, 1989–1990, the Excellence in Scientific Achievement Award, Vancouver Hospital, 1991, the Roy Patterson Lectureship, American Academy of Allergy and Clinical Immunology, 1993, and the Charles Reed Visiting Professorship, Mayo Clinic, 1995.

Dr. Yueng has had over 215 refereed publications in Journals from 1968 to 1999 and has written over forty textbook chapters. She has been the invited speaker on more than 100 occasions from 1980 to 1995 in Canada and the United States, China, Columbia, Cuba, England, France, Germany, Hong

Kong, Italy, Korea, Sweden, and Switzerland. She is active in Continuing Medical Education at UBC; one of her lectures at Medical Grand Rounds was playfully titled, "On Mites and Men."

1971

DR. MARY MARSHALL BAILEY
(1911–1999)

Dr. Mary Bailley, one of the early pioneers in psychiatry, graduated from the University of Toronto in medicine in 1935. A clergyman's daughter, she had never considered any career other than medicine after spending her formative years listening to Canadian missionary doctors telling of the wonders of life in foreign countries.

As a seventeen-year-old medical student, Mary lived in a rooming house in Toronto, working hard and taking extra classes in sociology and philosophy. She interned at the Hospital for Sick Children in Toronto, and met her classmate Allan Bailey during her first year at medical school. They married six years later and began their post-graduate training as "fellows" at the Mayo Clinic in Rochester, Minnesota, in 1937.

In the 1930s, psychiatry was not a specialty, and the training was very eclectic. There was no formal training in psychoanalysis. Although electroconvulsive therapy was used, anti-psychotic medications such as chlorpromazine had not yet been discovered.

After the birth of their first child in 1940, the Baileys returned to Canada and began to practise in Ottawa. Allan, a neuropsychiatrist with the Army, was eventually stationed in Montreal at St. Mary's Hospital (the receiving centre for the emotionally and neurologically crippled from overseas). Mary was one of the two psychiatrists working in Ottawa—the hub of the war depot and training centre.

Two more children were born to the Baileys in Ottawa and a fourth in Montreal during a postwar sabbatical. In 1947, Mary and Allan returned to the Mayo Clinic; she to continue her fellowship training and he to accept a staff appointment.

In the ten years since the Baileys had left, the Mayo Clinic established a fully-developed Department of Psychiatry. Dr. Adelaide Johnson, the department's chief analyst, and Dr. Lawrence Lolb were most influential in Mary's training. Although psychoanalysis was already considered a speciality at that time, few were using analysis techniques.

The clinic was very good to women residents, allowing them to work part-time to complete their program so that they could be at home with their children during school vacation. Mary cannot remember an uninterrupted Christmas. Perhaps that was why none of their four children (an historian, a musician, a ballet director, and a sociologist) chose medicine.

In 1954, the Baileys moved to Saskatoon. Allan became Head of the Department of Neurology and Mary a clinical teacher at the medical school of the University of Saskatchewan. As the only psychiatrist in private practice, Mary was extremely busy. She was not able to spend time in long-term psychoanalytically-oriented psychiatry until more physicians arrived.

For five to six years, Saskatoon was the centre of attention because of the experimental use of LSD (lysergic acid diethylamide) as a cure for schizophrenia and alcoholism. Mary experimented with the drug's effects before using it therapeutically in hospital settings in her private practice. She spent hundreds of hours treating patients with LSD. Although the use of LSD shortened psychoanalytic therapy by months, the cost of supervising patients who were deeply involved in reliving childhood memories outweighed the benefits.

After Allan's death in 1971, Mary moved to Vancouver to live with her sister. She practised in White Rock, B.C., until 1980. In her spare time, she played the cello and was a member of the White Rock Community Orchestra.

Mary was most grateful for the support given by her husband and her colleagues who helped her to face the many challenges that circumstances (including the war) had placed in her path. "My children and their basic naivete and joie de vivre helped keep me sane," she claimed.

Mary died on June 3, 1999, aged eighty-eight. Her obituary stated: "She was an inspiration to her family, a warm and stimulating friend, and an indefatigable voyager of the mind and spirit."

(Written by Dr. Frances Forrest-Richards for the FMWC Newsletter, *Winter 1992–1993.)*

DR. HEDY FRY

Most people who have heard of Dr. Hedy Fry think of her as being politically active, first in the British Columbia Medical Association when she became President in 1990, and later as a Liberal member from B.C. in the Federal Government. But before she became politically known, she was a much loved and popular family physician in Vancouver for nearly twenty years.

She was born in Trinidad of progressive parents and remembers fondly her grandmother who was active in improving society's problems. Dr. Fry was trained as a teacher and later received her medical training at the Royal College of Physicians and Surgeons of Ireland, graduating in 1968 with LLM, RCP & S (Licentiate, Licentiate in Midwifery). At graduation she was the recipient of the Silver Medal in Applied Physiology. She registered with the British Columbia College of Physicians and Surgeons in 1971 and was involved in many BCMA committees: the Subcommittee on Midwifery, the Council on Health Promotion, the Nutrition and the Native Health Committee, Convention Committee, and the General Assembly.

Dr. Fry has served as BCMA representative to many outside organizations, was representative to the CMA Council on Health Care, and was Chair of the Obstetrics Subcommittee. She was a member of the BCMA Speakers Service, the Victoria Contact Group, and the Advisory Board, Physicians Against Nuclear War. President of the B.C. Branch of the Federation of Medical Women in 1977 and Editor of the FMWC *Newsletter* for three years, she later became President of the Vancouver Medical Association. She was a member of the *Medical Post* Editorial Board, and was featured on the Doctor Doctor television program during its three years of production.

In 1990 Dr. Hedy Fry became President of BCMA, the second woman to be elected President of the nearly ninety-year-old association. The first woman President was Dr. Ethlyn Trapp in 1946.

At her induction as President of BCMA, on the eve of Health Minister John Jansen's address to the 340 doctors attending the annual business meeting, Dr. Fry bluntly told Mr. Jansen that contrary to what he may say it was evident that the Social Credit government was rationing health care and it would destroy the health care system in British Columbia. Dr. Fry had entered her presidency with enthusiasm and with a promise to make the BCMA more aggressive. She was a strong advocate of the role of communication and public relations in promoting the aims of the profession. From the *B.C. Medical Journal* of August, 1990, in an interview she describes her hope that during her presidency "the negotiation farce with the government will be over and we will have a settlement that we can all agree on, so we can forge a satisfying relationship." Her goal was to start building a good strong relationship with other health-care providers and with the government so that at the same time next year she would be able to say, "We did it—we saved medicare."

Dr. Fry considers that her greatest accomplishment while President of BCMA was her role as chief negotiator when she was successful in getting an agreement within three months after three years of failed negotiations, and got the first ever RRSP plan for doctors in Canada.

She chaired the Council of Health Promotion and later became the chief negotiator lobbying for the doctors' fee contract, which was under siege by the B.C. government, leading the BCMA membership through a tumultuous and challenging time.

It was no surprise to those who know Dr. Fry that she decided to run for the Liberal seat in her riding of Vancouver Centre in 1993 in the Federal election, the same riding held by the Progressive Conservative leader—and Prime Minister of Canada, Kim Campbell. Her victory was unexpected—even to her. She strongly believes that the only way you can make changes is by getting involved. Prime Minister Jean Chretien and appointed her Parliamentary Secretary to the Minister of Health, later she became Secretary of State for Multiculturalism and the Status of Women. Despite her busy life, she kept in contact with the Federation of Medical

Women of Canada through interviews, and when possible attending the Annual Meeting and taking part in the program. Dr. Fry is a great promoter of the status of women in Canada, tackling problems with frankness and courage.

DR. MARY TROTT

I was born in Bermuda in 1943. When I grew up, I expressed an interest in being a nurse, but my parents said that I was too bossy to become one, thus I should become a doctor instead. (They obviously didn't know any OR nurses!)

I started my medical education at McGill University, Montreal, in 1965 and graduated with MD and CM in 1969. During my postgraduate training, I realized that I had spent eight years in Canada and hadn't travelled further east than Toronto. Past graduates who had gone to Vancouver seemed to be enjoying themselves much more than those who stayed in Montreal, so I decided to go west.

My plans for specialising were influenced by Dr. Heidi Patriquin, a radiology resident whom I encountered at the Montreal Children's Hospital and at the Montreal General. I was impressed with the fact that the radiologist seemed to be the consultant's consultant. I was captivated by the pictures of a barium study of the colon, and thus my interest in radiology grew. I did not know at the time how the pictures were obtained!

I began my internship at St. Paul's Hospital, Vancouver, from 1969–70. The nuns were still a presence in the hospital and there were prayers over the PA system daily. Female staff was housed up in the convent area on the top floor, until one particularly rowdy party at the men's residence across the street so upset the 'powers that be' that they thought moving the women into the men's residence might tone things down a bit—a remarkably progressive point of view for the times. There was a myth 'up the hill' at VGH that things shut down at St. Paul's at midnight. Folks at VGH had no idea that most of the street people from the Hastings area were brought nightly to St. Paul's as it was closest. The ambulance guys wanted them out of the vehicle as soon as possible because some of them smelled pretty ripe. One of the orderlies at St. Paul's was an Englishman, Mr. Harvey. He had the air of a butler at a grand residence and had a real way with the street people who at that time were mostly alcoholics; they never gave him too much trouble.

He was also very good at putting on casts. Observing him at every opportunity taught us a lot.

One morning at 3 a.m. while assisting at a C-section, I was invited to apply for an Obs-Gyn Residency, but I declined, mumbling that "I like to sleep at night." This remark caused great laughter because I was talking back to the Chief of Obs-Gyn who as a rule had no use for interns. Eventually, I chose Radiology. During this time, Dr. Patricia Rebbeck became a friend and mentor and has remained so to this day.

During my first year of Residency, I did barium enemas all day, then went home and did them again in my sleep at night. I was amazed when I saw the first mammography machine which had a big latex balloon for compression. During my training at St. Paul's, I requested for a platform built for doing myelograrns because the X-ray table was so high. I was proud to say that my request was finally accepted.

As the only female resident I became very good at doing chain cystograms on women with incontinence problems because the male staff never had to do these procedures as long as there was a female staff person around. I was very fortunate to have Dr. Martha Grymaloski, Dr. Kathleen Elliott, and Dr. Pat Chipperfield as my mentors, all very skilled radiologists.

During my first year of Residency, I did barium enemas all day, then went home and did them again in my sleep at night.

My second year of Residency took place at VGH. The Head of the Department was Dr. J. S. Dunbar who came from the Montreal Children's Hospital where he had been Professor of Pediatric Radiology. He spurred his residents to write papers and did a lot of teaching. We had lots of visiting professors from North America and overseas. I went to the Armed Forces Institute of Pathology in Washington, D.C., for a two-month fellowship; it was an intensive course in radiologic-pathologic correlation. Part of the time at VGH was also spent in the Health Centre for Children with Dr. Betty Wood, an excellent pediatric radiologist and another great mentor. This was before the Shaughnessy site had been transformed and the pediatric service transferred there.

My third year of the Radiology program was spent doing six months of Internal Medicine and six months of Pathology at Shaughnessy Hospital, where I also spent a few months doing Radiology. My fourth year was divided between St. Paul's and VGH. Between Internal Medicine and Pathology, I found time to get married. Since my husband, Bernie Littlejohn, was a Maintenance Engineer at Howe Sound Pulp on the Sunshine Coast, it meant that I had to commute home on my free weekends by ferry. The Friday night line-up for the ferries from Horseshoe Bay was usually hours long, and the ferry trips became my opportunity to study for the Fellowship exams.

I had originally intended to take the baby to work with me while I was nursing, but the chief of staff begged me not to because the nurses might get ideas.

During the summer between third and fourth years, my husband and I spent our holiday travelling through much of the province, trying to decide where we would like to live. We decided that small town life appealed to us, and that we wanted to get out of the Lower Mainland. On that basis I made applications to some smaller community hospitals to see if they would need a radiologist on site. The level of remuneration was secondary compared to the lifestyle a small town could offer. Williams Lake seemed to be the right size, and the incumbent radiologist Dr. Peter Devito needed help, as he was covering 100 Mile House, Williams Lake, and Quesnel. His duties kept him travelling up and down Highway 97 quite frequently, and he was ready to hand Williams Lake Cariboo Memorial Hospital over to someone else. I did a locum tenens in July 1975, and when I finished the written part of the Fellowship exam, he invited me to take over Williams Lake in November 1975. Thus began a ten-year association with one of the province's best community radiologists who, unfortunately, left the Cariboo for Powell River and subsequently died an untimely death. I still miss him as a friend and colleague.

Our first step to taking the job was to buy a mobile home and have it set up in a park overlooking the lake. It was an inexpensive way to acquire a home with a view. I started working in Williams Lake on November 5, 1975. The trip up Highway 97 was a bit hair-raising as the highway north of Cache Creek was covered in snow and quite icy. This introduction to treacherous driving conditions has remained part of my professional and personal life for twenty-five years. I was temporarily free from the worry of accidents when I recently did a locum tenens in Yellowknife, NWT. There were few roads in that community, thus the caseload was almost devoid of road traffic accidents!

The medical staff at Cariboo Memorial Hospital was on the whole quite supportive of their new full-time radiologist and first woman specialist, although at times they were so busy that they hardly noticed my presence. Some of the male physicians had to be handled carefully, though. In one case, discussions had to be tailored so that the physician in charge would feel the decision was his alone. Surgeons soon learned that rudeness would not be tolerated in my department, and apologies came voluntarily when bounds were overstepped. Some nurses also had to be taught that the radiologist was in fact a real doctor.

One feature of working in a ranching community was the presence of several rodeo injuries on the day sheet during the spring and summer months. Throughout the years, we have accumulated enough material to write a paper on rodeo radiology, which I always vowed to write but still haven't found the time!

When Medical Staff Committee elections came up shortly after my arrival, I was immediately nominated as secretary. As the only female on staff, I had vowed that I would not take that position, and firmly declined. I later did a stint as the Vice President of medical staff, but never had any aspirations to higher posts. One needs a wife to do that sort of thing.

My pregnancy in 1979 caused a little consternation. I had originally intended to take the baby to work with me while I was nursing, but the chief of staff begged me not to because the nurses might get ideas. I obliged by leaving my daughter at home with expressed milk, which was one decision I have always regretted. The pace in those days was leisurely enough that there would have been time to care for her during the day, especially in the first three months.

In 1982, I spent time in Vancouver at VGH and Lion's Gate Hospital and also at Royal Inland Hospital, Kamloops to learn ultrasound before a machine was installed in our hospital. It was a good opportunity to be in the company of other radiologists and back in the world of academic medicine for a brief period.

Mammography was another development which occurred shortly after my arrival in Williams Lake. The Barrett government was making these machines available to community hospitals throughout the province, and Williams Lake, as the geographic centre of the Cariboo region, was a logical location. This also occasioned a trip to BCCI in Vancouver, which enhanced my proficiency in reading these films.

In 1978, my husband began work on our underground home, and that became his occupation for several years in addition to being my practice manager. We moved the mobile home in 1976 on to the fifteen acres we had bought, and we finally moved into our new home in 1983. The house attracted considerable attention as a new concept in housing, and Bernie did most of the building himself. Life in the country was a pleasant retreat from the increasing work demands in town.

In recent years, the X-ray Department has moved to a different area as the hospital has expanded. It has also become busier, since we have to travel to 100 Mile House twice a month. For the past year we have been able to benefit from the Northern Isolation Travel Allowance Program for these trips, but for twelve years we made trips in all kinds of weather without any compensation other than the fee we received for our service there. Of course, if the machine broke down, we only got paid for the pile of films we read while we were there.

In 1990, one of the Kamloops radiologists decided that he would like to semi-retire, and so Dr. Ken Macdonell moved up from Kamloops to share the practice on a fifty-fifty basis. This change gave me time to spend with my growing daughter and my husband.

Recently, there is increasing pressure to have CT scanning services in the region. Certainly if there is to be a successor to the two incumbent radiologists, this service must be available. It would also be advantageous in the retention and recruiting of surgeons, be they general, orthopedic, or otherwise. So at the close of my career I may be travelling again to Vancouver or elsewhere to learn to use this modality. At the time of writing I am also preparing to lobby for equipment to enable us to use telemedicine in Williams Lake to gain access to specialists and to help physicians in the smaller communities. New developments in radiology in the next decade will make it possible to provide more services for rural patients without their having to travel long distances on icy winter roads for five or six months of the year. The age of teleradiology conjures up visions of someone hundreds (thousands?) of miles away looking at Williams Lake's films on a monitor. I don't think, however, that the other physicians will be coming to socialize with a workstation monitor, and someone is still needed on hand who can advise the techs on the spot, calm patients' fears about the machinery and their illness, and act as an interface between the techs and the other physicians. A real live radiologist is ideal for those tasks, even if a lot of the film reading work were being done elsewhere.

Practising in a small interior community hospital is very different from working at hospitals in the lower mainland. After twenty-five years of practice, I have been the one constant in some patients' encounters with physicians, and have known some of them since before they were born! One's life is an open book in a small community, and being honest and humble and having a sense of humour helps one to keep a modicum of self respect, especially if things are not going well. A good collegial atmosphere is one of the great blessings I have been fortunate to enjoy here. A rural lifestyle is great for raising children as well. It is not hard to teach them to have the common touch in a small world. They rub shoulders with all walks of life on a regular basis, and the 'whole village' tends to be involved with them one way or another as they grow.

1972

DR. ROBERTA C. ONGLEY

In retrospect, I chose medicine because my father, a lawyer, was not enthusiastic about the law firm title, Ongley & Daughter. Having been discouraged in my early ambition to enter law, I chose medicine as my next logical choice. As Toronto was home, I applied to and was accepted by the University of Toronto, School of Medicine, in 1961. At that time, U of T had a two-year non-degree pre-med course, which shortened the program to six years overall. I still remember my early days in pre-med; there was an unspoken quota for women in med school and I was one of only sixteen females in a class of one hundred and eighty medical students—quite overwhelming for a graduate who had never shared a classroom with males.

Having mastered bridge at every break and acquiring an MD in the process, I applied to the Vancouver General Hospital for internship. I chose Vancouver for two reasons: I had never been west, and VGH paid the highest salaries in Canada—the princely sum of $400 monthly. My first rotation was Emergency, and it was frightening. In 1967 Emerg was staffed only by interns with a supervisor, a first-year resident, who floated between Emergency and the Outpatient Department, and general practitioners, who did an evening rotation—a far cry from today's well-staffed Emergencies. I am still amazed at how well we coped and how many patients actually survived our care.

Before long, I had decided to settle in Vancouver—no way was I leaving this paradise! I became interested in dermatology, a subject which we had little exposure to in med school. While on a medicine rotation at VGH, I had the good fortune to meet one of the first residents in dermatology. His enthusiasm for his subject was infectious, and dermatology won out over my other considerations for practice.

After a year of residency in general medicine and one in pathology, I finally entered the Dermatology residency. I was very fortunate to acquire two excellent mentors: Dr. William Stewart, Head of Dermatology, and Dr. Peggy Johnston, who started the first pediatric dermatology service at VGH. Bill guided me into the arenas of teaching and research, and Peggy introduced me into the Federation of Medical Women of Canada, which marked the start of my political interests.

Teaching has been a significant part of my career. On completing my fellowship in 1972, I became a teaching fellow and joined Bill Stewart in practice. Shortly afterwards, the two of us moved into university space near VGH and established the official Division of Dermatology with teaching practices, expanded the residency program, and attempted to increase undergraduate exposure to dermatology. Our efforts proved to be more successful in Pharmacy than Medicine. Thanks to an enthusiastic pharmacology professor, we began a course that provided more hours of training in dermatology to the pharmacy students than we were able to provide to medical students. For the next ten years, UBC-graduated pharmacists became more knowledgeable than doctors in dermatology. I remained on geographic part-time faculty as Associate Professor until 1989 when I relocated my practice out of the Division of Dermatology space, but I still continued undergraduate teaching activities.

My favourite aspect of teaching has always been the office preceptorship program, whereby medical students and residents spent time in my office. Patients were remarkably accepting of their presence, seeing as I had a student observer every day for almost twenty years. On the odd occasion when the student cancelled or missed, patients would often comment on their absence in a tone of voice that questioned whether I could function on my own!

Lecturing has continued to be a fun part of my teaching life as well. It seems that once you are on the circuit it is hard to get off. Dr. Stewart and I initiated an annual dermatology review course in 1976, which has continued to this day, and I am still trying to get off the organizing list. Actually, I now feel like an emeritus chair, as this course is ably run by two members of our Division, but they refuse to let me off the program. Gradually I have managed to reduce other presentations down to the most enjoyable, especially the two courses that are held at ski resorts each year—a great excuse for a holiday.

Shortly after I started in practice, Dr. Peggy Johnston coerced me into attending the annual meeting of the Federation of Medical Women of Canada (FMWC) Vancouver Branch, with the very sensible reasoning that meeting a number of female practitioners would be good for my practice. Little did I suspect where that meeting would lead. I was promptly nominated and elected as treasurer (the nominator noted that I would be a good choice as I was then married to an accountant!) and then promptly received a congratulatory note from the secretary in Ottawa, asking if I would also consider joining the Federation and paying my dues. It is illustrative of the camaraderie and informality of FMWC that the Branch would elect a non-member to office.

Having climbed the executive ladder of the Branch to president, I was appointed representative to the CMA Council for FMWC in 1979, and a new political world opened up. The next step was to the BCMA as vice-delegate in 1979, and subsequently as delegate to the Board. Partisan politics were very active in BCMA in those days, and it was easy to get caught up in the fervor of the traditional moderates versus the reformers. As a result, I found myself as Secretary-Treasurer of the BCMA in 1982, then Chairman of the General Assembly in 1983. My bid for the presidency was unsuccessful, but before I had time to rest and catch my breath, I took on the Presidencies of the Vancouver Medical Association (VMA) and the Pacific Northwest Dermatology Society. This was followed by several years on the Medical Advisory Board of the G.F. Strong Rehabilitation Centre, including President of the Medical Staff, Presidency of the Canadian Dermatology Association, and Vice-Presidency of the Pacific Dermatologic Association.

In 1989, I was thrilled to receive the *Primus Inter Pares* award of the VMA and must admit that it is the only certificate I have ever framed (the rest have sat in a drawer all these years while my patients search the walls in vain for proof that I really am a doctor). One of the most interesting positions I have held internationally was that of Chairman of the Committee on Diversity for the American Academy of Dermatology. The name of the committee was not very indicative of its mandate—when I took it on it was called the Committee on Minority Affairs. It's mandate is to be an enabler for members of minority groups to enter dermatology, and it was wonderful to discover that women are no longer one of those minorities. At least in Dermatology we have come a long way.

In 1994, I made a major change by leaving Vancouver for rural Abbotsford and semi-retiring from everything. I now practise two days a week, garden five days, and lecture only six or seven times a year. I haven't quite been able to leave the political arena. I am currently President of the Pacific Dermatology Association, but hopefully that will be my last position, and I will be able to concentrate more on the posies than the politics.

DR. ALICE CAROLINE PATTERSON

As a child I was famous for being terrified of doctors (still am), and indeed on one occasion I ran away when my mother's GP (female, of course) came to call. Thus it was with some surprise that my family received the news of my intended application to Medical School. I thoroughly enjoyed my time at the University of Manchester Medical School. The thrill of dissection stays in my mind as it was truly a path to know the human body, and although students these days do not have that grind, for me it was a big step along the path of becoming a doctor. The camaraderie and fun we had endures even now as we plan a thirty-five-year reunion in Sydney, Australia where one of our 'year' lives on dialysis now, so we are all off to see him there rather than miss him in the U.K.

After the final exams came the house job lottery, when I experienced for the first time discrimination based on gender. A prospective boss opined that he never took female housemen as they would likely be "in love, menstruating, or pregnant." I suggested that I thought I could do a good job and that if he was not satisfied, then I would like to be the first to know. After six months he was gracious enough to say that I had been the best houseman that he could remember. When I had obtained the MRCP in 1969, I married a man I hardly knew and came to Vancouver, Canada, where a job as Fellow in Rheumatology awaited me. I have to say I took the job because it did not involve as much night call as did Internal Medicine, and hardly having spent any time with the aforesaid husband, I thought being at home most nights would be a good idea.

In 1970 all the Chief Medical Residents were female; we were Mirian Schaffrin at Vancouver General Hospital, Vicki Bernstein at St. Paul's Hospital, and myself at Shaughnessy Hospital. By year's end I was ready to embark on some sort of career, and was lucky enough to be taken under the wing of Dr. Harold Robinson at the Arthritis Centre, now the Mary Pack Arthritis Centre. This place was and still is a world leader in the care of people with rheumatic diseases. Dr. Denys Ford was totally dedicated to finding the cause of Rheumatoid Arthritis and Dr. Harold Robinson to taking care of people who had it. At the Centre were professionals with expertise and compassion, so that arthritis became an exciting challenge, not a boring illness for which nothing could be done.

I was the first Rheumatology Fellow and consequently the first female rheumatologist in British Columbia. As there were way more female than male patients, I did feel that I had something useful to offer, although Dr. Ford soon saw that I was not going to be the one to find the cause of arthritis. We used to meet every Friday for lunch at the Arthritis Centre, and there would be Rounds and a great opportunity to learn, which was an urgent matter for me after my one-year Fellowship. The interactions and bonding that happened at those Rounds continue today, although by now we have five or six Fellows, not to mention Residents, medical students, and sundry visiting firepersons. Now, too, we must have goals and objectives and learning outcomes, but the end result is not much different and is positive. Then, I must say we all had brown bag lunches, while now we have a delicious lunch provided by a pharmaceutical company. It tastes good, but it's vaguely immoral. The amazing leaps forward in the treatment of arthritis have been in large part due to the development of new and powerful drugs, but the bottom line remains that people who cope best with this terrible affliction are those with education, wealth, and strong social support.

A prospective boss opined that he never took female housemen as they would likely be "in love, menstruating, or pregnant."

In 1978 I moved to Shaughnessy Hospital and opened a small practice in the Jean Matheson Pavilion, as well as participating in the Medical Wards and student and Resident teaching. It was tough to raise three kids, run a practice, and try to teach. Thus I found that research was not really an option for me. For those who succeed in all three areas as well as at home, I salute them. I suppose it is a matter of choice, although I did not feel I had much choice at the time. I did manage to present a paper at the American College of Rheumatology in 1979 and to write a few minor papers, but it was not enough to permit promotion to full clinical professor.

By 1985 I felt ready to take on the challenge of returning to the Arthritis Centre to become Associate Medical Director, which allowed me to find out a bit about organising committees and working with allied health professionals and volunteers. I found that I enjoyed all this, and in 1989 I became Medical Director of the Mary Pack Arthritis Centre. Mary Pack was *the* pioneer of arthritis treatment in British Columbia as she was the one who saw the need through her work as a teacher for home-bound children, and her legendary energy and persuasiveness led to the establishment of treatment facilities for people with arthritis. As a Medical Director I was sent off to learn about management, financial statements, organisational psychology, and leadership, to name but a few of the skills needed. Around this time we began to feel the winds of change and to feel threatened by them, making the job of any medical manager very tough. I felt proud that I helped to launch the Arthritis Telephone Information Service, the Arthritis Self-Management Program, and other programs designed to help people help themselves. Empowerment of these people is very important to me, and I enjoy tremendously referring them to these programs that let them take control when loss of control, inherent in having a chronic illness, is almost the worst part of the illness.

From 1991 to 1995 I was Acting Head of the Division of Rheumatology at the University of British Columbia. Perhaps my greatest achievement in that position was to hold the Division of Rheumatology together and to be part of the successful search committee to recruit Dr. John Esdaile to the Division as Professor and Head in 1995.

Since 1995, I have been in private practice in rheumatology. Along the way I have spent many years associated with the Arthritis Program at the GF Strong Centre, where it has been a privilege to work with many nurses, physiotherapists, occupational therapists, pharmacists, and social workers to provide a program that is the envy of arthritis caregivers the world over. However, the major player in all of this is always the person with arthritis whose incredible resilience, indomitable spirit, and courage to go on are a wonder to us all. I have enjoyed learning of the big disease of the '90s, osteoporosis. When it was just a disease of old women it was considered very dull, but as effective new drugs began to be available, it became increasingly recognized as important in many settings, such as in runners, in people with chronic inflammatory diseases on long term corticosteroids, and in men. I was invited to work at the Pain Clinic where my interest in motivating people to help themselves was greatly strengthened. It seemed to me that for most of the 'clients' at the Clinic this was the first experience they had had of being in a totally supportive environment.

The dysfunctional, and in some cases non-existent, coping skills that they had were a direct result of the difficult childhood and adulthood they had experienced. I already knew that I was blessed with a wonderful family, but the clinic really made me realize how crucial this type of support is for all of us. If only governments would remember this when they think about cutting family support, daycare, and other services, which if properly used could help to prevent so many later more expensive problems, including ill health.

One of the most fulfilling and interesting aspects of my life in Rheumatology has been the provision of rheumatology service to the Peace Country of British Columbia. The Travelling Consultation Service in Rheumatology was set up by the Arthritis Society almost forty years ago and continues to this day. My trips north provide me with a glimpse of the real British Columbia and its people, from the farmers and miners to the amazing physicians, many of whom stay there for years dealing with illnesses and crises the like of which those of us in downtown Vancouver would never dream. The approximate 60,000 people living in the Peace Country create a need for almost half a rheumatologist, thus the four to five weeks I spend there a year are more than filled with interesting people with fascinating illnesses. After clinic hours the glorious open country, hot springs, and wonderful golf courses beckon.

Now I am in the final phase of my life as a physician and can enjoy seeing people with various rheumatic diseases, most of which I have seen before. But there is often a new problem never seen before, and there are always new young doctors whose insightful questions force a new look and a new thought about an old disease. It truly is a privilege to be a physician and to share in such a private part of a person's life.

No biography would be complete without a word about significant others, especially family. I must mention my parents who gave me my education and made me think that all things are possible. I always tell my husband, Dr. Michael Patterson, pediatrician, that he was picked from a cast of thousands, and he truly seems to be that. Raising a family and pursuing a career for thirty-two years from 1969 could not be attempted without a totally supportive spouse, and one who could get by with dust bunnies on the floor and plain food on the table. However, my sons do not think this is anything unusual, and indeed they expect to be sharing the caring with their partners. I am proud of their attitude, and indeed of their skills and readiness for the task. My daughter has been a big help and inspiration too, with her energy and dedication to any task at hand.

In conclusion, I can say that I have had and continue to have a truly wonderful job, and I think the next generation of physicians can too if they keep their sights on the main thing, which is not the hassles of practice, not the lack of resources, not the pain of being on call, not the poor remuneration, not the few trying patients, but the sick person who will always need a real doctor.

DR. MARGARET PENDRAY

Margaret Pendray was born in the U.K. and received her medical degree from the Royal Free Hospital University of London in 1966. She took pediatric training in Exeter, U.K., London, Ontario, and Vancouver (1966–1970), and Adult and Pediatric Nephrology at St. Paul's Hospital (1971–1973). She joined the UBC Department of Pediatrics in 1973.

Since then, Margaret has had a major influence on pediatric care in the region. From her experiences in renal medicine she developed an interest in parenteral nutrition, which she adapted to the needs of the newborn. She has also been instrumental in the education of many pediatric residents and developed the Neonatal-Perinatal sub-specialty program, accredited by the Royal College in 1995. She also developed the neonatal infant transport team and service, and the provincial neonatal resuscitation program.

Margaret's major contribution, however, has been in Neonatal Intensive Care within B.C., the sub-specialty of which is synonymous with her name. Not only did she design the special care nursery for both the old VGH site and the sixty-bed unit currently operating at BCCH, she also facilitated the development of regional neonatal special care areas. Margaret introduced co-ordination and discipline into this challenging area, and protocols of care developed by her team are now in use province-wide.

Hundreds of children in B.C. owe their good health and well-being to the start in life afforded them by Margaret's hard work and dedication.

(Dr. Steven Tredwell presented Dr. Pendray's story to the Medical Alumni Division of UBC. She received an Honorary Alumnus Award on May 26, 2001. Dr. Tredwell and Dr. Pendray have given permission to print this story.)

1973

DR. JUNE ESTELLE STEINSON
(1935–1975)

Dr. June Steinson was born in Illinois and had her early education in Burnaby and Vancouver, B.C. In 1959 she graduated from UBC Medical School. She took post-graduate work in Psychiatry and obtained the FRCP(C) in December, 1972 in the specialty of Psychiatry. Dr. Steinson was a teaching Fellow in the Department of Psychiatry at UBC and since 1973 had been on the staff of the Mental Health Centre in New Westminster. Sadly, she died on February 26th, 1975 at the age of forty, leaving her husband and three children.

DR. JIRINA (STRAKATA) VAVRIK

Jirina Strakata Vavrik was born in Ostrava, a coal-mining town in the northern part of Moravia in Czechoslovakia, near the German and Polish borders. Her father was a mining engineer. She attended Charles University in Prague. When the Germans occupied the country in 1938 they closed the universities and this closure lasted until 1945. The medical schools were opened when the Germans left and the Czech government offered free tuition and living quarters to those who wanted to study medicine. At first 3,000 medical students were taught in a large hall. There was a shortage of professors because many Jewish professors had been killed by the Nazis. Later, during this time of freedom from 1945 to 1948, the students were divided into four different medical schools. An American Ambassador of the UNRA helped organize equipment and supplies for the medical schools, as there were very few resources and no medical books remaining.

Living quarters for the medical students were the former barracks that the German soldiers had used. There were no showers, only cold water sinks like troughs, and heating the quarters was by coal. Jirina's father sent coal to her to help with the heating of the barrack.

In 1948 the Communists took over Czechoslovakia, and some professors left for England. Jirina graduated in Medicine from Charles University in 1951. In 1953 she married a man she had known since the age of fifteen and who was now also a doctor. The young doctors were ordered to go into general practice. In 1955, her son Jan was born. She hated her job, applied for a research position, did two years of Internal Medicine in a Prague hospital, and obtained a PhD in Nutrition and Diabetes. There was a request from Cuba via the Communists to Czechoslovakia for an expert in Nutrition. Jirina was assigned the job in 1967. Her husband was a Cardiologist and returned to Prague after several weeks in Cuba.

In Cuba, where eventually her son joined her, she did research of the local available foods. In Cuba young teenagers had to live in group homes for education and military training. Jirina and a dietician were working on setting nutritional allowances for these groups with a rather limited variability of the local food. Jirina enjoyed Cuba and did not have to work too hard. She was allowed trips into the country, and snorkeling was exciting to her. Eventually she worked with Hungarian chemical engineers, then ended up working on nutritional standards for the production of canned baby food for Cuba.

After Dubchek, the moderate leader, opened the borders of Czechoslovakia for those who wanted to leave, her husband went to Vienna where he had a cousin. Jirina decided in August, 1968, that she and her son, who was on vacation in Cuba, would emigrate to Austria. She didn't want to wait for permission from Cuban authorities which took time. Knowing that a ship from Europe with a Czech Captain was in port, she got some of the crew to smuggle her and her son onto the ship to go back to Europe. The Cuban police learned of their escapade and took them off the ship.

Jirina was then allowed to arrange tickets one-way to Prague, via Gander, Newfoundland. In Gander she and her son got off the plane during the stop-over for refueling, but did not get back on the flight. She tried to buy two tickets to Vienna with Cuban money and was told that it was worthless paper. They were sent to Immigration with no real knowledge of spoken English, dressed in light clothing, discouraged, and with no money. Jirina wept while her son, age thirteen, was in great spirits and excited that he might see bears! The Immigration Department organized a flight for her and Jan to the Halifax headquarters. She was very anxious, but the immigration people were kind to her. She was interviewed and eventually it was learned that the cousin in Vienna had a friend in Toronto, a dentist, who was married to a Danish pediatrician. This lady, Johana Mraz, had helped many Czech doctors to immigrate. It was arranged by Dr. Mraz that Jirina and her son would go to Toronto by train where they were given living quarters with a very kind family who had a son the same age as Jan.

During the first year in Toronto, Dr. Vavrik worked in Diabetic Research as a Fellow at the Best Institute with Dr. Fritz as her boss. She had to write her reports in English, which she found frustrating. When signing the contract for a year, she asked if she should "sin" here, and everyone had a laugh. In her second year in Toronto she had Residency training in Sunnybrook Hospital. Her husband had emigrated to join her and their son and they bought a little house.

For the LMCC exam requirements, Jirina had to have a rotating internship, which she did at Women's College Hospital. Her poor English continued to humiliate her, and she felt very insecure being on call every second day and every second weekend, often feeling that she was too old to start again doing Obstetrics and Surgery.

Her father was ill with bladder cancer and she longed to see him again. Jirina arranged to have her parents visit her in Toronto. Her father spent most of the visit sick in bed. Her parents wanted to go home to Prague earlier than planned, two weeks before Christmas. Jirina felt very sad, in addition to being exhausted from the hospital schedule.

The most encouragement she had was from the Dean of Medicine of the University of Toronto, Dr. Jan Steiner, an earlier immigrant from Czechoslovakia, who organized special language tutorials in English for the 150 Czech doctors who arrived in Toronto after Dubchek opened the borders. He arranged oral exams in Internal Medicine, Surgery, and Pediatrics. The Immigration Department organized courses in medical English. One of the teachers was Estelle Reed, herself an immigrant from Estonia, who was very kind and became a close friend of Jirina. She helped many of the foreign doctors in a personal way and entertained them at Christmas. Two professors of physiology, Drs. Anna and Otto Sirek, also Czech, were very helpful. Jirina's English improved. She did a year of Residency in Internal Medicine at Sunnybrook Hospital, along with other doctors from Czechoslovakia. The medical staff at Sunnybrook was very good to them.

Her son learned English quickly. He had read the books *Tom Sawyer* and *Huckleberry Finn* in Czechoslovakia, and when he arrived in Toronto he learned how to translate the stories from English.

Jirina had finally finished the two years of training in Canada required of foreign graduates before taking the LMCC exams, which she passed.

Her first practice was in North York in the Toronto area, and in addition she looked after the nurses at the hospital. Her practice built up quickly; her husband joined in her practice after he had interned a year and finally she was financially secure. Jirina practised for a few years in North York.

Eventually she decided not to stay in Toronto as her marriage was breaking up. She sold her practice to her husband for $3,000, and she and her son drove to Vancouver to look for a practice. Jirina was very discouraged after arriving in Vancouver as there didn't seem to be any opening for her. One day, however, she and her son were walking along Broadway and saw an office for rent which had been the practice of a Ukrainian doctor who had died. Being familiar with Slavic languages, she phoned the doctor's widow who was asking $5,000 for the practice. Jirina told her story and explained that she had only $3,000, and the doctor's widow graciously agreed to the $3,000 price.

Mother and son returned to Toronto to settle any business and within two months returned to Vancouver by train in time for Jan to begin his studies. At the Slovac Church it was announced to the congregation that Dr. Jirina Vavrik had taken over the practice of their well-loved Ukrainian doctor. Her practice was secure.

Dr. Jirina Vavrik sponsored her widowed mother to come to Canada. After many years in practice in Vancouver she found her dream retirement location on the Sunshine Coast in B.C. She built a small home; the view continues to delight her, and she is only a ferry-ride from her son and grandchildren. Her former husband later moved west, and occasionally they enjoy baby-sitting their two grandchildren together.

DR. ELIZABETH WHYNOT

To this day I still don't understand how I decided to apply for medical school. There have never been any doctors in my family, and the closest connection to health professions was my mother's quite short experience as a nursing trainee in an English hospital in the early forties, which I recall she didn't quite enjoy. I did read all of the books written by the American doctor, Tom Dooley, about his adventurous work in Laos, and I was perhaps inspired a little by that, though if so not consciously. I think I applied largely because of the challenge, and in my narrow experience at that time (forty years ago!) the other options for women seemed dull to me.

I applied to two Universities, Queen's and the U of T, and was accepted to both. I decided on Queen's because at that time admission to the two-year pre-med course guaranteed admission to medical school on successful maintenance of a pre-set academic standard. This seemed like a good deal. I started the program in September 1966, three months before my nineteenth birthday, and graduated in June 1972, six months before my twenty-fifth. In retrospect, I think it is pretty surprising that I managed to complete the course, considering my naiveté on entering in 1966 and how much 'adolescing' I had to do in those years.

As everyone knows, the late sixties and early seventies were a time of social unrest, especially among young people. Queen's was to some extent a backwater, but especially in the early seventies, some of the unrest managed to erupt even there. I was certainly affected by this. I lived in and eventually helped manage a housing co-operative where I had the benefit of rubbing shoulders with some of those rejecting the status quo. The rejection took many forms: for some, dropping out; for others, experimentation with drugs, political action, or a re-examination of accepted norms, such as women's role in society or conventional sexual morals. Although my main struggles through that period were growing up and getting through medical school, I was undoubtedly affected by the iconoclasm of the times. I had begun to feel quite ambivalent about being a doctor, and I had become involved with a woman who showed me books on feminism and social theory—a relationship which remained a secret throughout my remaining three years at medical school, because the challenge to social norms had yet to encompass same-sex relationships.

I am writing this on June 8, 2003, thirty-one years almost to the day after my arrival in Vancouver. I had bought a '67 Volvo 122, washed it, and jumped into it one day after competing my LMCC. I drove west on my own in four days to start a rotating internship at St. Paul's Hospital on July 1, or thereabouts. I met my friend who took me immediately to Long Beach and then on a trip down the coast to Oregon. That was enough for me: the west coast was better than Ontario and I was definitely staying here.

I was lucky enough to get my first choice in the intern matching service, i.e. St. Paul's. I had chosen this on the advice of Dr. Pat Kinahan whom I had met during an elective in my fourth year, which I had done at Vancouver General. In those days, St. Paul's was a much smaller facility, physically. The medical student residence was located where the new tower is, and the emergency was in a small area just off Comox Street. There was also still a small pediatric ward. The rotating internship involved spending time in all of the major acute care areas of course, including ICU, emergency, pediatrics, surgery, urology, medicine, obstetrics and gynecology, but no family practice or psychiatry. On call was one in two or one in three, and we spent a lot of time making toast in the residence when we weren't being overwhelmed by the work we were learning to do on the wards. I don't know whether others would say the same thing, but the intensity of that year, the exposure to life and death situations in circumstances where I wasn't at all sure what I was doing, left deep impressions. I still seem to remember almost everything that happened, almost all the most severely ill and dramatic patients, and certainly all the other interns and residents who helped me and suffered alongside.

I also encountered some of the role models who made me realize that it was actually possible to be a woman doctor. Some of these women probably have no idea that I was watching them, and benefiting from their wonderful examples. I particularly recall watching Dr. Pat Rebbeck perform surgery, Dr. Vicki Bernstein teach clinical cardiology to us, and Dr. Doris Cavanagh-Gray provide leadership. St. Paul's also offered me my first experience of the marginalized in this city, many of whom got most of their medical care in the outpatient clinics or at the emergency. I did an extra rotation in the emergency because I was so enthralled with the crazy environment there.

Although I had many important and educational experiences in that year, I was still pretty ambivalent about whether or not the medical profession was the place for me, and I decided not to apply for a residency because I was in a big hurry to escape the hospital setting. I had no idea what I was going to do next until, at the going-away party for the interns and residents, I struck up a conversation with Dr. Hedy Fry who told me about the Vancouver Women's Health Collective. She and several other doctors, including Fran Wilt and Diane Watson, provided medical back-up for the collective's self-help clinics. Hedy recruited me to join them in this volunteer activity. It was an important first step in the development of my still unintentional career path.

At the Heath Collective, which I later joined, I met some women who were working at the Pine Street clinic. They told me that the doctor there needed help and they were actually looking for someone to work several days a week. I arranged an interview with the doctor, Art Hister, and showed up dressed in my best short skirt outfit and nylons, the last time I did that, and barely had my mouth open before he said you're hired, call this number and they'll sign you up. He was desperate, I guess. Luckily, he was also quite good at his job and able to hold my hand through that awful introduction to real medical life. I worked at Pine Street, now just called Pine Clinic, for four or five years. There I met many other people who I still get to work with, including Perry Kendall, the Provincial Health Officer now, John Blatherwick, and several wonderful community health nurses. The Pine Street clinic was organized to serve the street youth of the time, some flower children, a lot of whom were, as I came to realize later, victims and runaways. We did lots of primary care of course, and saw some pretty sick kids: hepatitis, skin infections, bad, bad PID.

I continued to volunteer with the Women's Health Collective. It was there that some of my basic education about reproductive health and reproductive rights took place. The women were pioneers in the women's and consumer health movements. The issues for those of us working there were providing women with as much information as possible about their bodies, and supporting as much choice as possible for them in looking after their bodies. For example, we all learned and taught self-examination of the vagina and cervix, learned how to fit diaphragms, and advocated for abortion rights.

In the mid-seventies, it was just possible for a woman in Vancouver to get a therapeutic abortion in a few hospitals, but if you were young, that involved jumping hoops. We were lucky in Vancouver at that time that there were several gynecologists who supported a woman's right to choose this procedure. However, the anti-choice movement was very strong. Both through the Women's Health Collective and the Vancouver Status of Women, I became involved in the struggle to maintain access to the existing services. Many hospital boards were elected at large by people who bought memberships in the hospital society. Therefore it was possible to stack the annual meetings and elect a single-issue board. We spent several years fending off this eventuality by flogging memberships to VGH. The issue was so hot that the last AGM of the board had to be held in the Hyatt Regency Ballroom, and the subsequent year the Ministry of Health appointed a public administrator. It was over this issue that I made first made a few speeches and spoke to the media.

In the mid-seventies, it was just possible for a woman in Vancouver to get a therapeutic abortion in a few hospitals, but if you were young, that involved jumping hoops.

In 1977, I left Pine Clinic. I was still uncertain whether medicine was the place for me, so I took a sabbatical to think about it. I tried acting classes, which were a lot of fun, and which taught me some things about voice projection and about my limited talents. It was a good year, but at the end of it when I was offered a couple of locums by my old friend, Art, and by the St. Paul's Outpatient clinics, I took them. Then the Vancouver Health Department, which had taken over the Pine Clinic, called to say they were looking for a medical health officer to work in their Mid-Main offices at 25th and Main. Once again, I took on a job for which I wasn't really trained, and once again I found people to help. This time it was the person I consider to be my most important mentor, Dr. Anne Vogel. Anne (Patty, then) was the Deputy Medical Health Officer for the city, and I've had the pleasure of working with her on and off for more than twenty years.

The best thing about being a medical health officer in those days was the exposure to the community through its schools and homes. In that first two-year stint with the Health Department, I learned a lot about the diversity of the city from both cultural and socio-economic perspectives. I got to visit the elderly and isolated individuals who were struggling to stay at home and independent, and saw many areas of the city that had been completely unknown to me.

I left this job after two years to join my old friend Art Hister in his family practice on Fourth Avenue. I stayed in this partnership, which ultimately included Ellen Coburn and Georgia Immega, for eleven years. I loved family practice. I liked getting to know people gradually over the years, and when I decided to leave the practice in 1990, it was a terrible loss for me in many ways.

Shortly after I went into practice, I had a call from the Vancouver Police Department asking if I would be willing to provide medical examinations for rape victims. The call came to me because I had expressed some interest in the issue while I was working for the health department at Pine and later as an MHO, and had participated in committees discussing the lack of services for rape victims. Because I had heard that Dr. Carol Herbert was also interested in this issue, I called her up to discuss it. At the same time, I became involved with a society developing services for street kids, and began to learn about sexual victimization of children. Leslie Arnold from the Ministry of Social Services approached me about whether I was interested in providing examinations for children who may have been sexually abused. To make a long story short, Leslie agreed to support Carol and me to set up the Vancouver Sexual Assault Assessment Service, which began in late 1981. The service included both provision of acute medical care for adult rape victims as well as a clinic for children who may have been victimized. Carol, Georgia Immega, and I provided the care at the clinic for children; several other women physicians joined us on an on-call roster for the adult part of the service which happened at St. Paul's first, but soon moved to the old Shaughnessy hospital emergency department.

Right from its beginning in 1982, the Shaughnessy Sexual Assault Service operated as a partnership among the physicians, the hospital emergency staff, the police, and the community-based Rape Crisis Centre. The first roster physicians participated as volunteers except when the victim agreed to our providing forensic evidence and a report to the police, in which case there was a report fee. The Service's protocols were developed from a patient-centered perspective, emphasizing the patient's right to decide what she wanted to have done. The doctors' first duty was to the patient, not to the police, which was a big change from previous procedures in which the MD's role was primarily forensic. I participated as the Co-Director of this service for about eight years, sharing the role with Carol and then with Ellen Wiebe. The Vancouver Sexual Assault Service was the first of its kind in Canada; it is now an important program of B.C. Women's Hospital. The Sexual Assault Services are still offered by a team of physicians and nurses at the Vancouver General Emergency, and the program has supported the development of resources across B.C., as well as training practitioners, counsellors, and police from all over the country.

In 1990, I left my practice to take a job with the Vancouver Health Department again, this time as the Medical Health Officer for the North Health Unit, i.e., the northeast sector of the city. As usual, I'm not really sure why I made this move, though it was at least partly because of my interest in the community and in working with the 'system' rather than seeing patients one at a time. Whatever the reasons, I do not regret the decision, though I certainly found myself in the soup once again.

This area of the city was characterized by many classic public health problems: poverty, poor housing, poor nutrition, and especially epidemics, i.e.: tuberculosis, HIV, and hepatitis. Plenty to learn, anyway. Once again I was able to work with Dr. John Blatherwick and Dr. Anne Vogel, as well as a wonderful cohort of medical health officers. With the VHD's support, several of us were able to complete Masters' degrees in the Department of Health Care and Epidemiology at UBC. And I had the great good luck of working in the most organized community in the city, with the many community health nurses, community activists, committed physicians, community agencies, and politicians who were all trying to reduce risk and improve conditions in the area. In spite of us all, in 1996 the community was beset with the worst HIV and Hepatitis C epidemics among drug users in North America, and we had horrible numbers of deaths from overdose, death, and violence. For me, it was a privilege to work in the area, but often very frustrating and sad.

Shortly after I started, I was introduced to the YWCA Crabtree Corner and to Dr. Christine Loock, a well-known expert on fetal alcohol syndrome and an advocate for services to reduce risk for substance using women and their infants. She and others had been working to develop a proposal to provide intensive prenatal and postnatal services for pregnant women in the area. Eventually, we were able to develop core funding for this project through a partnership with B.C. Children's Hospital. This was the beginning of the very successful program known as Sheway, an intensive outreach program for pregnant women using street drugs and/or alcohol, and their infants. This program was another partnership, including the Vancouver Health Department, the YWCA, The Vancouver Native Health Society, B.C. Children's Hospital (and eventually B.C. Women's), the Ministry for Social Services, and alcohol and drug programs. Over the years, it has provided support and reduced risk for thousands of women and their infants. Recently, B.C. Women's has been able to open a specialized unit for the inpatient care of women and infants, another part of the continuum.

Another organization that developed tremendously in the early nineties was the Vancouver Native Health Society, led for most of this time by Lou Demerais. Working on various projects with this agency was the first chance in my professional life to learn about Aboriginal communities and their issues. Under Lou's both principled and pragmatic leadership, VNHS has become a comprehensive community health centre, incorporating everything from jobs training and supporting foster parents to the provision of specialized care for HIV patients.

In 1998, I left what was then the Vancouver Richmond Health Board to take a job at B.C. Women's Hospital. Through a variety of committees in the preceding years, I had come to know Dr. Penny Ballem in her role as the leader of B.C. Women's and an inspired advocate for women's health. As I had grown more disenchanted with the government politics impeding improvement in conditions for people in my health unit area, I had spoken to Penny about the possibility of working at B.C. Women's. Much to my delight, she was able to find a role for me at B.C. Women's, then part of the Children's and Women's Health Centre of B.C. From 1998 to 2000, I provided support for several women's health programs such as the Aboriginal Health, Youth Health, Sexual Assault and Relationship Violence, and Reproductive Mental Health. In many ways, this change felt like coming home. It had been almost twenty-five years since my work with the Vancouver Women's Health Collective and almost twenty years since the beginning of the Sexual Assault Service, and for several years I had been involved with both B.C. Women's and C&W because of shared interests in reducing risk for mothers and children.

B.C. Women's is an academic, acute care institution, a world very different from the community environment I came from. I spent a lot of my first two years there just learning some of the ropes. When Penny resigned her position as Vice President, I applied and was eventually offered that job. This was a big leap both for me and for the organization. Almost three years later, I find I am still often negotiating the gap across this leap, although I am more comfortable than when I started. Never an academic, I have a lot to learn about the current knowledge and emerging evidence about women's health. Budgets, human resources, projects, organizational change, and development are all areas that have been new to me in the last three or four years, not to mention maternity and newborn care. I am still sobered by the knowledge that B.C. Women's delivers more babies annually than any other centre in Canada, more than 7,000.

Meanwhile, the health care system as a whole continues to change in large ways, frequently. For example, B.C. Women's has become part of the Provincial Health Services Authority, appropriate because so many of our programs serve people and communities across the province. This means that I get to have contact with people in many regions across B.C. Playing this and the other roles assigned to me as the President of B.C. Women's is fun because I am so proud of what the organization does and can do, and because of the many stimulating people, women and men, who work here.

I consider myself to be a very lucky woman. My wonderful life partner Linde and I have been living together for twenty-three years so far. We have children and grandchildren and pets. I have been able to pursue a varied professional life, supported by them, my family, and by many mentors and friends. Really lucky, I'd say.

1974

DR. KIRSTEN EMMOTT

When I arrived in B.C at the age of seventeen, I had little idea what I wanted to do with my life. I had had two years of college in California where my father (who had been in the RCAF) was stationed, and I wanted to return to Canada. I loved UBC, and got involved with the student newspaper, the *Ubyssey*, where I met Tom Wayman, who was then the editor. He has been a mentor to me ever since. I began to write, and became a student activist. These were two factors that might have led the admission's people to consider me when I applied to medical school later. I dropped out of school for a while, became a reporter for the *Vancouver Sun*, wore hippie clothes, and grew my blonde hair down to my waist. I hung out with the young poets and activists, went back to school, took science courses, and became one of the first three students elected to the academic senate at UBC (one of the others, Gabor Mate, was then a wild and crazy leftist who eventually became a doctor too).

On the day medical school began, while I was waiting at the lobby of the anatomy building with the other students, I noticed a handsome boy leaning against the wall. He was later to become my second husband.

I graduated from UBC in 1974, married, and interned at Dalhousie University in Halifax. Internship was really hard for me. When I miscarried in the middle of the year, I had to spend some time in the hospital as I was very anemic and weak. It was difficult to do the work and I wrote a poem about it in the medical student journal. Tom Wayman saw the poem and invited me to join the Vancouver Industrial Writers' Union (VIWU), a group of people interested in writing about the work experience. Thus began my fifteen happy Vancouver years of an increasingly active writing career, which has so far produced two books of poetry and contributions to fourteen anthologies (three of them produced by VIWU). Our group joined forces with the folk song quartet Fraser Union, and we performed at the Vancouver Folk Festival and Seattle's Bumbershoot Festival.

At a labour arts festival in San Francisco, some of us were present at a performers' after-party where, as the custom was, the guitar went around and everyone was expected to sing. When it was my turn, I explained that I could not play or sing, but I recited from memory my poem about a woman's work ("in the infertility clinic sit the chronically unemployed . . . "). It was well received.

Meanwhile, I became a GP, moved to Victoria with my husband, bore two children, spent a couple of uneventful years as an obstetric resident, and returned to general practice. I spent several pleasant terms teaching medical students in my office.

When Sono Nis Press published my first solo book *How Do You Feel?* in 1992, I became known as "one of a surprisingly large group of physician writers," and began to appear regularly in the *Medical Post* and in American anthologies.

I had once written an essay for an epidemiology course at medical school about the image of women in medical journal advertising. Needless to say, the image of women was often negative, a continued projection of male fantasies and stereotypes, such as the ads for *Premarin*, which invited doctors to prescribe hormones to shrieking, miserable menopausal women in order to make the husbands' lives more pleasant. Other examples could also be found in the dermatology journals, which often showed a lot of bare skin on nubile young models without any skin diseases. There was an ad for prenatal vitamins that showed a pregnant woman holding a vitamin pill and wearing a dopey grin; the caption was: "Don't let her forget this one." Medical textbooks also had some scary sexism. How times have changed! This essay of mine was extensively quoted in an early publication by the Vancouver Women's Health Collective. I taught the staff at the Collective how to fit diaphragms and do speculum examinations, and I also worked at those early clinics.

I was a supporter of midwifery and natural childbirth at a time when it was unpopular among most doctors. Women, on the other hand, welcomed these views. Soon after, I opened my practice in Victoria in 1976, and I was delivering more babies than any other GP in town. Now, twenty-five years later, it is amusing to see that my pro-nature, anti-episiotomy views have been adopted by everybody. As the saying goes, "When the people lead, eventually the leaders will follow."

I was always interested in evidence-based medicine, and have continually spoken out against quackery. I contributed to the *Rational Enquirer*, the *BC Skeptics* newsletter. Here in Comox, I have contributed a few articles on evidence-based medicine to local publications, and hope to teach a night school course on the subject.

I got divorced in 1992 and moved to Comox to be with my current partner, also a GP. General practice here is even more rewarding than that in the city; and, to my delight, Zoe Landale, a dear friend and a VIWU member from Vancouver, moved here too. I am content, with the beautiful gardens, mountains, and ocean. At present, when my evil devil computer decides to work properly I work on pulling together another manuscript of poetry, and have also tried my hand at some other genres. My writers' group meets regularly to critique and edit each other's stuff, and we do occasional public readings.

My son and daughter are everything a mother hopes for—intelligent, healthy, attractive, sensible, and employed! Both are in the computer field, and live in Vancouver. I see a lot of my two stepchildren, who are younger. So all in all my life has been a good one.

DR. ELEANOR PAYNE
(1944–1975)

Dr. Eleanor Payne was born in Montreal and graduated from Laval University, Quebec in 1968. She then came to Vancouver and did her internship and residency training in both anesthesia and obstetrics and gynecology at the Vancouver General Hospital and St. Paul's Hospital. In 1972 she was a resident in medicine at Shaughnessy Hospital. Tragically, Dr. Payne did not have time to use her extensive training for very long, as she died January, 1975.

DR. LORNA SENT

My life has been a journey that has taken me across the Indian and Atlantic oceans, from Asia to Africa, and to North America. Starting in Hong Kong, I have travelled through the rainbow nation of South Africa to the ethnic diversity of Vancouver, my home. My interests, activities, and beliefs are very much the product of my background and experiences.

I am of Chinese descent with Hakka as my spoken dialect. The Hakka people, known as the gypsies of China, originated from Western China and spread out to settle in villages in the south some twenty-five generations ago. They were a hardy folk who worked the soil as they migrated; this probably accounts for the fact that Hakka women were never subjected to the ancient tradition of footbinding to transform their feet into "precious lilies."

My father, Line Fong (Lionel) Ching Sent, was a young boy when a guardian uncle took him to South Africa in the 1920s. He gained experience as an assistant in a grocery store, and, after his uncle died, took over management of the store at the age of thirteen years. The scarcity of young single Chinese women in South Africa led to his return home to seek a bride. With the post-war devaluation of the Chinese yen, the South African currency that my father carried with him made him an eligible man. He soon married the lovely Lim Tzao Fa (Jeanette), my mother. The young couple honeymooned, and I was born in Hong Kong whilst they awaited completion of the immigration process to South Africa. I was oblivious to my first experience with Chinese tradition, when my father was advised to take a substitute boy-child to South Africa instead of wasting the opportunity on a girl. Lionel disregarded this sage advice and embarked upon the slow boat journey across the Indian Ocean with his new family. After living on crowded public decks for more than a month, my mother, babe in arms, disembarked at the South African port of Durban, to a Western and alien environment. As Hakka was her only spoken language, she was unable to communicate verbally with the locals, and this came as a distressing shock to her. However, her independent spirit and resilience saw her through this difficult period of adjustment.

The apartheid laws that were introduced in South Africa in 1948 impacted every facet of life. The Chinese community did not conveniently fit into any specific category of "race" and had to contend with the arbitrary whims of apartheid officials who enforced the laws of segregation, including those dealing with residential and business areas, hotels, buses, post-offices, schools, and recreational activities. There were few rights for those who were not White. During the 1950s, all Chinese were regarded as potential Communists and lived under threat of deportation for any infractions or suspicion of Communism. The foreign-born were classified as "aliens" and were not allowed to apply for citizenship. I remained forever "alien." It was only during the more liberal and "verligt" (enlightened)

When I was accepted to medical school for the six-year post-secondary degree, members of the local community were aghast that my father would squander so much money in sending a girl to university, let alone to medical school.

period of the 1980s, some forty years after arriving in South Africa, that my parents were finally granted their citizenship. These circumstances contributed to the Chinese being a reserved, apolitical, and law-abiding community. Ours was a small but thriving business community with an extraordinary rate of first-generation university graduates. My family lived in the coastal city of East London, a relatively more liberal part of the country. We were treated as a shade more "white" than others, and we were consequently accorded a few extra "privileges." For example, while I was not allowed to attend a white public school, I was able to attend a white private Catholic school.

Being daughter number-one and the eldest of nine siblings, I became an expert baby-bather and nappy-changer from an early age. My other big responsibility was helping in the family store from the age of five. Fortunately, daughter number-three was more interested and skilled in cashing duties and soon took over. She went on to become the first of four accountants in the family, while my other siblings qualified as a social worker, an actuary, and a computer programmer, respectively. Tragically, son number-one contracted rheumatic fever and died at the age of sixteen from acute bacterial endocarditis. The years between my birth and that of my

youngest sibling span some twenty-one child-bearing years. I had already left home to attend medical school when my mother phoned on two occasions with the news that she was expecting another baby, my youngest brother and sister. Being the eldest child of immigrant parents, Chinese was my first spoken language, but this changed when I started kindergarten. Now I speak only a little Hakka, and with a strong English accent. I was a diligent student with high academic achievement—this was expected and taken for granted by parents who were dedicated to the education of their children as the best defense against the travails of racial discrimination. When I was accepted to medical school for the six-year post-secondary degree, members of the local community were aghast that my father would squander so much money in sending a girl to university, let alone to medical school. Lionel was a slow learner.

How did I decide on a career in Medicine? To be honest, I had no burning desire to heal mankind when I entered the program; I was only sixteen years old. There were very few career choices for women in those days. I preferred the sciences, and Medicine was the highest achievement possible in the sciences. So I went into it naïvely. Fortunately, I have found great satisfaction in interacting with people, and I love clinical work.

Medical school itself was another life. It took me a while to adapt to living in a big city and at the University of Cape Town. There were the usual practicalities of finding suitable living accommodations because, according to the Group Areas Act, residential areas were segregated by race: White, Coloured, Indian, or Black. It was following a personal hearing with the Vice-Chancellor during our fourth year at university that a fellow Chinese student and I became the first non-Whites to be permitted to live in a university residence. In the 1960s, the culture of medicine, at least in South Africa, was patriarchal. Male and female students were separated for certain blocks such as anatomy and obstetrics. We were further segregated as White and non-White students for all clinical training at the Groote Schuur Hospital, the site of the world's first heart transplant. The training program for me was even more difficult, as I was one of five non-White females and the only female amongst four Chinese students; I did not easily fit into any of the assigned four-student tutorial groups. Consequently, I was assigned to different groups at different times: White female, non-White female, or Chinese male and female. Fortuitously, this resulted in the unexpected opportunity of interacting and socializing with diverse individuals and making many friends in the process. Our friendships were rekindled at a memorable twenty-fifth anniversary class reunion a few years ago.

When my husband, Clifford Chan-Yan, passed the Fellowship examination in Internal Medicine, the head of the department of Medicine at the University of Cape Town approached him with an offer of a staff position at the Groote Schuur Hospital. What an honour. This would have been the first staff appointment of a non-White doctor at an institution where the medical staff was exclusively White. Lengthy negotiations with the hospital administration and the provincial health authority ensued. After six months, permission was granted with two conditions attached: Cliff's work would be confined to non-White patients, and he would be paid as a Coloured senior registrar, i.e., on a lower salary scale. The next leg of my journey was thus determined. Three months later, in June of 1973, armed with a special immigration minister's permit, we arrived in Canada at Montreal's Dorval airport, en route to Vancouver.

We chose Vancouver as we had heard how the beauty of the city rivaled that of Cape Town. Moreover, Cliff's brother, sister-in-law, and young family, who had immigrated eight years earlier to start a business, were especially thrilled with the prospect of having some family around, and were instrumental in getting residency application forms to us in quick time. Thanks to them we could wait for a few months' salaries to buy a bed. Our sadness over the circumstances of our departure from South Africa dissipated with the warm reception we received from everyone we met in Vancouver. We were fortunate to land residency jobs at short notice: Cliff at St. Paul's Hospital and I at the old Shaughnessy Hospital. These jobs at separate hospitals facilitated our integration into our new community and gave us the opportunity of quickly establishing a network of friends and colleagues. Residency and hospital life was particularly lively because of the house-staff living quarters and lounges at these hospitals. We were introduced to Canadian culture—hockey night in Canada and peanut butter and jam sandwiches, and driving on the right-hand side of the road. There were slight twinges of homesickness, but a hectic pace ensued with the LMCC exams, my residency at Vancouver General Hospital, and Cliff's Canadian

Fellowship exams and subsequent commencement in private practice.

Unfortunately, pregnancy with its attendant physiological changes began to conflict with the demands of my internal medicine residency training. One in three ICU and CCU calls met with overwhelming first trimester fatigue and somnolence. My fellow residents often carried my pager and dispatched me to the house-staff quarters for lunchtime snoozes. This was ultimately unrealistic and unfair to my colleagues, so I quit. For the first time in my life I found myself at a loss. I was home alone while everyone I knew was at work. Fortunately, I adapted to the change and discovered what my neighbourhood was like during the day and what other people did with their time. I registered for an array of courses, from accounting to weaving, macramé and pottery—the popular crafts of the seventies.

Our daughters Debbie and Sharon arrived in 1975 and 1977 respectively, and my life began to revolve around feeds and diapers, the milestone events of teething, crawling, walking, and wipe-outs. I yearned to get back to medicine, and six months after Debbie was born, I started with part-time practice. Not having the luxury of family help, we had to deal with bundling up the babe and dropping her off at the sitter every day. This, with obstetrics call, became unsettling to our family life, especially as Cliff had to spend very long hours in establishing his practice in Internal Medicine and Nephrology. Thus, towards the end my second pregnancy, I reverted to being a full-time mother and housekeeper for a year, and wondered whether Lionel's advisors were right after all.

Fortunately, time passed quickly and I again ventured back into medicine, starting with Planned Parenthood clinics, locums, and sessions with the practice in which I am now a senior partner. A focus in Geriatrics with patient visits at home and in nursing homes allowed convenient work hours while the children were at school. Life was hectic but fun-filled, and there were tears and laughter. I had to learn the art of time management and priority management. On non-office days, I shared babysitting with other mothers, carpooled for school, music lessons, and athletic activities, and volunteered in the library at the school and other programs. I enjoyed city-league team tennis and fitness classes, and gained some knowledge of plants in the garden. This was a valuable period of my life when the common bond I shared with other mothers resulted in lasting friendships. It was rather late that we found out the benefits of live-in help, but this finally enabled me to ease into full-time family practice with no obstetrics.

As our daughters grew up, the constant busy-ness of our household subsided, and I found time for other types of volunteer activities. Although my upbringing was Western and my Chinese language skills were rudimentary, I began to develop a sense of my Chinese roots, which became heightened with the influx of Chinese immigrants to the Vancouver area in the 1980s. I joined the local and national Chinese Canadian Medical Societies and, during my term on the board and as president, we tried to assist the newcomers in health education and in accessing health care resources by media promotion and presentations at Health Fairs.

As an extension of this involvement, I became interested in Chinese women's health. My interest gained impetus when I became aware of a

When I joined a women physicians' goodwill delegation to China, I came face to face with some of my roots, which had first sparked my interest in the health of Chinese women.

study, published by the British Columbia Cancer Agency in 1990, which revealed a four-times higher incidence of invasive cervical cancer amongst Chinese women in British Columbia compared with women in the general population. A low rate of presentation for Pap smear screening was noted, and this was attributed to factors such as language and cultural barriers, and a lack of knowledge about cancer screening. Cultural barriers are still significant today, not only for Chinese women, but also for some Chinese physicians. Many traditional Chinese women and physicians are not comfortable in discussing sexuality, including breast and gynaecological matters, and many Chinese women express embarrassment about having "private" pelvic examinations performed by male physicians. Therefore, Pap smear screening and information about cervical cancer are frequently neither offered nor requested.

I thus became a founding member of the Asian Women's Health Clinic (AWHC), the first Pap smear clinic in North America, and I served as volunteer medical director from the clinic's inception in 1994 to July 2000. Prior to the opening of the clinic, a survey amongst Chinese physicians regarding the need and the feasibility of a Pap smear clinic was undertaken. This was met with only modest support. However, community groups enthusiastically supported the concept, and we proceeded to launch the AWHC as a community partnership between the British Columbia Women's Hospital, the Vancouver-Richmond Health Board, SUCCESS (a Chinese social services agency), and the Chinese Canadian Medical Society (CCMS-B.C.) in January 1994. When the clinic outgrew its space at a public health clinic, it was relocated in 1997 to the Mount St. Joseph Hospital (MSJH), becoming one of that hospital's community service programs. Around this time, a realignment of partnerships took place to include MSJH while the CCMS withdrew.

The clinic is centrally located in Vancouver and, in order to accommodate the schedules of working women, is open in the evenings three times a month. To address the cultural and linguistic barriers that were identified, all the staff are women and are fluent in Cantonese or Mandarin as well as English. The clinic has provided many women with their first ever Pap smear and breast examination. Breast self-examination (BSE) teaching became an additional mandate of the clinic when it became apparent that a large number of the women were not familiar with BSE. A clinic visit includes the viewing of educational videos on Pap smear testing and BSE, a one-on-one education session with demonstrations on pelvic and breast models, followed by a pelvic and breast examination by the clinic physician. The clinic remains exclusively a screening and education clinic, and it is hoped that this arrangement will encourage the support of community physicians by not 'competing' for their patients. Educational materials developed by the clinic include pamphlets and videos on the Pap smear test and on BSE, in both Cantonese and Mandarin. Education workshops using these teaching aids have also been conducted in the community. The clinic appears to enjoy a unique sense of camaraderie, with patients frequently accompanied by a supporting spouse, boyfriend, mother, daughter, sister, or friend.

It was a challenge to develop this program, from the basics of creating documentation and history forms, protocols and job descriptions for the clinic, to the development of educational tools in the form of pamphlets, videos, and slides on Pap testing and BSE, and then to the realms of designing and renovating the clinic premises. The greatest challenge was the fund-raising aspect as there has been no specific budget for the development of the program. We were fortunate to be invited to co-plan and be a co-beneficiary to a major fund-raising fashion show. I was introduced to corporate business and event planning, and learned how to cajole friends into buying tickets for the event. It was hard work and stressful, but the networking and the results were well worth it. Community donors have been generous in funding the new clinic premises, and physicians who have volunteered their expertise and time in developing the educational materials and the patient database have done a tremendous job. The clinic staff, the physicians, the nurses, the receptionist, and the volunteers also need to be commended for their dedication in working at the clinic and in the promotional and educational programs outside of clinic hours. They have all made this venture a reality.

I am both proud and pleased to have brought the clinic from a predominantly volunteer-based service to a level where it is now a formal community service program of the Mount St. Joseph Hospital. The Asian Women's Health Clinic now requires stable funding from its community partners as well as the province of British Columbia. The program needs continued growth and expansion in order to reach more Chinese women and other Asian women who may be encountering similar barriers to accessing the kinds of services provided by the AWHC.

When I joined a women physicians' goodwill delegation to China with representatives from the Federation of Medical Women of Canada and the American Medical Women's Association in 1998, I did not anticipate the immense effect that this trip would have on me. I came face to face with some of my roots, which had first sparked my interest in the health of Chinese women. We were hosted for a series of workshops on Woman and Child Health, and we were able to observe both Western Medicine and Traditional Chinese Medicine in China. However, the highlight of the trip was a meeting with a special uncle, a semi-retired physicist at the Beijing University. My father had been adopted out when he was a child and had very little contact with his birth mother thereafter. He did not meet his younger brother until a recent visit to China. My parents provided me with instructions on how to contact this uncle, and I was warmly received by his family and treated to an extraordinary dinner at their home in a social housing complex. We were fascinated with each other and communicated in snippets of Hakka, Mandarin, and English with the aid of a Chinese-English dictionary. My treasured gift from this visit is a computer-generated copy of the only photograph in existence of my father's birth mother, my grandmother.

I have been fortunate to be able to combine my professional knowledge with my community interests, and this has led me to become involved with a variety of interesting and challenging projects. As a member of a Breast Cancer Information Project for three years, I participated with other health-care givers and breast cancer patients in promoting breast cancer awareness and in striving to enhance care. Two years on the Vancouver YWCA Board of Directors made me aware of much broader issues facing the women of today. I scratched the surface of issues of poverty, day-care, single-parent housing, career counselling, women's shelters, government lobbying, and fund-raising. It was both an education and a privilege for me to have met women from different walks of life and to see things from the diverse perspectives of sociologists, lawyers, bankers, social workers, CEOs, fitness leaders, fund-raisers, and philanthropists. Four years on the Board of the Federation of Medical Women (Vancouver) gave me the opportunity to work with other women physicians at both the local and national levels. Locally, a project that I enjoyed managing for two years was a mini-mentor matching program in which woman medical students were matched for their area of interest with woman specialists.

The well-being of medical students has always been a special interest. My husband and I have been participants in the University of British Columbia (UBC) Medical School's mentor program since 1989. We have had the pleasure of learning about the students' individual personalities,

As a member of a Breast Cancer Information Project for three years, I participated with other health-care givers and breast cancer patients in promoting breast cancer awareness and in striving to enhance care.

talents, uncertainties, and aspirations over dinner and BBQs at our home. I am also a Clinical Instructor with the Department of Family Practice, and taught Clinical Skills to first-year students from 1987 to 1994. I was thus delighted when I was elected to the UBC Medical School Admissions Selection Committee for a four-year term. With the benefit of years of personal interaction with medical students at all levels, I felt that I could assess applicants with good insight. I took this responsibility seriously and, with my colleagues, endeavored to select the finest candidates for our profession.

Thanks to the advice of a few friends, the last year of the twentieth century marked a new milestone in my life and also a slight career shift with my election to the Council of the College of Physicians and Surgeons of British Columbia. My first year on Council and on the Quality of Medical Performance Committee has been an eye opener. I had not previously appreciated the complex role that the College plays in regulating the profession and in protecting the public from us, the doctors. Work on the Ethical Standards and Conduct Review Committee and on the Legislation and Policy Committee is destined to be an even greater education. I am looking forward to working at the College as it faces the challenge of a technologically changing world and an increasingly diverse and knowledgeable society.

On a more personal note, I continue to enjoy physical activity and time with family and friends. Shortly after our arrival in Canada, Cliff blew our bank account when he signed us up at a multi-facility family athletic club. It turned out to be an excellent investment as we had a focus for our family physical activities and the opportunity to make new friends. My tennis improved and I was a city-league and tournament participant for many years, until the advent of middle age diminished some of my competitive fire and ability to hustle. I currently enjoy social tennis and workouts in the gym, having discovered the benefits of the exercise ball and cross-trainer machine. I have also begun the quest of unravelling the mysteries of the golf swing, a physical movement whose mythology and methodology necessitates a twenty-four-hour TV golf channel.

I feel so fortunate in my family life too. My husband is happy and successful in his career; he is in private practice, and continues to teach clinical medicine and to participate on hospital committees. He shares the household chores and thankfully, he actually enjoys grocery shopping and is a wizard in the kitchen and on the BBQ. He has accumulated a mountain of 'how-to' golf books and magazines, and the dents and scuffmarks on the downstairs fireplace and ceiling are testimony to his diligence in practising. But, he claims, he is not obsessed.

We are proud of our daughters who have grown into intelligent, independent, and globally-minded young women. Debbie has a degree in Civil Engineering from Queen's University and her Masters from the University of British Columbia. To spend four years at medical school, four years in residency, and then a few more years in a sub-specialty fellowship was something she thought would be quite crazy. She is now a Water Resources Engineer for a consulting firm in Calgary. Sharon has a Bachelor of Science and a Bachelor of Physical Health Education degree, also from Queen's University. She is currently exploring different career paths and expresses an interest in working in the health field; she has no qualms about the number of years that further studies may entail. Both young women are physically active, love the outdoors, and have found the time and opportunity to travel extensively. Their fascination with people and places has facilitated their interest in several languages, and they already have an admirable history of volunteering abroad and in our local community.

My journey has been enriching and rewarding. I have learned so much, and I am optimistic about future challenges and experiences. We have planned a family trek in the Himalayas of Nepal for this fall, when Cliff and I are still physically fit and before our daughters move on with their own lives. Our plans are coming to fruition; we are packing and are eagerly looking forward to our adventure—a new experience, a physical challenge, a family time, and time to reflect on nature's timeless beauty, on the rooftop of the world.

DR. EMILY STERBAK
(1924 – 1982)

Dr. Emily Sterbak graduated from Charles University in Prague, Czechoslovakia, in 1952 and specialized in Child Psychiatry. She came to Canada in 1968 with her family. She was Resident in Psychiatry at Vancouver General Hospital and Health Sciences Centre and was on

Fellowship in 1974 at the University of British Columbia. She then joined Woodland School's staff.

Dr. Sterbak was ill for several years, and continued to work until the time of her final hospitalization. She died on December 31st, 1982, aged fifty-eight. She is survived by her daughter Jana, an artist in Toronto, of whom she was very proud.

(The above was prepared by the Woodlands' Medical Staff and written by Dr. Bluma Tischler, Medical Director of Woodlands School.)

DR. JOAN R. STOGRYN

I was born Joan Wilson and grew up in Edmonton as part of the Baby Boom generation. My family was quite overwhelmingly medical in that both grandfathers, an uncle, my father, and my older brother were all doctors, all of them university-based specialists. In fact, I am the sixth generation of my family to be a doctor. I attended high school at Strathcona Composite and went on to do my undergraduate work at the University of Alberta, winning a City of Edmonton full scholarship for three years. Before entering medical school, I took a year off and worked as a research technician at the renal dialysis unit at the University of Alberta Hospital, and then went travelling across Europe for six months in the approved mid-sixties student fashion: alone, hitch-hiking, staying in youth hostels, living on less than $5 a day, and dressed in bell-bottoms, flowers, and beads.

I returned to begin medical school in 1969, three days after my twenty-first birthday. There were twelve women in my class of 112 students. This was just the beginning of the influx of large numbers of women into medical school. There I met my husband and classmate, Dale Stogryn, and we were married at the beginning of third year.

During medical school, I did research in the summers. One project was on ARDS and lung biopsy techniques. This project earned me a trip to Atlantic City in the United States to present a paper. My other summer project was more interesting. This was in 1970 when tissue typing and transplantation were in their early days. My supervisor was an immunologist who was interested in tissue inbred populations. I spent the summer in Inuvik,

Aklavik, and Tuktoyatuk researching the family trees of all the Inuit families to select individuals for study. I researched municipal and church records, but mostly spent many hours drinking tea with Inuit elders and listening to their stories of the Inuit families of the Mackenzie Delta area. This project and the resulting publications won the University of Alberta Student Research Award, and earned me a trip to Galveston, Texas to present at an International Student Research Forum.

My only other research effort was an elective in 1972 when my husband and I spent a month studying mountain climbers at Mt. Rainier in Washington for the effects of altitude sickness. However, I have to confess that we probably spent as much time hiking and climbing as doing scientific research. The highlight of the project came when we actually climbed Mt. Rainier ourselves and my husband got to experience, firsthand, some of the effects of altitude sickness.

I graduated from the University of Alberta Faculty of Medicine in 1973, the first woman to win the John W. Scott Gold Medal for "the graduating student who has evidenced to an outstanding degree those qualities of scholarship, leadership, and character that may be expected to lead to a distinguished standing in the medical profession." I narrowly defeated my husband, Dale, for the award. He had to settle for the Mewburn Gold Medal for surgery and the Schaner Medal for service to the medical student population.

Following graduation we moved to New Westminster, B.C. to do a rotating internship at the Royal Columbian Hospital, attracted by its reputation for packing the maximum amount of experience possible into a one-year program. There were no medical students and very few residents there, so we were given tremendous opportunity to get hands-on experience, especially in Emergency, Obstetrics, and Critical Care areas. I was president of the intern group that year, the first woman to fill this role.

It was 1974 when we finished. The NDP government of Dave Barrett was newly in power. The Fishermen's Union had backed the NDP strongly and, in return, were agitating for better medical care for the fishing fleet when they were congregated in remote areas of the Coast. This demand was strengthened when a high-ranking union man infarcted, arrested, and died in Rivers Inlet, far from any medical intervention.

The newly formed Emergency Services Commission decided to send a medical team with the fleet to Rivers Inlet in July and to Port Renfrew in August when there were large numbers of boats fishing. They recruited us because RCH grads were considered to have the best training in emergency and critical care work.

So, in July, 1974 we flew up to Rivers Inlet in an old Goose amphibious plane, along with five crates of medical supplies, including a defibrillator and a wide range of medications. While in Rivers Inlet we were housed at the Canadian Fishing Company camp at Goose Bay, a former cannery. It was truly an educational experience for two kids from the Prairies. We spent many hours sitting on fishing boats, learning about the fishing industry, playing poker and drinking tea (or stronger stuff) with the fishermen who came from a wide variety of ethnic origins. On non-fishing days we learned to catch salmon, red snapper, halibut, and squid, dove for abalone, dug for clams, and generally acquired a gastronomic education from the Japanese, Scandinavian, and Greek fishermen we met.

I researched municipal and church records, but mostly spent many hours drinking tea with Inuit elders and listening to their stories of the Inuit families of the Mackenzie Delta area.

In August we travelled by treacherous switch-backed gravel roads to Port Renfrew where there was a fleet of seine boats, an active logging operation, and some tourist trade from the West Coast Trail. We were housed there in a small travel trailer provided for us by B.C. Packers. The trailer doubled as our home and our treatment centre.

For the most part, the medicine we practised was minor emergency stuff, everything from blood pressure checks to fish hooks in eyes, "fish poisoning" (cellulitis due to a spirochete found in fish slime), and pulling abscessed teeth (we had a quick course in dental blocks and extractions from a dentist friend before we left). We did see some major trauma in Port Renfrew, both from the seine fleet and the loggers. Our most serious incident occurred when a seine worker sustained a depressed skull fracture while the boat was working out in heavy seas. Dale went out on a Coast Guard cutter to get him stabilized and bring him in to shore; I flew with him in a helicopter to Victoria. We had two other emergency evacuations, a

back injury and a compound fracture-dislocation of an ankle, but everything else we managed on site.

We did the fishing fleet job for two summers in 1974 and 1975. In between we worked as GP locums in the Tri-Cities areas, saving our money for a year's travel, which we undertook after our fishing job in 1975. We spent three months in various South Pacific countries—Hawaii, Samoa, Tonga and Fiji—landing up in New Zealand in November. There we were able to get work permits and were hired to look after an eighty-bed cottage hospital in Kawa Kawa in a tourist area called the Bay of Islands in Northern New Zealand. It was normally staffed by an internist who was sick in hospital in Auckland and a surgeon-obstetrician who was due to go on holidays for a month. It was a wonderful experience both socially and medically. Medically we coped with a wide variety of things with minimal equipment and lab support. We rigged up our own underwater drainage for a pneumothorax, resuscitated a multiple trauma motor-vehicle accident patient with a transected larynx, coped with a malignant hypertension case, and learned how to use vacuum extractors in OB cases twenty years before they were re-popularized in this country. We also experienced the trailing end of a tropical typhoon with torrential rains which flooded the town and access roads. We were high and dry in the hospital which was strategically built on top of a hill, so we spent the time praying we wouldn't have any surgical emergencies as we had no way to evaluate them, and neither of us had any more than a month's elective experience in anesthesia!

The hospital staff took us under their wings, helping and supporting us, feeding and entertaining us, and instructing us in New Zealand and Maori culture. When we left they outfitted us with camping gear for the rest of our travels around the country.

From New Zealand we went on to spend three months in Australia, then a month in Papua, New Guinea. There we stayed with a Canadian, Dr. John Millar, who later returned to Canada and became B.C.'s Medical Health Officer. At that time he was working in a small hospital in Mendi in the southern highlands area. From Mendi we were able to go into more primitive areas with travelling health teams. It was a fascinating taste of third-world medicine. The doctors in Mendi had to cope with everything and anything. They often performed surgery with the GP anesthetist holding the surgical textbook and talking the GP surgeon through surgical procedures. They performed symphysiotomies instead of C-sections for obstructed labour because patients would not return for subsequent pregnancies and often died with a ruptured uterus in the bush. Patients were hospitalized on wooden pallets for beds in cement-floored rooms which were hosed out daily. Leprosy was common and perinatal mortality appalling. It was all a far cry from our comparatively luxurious health care system.

From Papua, New Guinea we had an abbreviated trip through the Orient, the Philippines, Taiwan, Hong Kong, and Tokyo, abbreviated because I was twenty-eight weeks pregnant and it was summer and unbearably hot and humid. We arrived home in September, 1976. Dale went to work as a locum (we were totally broke by then), and I settled to await the birth of our first child. I returned to doing locums after she was born, and in 1977 started my own family practice in Coquitlam.

Since then, we have been engaged in more mundane pursuits. We both elected to stay in family practice. For myself, that decision was made primarily because I was unable to find a specialty that I thought could keep me interested and entertained for thirty years of practice. I also truly enjoy the ongoing involvement in the lives of families from the cradle to the grave, and find my involvement immensely rewarding, whether the medicine is complicated or simple. My own practice was, for many years, heavily weighted with obstetrics, pediatrics, and adolescent medicine (inevitable when you are the only female in a group practice). I work out of the Royal Columbian and Eagle Ridge Hospitals and have served for many years as a GP representative on the Department of Obstetrics, the Education Committee, and the Credentials Committee. I was also the first woman President of the New Westminster Medical Association. I have a part-time family practice, and also work on a sessional basis for Tri-Cities Mental Health Unit and the Ministry of Children and Families, treating adolescent and adult eating disorders in association with St. Paul's Hospital and B.C. Children's Hospital. In addition, I do some work for the College of Physicians and Surgeons involving disciplinary investigations. My husband Dale is in family practice, a Director of Medical Education at the Royal Columbian Hospital, and a Clinical Associate Professor of Family Practice at UBC.

We have three children, the oldest now applying to medical school, the second, at the University of Victoria in Biology, and the third graduating from Grade 12 and aiming for Veterinary Medicine.

On the personal side, I have satisfied my yen for adventure by returning to a passion of my youth: horses. I am re-teaching my middle-aged body to fly over fences on the back of a 1,500-pound horse in the show ring. We also have a wonderful water-access only property on Nelson Island outside Pender Harbour which is our sanctuary and retreat.

It has been thirty years since I entered Medical School, and of course, there have been many changes over those years. I entered Medicine during an era which paid increasing lip service to the equality of women, but did not always carry through when it came to applying those principles. Medicine was probably first among the professions to accept women on an equal basis. However, it was still considered quite legitimate to question a young woman such as I as to whether I didn't feel guilty about "taking the place of a man" in medical school. Within the profession itself, I met with amazingly little prejudice against women in medicine on a day-to-day basis with the physicians I encountered. However, occasionally incidents did arise where blatant prejudice occurred. I was always so flabbergasted when they happened that I never quite knew what to do, and in most circumstances found that my colleagues and classmates rose most vigorously in my defence. As president of the intern group I was expected to organize the medical staff and intern golf tournament and dinner. I was informed that unfortunately the golf tournament was to take place on a day on which women were not allowed on the Vancouver Golf Course. I declined to organize the event and my intern group, who were all male but one (me), categorically refused to play in the tournament. Fortunately, such incidents were few and far between, and never placed any impediments on the pursuit of my career. I have enjoyed my medical career enormously and continue to do so. I appreciate that I am able to function on a totally equal basis with my male colleagues, and I love the flexibility that I have had over the years to tailor my practice life to the needs of my family life, and to continue to evolve and change what I do to keep myself stimulated and intellectually challenged.

DR. JEAN SWENERTON

Dr. Jean Swenerton was born in Regina, Saskatchewan, in 1944 and lived in Meadow Lake until she was ten. Jean's father was a general practitioner. She completed her BA from the University of British Columbia in 1965 and went on to the UBC Medical School. At the end of third year in medicine, Jean married a classmate. From 1969 to 1970 she did a rotating internship at St. Mary's Hospital in San Francisco, and began an anaesthesiology residency at UBC in 1970.

Jean lived first-hand the trials of trying to juggle the demands of family, babysitter/nanny uncertainties, the day-to-day rigors of residency work, and finding adequate study time to prepare for the FRCPC exams. Her two children, Doug and Anne, were born while she was still a resident. From 1975 to 1983, Jean lived in fits and starts—work, home, family, study, and 'catch-up.' She passed the written part of the anaesthesiology fellowship in 1979 and continued to do anaesthesiology locums at the Children's Hospital. After a refresher year of anaesthesiology residency to prepare for the oral exam, she completed the FRCPC in November, 1984.

Since then Jean has been an obstetric-anaesthetist at the Grace Hospital (now Women's Hospital) in Vancouver. She was the Chair of Medical Quality Assurance (QA) at the Grace for three years and was Chair Anaesthetist of the Interhospital Anaesthesia QA Committee of the Grace and University hospitals.

Jean's loves are the piano, skiing, golf, travel, cooking, gardening, and keeping up with her children's pursuits. She is very active in the Federation of Medical Women and was president of the B.C. Branch from 1987 to 1988. In April of 1989 she organized an event, "A Night of Tribute to B.C. Women Physicians." Jean was the National President of the FMWC from 1991 to 1992. From 1995 to 1997 she was the Vice President for North America of the Medical Women's International Association.

DR. MARY CONLEY

I was born in a fishing village in New Brunswick in 1944, the fourth child born in five years. My father died when I was eight.

I loved school, and went to the University of New Brunswick on scholarships. In 1966 I received a BSc with honours. My thesis was on "The Effects of Barometric Pressure on Sawbugs." (There was none.)

I went to UBC and studied medicine. I was one of the "token ten," as there was a quota on women in the '60s. The only person I knew in Vancouver was my alcoholic uncle who lived on skid row. Needless to say it was quite an education! After first year I was short of funds and dropped out of school. I worked in the surgery department doing research measuring the surface area of the hand in various positions. Dr. Robert Cowan and I published a paper in the *Canadian Journal of Surgery* on my findings. At night, my girlfriend and I ran Vancouver's first art boutique. We made a lot of crafts in our spare time and sold them out of a rented store, "The Purple Gherkin." My brother arrived from N.B., unemployed, and ran the store during the day. Our story made the newspaper, and hordes of shoppers arrived and bought everything. We had to close for three days to replenish the shelves!

I continued to work at UBC as a research technician and to take art courses at night. I went to art school in Hawaii for a year and painted nudes, and then returned to medical school. In all it took me nine years to finish medicine. The Dean shook my hand and said, "Thank God we're finally getting rid of you!"

After interning in Ottawa, I returned to the west coast and started general practice in Victoria. Many of my first patients were young women with unplanned and unwanted pregnancies. At first I referred them to a gynecologist for an abortion. But soon it was clear that their experiences were laced with bitter criticism from the hospital staff. I started to accompany them to the OR to buffer them against verbal abuse. Then it occurred to me, since I was there anyway, I would train to do the abortion myself. After a few months under supervision, I began on my own.

I read an interview by Dr. Morgentaler in the *Medical Post* and was surprised that his complication rate was so low, so I arranged to meet him when he was visiting Vancouver. We met in the Garden Cafe in the old Sylvia Hotel. I wanted to know how he could do abortions in his clinic since it was against the law. It was clear that he thought the law was wrong and it was a matter of necessity to do the abortion as soon as possible for medical reasons. I flew to Montreal to train in his clinic. I was now launched to fight for a woman's undeniable choice to an abortion.

My first public speech was to the Minister of Health, demanding sex education in the schools. I was so nervous, my tongue kept sticking to the roof of my mouth. But the speech was a hit, making the front page of one paper and the editorial of another. In time I got over my fear of public speaking and became the spokesperson first for CARAL, and then for the Coalition for Choice. I was front and centre for every crisis concerning abortion issues. When I went from door to door to sign people up for the hospital society to ward off the takeover by the Pro-lifers, CARAL made me an honorary director. I marched in parades, gave many speeches, and appeared on TV and radio. I took on Premier VanderZalm on the evening news when he tried to cut funding for abortion services. I was the key speaker for a rally in front of the Legislature attended by over 3,000; SWAG presented me with a huge bouquet for my efforts. I gave one of the first lectures in Vancouver in support of the abortion clinic, and was one of their main supporters. When they were short-staffed, I commuted to Vancouver to work in the clinic for six months and continued my practice in Victoria at the same time. I worked as a medical director for the birth control clinic, taught many interns about contraception, and gave lectures at Camosun College, University of Victoria, and community centres on women's health issues such as contraception, PMS, and menopause. In 1996, the YWCA gave me the Woman of Distinction Award for Health, and in 1998, UBC notified me that I had been voted as a leader by my peers for being an educational influence.

I continued my interest in art, which was focused on lettering art twenty years ago; more recently I have concentrated on paper maché sculpture, and making pop-up books. I have been in a dozen or so art shows, have given a number of workshops, and had some of my work published.

I think I have had a wonderful career as a family doctor, as an abortion rights activist, and as an artist. I have met so many extraordinary people—I wouldn't have missed any of it for the world!

DR. MILLIE CUMMING

I wanted to be a doctor when I was seven. I worked in a nursing home for one summer and as a nurses' aide in a small hospital in Ontario for three summers. My father suggested that if I could make it as a nurses' aide, then I probably could make it as a doctor. So I attended the University of Western Ontario, doing a BSc in Mathematics (1970), an MD cum laude (1974), and a two-year Family Practice residency at St. Joseph's Family Medical Centre in London, Ontario, CCFP (1976).

During my fourth year of Medicine, I spent two months interning at Wrinch Memorial Hospital in Hazelton, B.C. This wonderful experience introduced me into the variety of family medicine. In Hazelton, I began to feel like a real doctor as I did my first deliveries, removed my first fish hook, and witnessed my first case of delirium tremens. I decided to return there to work in 1976.

Wrinch Memorial Hospital is one of the United Church Hospitals, staffed by physicians who had a commitment to maintain quality care and ongoing medical education. There were also ongoing opportunities to teach medical and nursing students as well as Family Practice residents. It was great to have the full support from very competent colleagues. For example, on one Christmas day when I was on call, an ambulance arrived right at dinner time. I called the cardiac arrest team, and within a few minutes four other physicians came to assist.

In the years from 1976 to 1988, there were many great memories and some painful ones. Obstetrical cases were important for me, especially in the first few years of my practice. By attending some of my patients from remote, small towns, I became skilled in keeping childbirth as natural as possible through working closely with the patients and listening to the concerns of their partners. This approach was less common at that time. We often did our best to accommodate our patients, whether this meant delivering on all fours, or not on a delivery table, or with siblings present. Delivering babies could be difficult at times. Patients with the most insistent requests (or demands) often ended up with the most difficult deliveries, including Caesarean sections. I particularly remember my first devastating experience of losing a baby in labour (from a prolapsed cord), and the tremendous comfort given by the parents of that baby, who told me the next day that I was a wonderful doctor and that they wanted me to deliver their other babies (I did deliver three more).

There were other times in the practice you would never forget, such as waiting for your good friend and colleague to arrive by ambulance from an accident and failing to resuscitate him. There were also times when you felt you knew your patients well, having known them over a number of years, only to find out that they had been suffering from continued abuse you had never suspected. There were those sad, special moments of accompanying your patients through the period from cancer diagnosis to surgery and chemotherapy, and to their eventual deterioration. Sometimes I would play the organ for the funerals of my patients. I remember at one such funeral, as I looked out on the congregation, I began to realize how privileged I had been being able to take part in the lives of many people—the births, marriages, separations, death, life-threatening illnesses, and day-to-day medical events ranging from chicken-pox to contraception.

I also remember many funny incidents, such as dealing with bats in the labour room, trying to suture a small scalp laceration for a drunk and belligerent person at two in the morning, and doing sex education at local high schools and consulting with my colleagues about some anonymous questions submitted ahead of time by the students. I did not mind being single in a relatively remote area, for I could afford to do deliveries on my off days, or to stay late finishing all my charts before going home. And I could also enjoy the strong friendships and the terrific outdoor activities, like white-water canoeing and kayaking, hiking in the mountains, skiing, and snowshoeing. I jogged along the road each day, and I would often get comments from the logging truck drivers when they came in for their physical examination.

I might have stayed in Hazelton for the rest of my medical career, except that in 1988 I married Graham Chalmers, a UBC professor who could not do his work in Hazelton. After moving to Vancouver, I worked as a locum, but did not find family medicine nearly as exciting as up north. In May, 1989, I started as the third Palliative Care physician at the St. Paul's Palliative Care Unit, which was funded to serve both cancer and AIDS patients. Having not treated any AIDS patients before, I quickly learned how to look after the far too many courageous young men dying with this disease. What I miss most are the friendships developed with their wonderful partners and families, but definitely not the numerous nights of lost sleep.

I became a mother at the age of forty-one, experiencing the joys and tribulations of the complicated delivery that "elderly primip" medical people would usually experience. Nonetheless, this was an experience I am really glad to have. Even though I now work only part-time, I have to struggle between fulfilling my responsibilities as a doctor, a mother, and a wife. Having practised medicine as a single woman for all those years, I now have tremendous respect for women who can maintain a good balance between work and family.

As I grow older, and particularly since I have become a mother and have been working in Palliative Care, I have come to realize what is more important, and my career is no longer the first priority in my life. But I do value and admire those physicians who devote all their lives to medicine, to become the "Complete Physician."

DR. SHELLEY NAN ROSS

I was told that I had made up my mind to become a doctor at the age of two. My maternal uncle, who had wanted to be a doctor all his life but could never afford to go to university, gave me a doctor's kit for a birthday present and thus determined my destiny. During my school years I was always a good student, but I particularly had a flare for math and science. At one point in high school, I remember some teachers telling me that girls should not aspire to become doctors, so I wavered for a moment about going into medicine, but soon came to my senses.

I graduated from James Fowler High School in Calgary, Alberta, and received the award for the top student of my graduating class. During my school years, I also had time to be a Highland dancer and a snare drummer in the Brig 'O Doon Girls Pipe Band.

I did two years of pre-med at the University of Calgary from 1968–1970, and was accepted to both the University of Alberta (Edmonton) School of Medicine and the University of Calgary School of Medicine. As this was Calgary's very first class, and also because it was a shortened program of three years with eleven months per year, I chose to go to Edmonton, where they had 'done it before.' I was one of only twenty females in a class of 100 students. Nonetheless, I had a great four years in medical school, and graduated in 1974. I made many lasting friendships with classmates, which began with the dissection group hovering over the cadaver in the anatomy lab, and with whom you spent your clinical rotations doing histories and holding retractors. In 1999, our class had its twenty-five-year reunion, and it was almost as if we had just seen each other yesterday.

After graduating *cum laude* from medical school, I had to decide which residency to pursue. It was a tossup between ophthalmology, obstetrics, and family practice. A decision was made during a complementary wine and cheese party given by the Family Practice department to attract residents. I spent my Family Practice Residency in Vancouver from 1974 to 1976, and then wrote the certification exam for the College of Family Physicians of Canada. I remained a minority as one of only two women in a program of twelve residents.

It was during my residency that I was first introduced to the Federation of Medical Women of Canada. The only other female family practice resident at the time asked me to come and help her make coffee for a public forum presentation on the topic of women's health. Dr. Hedy Fry was going to speak, and refreshments had to be served. The rest was history, of course; Dr. Hedy Fry is now in parliament and I am still making coffee!

I did one month of locum work after finishing the residency program, but I quickly decided that this was not my cup of tea. I joined a group in Burnaby, and began to practise in B.C. in 1976. Once again, I found myself the only woman in a group of eight. Not surprisingly, the women patients were flocking to see a woman doctor and many of them were pregnant. I soon found that my love of obstetrics helped me develop a large obstetric practice, in addition to doing all the regular family medicine work that my partners were doing. Other than changing offices, nothing much has changed in my practice except that I have done more deliveries and have had the pleasure of looking after the same patients for twenty-four years

since I first hung my "shingle." It has been a joy to work with families that have four or five generations all calling you their doctor.

I have never learned to say no fast enough. This has landed me on more committees than I can remember and left me with such responsibilities as Head of the Department of Obstetrics at Burnaby Hospital, Chair of Credentials and Manpower, and finally Chief and President of the Medical Staff, the first woman ever to have held this position at Burnaby Hospital.

I have been President of the Vancouver Branch of the Federation of Medical Women of Canada twice, once in the 1970s and once in the 1990s, and President of the National Federation of Medical Women of Canada in 1984. I also represented Canada and the U.S. at the Medical Women's International Association from 1987 to 1993. I am currently President of that organization. Both the Federation of Medical Women of Canada and the Medical Women's International Association have a two-fold mandate: first, to promote the personal and professional life of women physicians; and second, to be advocates for women's health.

These organizations have allowed me to meet wonderful colleagues from around the world and to cement friendships that otherwise would

The prevailing idea was that women would never stay as committed to the job as men would, so it was probably a waste of money to educate them.

never have been possible. They also have afforded me the opportunity to travel with an added medical component. I have visited a public obstetrics hospital in downtown Nairobi, where a woman needing a Caesarean section had to be carried up a flight of stairs on a stretcher due to the elevator having been broken for four years. I have seen the obstetrics hospital in Bombay, where forty deliveries a day is a slow day. I have visited a hospital in Naples, where a colposcopy came to an end when the equipment went missing somewhere between the clinic and the sterilizer. Throughout all these different scenarios, I have seen a common bond of caring shared by physicians throughout the world who have a genuine concern for those who are in need.

Through these organizations, I have also been given the opportunity to influence policies that will improve the health of others. I have represented my region of Burnaby at the British Columbia Medical Association as a board delegate and vice-chair of the board, and I chair the committee to encourage female participation in the BCMA. I also wrote a column in the *BCMA News* on issues in women's health. It was my honour when the College of Family Physicians of Canada made me a Fellow of the College in 1998.

I could not have done half of what I have been able to do throughout my career without the support of my wonderful husband, Don Stephenson. Don has done every job ranging from being "Mr. Mom" when our two boys were young, driving kids back and forth to school, to being the manager in my office. Any woman physician with a family certainly needs such a good support person behind her all the way.

When I reflect back on my career and how the practice of medicine has changed since my graduation, I ask myself if I would choose to do it again. The answer is a resounding YES, because I have had a wonderful professional and personal life. I began my career at a time when women in medicine were merely tolerated by the medical establishment. The prevailing idea was that women would never stay as committed to the job as men would, so it was probably a waste of money to educate them. As I look at my graduation class photo, however, I see only one woman who has not worked full-time for the last twenty-five years, and that was due to a debilitating illness. When you look at these modern times where the majority of the medical school classes are women, it shows how far we have come.

The only sadness I have now is seeing the graduating physicians focusing more on their salaried positions than promoting and delivering quality care to the patients. The lure of a salaried position with no extracurricular responsibility may seem inviting, but having had the opportunity to be involved in a rewarding family practice, my advice is to live your professional life to the fullest. Do not be afraid to 'give it your all' and say yes when asked to participate in some extra activities. Those of us who are in medicine have been given so much and we have so much to give in return.

Curriculum Vitae

Date of Birth: Nov. 1950.
Citizenship: Canadian.
Education: Primary and secondary school education in Calgary, Alberta, graduating from James Fowler High School with honours with distinction in June, 1968; pre-medical education in the Faculty of Science, majoring in Zoology, University of Calgary, 1968–1970; medical education, Faculty of Medicine, University of Alberta, 1970–1974, graduating with honours with distinction with BMedSci and MD degrees; Resident in the Family Practice Program at the University of British Columbia, 1974–1976; Certification in Family Medicine from the College of Family Physicians of Canada, 1976; Fellowship in College of Family Physicians of Canada, May, 1998.

Practice Experience: Locum for Dr. Conrad Mackenzie, June, 1976, Vancouver, B.C.; Private Family Medicine Practice with special interest in Obstetrics in Burnaby, B.C., from July, 1976 to present.

Organizations: Federation of Medical Women of Canada, since 1976; Medical Women's International Association, since 1976; College of Physicians and Surgeons of British Columbia, since 1976; British Columbia Medical Association, since 1976; College of Family Physicians of Canada, since 1976; Section of General Practice of the British Columbia Medical Association, since 1976; Canadian Medical Protective Association, since 1976.

Offices Held: President, Federation of Medical Women of Canada, British Columbia Branch, 1979; President, Federation of Medical Women of Canada, 1984; Vice-President for North America for the Medical Women's International Association, 1986–1992; Vice-Chief of Staff, Burnaby Hospital, January, 1987 to December, 1989; Chief of Staff, Burnaby Hospital, January, 1989 to December, 1990; President, Vancouver Branch, Federation of Medical Women of Canada, 1996–1997; President of Medical Staff, St. Michael's Long Term Care Hospital, 1996 to present; President-Elect, Medical Women's International Association, 1998–2001; Mother, 1981 to present.

Committee Positions: Chair, Education Committee, Burnaby Hospital, 1977–1981; Member, Medical Audit Committee, Burnaby Hospital, 1988; Member, Utilization Committee, Burnaby Hospital, 1983, 1987 to 1988; Member, Perinatal Morbidity and Mortality Committee, Burnaby Hospital, 1988; Department Head, Department of Obstetrics and Gynecology, Burnaby Hospital; Member, Board of Directors,

Burnaby Hospital, 1989 to 1991; Member, Finance Committee, Burnaby Hospital, 1989 to 1991; Chair, Manpower Committee, Burnaby Hospital, January, 1991 to December, 1992; Chair, Credentials Committee, Burnaby Hospital, January, 1991, to December, 1992; Member, Burnaby Hospital Foundation Board, January, 1992 to present; Member, Finance Committee, Burnaby Hospital Foundation, January, 1992 to present; Member, Manpower Committee, Burnaby Hospital, January, 1993 to present; Member, Credentials Committee, Burnaby Hospital, January 1993 to present; Member, Planned Giving Committee, Burnaby Hospital Foundation, April, 1993 to present; Local Action Committee Chair for Burnaby-Willingdon since the beginning of the program to present; Member, Scientific and Research Committee of the Medical Women's International Association, 1995–1998; Vice-Chair, Burnaby Foundation Picture of Health, $4.5 million fund-raising program, 1995 to 1997.

DR. ELLEN WIEBE

Growing Up
I was born into a wonderfully warm family of four girls in Abbotsford, British Columbia. Dad taught high school and Mom stayed at home sewing all our dresses, baking, cooking, canning, and gardening. We lived in Nigeria and Singapore in the 1960s when Dad taught for CIDA, and had an exciting childhood with lots of travel, music, books, love, and laughter.

One Saturday morning when I was about twelve years old, Dad found a recently killed cat on the road in front of our house. Knowing of my interest and of an impending school science project, he brought it home and woke me up. I was thrilled and did my first dissection on the ping-pong table in the basement. I remember how excited I was as, dripping blood to my elbows, I recognized the cat's liver and kidneys from my science book and imagined what it would be like to be in medical school.

In 1971 when I applied to medical school, the quota for women applicants had just been lifted and the acceptance rate had risen to an unprecedented twenty-five percent. It was therefore easier on us than our predecessors, but I well remember the male teachers with their sexist jokes.

Abortion Care
I always planned to be a family doctor with a strong interest in women's health. When I started practice in 1976 in Vancouver at the age of twenty-four, I already had my first child. My practice quickly grew with mostly young women, and I did lots of obstetrics. I got my D&C privileges at the hospital as quickly as I could because I wanted to offer a full service to my patients. In those early years I only did abortions for my own patients and a few other doctors. I perceived no danger. In Vancouver, abortions had been freely available on demand since the 1969 change in the law because Vancouver General Hospital and Shaughnessy Hospital established Abortion Committees of pro-choice doctors who approved every application.

It was only after I started to work at B.C.'s first free-standing abortion clinic that I encountered anti-abortion protests aimed directly at me and my patients. Before that, I had always believed that the principles of free speech meant that people who disapproved of abortion should be able to protest. When I saw my patients in tears, devastated by the cruel taunts of the protesters outside the clinic, I realized that free speech needs to be limited. I started to attend the National Abortion Federation where security is extreme, and I got to know people who were victims of anti-abortion violence. On November 8, 1994, my colleague, Dr. Garson Romalis, was shot in his home and almost died. The following year, there was a protest just for me in front of my office with about twelve protesters who had placards with "Dr. Ellen Wiebe murders babies," etc. The office building was doing some renovations and so the only exit was through the protesters. I thought I was calm as I wheeled past the protesters and the TV cameras. As I drove from the office to the clinic on my usual route, I suddenly found myself driving the wrong way down a busy street! I survived, but I realized I was not exactly calm and that the protesters don't have to shoot me; I can easily get myself killed by just driving when upset.

Most abortion providers have kept quiet about their work to avoid both the nuisance and the dangerous anti-abortion activists. I feel that for myself, I need to speak out when the issues are in the media and only the anti-abortion side is being heard. The majority of Canadians are pro-choice and yet most avoid using the "A" word. This silent majority allows the problems of limited access to continue. Living with the fear of bombs and snipers has not been easy for me or my family, but I have never even considered quitting because this service is needed by desperate and very grateful women.

Research

My first research project was sparked by the anguish of my first malpractice suit. A teenager on whom I had performed one of my very first abortions remained pregnant with twins and sued me for the costs of raising them. The court found me partially responsible for the "pain and suffering" because I had not tracked her down when she failed to return for her follow-up appointment, but not for the "wrongful birth." As I prepared for the court case, I had to know if I was really competent or not so I could decide whether I should quit. I did a chart review of my last 100 cases and found that my complication rate was slightly better than the published rates. This review allowed me to feel confident enough to continue doing abortions.

When I saw my patients in tears, devastated by the cruel taunts of the protesters outside the clinic, I realized that free speech needs to be limited.

Other questions needed to be answered, and I loved the challenge of trying to figure out how to do it. Many of my projects have failed, but others succeeded, and to date I have twenty-six research publications. For example, one day the clinic manager came to me and said, "Why do you use the more expensive carbonated lidocaine instead of the plain that the other doctors use?" The answer that it was recommended by a doctor didn't seem good enough. That question led to my first randomized controlled trial and the first of many pain control studies.

One morning I was reading the *Globe & Mail* with my breakfast tea and saw an article about Mitchel Creinin having induced ten abortions using methotrexate and misoprostol. I was so excited that I had my Ethics application in to the University within four days and my first patient enrolled in the study within two months. I had followed the RU 486 story with great interest and so was thrilled that we finally had a non-surgical option for Canadian women. Surgical abortion is still the choice of most women seeking abortions, but for some women, it is so important to avoid surgery.

Disability

When I turned forty, I had a big party for myself, burning my mortgage papers in the fireplace and then leaving on a trip to Central America. The next month I was on a cycling and camping trip in the Gulf Islands and found that when I tried to catch up to my kids cycling up the steep hills, I got chest pain. It went away when I coasted downhill, but returned on the next hill in a totally predictable pattern. I ignored it after the trip and told no one. Then I noticed chest pain when running one day. I was planning a very strenuous summer, doing a locum up in Iqualuit. I decided to have a stress test before I left. I did not see my doctor, but just booked it myself. When it was grossly abnormal, I did not panic. I called my father to say I had inherited more from him than just his myopic eyes and flat feet. He had started getting angina in his forties and was still going strong in his seventies. The diagnosis was microvascular angina or Syndome X.

A few months later I was deteriorating quickly. Each week I would discover yet another thing I could not do without disabling chest pain and shortness of breath. September 1992 was extremely difficult as I started a merry-go-round of trying all the angina drugs available and trying to decide whether to sell or renovate my three-storey house because I could no longer cope with stairs. One of my colleagues met me after I had done hospital rounds one morning, and I was unable to speak for ten minutes despite nitroglycerin. She told me I should get a scooter to do rounds. I was outraged at the suggestion. I was smart enough to think it over and by February of 1993, I had my new elevator installed in my house and was doing hospital rounds by scooter.

Being a disabled person required me to rethink almost everything I did or felt. I am tall, but now I have to look up at everyone from a chair. I had to reorganize much of my work. For example, I found it too difficult to continue to deliver babies. Sometimes one just sits there and watches a medical student do the delivery; other times it is an emotionally and physically strenuous vacuum extraction for fetal distress, and I no longer had the necessary strength. The worst adjustment was figuring out how to have fun on weekends and holidays. I had always been so active—biking, hiking, skating, swimming, and camping. After I had played a card game with my five-year-old and read him a story, I didn't know what to do next. Luckily, I love reading and music, and I discovered that my addiction to exercise could be overcome.

I had a new group to join: people with disabilities. Every time I was blocked by some barrier, I would remind myself that I have more ability to get things changed than the majority of disabled people, so another letter would be mailed. The people at the B.C. Human Rights Commission know me well by now, and little by little my environment is becoming more wheelchair-friendly.

Family Life
There were two good things about my marriage to a charming, abusive, sociopathic alcoholic: one was that it was brief, and the other was that our son, David, has grown up to be a fine young man who graduated from medical school in the spring of 2000. After that marriage was over, I did not have the courage for another, but I was not ready to give up having children. Michael was born in 1980 and Robert in 1986, and raising the three boys has been the best part of my life so far.

Epilogue
So far, life has been very exciting and challenging, and I have lots more planned for the future. I have been so lucky to have a profession I love, three healthy sons, and lots of friends and family with whom to share my life.

1977

DR. WEDAD THERESA ABRAHAM
(1930–1982)

Dr. Abraham was born in Egypt. She obtained her MB and ChB from Ein Shams University in Cairo in 1955 and Diploma in Anesthesia in 1961. She practised in England and passed the FFA of the Royal College of Surgeons in 1967 and the LMCC in 1977. In Canada she studied and practised for fourteen years in training positions in anesthesia and internal medicine respectively at the Saint John General Hospital in New Brunswick, the Regina General Hospital, and Veterans' Hospitals in Victoria and Vancouver. In 1972, she joined the staff of Riverview Hospital in B.C. and continued her duties as a general practitioner until her illness debilitated her.

Dr. Abraham had two nieces whom she looked after, and a younger sister and brother in Canada. On July 10, 1982, she died of a lung infiltrating disease, aged fifty-two.

DR. GILLIAN ARSENAULT

My name is Gillian Rolande Arsenault. I was born in Fort Churchill, Manitoba, on May 2, 1952 in a blizzard—so my mother said. My father was a doctor, but I rarely saw him. He was in the army, and served with a MASH unit in Korea. Unfortunately, he smoked and drank to excess. The smoking ruined his health and the alcohol sabotaged his life. Once he left the army, because of his drinking, he was never able to complete an internship, and was thus not able to carry out civilian practice. He left home when I was around eight years old, and I never saw him again. When I started my medical training, I used to worry that some of my teachers might have known him, and therefore be suspicious of me. In fact, the only person I encountered who had known my father was a very nice woman whom I was admitting to hospital. It turned out that she had been my father's lover!

I was a very serious, intense child, and those who know me tend to comment that I have not changed a whole bunch. I decided around age four that I was going to be a doctor. Every adult except my mother in whom I confided my ambition invariably responded, "Oh, no, dear—you don't want to be a doctor, you want to be a nurse!" My mother, on the other hand, said, "You can be anything you want to be as long as you're prepared to work at it." Naturally, I listened to my mother. The other defining influence in my life was my stepfather, a mechanic who had emigrated from Poland. I remember him at first as being very warm and a good teacher, but then he had a period of illness, after which his personality changed and he was unable to work. Looking back now, I wonder if he had a series of small strokes, as he too was a heavy smoker. Afterwards, nothing my younger brother and I did was right. Punishments included confinement in the six-foot square dirt root cellar under the house, and being beaten with a one-inch diameter stick. As a serious, intense child, I tried my best to work out what my stepfather expected of me, but I always failed. He summed up my efforts by his often-repeated comment, "You're stupid, fat, dumb, and ugly. The only thing you're good for is book learning, and book learning ain't worth shit."

On the positive side, even though we were dirt-poor, he kept us fed. He hunted and brought home a moose each year while mother grew all our vegetables. My stepfather also had great respect for schoolwork, and as long as I was doing homework, I was safe. Needless to say, I did as much homework as I possibly could, and was a straight-A student, despite having skipped Grade 2 and being the youngest student in my class.

I was flabbergasted when I was accepted for entry into the UBC medical school class of 1976. Of 800 applicants, eighty were accepted, of whom ten were female.

At Grade 11, I was getting very tired of being beaten, and decided to run away from home. I casually mentioned this to a teacher at my school, George Elliot Secondary. The school quickly helped me to apply for early entrance to Simon Fraser University and a bursary to cover tuition and living costs for the first two semesters. I was accepted and started first year Biology in 1968.

University was wonderful! I was on my own with nobody telling me how stupid I was and nobody beating me. As I had no money to spare—I hiked up Burnaby Mountain to class in order to save bus fare—I had a great deal of time to do my work and was able to maintain my A average despite having skipped Grade 12. In 1969, I was able to get work, at first doing dicta-typing for Burnaby Hospital, then typing in computer-assisted instruction (CAI) programs for Dr. Lower, a professor of chemistry. The latter job quickly evolved from testing the programs and fixing problems to programming and writing manuals to assist other people writing CAI programs. In time, I had enough money to buy my very own vehicle, a Honda 100 motorcycle, which I gleefully rode up Burnaby Mountain.

In my third year of university, I decided to apply to the University of British Columbia medical school for the practice. I knew I would not get in the first time around because very few medical school applicants were accepted without their degrees, and the word was out that the standard was higher for girls. (Yes, "girls" was the term we used back then.) I did well on the MCAT, although I did not think I did very well on the screening interview. The professor interviewing me kept asking, "Why do you want to go into medicine?" My only answer, which I repeated about four times, was, "Because I think I'd be good at it. And, I did vocational testing that said I should go into medicine." He did not seem to find this a particularly good answer, so I decided I should spend the next year thinking the matter over in greater depth.

I was flabbergasted when I was accepted for entry into the UBC medical school class of 1976. Of 800 applicants, eighty were accepted, of whom ten were female. Medical school was fascinating and all-consuming. Because I could not afford to buy many textbooks, I never missed a class and was very, very thorough in my note-taking. Our class was, I think, a particularly good one. As a group, we were interested in medicine and very supportive of each other. Our number included a few older students, who provided quiet mature guidance. We also had our fair share of genius types and talented eccentrics. Our Beer and Skits Nights presentations were, I think, unparalleled. (I have the photographs to prove it. Some of them probably have splendid blackmail potential, as the class rowdies have now gone on to become distinguished and eminent physicians.)

The clinical clerkship was a black hole of a year for me, as for some other members of the class. In my case, long hours and sleep deprivation combined with isolation from classmates and friends made the cavalier and sometimes cruel treatment of patients hard to handle. Added to this were sexual harassment from a few of the residents and the sudden death of my roommate, who was my boyfriend's sister, in a plane crash. Their mother, with whom I was very close, developed cancer and died shortly thereafter. I developed clinical depression, but did not tell anyone until we had a group session with classmates on our psychiatry rotation. A psychiatrist then saw me for two visits. His conclusion was, and I quote, "Given your childhood, it's remarkable that you're not even more screwed up than you are." No treatment was offered, and the depression went away of its own accord after about a year. I will never forget the first lifting, the first return of normal mood, which happened while I was riding my motorcycle to UBC in the spring sunshine. It lasted about fifteen minutes. Even though the dark despair dropped back, I knew then that it would eventually go away, and I would get my normal brain back. I have never been depressed since, thank God!

Because I had been planning to kill myself, I did not apply to the internship match. However, one of my classmates, who was in the military, was matched to St. Paul's Hospital. As she was paid by the military, St. Paul's therefore had an extra internship salary. Dr. Angus Rae, who was in charge of the internship program, offered me a position. I owe him my career in medicine: if it had not been for him, I would not have continued into practice.

My internship included a rotation out to Maple Ridge Hospital, where I fell in love with general practice. For the first time, I felt I was doing something to help people. I tried to get as much experience as possible in areas that I thought I would need as a general practitioner, particularly in delivering babies and in doing any minor surgical procedures that the attending would let me carry out myself. For a while, I was known as "the D&C intern."

Some of the Maple Ridge physicians were very involved in student teaching and were very good at it. One of them, Dr. Chris King, noticed how intense, even scared, I tended to be. He told me not to be worried about being frightened, that it was appropriate and even necessary when first starting practice. "You'll be scared for the first ten years until you know what you're doing," he said. "Then, watch out, or you'll get too cocky and kill someone!"

After internship, I did a few locums in Vancouver and in Maple Ridge. I was amazed at how much I could not do in Vancouver. One practice had no specula at all, and another, of a physician who prided himself on practising real family medicine, had three: small, medium, and large. The latter did, however, have an ear syringe, which the other Vancouver doctor did not. The final indignity, however, came about as a result of a routine visit to a nursing home, where I saw one patient who had massive diffuse lymphadenopathy. As her physician, whom I was replacing, had admitting privileges to St. Paul's hospital, I naively assumed that I could admit the lady and do the workup with consultation as indicated. My plan met with total amazement on the part of St. Paul's Hospital, which assumed that admissions of interesting cases were always done by consultants. When a lymph node biopsy was booked, I again amazed the St. Paul's OR by assuming that I could and would be there for the procedure. I was, in fact, hoping that the surgeon would be willing to teach me, and maybe even let me do some of it. In the end, the OR time was changed four times. I was able to rearrange my office to accommodate the first three times, but the fourth time was too short notice. After that, I set up practice in Maple Ridge.

Having my own practice was different from doing locums in many ways. For a start, I used from ten to fifteen specula a day! I had to learn a great deal about common things that did not get covered in my specialty-oriented training. Recognition and treatment of diaper rash came to mind as one such revelation; others included low-tech removal of foreign bodies from children's noses, and taping small cuts on small faces so that the tape would stay on. That was the easy stuff. Much more difficult were all the things you found out when patients decided you could be trusted: anorgasmia, dysfunctional relationships, parenting, drug and alcohol abuse, and general misery and inadequacy.

Patients generally have far higher expectations of female doctors than they do of male physicians: they expect you to be interested in everything, to listen longer, and to be more sympathetic.

I learned about parenting from my patients who were successful parents and took courses in parenting skills. This was very helpful in advising people with parenting problems, as well as providing wonderful training for raising my own children! By the way, the best approach I have ever seen to dealing with difficult children is described in Dr. Thomas Millar's *The Omnipotent Child*. His thesis is twofold: firstly, that discipline of children is essential, and, secondly, that discipline does not have to hurt to work. In fact, it works best when it does not hurt.

I also quickly found out how much I did not know about breastfeeding— and did not know how inadequate my knowledge was in this area. My two best friends, one of whom is a midwife and one a La Leche League Leader, took me in hand and made me aware of my ignorance, which took considerable study and searching of the medical literature to remedy. Information about breastfeeding is slightly more available now than it was then, but not much more. I cringe to think how many breastfeeding mothers I sabotaged with bad advice that I honestly thought was helpful but actually made things worse.

As I continued to work in general practice, I gradually became more comfortable. I learned from other physicians, my patients, and from experience. Practicing medicine took on a whole new angle for me when I sent in an article to the *Medical Post* in 1984 on why the thesis that nurses could provide more cost-effective medical care than doctors was highly dubious. I thought then, and still do, that good Canadian physicians are a bargain. To my delight, my article was accepted and printed. Then, to my shock, I received a cheque in the mail for $180! Needless to say, I have been writing articles for the *Medical Post* and an occasional few for other publications ever since. I have even written some science fiction novels, but have not yet nailed a publisher for any of them, so I am not about to quit my day job.

The *bête noire* of general practice, as far as I am concerned, has to be treating patients with major psychological issues. I was trained in treating classic psychiatric illnesses with medication, but I knew very little about managing difficult patients with difficult lives. Furthermore, patients generally have far higher expectations of female doctors than they do of male physicians: they expect you to be interested in everything, to listen longer, and to be more sympathetic. Some patients were quite clear on this point: "Now, dear, I wouldn't dream of bothering a male physician with this, but I just know you'll understand. . . ." Then, out comes the list of between twenty to fifty problems.

There is a subset of female patients who have these expectations honed to a fine art. They will tell you that they really want a female doctor, and they stare at you, a female doctor, with an expression of hunger. It reminds me of the way Bela Lugosi used to portray Dracula looking at a potential victim. They are horrified if you suggest that it is more important to find a doctor who practices good medicine than it is to find one who is female.

These patients are trouble. They made up about ten percent of my practice, and were responsible for ninety percent of my stress. I attempted to deal with them in my usual obsessive-compulsive, perfectionist way by doing everything I could for them. This was a major mistake, as they would happily soak up all my attempts to understand, treat, and work with them on problem-solving. Some did benefit, I think, but most just enjoyed the attention and found it made their lives more bearable, so they did not have to make any changes.

Interestingly enough, when I left practice to go back for training in community medicine, these were the patients who left as soon as they were informed without even bothering to see if they liked my locum, who was also female. Needless to say, the office staff was dancing in the halls with delight. Since then, I have been introduced to the BATHE system of office stealth psychotherapy, and that is what I would use with such patients were I ever to return to general practice.

For those of you unaware of the BATHE method, it is set out in a book entitled, *The Fifteen Minute Hour*. "B" stands for asking patients what is Bothering them, "A" for how they feel about it (Affect), "T" for what Troubles them most about it, "H" for how they have been Handling it until this point, and "E" for expressing Empathy. ("I can see this is very distressing for you.") No word of advice is given. The beauty of this method is that the patient feels understood, at the same time as they are being led through an analysis of their situation and the realization that they have, indeed, made choices on how to handle the problems. Sooner or later, it will occur to them that they could, if they wished, make alternate choices. This method can, of course, be used on friends, family, co-workers, or even on oneself—the last application being particularly illuminating.

Going into residency training in Community Medicine at UBC after fifteen years in general practice was sheer, unalloyed joy. The first year is completely academic during which one earns a MHSc or Master of Health Science. The remaining years involve placements in health units and occupational health or other settings. I was told that the Masters' year was "a ball-buster" of a year and it certainly is intense. However, you get to sleep at night, every night. Difficult assignments may be hard, but I found them much more satisfying than working with difficult patients!

In 1996, I sat for my Fellowship exam in Winnipeg. The pass rate was not very high for community medicine, and the three of us from UBC worried and studied our brains out. I am delighted to report that we all passed. My first job as a newly minted Community Medicine Fellow was as medical health officer for East Kootenay. I was still living in Maple Ridge, and was on-site in the East Kootenay Health Unit only one week a month. The public health staff were wonderful people to work with, and the work was fascinating, but being a remote medical health officer was not ideal.

In 1998, East Kootenay hired a new medical health officer, and I became the medical health officer for the Fraser Valley region, which runs from Mission to just beyond Hope. In this position, I am both medical health officer and the manager of the public health service. The second part of the job has required me to learn a great deal, very quickly, about administration. It has given me a new respect for administrators: like medicine, administration is fairly easy to do poorly, but a challenge to do well. Similarly, as our Regional Medical Advisory Committee has come together and begun work, I think the administrators of our region have also developed an increased respect for physicians and the role we can play in helping to manage an integrated Health Region.

Meanwhile, I have been extremely fortunate in my family life. My first marriage did not last. However, on the second time around for both of us, Ray and I have been together for eighteen years. He has two sons from his first marriage, now grown and living on their own. We have two children between us, Eric, now graduated from high school, and Matthew, just finishing elementary school. As both Ray and I are doctors, we have relied upon live-in nannies to hold our lives together. Our last nanny came thirteen years ago before Matthew was born. Since then, she has married, and she and her husband have two children. Recently, we have been joined by a foster child, Matthew's friend John. All nine of us live together in one house, with the boys' friends coming and going. It is rather like living in a small village. Of all the challenges I face in life, making time for my family has to be the hardest. I modestly think that our boys are incredibly wonderful people, and I resent being taken away from them and from Ray. This requires constraining the time I spend on medicine, and was one of the goals I hoped to accomplish by going into community medicine. Unfortunately, just as I finished training, regionalisation

happened, and the workload of medical health officers increased by at least fifty percent.

Obviously, my life has not ended yet, and, God willing, will not for a long time to come. Like most working moms, I feel a particular resonance with the T-shirt slogan that reads: "God put me on this Earth to do a certain number of things. I am now so far behind that I will never die!"

Curriculum Vitae

Post-Secondary Education: 1968–72, Simon Fraser University, BSc Biology; 1972–76, UBC, MD Medicine; 1976–77, St. Paul's Hospital Rotating Intern; 1992–93, UBC, MHSc Community Medicine. Thesis: Breastfeeding and Breast Cancer: A Meta-Analysis; 1992–96 UBC, FRCP(C), Community Medicine, Resident.

Special Professional Qualifications: 1977, Registered with the College of Physicians & Surgeons of B.C.; 1988, Certificant of the College of Family Practice (CCFP); 1988, International Board Certified Lactation Consultant (IBCLC); 1991, Acute Cardiac Life Support certification; 1996, Fellow of the Royal College of Physicians & Surgeons of Canada (Community Medicine) (FRCP(C)).

Academic Affiliation: University of British Columbia Department of Health Care & Epidemiology: recommended for Clinical Assistant Professor, Division of Public Health Practice (in process).

Employment Record: 1970–72, Simon Fraser University, Computer Assisted Instruction Centre Co-ordinator and Programmer; 1977–92, Maple Ridge Hospital, Family physician; 1992–1996, University of British Columbia, Internal Residency Committee; 1993-94, Chief Resident; 1995, Community Medicine Resident; 1996 to present, B.C. Ministry of Health, Medical Health Officer (East Kootenay).

Membership in Professional and Learned Societies: Maple Ridge-Pitt Meadows Medical Association, 1997 to present; Medical Staff Liaison to Laboratory, Physiotherapy, and Radiology, Maple Ridge Hospital, 1980–81; Medical Staff Liaison to Pharmacy, Maple Ridge Hospital, 1981–84; Communications Officer, Maple Ridge-Pitt Meadows

Medical Association, 1981–88; Member, Obstetrics Committee, Maple Ridge Hospital, 1985–88; Member and Certificant, Canadian College of Family Practice, 1988–97; B.C. Association of Lactation Consultants, 1988 to present; Member, International Lactation Consultants Association, 1993 to present; Fellow, Royal College of Physicians and Surgeons of Canada, 1996 to present.

Service to the Community: Medical consultant for Maple Ridge School District, 1978–82; Medical consultant in establishment of and subsequent sessional work in Haney Place Clinic, Maple Ridge (a gynaecological clinic for young women), 1979–81; Medical consultant for Community Services Centre, Maple Ridge, 1979–82; Member, Board of Education, B.C. Association of Adlerian Psychology, 1981–82; Member, B.C. Medical Association Speakers' Bureau, 1985–1988; Member, West Coast Advisory Board, *Medical Post*, 1986 to present; La Leche League Medical Associate, 1991 to present; author, medical column, *Ridge-Meadows Times*, 1991–92; College of Physicians and Surgeons of B.C. Medical Library Committee: Member 1992 to present; Deputy Chair 1996 to present; International Christian Aid Canada: Board member 1993 to present; Chair 1996 to present; Member, B.C. Medical Association Committee on Breastfeeding & Infant Nutrition, 1994 to present; Member, Human Milk Banking Association of North America Advisory Board, 1996 to present.

Teaching: Family Practice: Special interests: doctor-patient relationships, combining the art and science of medicine; Clinical teaching of medical students/residents in family practice, 1986–1992; Keynote speaker, Family Practice Residents' Day, March 1995: "Things to know when you're starting practice"; Clinical Epidemiology: Medical student small group sessions spring 1993,1994; fall 1994, 1995; Clinical Decision Analysis: Co-instructor for HCEP 529 with Dr. Elizabeth Peter, spring 1994 and 1995. Developed computer teaching materials. Fourth-year medical student CDA lecture for 1996 and 1997; breastfeeding: numerous seminars on various aspects of breastfeeding to lay audiences and to practicing physicians and nurses. Clinical instruction of public health nurses in breastfeeding medicine; Ethics: tutorial assistant for selected sessions of Ethics 400, 1995. Lectured on ethics and health care information; Injury prevention:

seminar on the use of Haddon's matrix in injury prevention to provincial Environmental Health Officers, 1994, 1996.

Awards And Distinctions: S. Stewart Murray Prize, Department of Health Care & Epidemiology, UBC, 1993.

Refereed Publications:

Arsenault, G.R. "Toxic Shock Syndrome Associated with Mastitis: A Case Report." *Can Fam Phys.* 1992; 38: 399, 401, 456

Arsenault, G.R. "Video Reviews: Breastfeeding and Family Planning: Mutual Goals, Vital Decisions, and Guidelines for Breastfeeding, Family Planning, and LAM." *J Human Lactation* 1995; 11 (2): 151–152

Arsenault, G.R. "Video Reviews: Early Breastfeeding: How to Keep It Going." *J Human Lactation* 1996; 12(3): 255

Arsenault, G.R. "Birth control: LAM really works." *B.C. Medical Journal*, 1996; 38(9): 472

Povey, W.G., Arsenault, G.R. "Re: Case-Control Study of the Effectiveness of Different Types of Helmets for the Prevention of Head Injuries among Motorcycle Riders in Taipei, Taiwan." (letter) *AJE* 1996; 144(7): 709–10

Arsenault, G.R. Book Reviews: *Lactation: The Breast-Feeding Manual for Health Professionals. J Human Lactation* 1997; 13(3): 25–251

Arsenault, G.R. "Practice tips: Using a disposable syringe to treat inverted nipples." *Can Fam Phys.* Sept. 1997; 43: 1517–1518

Non-Refereed Publications:

Arsenault, G.R. "You Learn The Darndest Things When You Have Kids, or, What I have Learned About Breastfeeding." *B.C. Health and Disease Surveillance*, 1993; 2(1): 94–103

Arsenault, G.R. "Breastfeeding in the Workplace: Safety Considerations." *B.C. Health and Disease Surveillance*, 1994; 3(2): 18–24

Arsenault, G.R. "Outbreak of Probable Spider Bites at Boulder Bay Camp." *B.C. Health and Disease Surveillance*, 1994; 3(5): 50–53

Other: Regular short articles in magazines oriented toward the medical profession: *The Medical Post, Family Practice, Stitches*, and others; Video/film and book review, *Journal of Human Lactation*, 1994 to present

Medical Consultant to: Rosenthal, M.S., *The Pregnancy Sourcebook*. Lowell House, Los Angeles, 1994, 1995, 1996.

DR. EMILIA BARTON
(1938–1998)

Dr. Emilia Barton, a much-loved and respected East Vancouver family physician, died on 28 February, 1998, three years after breast cancer and a succession of complications of increasing severity forced her to give up her practice in January, 1995.

Emily, as she was known to her friends, was born into a large farming family in Vozokany, Czechoslovakia, on 9 December, 1938. She began her study of pediatric nursing in 1956 and graduated with honours in 1957. She worked in this field for the next two years. Compelled to further her knowledge of medicine by a keen desire to serve her young patients better and to respond to their mothers' concerns, Emily entered medical school at Comenius University, Bratislava, graduating in June 1965. She married while a medical student, and her daughter, Anna, was born two months after her graduation. For the next three years, she served as staff pediatrician at two hospitals and one polyclinic near Bratislava. In December 1968, four months after the Soviet invasion of Czechoslovakia ended the all-too-brief 'Prague Spring,' Emily emmigrated to Canada with her husband and daughter.

Their first five years were spent in Winnipeg, where she restarted her medical career from the ground up as a nurses' aide while preparing for her examinations to obtain a Canadian medical licence. Emily interned at Winnipeg's Grace Hospital from 1970 to 1972, and served at Winnipeg Health Sciences Centre for Children as a pediatric resident from 1972 to 1974, where she was presented with the F.W. Horner Award for highest proficiency and aptitude in their Comprehensive Family Care Program.

Shortly after a summer holiday in B.C. the Bartons relocated to Vancouver. In July 1974, Emily began a residency at the Vancouver General Hospital. There she remained for the next two years, training under Dr. Mavis Teasdale in pediatric oncology from 1975 to 1977.

Emily joined a private practice in July 1977, keeping her focus on treating young people. Over the years she developed a loyal patient following, who unwaveringly awaited her return even as cancer forced her to stop practising in January 1995. Happily, there were a few brief interludes of relative good health in between the relapses of the last three years. Not well enough to return to work, she managed to visit family and friends in Europe and in North America. Her vivid reminiscences of people and places she loved, whether from her early years or from more recent times, were a joy as much for her daughter and friends as for her, for she recreated the magic she had lived.

Patients and friends alike sought her advice and support on issues emotional as well as medical. She adored babies, children gravitated to her, and she gained the trust of many of the adolescents in her practice. When she could no longer nurture the many she had seen grow through childhood, she turned her attention to her small garden at home, and almost everything flourished under her care.

Emily will be remembered both for her caring and for the inner strength that saw her through many difficult times and empowered others through theirs. She is survived by her loving daughter, as well as by three sisters and one brother. She will be dearly missed by her large, close-knit family abroad, and by an extended family of patients and friends here.

(Written for BCMJ, *Volume 40, Number 4, April 1998, by Dr. Mukul N. Vyas.)*

DR. ESTHER BROWN
(c 1921–1987)

Dr. Esther Brown was born in Moose Jaw, Saskatchewan. She received her MD from the University of Manitoba in 1945 and she served as Captain in the Canadian Army Medical Corp. After her training in radiotherapy at the Saskatoon Cancer Clinic, she became one of the first Canadian oncologists. For twenty-three years, she worked as a radiation oncologist at the Saskatoon Cancer Clinic, during which time the use of Cobalt 60 in radiotherapy was pioneered.

At age fifty-two, Dr. Brown obtained a Masters degree in Business and Health Care Administration at the University of Saskatchewan. In 1977, she joined the Cancer Control Agency of British Columbia and played a significant role in the division of radiation oncology. Besides her role as an oncologist, she was also a pilot, an accomplished figure skater, a speed skater, a badminton player, and the wife of Dr. Dougald Blue, a urologist. She retired four months before her death of cancer in May, 1987.

(Written by S.M. Jackson M.D. and V.E. Basco M.D. in Vancouver, for the BCMA Journal of July, 1987.)

DR. DIANA HO YUEN

I was born in Kimberley, South Africa in 1945. My parents had seven children and I was the fourth. My mother was born in Port Elizabeth, South Africa, and returned to China as an infant after losing her mother in the 1918 influenza epidemic. She was raised there by her grandmother and returned to South Africa in 1938 to be married to my father, who came to Kimberley in 1936 from Kwangtung Province, China. With very little formal education and very little materially, but endowed with the guidance and teachings of their elders whom they left many miles away, they set out to work hard in a grocery store to build their future together. They raised and educated their children through very difficult times. On the positive side, these difficult times built strong families and strong communities. My parents came to Canada to join their children in 1978.

We were grateful to our parents' dedication and their vision, for today three of my brothers and myself are physicians, and my two sisters a teacher and a hair stylist, and a brother an accountant. We were educated in South Africa. We are all living in and working in Canada, our new homeland, except for one brother who still lives in South Africa. The next generation in Canada continues the vision of my parents: two of their grandchildren had the privilege of recently becoming a Rheumatologist and an Ophthalmologist.

My ideals of becoming a doctor began at, I believe, age eleven, when I decided that this was indeed what I wanted as my career. Through the grace of God and the foresight of my parents, and the wonderful people responsible for my education from an early age to the present, I have been able to fulfil my childhood ambition.

I attended the University of Cape Town, in Cape Town, South Africa, where I obtained a Bachelor of Science degree. Then I proceeded to Medical School at the University of Witwatersrand, Johannesburg, where I was in the graduating class of 1974. From my graduating class picture I counted a total number of 140 students, of which twenty-two were women.

My years as a medical student were most memorable. We were taught by excellent teachers at some of the greatest teaching hospitals in South Africa. Often we would meet students from North America, Britain, Europe, and other countries.

One of my best experiences was to go to mission hospitals during our electives to work. Another unforgettable occasion was after our final exams in our second year (the year of anatomy and anthropology), we joined Professor Phillip Tobias, our esteemed professor of anatomy and anthropology, on an excursion to the caves at Sterkfontien and Makapansgat where he has worked and done research. He is noted internationally for his contribution to Human Anthropology.

Internship followed at the Coronation Hospital and Baragwanath Hospital in Johannesburg. The next step was coming to Canada and leaving the land of my birth, at a very traumatic time in South Africa's history–the 1976 Soweta riots were to change the course of the country. These were difficult times; many of my classmates and colleagues left for the U.S.A., Australia, and Canada.

I arrived in Canada to join my family in 1976. My first stop was Vancouver General Hospital where I entered the Obstetrics and Gynecology program, then licencing exams and preparation for family practice. Adjustment to a new country was accompanied by many ups and downs, but with the help of family and friends this was soon overcome.

I began solo family practice in Coquitlam, British Columbia, in 1978. My practice was comprised largely of primary care obstetrics, pediatrics, and general practice. My work was very interesting and satisfying, but long hours were often the norm in solo practice. In 1990 I gave up my obstetric practice, which I still miss greatly.

I continue to practise in the same office, and continue to have hospital privileges at the Royal Columbian, Eagle Ridge, and St. Mary's Hospitals. I plan to continue to serve my community as long as I am able. I look forward to new opportunities to serve in the future; in particular I plan to go with groups to medical missions abroad to countries where medical care is greatly needed. As I approach my twenty-third year of practice, I continue to look to all my wonderful friends and colleagues for inspiration to make the journey into this new millenium, where many changes appear inevitable for us as citizens and medical practitioners. Thank you to all my educators and all who have been an inspiration over the years.

DR. BETTY KLEIMAN

I was born in 1940 in New york City, the oldest child in a large Jewish immigrant family. When I went to high school, a young woman went to university to get her "Mrs." The most exalted training my mother could think of was for me to become an executive secretary. My father wanted me to marry a man who could bring another store to his fruit and vegetable business.

I took my undergraduate degree in art/teaching. I loved painting figures, but this was the era of abstract expressionism, and my work was scorned by my painting teachers. I wasn't mature or strong enough to ignore this. Then I worked for several years in state mental hospitals as an Occupational Therapy Aide, teaching pottery, drama, drawing, poetry, and woodworking. I knew nothing about woodworking and was coached by a long-term inmate named Herman who constructed beautiful boxes and bright-coloured, sturdy furniture for children while talking to his voices! Thorazine had just been released, and I helped re-educate chronic schizophrenics who after years of incarceration suddenly were to live in the community. We taught them how to answer a telephone, use money, board a bus, make 'polite' conversation, etc. The wards were emptied and were shut down one by one. It was so exciting. Sadly, Herman could not make the adjustment to living 'outside.'

It was the start of the 'sexual revolution' and the 60s didn't help women very much. The only birth control was condoms or the diaphragm, a pretty risky business. Two close friends got pregnant. One tiny elf of a woman married her lover, who beat her frequently, blaming her for the pregnancy and forced marriage. The other had an illegal abortion; I was with her as we looked for an abortionist. Would she live and survive this? Would she be able to have children? How could we keep the terrible secret from her single parent mother and aunt who were proudly supporting her in college, each working two poorly-paid menial jobs? A more distant friend had a baby girl and gave it up for adoption, then spiraled into years of depression because she could never talk to anyone about her baby. She had been sent away from her family to a shelter, so as not to shame them. The men involved deserted the women who were left to deal with these decisions. After these informative experiences, I became very involved in women's access to birth control and then to feminism.

I wanted to have work that was meaningful to me and decided on medicine. I was the second person in my extended family of about forty people in North America to finish college. An earlier generation had one who graduated from university two years before I did. She was a WAVE in the second World War and used GI bill funds to attend a college while raising three young children.

I returned to Columbia University's General Studies to study pre-medical subjects. This was a wonderful school, because all students were at least in their twenties, most older. All had purpose in being at the University. My classes were often with Ivy League students, and I was pleased and surprised when I competed with them and achieved As.

Both my parents were against my attending medical school. So was my beloved Grandpa Jake who said to me, "How will I ever get 'naches'?" Naches are little gifts, but he meant great-grandchildren. My stepgrandmother, Sarah, who was so proud she graduated from high school in Russia, said to him severely, "Jake, she can always have children, but she has only one chance to go to medical school." She and my sister were the only family members to support me emotionally.

I couldn't bear to leave the ocean or New York City which I loved for the energy and vibrant art and music scene. Most medical schools had quotas for women (usually below ten percent) and for minorities. Columbia still did not accept women to its medical school. Though I was accepted in a 'better' medical school in Chicago, I chose to attend Women's Medical

School in Philadelphia. I was surprised to be accepted at any school, but was accepted at three. Women's Medical School was a good choice.

Work was very hard. There was so much to learn and I was not always aware of the purpose for learning some things. My favorite subjects were biochemistry and human physiology. During first year, my friend Nancy Coyne and I started the first medical student newspaper in Philadelphia. We called it *Vital Signs* and as editors, decided to publish anonymous articles. In those days medical students were not vocal. I remember the head of Biochemistry screaming at me in the corridor: "Who wrote that scurrilous piece of trash about my department . . . ?" I suavely said, "This is why we allow anonymous articles, so there is no retribution." He kept demanding to know the author and I repeatedly refused. I wonder if he suspected I was the author!

My step-grandmother, Sarah, who was so proud she graduated from high school in Russia, said to him severely, "Jake, she can always have children, but she has only one chance to go to medical school."

I loved the intricate biochemistry of the body and the interrelation between mind and chemistry and was very proud of my research projects. In another school, I probably would have graduated as a PhD/MD researcher. But Women's Medical trained mainly General Practitioners.

In anatomy the first year, four of us shared a cadaver. We called her LOL for little ol' lady. She was a shriveled black woman in her eighties and her body told us that she had had a hard life. All the school cadavers were paupers and almost all were black. The biting smell of formaldehyde always reminds me of the dark basement and rows of bodies draped in dirty white sheets. Because LOL had little body fat, she didn't smell as bad as some of the other cadavers in the intense Philadelphia summer heat. But eventually her skin began to rot and developed maggots, so we had to strip her skin off, a gruesome task.

We were the least serious dissection group and liked to place stray body parts in strange places and call the anatomy assistant over to 'question him.' We laughed hysterically, but the assistant was rather blasé, probably having seen it before innumerable times.

During my second year, my father stopped sending me money, although he could afford to support me. Working was out of the question, because of our course load. The registrar was wonderful when I told her I must leave. She quickly arranged substantial loans so I could continue, and continued sending bills for tuition to my father (which he paid).

I was depressed by the lack of family support and lonely and stressed, so I helped start a medical student support group.

The Vietnam War was beginning and this changed my whole life. I became politicized and began organizing rallies and going to Washington D.C. and New York City for big marches. The U.S. public was decidedly for the war, supporting our boys who were dying and saving the world from Communism. A man screamed obscenities at me and spit in my face as I marched. Then the New York police began herding people into traps where police waited to beat them. The march was so small; I could see that everyone was peaceful and controlled. The newspapers next day reported that the marchers were breaking windows and had attacked the police.

In Washington at the Pentagon Marches, I was part of the medical team for the demonstrators. The National Guard was there and I saw a young woman who was standing behind the designated line pulled over by a Guard and dragged by the hair, screaming, to a paddy wagon. No one tried to help her because the other guards were pointing their rifles at us. This was the march when the well-known pediatrician, Dr. Spock, and his wife were arrested.

I watched while the army cleared the road to the Pentagon. I stood there in the road like a deer caught in a car's headlights, watching the troops goose-walk toward me, spraying a cloud of white tear gas in front of them. They wore huge insectoid masks so I couldn't see their faces. As a child who grew up on stories of Nazi and Cossack atrocities against my family, I was stunned and horrified. This was the land of the brave and free? I stood there transfixed, my mouth open. A young man bravely jumped on the road and shook me. "RUN! RUN! Get off the road," he screamed. "They'll gas you." He grabbed my arm and dragged me to safety.

At another march, while at the medical tent which was run mostly by medical students and a few Residents, I was chosen for an odd errand. We were in touch with the Pentagon medical team so that if a demonstator was badly injured, they could arrange to get an ambulance through (as we did for a boy with a severe head wound). We were running low on bandages (all donated) and were told to send two people into the Pentagon for supplies. A male medical student and I were chosen. We went around the side of the Pentagon, which is a huge concrete block with a few windows, gave a code word, and were admitted into the citadel. We walked through about two city blocks past uniformed men and women who sneered or glared at us. Through rooms with jeeps and guns and computers, we were escorted to sick bay and given some medical supplies, then led out.

I went back to the command post where we were treating the demonstrators and stood helplessly watching young people turn purple, doubled over with coughing from the tear gas. These experiences were a major part of my decision to leave the United States.

In the third year, we started work in the Emergency Room. We were on call at night to do simple laboratory tests like a CBC and any cultures. Because our Emergency Room was 'private,' not 'public,' patients who had no insurance were turned away or sent by ambulance to a public hospital. One Saturday night, our wards were full as were the overflow beds in the corridors. A black man came in who had been stabbed in the heart during an argument. He was stabilized and the Chief Resident made the decision to ship him to the public hospital. Because he had to be accompanied by a doctor, I was chosen to go. The ambulance had no oxygen, no medication, no defibrillator, nothing except a gurney with an intravenous pole and a chair for me. I stared at the chipped gray paint despairingly. I was terrified. The patient cheered me up with a line of chatter. When we arrived at the other hospital which was even more chaotic than mine, the Resident asked through clenched teeth, "How could you send a man with a knife wound to the heart in such an ambulance?" "I'm just a third year student, a peon," I said with angry tears in my eyes. "I didn't make the decision."

Saturday nights in Philadelphia were a 'zoo.' I remember one beautiful young woman, drunk and angry, who flung herself from a moving car. Even though she had two intravenous lines with blood, her blood pressure fell to almost nothing. We used the gravity system for an intravenous then and she was bleeding too fast for the lines to replace the blood loss. I stood there squeezing the two bags by hand and replacing them through ten units until she stabilized and the surgeons could even look at her.

Stabbings were common. Once another friend, Mary who was seven months pregnant, was working over a man stabbed in the chest. His drunken assailant decided to finish the job, came to the Emergency Room, and waving the knife, started into the cubicle. Mary was tired and said, "I've had enough, thank you." She sailed over to him, big belly distending her blood-spattered white jacket, held out her hand, and said, "Give me that knife *now*, or get out." Thankfully the man and his knife left. During her ninth month, I drove Mary to her home in rural Pennsylvania. She was having frequent contractions (luckily Braxton Hicks)—more terror for me as I had never delivered a baby nor rotated through Obstetrics. Drive fast? Boil water? I didn't know what to do. She had her baby about three days after I got her safely to her parents' home.

One summer I worked on the Manic-Depressive ward at Columbia University. Research with lithium as a new treatment was on-going and I was asked to be a control. Everyone who tests a new medicine takes it as a control, I was told. "We've all taken it." Okay, I would do it. I took lithium daily, but had to collect every drop of urine and have a daily blood test to follow my levels. I loved carrying my large 'pee bottle' to Columbia parties. Luckily I had to stop the medication because I developed diarrhea. Now, I think that was one of the daft side effects, etc. But as I tell my children and my friends, at one point in my life, I was considered 'normal.'

My father did not attend my medical school graduation. Instead he sent my new stepmother, Joan, and my biological mother Molly also decided to attend. They hated each other (probably why he did not attend). The graduation was large enough that they would not have to talk to each other. But what to do about dinner after? My friend Hazel did the seating plans to intersperse her family with mine so as to keep everyone happy, a sort of riddle of the missionaries and the cannibals crossing the river. The dinner went well enough. Hazel later became a psychiatrist.

My friend Nancy didn't take her internship immediately after graduation, but went to Taos, New Mexico, to sit on a hilltop and commune with nature. She eventually became interested in Wilhelm Reich's theories and conducted research into orgone boxes.

My Rotating or General Internship was at Riverside Hospital in California run by Seventh Day Adventists. Their emphasis on a vegetarian diet and exercise predated our current knowledge, but was considered very odd then. Hospital food was all vegetarian, but twice a semester they provided the Interns and Residents with steak.

During Pediatric Rotation, I was lucky to meet two pediatricians who exemplified caring for children. Their humanity and gentleness was in marked contrast to how I had seen children being treated. For example, during my medical training a little half-blind two-year-old was dying from a metastasized eye tumour. The attending physician ordered blood tests twice daily and Mary, my friend, had to have the toddler held down while she probed for a vein, because most were thrombosed. Finally after a one-hour session of screaming and thrashing, Mary refused to do another venipuncture and we students all agreed to support her. There was no information to be gained from the blood tests, no treatment, no purpose except that the textbook said to follow the serum levels. Grumpily, the attending physician agreed to just let the little girl die.

My friend Hazel did the seating plans to intersperse her family with mine so as to keep everyone happy, a sort of riddle of the missionaries and the cannibals crossing the river.

I remember another emergency room lesson. Parents brought an infant swaddled in a blanket to the ER because, they said derisively, "Grandma doesn't like the baby's colour." The baby had had one loose stool, but everything else was fine. I settled myself in a chair to start the detailed pediatric history, including the genetic history, when I noticed the baby's eyes were open, but she had not moved in her mother's arms. I unwrapped the little scrap and her eyes were sunken and her lips blue! She was dehydrated fifteen percent or more. I grabbed the infant and ran to the Pediatric Ward to start an intravenous line and give her fluids. She was so dehydrated we gave her serum albumin to expand her blood volume. Always, at least, listen to the grandma!

During Psychiatric Rotation I was fascinated by the very crazy people. There was something quite creative about their thoughts.

I originally planned to be a plastic surgeon. As an artist, I thought rebuilding children's faces would meld my talents. But surgeons believed women did not have the stamina, so I decided to specialize in Pediatrics.

My husband and I alternated years where one of us determined where we lived. I chose California for the internship year, and Jim decided the next year would be in Vermont helping establish a small printing press to print his books. He'd just won a prestigous prize for book design.

We drove from California to Vancouver, B.C. Thirty years ago, Vancouver was a blue jewel of a city cosy in its ring of mountains. The city was small, but had an active art scene. British Columbia was astounding—more trees and more shades of green than I had seen in my life. We continued through the Rockies, awed by the beauty of the natural scenery. Canada was unbelievable. What could the next few miles bring? Then we hit the plains, endless, monotonous, brown. I felt as if the sky was so huge that the small line of earth we stood upon would go spinning away into the void. I became nauseated by the blue bowl of the sky and the endless horizon.

When we arrived in Vermont, we found the couple running the press wanted Jim to print their work.

Racism in the United States was becoming unbearable. I had married Jim Adams, my art teacher, who happened to be Irish, African, Cherokee, and Seminole. Philadelphia wasn't too bad. But during my internship year, life became unpleasant. At gas stations people leaned forward in their cars to stare at us, the interracial couple. Once as we walked, young men threw beer bottles which shattered around us. A policeman threatened to arrest us for a triviality. Jim was inured and it didn't seem to bother him. He ignored taunts and stares while I became enraged. I wanted to kill people who treated me this way. Parts of me were dying—we decided to leave the United States. I wanted to live in Paris, work as a doctor, and live the Bohemian life among artists. I spoke Spanish semi-fluently, but neither of us spoke French.

We decided to drive back to Vancouver and emigrated with no trouble. We found an historic house near City Hall, a short walk to the Pediatric Hospital. I applied for a Pediatric Residency. When Dr. Sid Israels interviewed me, he seemed to be selling me on the Residency Program. He charmed me. I started work at the hospital. Jim found a job teaching art at Kwantlen College and remained there until he retired.

We decided to have a baby before I started Residency, and my daughter,

Anya was soon born. She was a miracle. Jaundiced at birth and skinny because she was post-mature, she looked like a wrinkled old Vietnamese amah. But, oh her smile! I was like any other first-time mother. The first time Anya rolled over, she rolled off the bed. Blood gushed from her mouth and nose. She was dying! I picked her up and ran through the house screaming for help. As I was alone, this was remarkably ineffective. I finally spoke severely to myself, calmed down, and turned her over. The bleeding stopped and once I stopped screaming, she stopped crying. Anya and my son, Jake, taught me more than my Residency or Fellowship at Yale Child Study Center about parenting.

Medicine in Canada was different than in the States: different medications, different protocols, different textbooks, and a very different culture. Proceedures which I did as a student were forbidden to me as a first year Resident. Everyone had a doctor—so there were no charity cases. It seemed like heaven (mostly).

Being a Resident and a mother was difficult. We were on call every third night. You were up all night and then worked the next day, usually in a semi-conscious state by then. One Christmas, I was in the Intensive Care Nursery, on call every other night instead of every third night.

Now I work two to three days weekly. My practice is in Developmental Pediatrics, and I often get the children who fall between Pediatrics and Child Psychiatry. Many are undiagnosable and I work with their problems. Work is still fascinating, and although I could retire, and don't make much money, I never know what is going to walk into my consulting rooms.

For about thirteen years, I have been an avid kayaker and travelled with my boat to camp in many isolated areas of Vancouver Island, including some solo trips. My favorite adventure was in Johnstone Strait where a pod of Orca whales including a baby swam across the Strait to us and dove under our kayaks (gulp), then turned around and swam back to look us over again. Another trip was to Nootka Sound where we saw bears every day—none habituated. We named the days—the six bear day, the four bear day, etc. I am studying to teach kayaking skills at a local kayak store; this will probably not occur, because I am older and not so strong as the much younger male kayak teachers.

Being on the water in my boat is a profoundly spiritual experience. I can't let my mind chatter, but must be in the moment, in my body, aware of the sea's power, the currents, the winds, my body strength and skills, and my companions. I like to meditate as well (on land with a mediatation group).

A few years ago, I started competing in six-person outrigger canoe races. We train twice a week. This year, I moved to lessons in white-water canoeing on the rapids of the Cowichan River. I doubt I will get good at this, because my reflexes are slower and I'm a chicken about being smacked around amid rocks by the current. I don't mind cold water; we practise kayak rescues in the Pacific Ocean currents every year.

My life as an artist was shattered abruptly seven years ago when I had laser surgery on my eyes. I waited quite a while before arranging surgery, but did so after losing two contact lenses on a trip to the Broken Islands Group. The surgery went awry and I am visually handicapped. I can't see lines, so faces and expressions are difficult. In fact I once walked past my son in a crowd because I didn't recognize him.

My paintings relied heavily on drawing, so painting was closed to me. I was angry, bitter, and despondent for several years. I tried writing—especially poetry and short stories, and had about five pieces published, but never felt the same right brain tingle and facility I had with visual arts. A friend let me use her studio and I began making pottery. Now I belong to a Victoria pottery studio, part of an artist's co-operative, X-Changes. I feel the line of my pots with my fingers and integrate parts of my painting technique into the glazes. I like working with other artists to validate and criticise my art, share techniques, and arrange thematic art shows which inspire me (the last one was 'erotic art').

Now, at sixty-one years of age, my life is coming into a wonderful balance with challenges at work and learning new physical skills, travelling to isolated areas, supportive friends and family, and a spiritual life.

Life is good.

DR. LIANNE LACROIX

My life began on April 27, 1943 in the village of Lapasse on the shores of the Ottawa River about one hundred miles northwest of Ottawa, Ontario. My parents were French Canadian farmers whose families had settled the land a hundred years before when the farms around Montreal could no longer feed the growing population. I was the oldest of six children and as I worked daily on the farm with my close-knit family, I always felt that my life would be different.

My parents encouraged education for both boys and girls. We were fortunate that a high school was built in the next town, and I was pleased to graduate at the top of my small class. My family could not afford to send me to university, so I chose a laboratory technology course which paid a small amount to cover living expenses. I would have to finish Grade 13 first, but fortunately an aunt offered to lend me some money to live near the larger high school in Ottawa. The lab technology course lasted eighteen months and was located in the hospital where we worked every day. I knew that this course was the first step to a career in science, or perhaps research like Madame Curie where I would advance humanity. I had read about the life of Dr. Schweitzer in Africa, but medicine seemed impossibly out of reach to me, so I did not give it a second thought. I knew no doctors except the next town doctor, but fortunately my good health had prevented any contact.

While working as a lab tech for one year after my course, I wondered very much about my path in life. I could see that I enjoyed helping people most of all, and I did not have the intellectual make-up or solitary dedication for research. Then suddenly the mist lifted and the road became clear. As I walked into the hospital cafeteria on a sunny winter day, out of the blue came a life-defining moment. I knew that I would be a doctor, just like that! Great joy filled my heart. I did not reveal this dream to anyone for several months as I investigated this idea, since I am a very practical person. I read through the description of the medical curriculum and did some psychological tests to find out whether this dream was possible. The answer was positive except for one thing—finances. This was 1964, when loans and bursaries for students were just starting, but I did not qualify since I was not a student but a working person. There was only one option. I would work for one more year, saving enough for the first year of university, then I would apply for the loans during the other years.

The director of the lab, Doctor M., an imposing, bald, pipe-smoking gentleman who only ever spoke to the head technologist, called me to his office. "I hear that you want to go into medicine and I would not advise this," he said. "Women doctors are not happy." He went on, "They give up medicine to have a family and are not happy, or they remain single to practice medicine and are not happy, so I would not advise this." "Thank you, Sir," I answered, "I will remember that." As I walked out of his office I thought that my other choice would be to remain an unhappy lab tech wishing to be a doctor. Doctor M. has long since passed away, but his signature still sits on my Medical Council diploma on the pink wall of my office.

At that time in 1964, I was offered a position as technician to start a lab at the twenty-bed mission hospital of Fort George in James Bay, home of the Cree people. I gladly accepted and left Ottawa for thirteen months of satisfying work, interesting contact with the local people, and wonderful fishing and camping adventures in the beautiful isolated sub-arctic. I was fortunate to return there for the following five summers between my years of university, thereby saving enough so that I did not have to work during the years of studies, for this is often a recipe for failure.

While working in Fort George, I collected blood groups from over 200 people whose blood I was testing already, as requested by our only doctor. It occurred to me that such information might be interesting to anthropologists, since the population was quite isolated and unchanged by outside contact. On my return to the university I went to see our biology professor to offer this information for publication. He was most interested and we co-authored a short paper called "Blood Groups of the Cree Indians of Fort George" which appeared in the *Journal of Heredity*.

In 1968, I graduated from Ottawa University with a pre-med BA, followed by my medical degree in 1972. There were fifteen women in our class of sixty-eight students. My marks sat somewhere in the middle of the class and I did not win any awards. Our top student was a woman, Sheila Carlyle, presently a forensic pathologist in New Westminster, B.C. In the audience sat my parents with my illiterate grandmother who had never had the opportunity to attend school at all. We were all very proud. I then did a twelve-month rotating internship at the Ottawa Civic Hospital and applied to work in the Arctic.

By August 1973, I arrived in Inuvik, Northwest Territories, hired by the Federal Government, and soon after was sent on a two-month tour of the eastern arctic, based out of Churchill, Manitoba. I visited the nursing stations that had not seen any doctor for several months. Then I returned to

Inuvik for four years, as part of a team of six doctors that included a general surgeon and two GP anaesthetists. We worked in a fifty-bed hospital serving a population of 4,000 townspeople, plus another 7,000 people in twelve other settlements. Every month each doctor travelled by plane to visit one or two nursing stations staffed by nurse practitioners-midwives. Serious cases were flown out to Edmonton. Many times I ran to the hospital at three in the morning under the midnight sun to deliver a baby. Somehow it made up for the sixty below twilight darkness of noon in early December. At this time I noticed the Federation of Medical Women of Canada name on the Canadian Medical Association membership request and joined in 1974. I was the only woman Doc in the area. One gruff bush pilot was heard to say that he flew 500 miles to the next city to avoid having his pilot medical done by a woman doctor!

During this time I met and married Ron Fehr, a bush pilot flying a Twin Otter and many other smaller planes. I had retained an interest in flying since my Fort George days and had attained a private flying licence myself, in the last two years in Ottawa. We bought a single engine plane called a Piper Commanche and flew from Inuvik to Montreal and back that summer. However, with an advanced pilot in the family, I was happy to hang up my wings and have not piloted since.

The north is a place where people come and go and your friends all move back 'south' within a few years. By 1977 we decided to move to Langley, British Columbia, close to my husband's family. Ron worked for Airwest which was evolving into AirBC, and I joined three other doctors at the Avalon Clinic. A nurse asked if I would like to work with Planned Parenthood, since contraception was my special interest, and I worked at the Langley and White Rock Clinics once a month. Our daughter, Annette, was born in April, 1979. I practised until thirty-six weeks pregnant. I remember one case where the delivering young woman was in the care of a five-month pregnant nurse and myself, the six-month pregnant doctor! I wondered if this was a first of some kind. I had found a locum and future partner, Vivian Paul, and took four months off. I breastfed for nine months, and will never forget the first time that I left my daughter with a sitter to return to work, for it was one of the hardest things that I had ever done. I felt that I could not financially afford to be off any longer.

I worked five half-days, and did much obstetrics and emergency coverage where you went home and were called back if a patient came in, sometimes three times during the same night! Since my husband left at 5 a.m. for his flying work, I had lined up two neighbours I could call over to stay with my baby should a fully dilated patient show up suddenly. On one occasion I dropped off my five-month-old daughter with the emergency nurses at 6 a.m. We had to improvise. It was a difficult time and I learned the meaning of burnout, and I wish this experience on no one.

In December, 1981 we decided to move out of the rain and the difficult lifestyle to a new city, Kelowna, B.C. At least this hospital was large enough to have full-time emergency doctors! My husband was planning to get another flying job, but the economy was taking a downturn and pilots were being laid off, so he never did return to aviation. We opened a video store and for seven months I looked after our small daughter and tried to help in the store. The store was not doing well so that by July, 1982 I returned to medicine by doing locums for many local doctors. This turned into full-time work four days a week at two offices with much obstetrics again. We sold the store by wintertime and my husband decided that he could stay home as house-Dad. This worked out very well for our daughter who played ringette (like hockey) and rode horses, English style. The close relationship with her Dad made her into a young woman with excellent self-esteem who is presently at McGill studying urban planning.

"I hear that you want to go into medicine and I would not advise this," he said. "Women doctors are not happy." He went on, "They give up medicine to have a family and are not happy, or they remain single to practice medicine and are not happy."

Life was very busy. Most doctors covered their own obstetrics call all the time so you could get called to the caseroom anytime, such as the middle of Christmas dinner, or from the depths of a store changing room, as you tried to buy your child some school clothes. I very much enjoyed caring for women in pregnancy and childbirth, and my practice grew. In 1989 I moved to my very own office with another woman doctor, Jan Fisher, and we covered each other's call on weekends. One day as I hurried to the hospital once again at three in the morning in the middle of a snowstorm, I felt stuck on a treadmill that could not slow down. As if in slow-motion I raced down the empty hospital corridors and wondered if the nurse's phone call had been a dream. I would get to the caseroom and it would be empty, and I would wake up back in my own bed away from the cold lonely night. This never happened, and the labouring women were all too real. I must be reaching the edge of burnout again, I thought.

Fortunately, I managed to find a locum for one month and visited my family in Lapasse where I was known not for my work but for my connections to numerous relatives. It was heaven, and on return my husband said, "Why don't you quit obstetrics?" It had been eighteen years since I had finished my internship, there were new women doctors in town, and perhaps I had done my share. I thought about it for a long time, then stopped accepting new pregnant patients and delivered my last baby ever in September, 1991.

The Vancouver branch of the Federation of Medical Women invited me to their spring retreat at Harrison Hot Springs. Talking with other women doctors made me more determined to improve women's health in our city. By this time, new assertive women doctors, such as Marjorie Docherty and Sheila Ferguson, had moved to town. They no longer stood silently like my generation of medical women who made a statement merely by their presence. These young women demanded and expected their full share of medical responsibilities within the male-dominated medical establishment. Marjorie became the first Department Head of Family Practice and Sheila the first Director of Extended Care. Their courage inspired my actions. By 1994 we had over six members of the FMWC and we started our own Okanagan Branch. I have organized a monthly dinner meeting with a scientific speaker ever since. These are sponsored by pharmaceutical companies, and we always invite all women doctors. There are now over forty of us including several specialists, which is twenty percent of the medical staff. We are slowly becoming more accepted and woven into medical life.

Finally I had time to start work on my pet project, trying to organize a Planned Parenthood branch which was very much needed. I joined the local Pro-choice group who formed a clinic group, and after many difficulties our clinic opened in February, 1995 to great publicity. Kelowna is the headquarters of the provincial Pro-life group who oppose contraception

for their own reasons. They picketed our clinic and posted my name in their phone hot line so that I felt threatened for my personal safety. I called the police. This hit the media, even making it to the second page of the *Province* newspaper. That day I cancelled my office and spoke to them all: newspapers, radio, even French CBC and two local TV stations, to explain this neglected subject of contraception and unwanted pregnancies. It was strangely enjoyable, and perhaps our cause has been helped.

Other projects followed. With the help of Cathy Clelland and Arja Moreau, we revised the protocol for the sexual assault examination kit and organized the team. Ellen Wiebe came to talk to our group several times. She sent me information and because of patient request, I decided to offer the service of frozen donor sperm artificial insemination in my office, so patients did not have to travel to Vancouver.

From the Pro-choice group we lobbied the authorities to organize a pregnancy termination clinic in our hospital, since we have 400 women who must travel out of town for this procedure. I spoke to all the family doctors at one of our department meetings, asking for their support on this project. This was not easy, but my tachycardia could not drown my resolve. "You have guts," one woman doctor commented after the meeting. The family doctors voted over ninety percent in support of this service at our hospital.

Starting in 1995, Marjorie Docherty and myself have been giving lectures on menopause that have become yearly events in our city. Our largest audience was over 700 women and men at the 1997 presentation in our community theatre. We have also spoken in five other towns and cities in the valley. Marjorie continued many speaking engagements on other topics, especially physician wellness. I remain in contact with the Vancouver FMWC, especially Shelley Ross, and have met many other inspiring women doctors over the years.

As a millenium project I sent one of my paintings to the *CMAJ* and it was published in their April 18th, 2000 issue. It shows a newborn child being held by the hands of a doctor and a nurse. It is called "First Breath," and some day I will paint "Last Breath," which hangs in my mind's gallery of life. I have always wanted to paint and managed to take several art courses over the years. My father passed away with Alzheimer's disease in October of 1998 at age eighty-two. At his funeral in the beautiful Lapasse church, a beam of sunshine fell on his casket, and a long moment of clarity followed as I sat with my close-knit family of three generations.

Life is a circle. I could see it whole from the beginning to the end. I understood that someday I, too, will join all my relatives and ancestors in the tree-lined cemetery of Lapasse overlooking the sparkling river. In the meantime I have paintings to complete, working as a Sunday painter in a spare bedroom of my house. I still have patients to see of course, for another ten years, in my full-time practice. I will continue to specialize in menopause, having joined the North American Menopause Society (NAMS), and in older people and palliative care. My practice is aging with me. Just as I helped them to be born, I am helping them to die. A doctor's life summarized, I could have made no other choice, and do not regret the path chosen for one moment.

DR. WAN CHING (REBECCA) WOO
(1947–1977)

Dr. Woo was born in Hong Kong and had her early education in that city, followed by graduation from the Hong Kong Medical School in 1970. In 1971 she came to Canada and did her training in Pediatrics at McGill University. She was awarded the certification examination of the Royal College in 1976. In April, 1977 she registered in British Columbia and began practice in her specialty in Vancouver.

Her untimely accidental death on November 6th, 1977 at age thirty was a great loss to her profession.

1978

DR. LOIS BLATCHFORD FULLER
(1934–1996)

Lois was born in Tarrytown, New York, in 1934. She obtained her BA from Wellesley College in Massachusetts in 1955 and her Master's degree in

Public Health from Yale University in 1956. She married George, her devoted husband, the same year. Four years later, she entered the Albert Einstein College of Medicine in New York where she received her MD in 1964. After interning and completing her first year of medical residency at Montefore Hospital in the Bronx, Lois transferred to Psychiatry, and obtained her residency through the University of Minnesota Hospital, New York Hospital, and the Bronx Municipal Hospital Center.

Lois continued to work in the Bronx until 1972. The family then moved to Edmonton, Alberta, where she assumed an academic position at the University of Alberta until 1975. After a year at the Seattle Veterans' Administration Hospital in Seattle, she came to B.C. and directed the psychiatric unit in Cranbrook from 1976 to 1979. In 1970, she relocated to Abbotsford, where she worked as a psychiatrist until moving to Vancouver in 1986, when she joined the Department of Psychiatry at St. Paul's Hospital as a clinical assistant professor in 1989. Lois also continued her own private practice as well as co-ordinating and providing outreach psychiatry services to Prince Rupert (1983–1987), Williams Lake (1988–1990), and Quesnel (1990–1995).

Lois and her husband George fought hard for marginalized sectors of society, and to many who knew them, this was their true mission in life. Lois refused to let her voice go unheard, and she involved herself with several organizations at the executive level, including the British Columbia Medical Association, the Federation of Medical Women of Canada, and the American Psychiatry Association. She valued accountability and challenged her colleagues in this regard. She completed her last specialty board exam in Geriatric Psychiatry only a week before her fatal diagnosis.

Lois loved exercise, the outdoors, nature, music, and life. In her final summer she contemplated purchasing a triathlon wetsuit so that she could swim in the ocean at their cabin. When her cancer presented as back pain, we all assumed that her symptoms were due to a maladjusted seat on her new mountain bike. Lois believed that her illness had deprived her of her best academic years. Her greatest frustration was that she had so much to share with her family and friends in so little time.

Lois recorded all her thoughts during her illness until she was unable to write. One of her last entries read: "Yesterday is history, tomorrow is a mystery. Today is a gift. That is why it is called the present." (Author unknown).

Dr. Lois Blatchford Fuller died on February 14, 1996 in Vancouver at the age of sixty-two, in the company of George, her daughters Therese and Jane, and her son Timothy. Lois's cancer was aggressive and merciless, but she battled her disease to the very end. She died in the Palliative Care Unit at St. Paul's Hospital, where she had served as a Psychiatric Consultant until overtaken by her illness.

(Dr. Gavin Smart of Vernon, B.C., wrote Lois's obituary for the BCMA Journal of December, 1996.)

DR. JERILYNN PRIOR

Dr. Jerilynn Prior grew up in Alaska and began her education in a one-room school. She first attended university in Oregon but completed medical studies at Boston University in 1969. She then did a residency in Medicine (sub-specialty Endocrinology) which was completed at UBC in 1977, and received her FRCP that year. In 1979 she became a Diplomat in Endocrinology and Metabolism.

At UBC she has been a highly committed teacher. As well as bedside teaching, she lectures and is involved in the Problem Based Learning component of the first two years of the undergraduate program, particularly in the Endocrine-Metabolism and Musculo-skeletal blocks. She has also offered a session for undergraduates on Careers in Endocrinology, has been involved in resident education, supervised a large number of graduate students and post-doctoral fellows, and been actively involved in continuing medical education. Dr. Prior also has been active in the public domain, participating in such programs as the CBC science series "Quirks and Quarks," Dr. Rhonda Low's segments on BCTV, and Dr. Art Hister's "House Calls" on CKNW radio. She is the recipient of numerous awards and recognitions, from the Nobel Peace Prize for Physicians Against Nuclear War in 1985 to the UBC Distinguished Lecturer award in 2002.

Dr. Prior has maintained a productive research program throughout her career and is the recipient of a large amount of grant funding, both as an individual and with various groups. She has published extensively, including many peer-reviewed journal articles and book chapters. Her main area of interest is in the physiology of ovulation and its disturbances, pioneering the importance of progesterone for the prevention and treatment of osteoporosis. She has also spoken on issues related to perimenopause, documenting for the first time that estrogen levels are variable and high during this transition and not low as was previously thought.

While working for several years in Native health settings in Alaska, Dr. Prior was involved with the WAMI program, a multi-state (Washington, Alaska, Montana, and Idaho) undergraduate outreach program of the University of Washington.

In the spring of 2002, the Centre for Menstrual Cycle and Ovulation Research was founded in Vancouver, with Dr. Prior as the Scientific Director. It is primarily a virtual centre, with scientific advisory council members from Hong Kong to Norway and England to Australia.

In October, 2003, a vibrant local advisory oversaw the launch of the website (www.cemcor.ubc.ca) which is averaging 5,000 to 7,000 hits a day. This website has been contacted by people from every country on every continent, except Antarctica. It provides woman-centred information for adolescent, premenopausal, perimenopausal, and menopausal women. Handouts and diary forms that Dr. Prior has used in research and clinical care for twenty years are now available for all. There are also sections for researchers and health care providers, including an article titled "Management of Menorrhagia without Surgery." The site is continually updated.

Dr. Prior is a valued University member, serving on such committees as the Senior Appointments Committee, which is central to the maintenance of quality in the institution, and she is now a member of the Clinical Research Ethics Board (CREB). A Professor in the Division of Endocrinology of the Department of Medicine, she served for a time as Acting Head. She has wide-ranging interests, finding time in her busy schedule to sing in the Vancouver Bach Choir for twenty-five years.

Dr. Prior has made a major contribution to the Faculty of Medicine at UBC through teaching, scholarship, and innovative research. In May 2004, she became an Honorary Alumna of the UBC Medical Alumni Association.

(Adapted from Dr. William Webber's presentation address to the UBC Medical Alumni Association in presenting the award to Dr. Prior, May 15, 2004. Both Dr. Webber and Dr. Prior gave their permission.)

DR. LANI ALMAS

Curriculum Vitae

Born: Vancouver, British Columbia, June 5, 1949.

Marital status: married, 3 children.

Education: BSc (Honors Zoology), University of British Columbia, 1974; MD, University of British Columbia, 1978; Internship, St. Paul's Hospital, Vancouver, B.C. 1978–1979; Family Practice Residency, UBC, July 19, 1979–April 1, 1980; CCFP, 1988, maintained active status to July 1992, associate status to Jan. 1997; Residency, Obstetrics and Gynaecology, University of Calgary, Alberta, July 1992–1994; FRCS(C), September 1996.

Professional Employment: May 1980–June 1992, full time Family Practice in Terrace, B.C.

Privileges: Active privileges at Mills Memorial Hospital 1980 to 1993; 1996 to present. Courtesy privileges at MMH 1993 to 1996. Active privileges at Burnaby General Hospital March 1990 to learn use of Ventous. July 1993–July 1996, part-time Family Practice in Calgary, Alberta.

Additional Appointments: Teacher for the Rural Practice Program UBC 1982 to 1992, had appointment of Clinical Assistant Professor before resigning to do residency; Preceptor for the National Clinical Training Program of Nurse practitioners, through Health and Welfare Canada 1989–1992; taught formal course 'Reproduction and Endocrinology' to first year medical students, University of Calgary; taught medical students and Ob/Gyn residents as senior and Chief Resident.

Professional Activities: member of College of Physicians and Surgeons of British Columbia since 1980; member of College of Physicians and Surgeons of Alberta 1993 to 1996; member of College of Family Practice 1980 to 1997; past secretary of the Medical Staff of Mills Memorial Hospital; past Chief of Staff of the Medical Staff of MMH January 1990 to June 1992; junior member of American College of Obstetrics and Gynecology since 1992; member of the Society of Obstetrics and Gynaecology of Canada since 1992.

Awards: 1993–4, Ortho Junior Fellowship Award.

Additional Information: ACLS 1988, 1991, 1999; ATLS 1989; NRP 1991, 1996, 2001; Alarm 1996, 1997, 1999, 2001.

DR. B. LYNN BEATTIE

Growing up in two mining company towns (now ghost towns) with only occasional forays into the city, I was branded early in life as a somewhat precocious tomboy: single–minded, curious, and eager for new challenges, preferring Tinker Toys to playing with dolls. Born on April 13, 1940 at Kootenay Lake General Hospital in Nelson where I later had summer employment as an admissions clerk during my university years, I was the first child of George and Lila (Christianson) Beattie. My father was a bookkeeper and my mother a stenographer working for Sheep Creek Gold Mines. They worked hard and made many sacrifices to ensure that my sister and I were well-educated.

We lived in Zincton B.C., a mine townsite built to accommodate the staff needed to operate the concentrator which processed millions of tons of low-grade zinc ore produced from the "Lucky Jim" mine. Zincton was located in a narrow valley midway between Kaslo and New Denver. My sister Dawn was born in New Denver in 1942. After the mine petered out in the late 1940s, we settled in Sheep Creek, south of Salmo.

As children in those innocent times we took advantage of the freedom (as both our parents were usually working) available in the mining camp—sledding pell-mell down the hill in winter, roaming the woods along the creek seeking out lady slippers and trilliums in spring and trout and huckleberries in the summer, playing endless games of "Hangman" and "Lucky Sevens" and "Red Rover" and "Prisoner's Base" on the bridge. We also spent a lot of time arranging and rearranging the makeshift wood crate "furniture" in the woodshed that was our playhouse.

I was eager to start school and, after turning six, was thrilled to be allowed to occasionally visit the primary classroom where Mrs. Dilling had her hands full with seven grades in one room. At that time you had to be exactly six before you could be formally enrolled in the following September. Lodore School was situated alongside Sheep Creek near the bridge and next to an abandoned mill; to play on the rusted mill machinery was definitely off limits, but we often did so anyway. I remember the annual lecture by the policeman from Salmo about what to do if you found a blasting cap in or near the schoolyard, but we never did find one. The bridge was the central playground for various games and pastimes requiring little or no equipment, such as skipping, hopscotch, and marbles. Lodore School had the only library in town: a cupboard in the back of the classroom filled with old readers. I loved to read and I devoured these books. Then my mother bought the complete set of the "Book of Knowledge" and my horizons expanded.

There were sixty students in the class, including seven women. We women became good friends and supported each other during the vicissitudes of our training.

We had one field trip while I was at Lodore School. We went to the mill to watch my uncle Walter pour the final gold brick that was to be produced from the mine. Sheep Creek Gold Mine was closed in 1951, but the company moved its office to Nelson, and we were moved there. My sister and I enrolled at Central School, I in Grade 6 and Dawn in Grade 4. We made new friends and attended St. Paul's Church Sunday School, choir, Explorers, and later Canadian Girls in Training (CGIT). With respect to the choir, it was interesting to note that the choir director, Mrs. T.J.S. Ferguson, was the same church organist who had trained my father and his brothers when they were growing up in Nelson. While the Beattie boys were well known for their musicality, I'm afraid I was not a very gifted singer, albeit I was a faithful attendee at choir practice.

In 1955, my father went to work for Newmont Mining Company and in the spring our family moved to Stewart B.C., a community with a population of about 400 at the head of the Portland Canal on the Alaskan panhandle. Stewart was an isolated frontier town with few amenities where the event of the week was the arrival of the Union Steamship boat on Saturday nights, bringing mail and groceries and the occasional curious visitors. We were back in a three-room schoolhouse with multiple grades in one room and a couple of senior students attending regularly but doing their work by correspondence. Our teacher, Mr. Joe from Vancouver, was enthusiastic about his profession and worked hard to meet the curriculum demands set by the province. Summers were spent working at the local drug store as a soda jerk. Time off was spent hiking the surrounding mountains. The mountains at Stewart are the highest rising from tidewater in the world. On rare summer days getting above the tree line and sliding on the heather was exhilarating. The wildflowers of the alpine meadows and the brilliance of the blue and green glacial lakes were spectacular. Provisioning the Granduc Copper Mine located under a glacier required significant logistics. I helped my father pack parachutes for helicopter drops of provisions for the mine. As Grade 10 approached, I left Stewart to board with relatives and friends of my family and attended Burnaby South High School for two years.

My father returned to work for Sheep Creek Mines (then known as Aetna Mines) in 1958 and the family moved back to Nelson where our house was almost next door to the high school, L.V. Rogers. I completed Grades 12 and 13 there, but was reluctant to go to UBC which was generally regarded as a giant unfriendly place, opting instead to go to Bishop's University in Lennoxville Quebec. Bishop's had been talked about by a French teacher at Burnaby South who had moved west from Montreal. When I wrote for the calendar I liked the picture of the quadrangle and the description of the University and its courses. I registered in science with three possible goals: nuclear physics, chemistry, or medicine. Once at Bishop's and despite my homesickness, it soon became apparent that nuclear physics was not for me—the math was just too hard! Hours spent in the chemistry lab were very lonely. Students were allowed to work at their own pace to complete the labs (by a set date of course!).

In the spring, a number of senior students were accepted to McGill University Medical School and I re-examined my goals. UBC Medical School seemed a good option, since it was closer to home. I applied to UBC for third year Honours Chemistry and was accepted. But what a challenge I faced when I got into it. Physical chemistry was difficult enough, but the course on crystallography was unreal. At the end of the year I was accepted into fourth year Chemistry, but was also accepted into UBC Medical School. The chemistry lab was abandoned for anatomy, biochemistry, and physiology labs. There were sixty students in the class, including seven women. We women became good friends and supported each other during the vicissitudes of our training. Dr Friedman said at the beginning of the year, "Look to your left and look to your right. One of you isn't going to be here in four years." That set the tone. Only forty-two graduated in 1965, of which seven were women!

Upon graduation in 1965, I applied for a rotating internship in Toronto and was accepted at Toronto Western Hospital (TWH). We were paid every two weeks and worked every other night and every other weekend. Part way through the year my biweekly salary went to three digits, $113. My first rotation was at Sick Children's where John McCreary, formerly of that hospital and now Dean at UBC, was remembered fondly. My first rotation at Sick Children's was in the Emergency Room and required every bit of pediatric knowledge I had and then some. Staff were very helpful and most of the time things worked out well, except for one incident where I carefully sewed up a dog bite on the shoulder of a young girl, unaware that it should have been left alone for a period of time. Subsequent rotations were at Toronto Western Hospital, a place where I felt very much at home with colleagues, staff, and patients. I applied for internal medicine at Sunnybrook and was accepted there. Bill McArthur, my husband–to–be, was in the military and doing a summer placement there and that was where we met.

My last rotation as an intern was on the renal service, and I applied for training in nephrology under the direction of Dr. George de Weber. This was a very early time in dialysis and transplantation; the first transplant was done at TWH in 1966. I was very involved in all aspects of the clinical service and at the edge of developments such as HLA typing, availability of hyper immune globulin, and the use of intravenous furosemide and ethacrynic acid for diuresis. On one occasion we diagnosed a patient with pneumocystitis carinii and had to requisition a supply of pentamidine isethionate from the United States. Nowadays such diagnoses are more common and the therapy is more easily obtained. For the second year of my nephrology fellowship I was paid as the Hurst Brown Fellow. At that time

the $8,000 stipend was tax free and I felt very well paid. (My father, at the time living in Fraser Lake B.C. and working for Placer, pointed out to me that the general practitioner at Fraser Lake was much better reimbursed than I, while I had all the expenses of living in the big city.)

In 1969, Bill was posted to Moose Jaw as Base Surgeon and I decided to do training in internal medicine at Saskatoon. This was an interesting experience with wonderful new people and time spent getting used to the prairies. Bill and I were married in Vancouver in July 1970 and I wrote my fellowship exams in September of that year. When I received the results of my success in the written exam in the mail I cried for a while, feeling overwhelmed by the thought of attending the oral exam in Edmonton. Nevertheless, I steeled myself, attended the examination, and was fortunately successful, having a case with lupus erythematosus, a disease I had had a lot of experience with in my days training in nephrology. I returned to Moose Jaw to start a consulting practice in internal medicine with a physician group there.

I learned I was pregnant and that Bill was to be transferred to Toronto to work at Downsview. We moved to Toronto in the summer of 1971 where we rented a home which I enjoyed decorating while awaiting the birth of Heather Lynn who arrived on November 8, 1971. Bill is from New Zealand and, when Heather was five weeks old, we flew to New Zealand to introduce her to her grandmother Heather McArthur. This was my first trip to New Zealand and Bill's first time back since he had left at eighteen years of age. We explored the islands; Heather was a very good traveller, returning to Canada twice as old as when she had left. My advocacy for breast feeding was confirmed.

When we returned to Toronto, I wanted to work, but wanted a position that I could manage with a young baby and a husband who was often travelling. Nephrology service required very demanding working hours. I went to see Professor Irwin Hilliard at TWH. He had been a professor there when I was an intern and resident. He welcomed me and suggested that I should consider three things: working in the Tumor Clinic, working on the geriatric ward, and involving myself with undergraduate education. I said that I didn't feel well prepared to work in the Tumor Clinic. That problem was solved by sending me to the Sloan Kettering Institute in New York for a week–long course. I learned a lot in this Clinic. My patients were those who didn't fit into the specialty organ clinics, and 5-fluororacil was the main treatment modality. The nurse with whom I worked was very efficient and helpful and we had some wonderful patients. Fortunately, after a couple of years, another more highly trained individual came on staff and took over the Tumor Clinic responsibilities.

I started clinical work on the geriatrics ward. This ward was developed in the early 1960s as a result of a special grant to accommodate individuals from the Metro Homes for the Aged suffering from acute medical and surgical problems. Soon I found myself in charge of the ward. There were thirty-six (or forty-two) patients, and I had two teams of house staff and made rounds with them on alternate days. This was where I learned geriatrics from a practical perspective. My association with the ward was also an opportunity: Dr. Robert Laird, Emeritus Professor of Surgery, was President of the American Geriatric Society and he invited me to sit on the Board of the Society. This was an incredible introduction to an emerging area of special recognition, and I became President of the Society in 1985. I valued the associations with colleagues throughout North America and the insight that I gained during my tenure. The contributions possible for a Canadian with responsibility in the Society were in the areas of educational, organizational, and administrative aspects, rather than pursuing political or policy objectives. The strong lobby and advocacy roles of the Society now in place are really American initiatives. I was the first female President of the Society and the third Canadian to be President (after Robert Laird and Irwin Hilliard). On the AGS Board I had the opportunity to travel to many American cities and in 1985 was involved with the International Association of Gerontology Congress held in New York City.

Our second child, John, was born on September 21, 1974 at TWH. Maternity leave seemed brief looking back, but I was very happy with my job and my responsibilities. In addition to my clinical duties on the geriatrics ward, I became increasingly involved with undergraduate education and with the local and national effort to promote geriatrics as a specialty. We purchased a farm near Trenton and often went there on weekends. As Bill was frequently travelling in Europe and the Middle East, the family was always glad to be together at the farm.

Bill left the military and in 1979 was appointed Chief Coroner of B.C. and we moved to Vancouver in July of that year. Our children grew up in Vancouver and both have since graduated from UBC, Heather in Science and John in Arts. Heather went on to graduate in Medicine from the University of Toronto in 2001, and John completed a Masters in Public Policy from the Kennedy School of Government at Harvard University and earned a Masters in Economics at Oxford, having received a Rhodes Scholarship in 1998 from British Columbia.

I didn't have a job at the time we moved to B.C., though I had met with John Dirks, Professor of Medicine, and some of the players at UBC. Because of my previous experience in geriatrics I was encouraged to consider a newly created position as Head of the Division of Geriatric Medicine. In October 1979, I was appointed to a part-time position as Medical Director of Purdy Pavilion Extended Care Unit. In 1980, I became acting Head of the Department of Geriatric Medicine at Shaughnessy Hospital and the UBC Division of Geriatric Medicine with the idea that another person would be recruited to fulfill the roles. This never happened, and I was officially appointed Head in 1981. I found myself pulled in many directions—administration, education, research, and practice. It was hard to do everything well by myself and in reality it was impossible. Recruitment was difficult because there were so few trained geriatricians. By 1984, there was recognized training for Geriatric Medicine and people like me could qualify by grandparenting to write the Certificate of Special Competence examination. This made Geriatric Medicine recognized as a sub-specialty of Medicine.

In light of the new legitimacy of Geriatric Medicine, I wrote the test and appeared at the oral examination. All the insecurities of being faced by a Royal College examination board reappeared and seemed to be just as intense as they had been fifteen years earlier. Happily the outcome was positive.

The added qualification in Geriatric Medicine brought with it the need to have a Specialty Society, and the Canadian Society of Geriatric Medicine was born. I was on the executive at the beginning of the early meetings, and the Society was formally registered in 1981. I was the first Secretary–Treasurer and from 1987 to 1989, the President of the Society. In Canada, we had begun to develop a group of Specialists in Geriatric Medicine, those with a fellowship in Internal Medicine and the Certificate of Competence in Geriatric Medicine, a relatively small number in an 'emerging specialty.' With the growing numbers of elderly people in Canada, it was not the intention that the specialists would look after all these folks themselves, but that primary care physicians would have the bulk of the responsibility, ideally with consultants available. Although the Canadian Society of Geriatric Medicine (CSGM) was not meant to be exclusive, it was not perceived to be inclusive, particularly by family physicians with a special interest in geriatrics. Recently the name of the society has been changed to the Canadian Geriatrics Society and initiatives continue to broaden the base of the Society.

The annual meeting of the CSGM was held at the same time as the annual meeting of the Royal College, and over the years until 2000, the content of the scientific presentations mirrored the development of academic geriatrics in Canada where an increasing number of papers and posters were presented in greater depth and quality by faculty and trainees. In 1991 and 1993, the CSGM supported the Summer Institutes in Geriatrics at UBC, which I organized with additional financial assistance from the National Health Research and Development Program. We recruited students from almost all the university medical schools across Canada and presented an intensive week emphasizing care of the elderly in a very positive way and including material that would be complementary to that ideally found in undergraduate curriculae. The hope was that students would pursue geriatrics as a career, or at least be sympathetic to the needs of geriatric patients as they practised other specialties. This program has continued every two years, first in Toronto and most recently in Manitoba.

It became obvious at UBC that we needed to have more people available to fill the service, education, and research mandate of the division. At length, we recruited some faculty. As well, the training program was reviewed and was the only clinical program to receive commendation by the accreditation team of the Royal College. (Of forty-two programs reviewed at UBC, three received commendation.) Gradually, with our UBC training program, more clinicians and clinical teachers came into geriatric medicine and the Division was able to accomplish more. Strong academic development in terms of research expertise remains a need, but the faculty have excellent reputations as clinicians and teachers. After eighteen years, I stepped down as Division Head at UBC and then Vancouver Hospital, succeeded by Graydon Meneilly. By then we had about fifteen faculty members including our trainees.

In 1984, I was involved in setting up the Clinic for Alzheimer Disease and Related Disorders. This is a multidisciplinary Clinic with a three–part mandate: to provide assessment for referred patients; to provide counselling and recommend management for affected persons; and to be involved in research, either in projects that the Clinic does independently or in projects that Clinic team members are involved with, nationally and internationally. Over the years it has been very fulfilling to work with highly skilled colleagues in neuropsychology, neurology, psychiatry, social work, medical genetics, and other specialties. We accommodate students at all levels— be they undergraduates, trainees in specialty medicine, or apprentices for physicians in practice. When the Clinic first started, there were no specific treatments for Alzheimer disease or other dementias, but we worked hard to listen to the stories of the challenges patients and family members were facing and to refer them to appropriate community services. Longitudinal follow–up is provided as possible. The Clinic has been involved with placebo control trials of potential new treatments, and in 1997, symptomatic treatment for Alzheimer disease was approved in Canada. This has given patients and their families new hope, but many challenges remain.

UBC and Vancouver Hospital have mandatory retirement at sixty-five years, and as I approach this number I look back on a career that has had a lot of excitement and challenges. For a number of years there was great responsibility and the dilemma of being spread too thin. At Shaughnessy Hospital we provided both inpatients and outpatients a full continuum of care with consultation, a geriatric day hospital, and long-term care. This hospital was closed in 1993, but the service needs to remain because it is

Since its inception in the late 1980s, I have been involved with the Canadian Study of Health and Aging, a study involving eighteen centres across Canada and over 10,000 Canadians over the age of sixty-five years.

based on a demographic imperative of increasing numbers of older persons. Jockeying for position in a health care system that is changing all the time and where the resources seem to be shrinking for those who need them most is an uphill battle, particularly for the geriatric clientele. Since its inception in the late 1980s, I have been involved with the Canadian Study of Health and Aging, a study involving eighteen centres across Canada and over 10,000 Canadians over the age of sixty-five years. This study has involved a network of Canadians from many disciplines and greatly enriched the gerontology landscape by giving us information about the citizens we serve. There remain many satisfying aspects of clinical practice, working with wonderful people and their caring families. As well, there are continuing challenges in research and education which must be met. There is always too much to do and too little time. But it is never dull or boring.

We have been remodeling a home on Bowen Island, and I enjoy gardening and other Island activities. Bill remains occupied with a variety of medical and other projects.

I look forward to embarking on our next project, which will be to take the Power Squadron Course and acquire a power boat for intensive coastal cruising. I suspect that this direction will not be dull or boring either.

DR. SUZANNE MONTEMURO

In 1979, I came to Vancouver looking for a job in general practice. My husband, Richard Longpre, had worked in my hometown, Thunder Bay, Ontario, for three years and had recently been transferred back to his hometown of Vancouver.

Fortunately his father, the late Dr. Leo Longpre, a well-respected urologist at Lions Gate Hospital, arranged an interview for me with Dr. Beverly Barron, who had a general practice in West Vancouver. I worked with her until 1982 when I moved to North Vancouver to practise as a solo family doctor. In 1996 Dr. Cara Wilson Haffenden joined me, and our shared practice arrangement has worked well. My affiliation with Lions Gate Hospital has provided a wonderful group of colleagues to work with and learn from.

Working for twenty-two years on the North Shore provided me with many opportunities to interact with this community. A full family practice, which included obstetrics for the first sixteen years, introduced me to many families. As time has passed and my original patients aged, obstetrics seemed less important than attending to the health of mid-life and older women. Cara, therefore, took over the younger side of the practice, including obstetrics, while I developed the North Shore Menopause Information Centre and became involved with the first wave of baby boomers entering menopause. As interest grew in mid-life health, I found that the demand for information was enormous. The Menopause Centre is a non-profit society, staffed by trained volunteers, physicians, and alternative practitioners. Thousands of women have received up-to-date information and a warm reception at the Centre since it opened in 1995. On reflection, it seems that I like to give talks. In the past three years alone I have spoken about women's health at seventy public and medical forums/seminars to over 6,700 people, not including several radio and TV interviews. An added highlight in 1998 was being part of the SOGC writing group for the consensus on menopause and osteoporosis.

If the last twenty-two years of practice have been rewarding, the first few years were fairly challenging. I graduated from Queen's University in 1973, trained in family practice at Foothills Hospital until 1975, and began a part-time practice in Thunder Bay in 1976. Finding a balance between work and family has not been easy. In medical school the balance was definitely 'off,' with considerable negative consequences. I married at the end of second year medicine (1971) and gave birth to my son Reg at the beginning of my fourth year (clinical clerkship). A three-week maternity leave followed by a full clerkship year, then writing LMCCs and starting a fellowship in internal medicine (in Calgary), were overwhelming. As a result the marriage ended and I switched from internal medicine to family practice. Both of these difficult decisions eventually proved fruitful. I moved to Thunder Bay where part-time practice at the Port Arthur Clinic allowed time to raise my son and pursue other educational opportunities. Over this time, women's health became a major part of my practice. Public awareness presentations on breast cancer and other female health issues as well as teaching in the Nursing Science Program at Lakehead University satisfied my love of teaching. The positive feedback I received provided encouragement to continue looking for teaching opportunities when I later moved to Vancouver, I was fortunate to have the opportunity to marry once more, this time to a wonderful understanding man, Richard Longpre. Together we raised Reg and added two daughters, Kate and Michelle. Thanks to Richard and the kids, my life has been more balanced with the medical practice I so enjoy and the love we share within our family. We have had many wonderful trips, summer cottage experiences, and skiing adventures together. All these memories we will always cherish.

Finding the right balance between work and family is a continuous challenge for virtually all working women. 'Burn-out' seems to lurk in the shadows. The ingredients that constantly help me to reset the balance are the following: firstly, having Richard who is confident enough to understand the commitment medicine requires without feeling unimportant. He shares a love of children with a willingness to be an equal partner in their care and education, and is interested in a balanced life as well, so that his work is not 'the only thing.' Secondly, having Reg (1973), Kate (1980), and Michelle (1981). They are all independent and self-confident and they understand that work at times interferes with their plans, but that I love them. They live their lives to the fullest and seemed to learn the importance of balance earlier than I did. Thirdly, having a wonderful group of friends whom I share a wide variety of fun with through hiking, skiing, snowshoeing, and running the notorious Grouse Grind.

I remember on a day in 1987 when Michelle, who was then five, told me she was going to be a doctor when she grew up. Thrilled with this revelation, I asked her what made her want to be a doctor. She answered, "Then I will get to see you more often." I felt deflated. I guess that, once again, the balance in my life needed to be adjusted.

The life of a woman practising medicine has changed significantly over my years. The attitude of most male doctors has changed. One example: when I was in medical school, I ran into the odd 'male chauvinist' who had not realized that women physicians were not 'lesser qualified.' One particularly difficult obstetrician liked to have me fetch him coffee on a regular basis. He was British and must have felt it was like having tea served by the nursing sisters in old England. Trying to be nice, I often brought him a coffee. Well, one day he paged me from the seventh floor to the Outpatient Clinic where I found him sitting with the other male residents discussing various cases. He looked at me and ordered coffee. I carefully poured the coffee and then slowly dumped it on his head. The ensuing chase around the Outpatient Clinic was reminiscent of a "Saturday Night Live" skit. The result was that he stopped asking female medical students to serve him. It was time!

Our children are at university, working and no longer living at home full-time. There is more time to spend with Richard and to explore interests like sports and travel. This has come at a time when slowing down does not seem so bad anymore. Indeed, it is very enjoyable—something I might not have said a few years ago.

Medicine still fascinates me. I see my patients getting older now. They will need assistance to age gently and with dignity. I still have a lot to learn about geriatric health and hope it will be my next frontier of interest.

DR. HOLLY STEVENS

In 1974, I went to medical school at the University of Toronto, having completed a BSc at McMaster University. I was a small town girl from Thunder Bay, Ontario in a class of 250 students, didn't know a soul, and was intimidated beyond belief. The first day of school there was a subway strike in Toronto, so I walked from the Danforth where I rented a room, across the Don Valley Parkway, and on to the University. It was a long walk and I worried all the way there.

Fortunately, being an outstanding student was not a prerequisite for making friends, and the next year I moved into a small four-bedroom house with three other women. It was on Berryman Street, which was in Yorkville. Yorkville was already an upmarket shopping area full of expensive boutiques and galleries, but the gentrification had not yet moved one block north to our street. We lived in a rundown house covered with tarpaper made to look like brick (remember that stuff?) and I paid $90 per month in rent. Nowadays it would cost twice that much to park there.

By the time I was a clinical clerk, we had a group of friends, all women slightly over five feet or less, and we became known as the Five Foot Club. Two of us did an elective in Ear, Nose and Throat at Toronto General

Hospital where we met Dr. Wilf Goodman, the Department Head, a physically imposing man of about six-feet-four, but gentle as a lamb. We all got along very well from the outset. In truth, I didn't have a clue what type of doctor I wanted to become. It was my father who had suggested ENT to me. I assumed that he knew better than I, hence the elective. However, Dr. Goodman was so enthusiastic about the idea I guess it made up my mind.

Since I had been a kid and heard my older brother and his friends romanticizing about Vancouver and Whistler, British Columbia, I wanted to go there. When I applied for an internship at St. Paul's Hospital, however, I never expected to get one. Even then there were far more applicants than positions, and they didn't even do interviews. Maybe that was to my advantage. I'll never know how I got lucky, but I did. I was accepted as a rotating intern.

Along with Mike Woods, a university buddy, and my old rusty skis, I got into my parents' old Camaro (my graduation present), and headed west. It was June, 1978. As things turned out my dreams of Whistler powder never materialized that year. I sustained a tibial plateau compression fracture on my first day downhill (not even at Whistler). I was hospitalized and operated on. Worse, I had to be replaced on the internal medicine rotation I was currently in. (I would later forfeit my holidays to make it up.) As a result, when I was ready to return to work sooner than expected, there was no place for me to go. Then, I got lucky again. There was room in ENT. I hobbled in one day feeling like a bit of a goof to discover that the head there, Dr. P.J. Doyle, had broken his arm and also sported a cast the full length of his limb. This 'commonality' probably had as much to do with me getting into ENT at the University of British Columbia as anything.

Sinonasal surgery does not provide much leeway for error. One is operating between the eyes and below the brain which are an eggshell away.

After completing my internship in 1979, I spent a glorious year doing general practice locums before starting my Residency in ENT in 1980. When I finished that I got a scholarship to do a Fellowship in ENT Allergy. I'd seen so many patients with rhinosinusitis, who allegedly had allergy, I was eager to learn how to treat it. Naively, I thought I could cure them all! I also desperately wanted to return to Vancouver, which I loved, and which fortunately happened to need a "sinus doctor."

I started practice in the summer of 1985 at good old Shaughnessy Hospital. ENT was its own department back in those days, headed by Dr. Nathaniel (Nat) Blair, who even then sub-specialized in allergy and sinonasal disease. Although his methods would be considered archaic today, he was a great sinus surgeon and he taught me well.

Almost by default and not entirely by choice, I became head of ENT at Shaughnessy Hospital. We had a wonderful albeit small department. I'm sure if you asked any of its members today, they would have fond memories of our time there. We had two fantastic, dedicated nurses, Ruth Fraser and Mary Witt, running our ENT ward and the ambulatory clinic respectively. The OR nurses were great, the hospital staff were familiar, friendly, and helpful. It was just a good easy-flowing place to work. I'll never forget the overwhelming dismay I felt that morning in 1993, getting dressed at 6:30 a.m. to go to work, hearing on the radio that our hospital was to be closed. Elizabeth Cull, the then NDP Health Minister, certainly left her mark. It was the first teaching hospital in Canada to be shut down.

The medical, nursing, and all other staff of Shaughnessy were scattered willy-nilly. In order to try to preserve as much of our ENT clinic as possible, I applied for the divisional head position at St. Paul's. I did go there with a couple of the other ENT Clinic staff, but the doctors were separated and we lost our nurse. The atmosphere of our old Shaughnessy Clinic was gone.

The closure of Shaughnessy had been a cost-saving measure and heralded a new period of consolidation, rationalization, regionalization, and cost-cutting. Transfer payments to the provinces from the federal government were being withdrawn to balance the national budget. The province reacted in the name of fiscal accountability, responsibility, and efficiency. In actuality, it was the beginning of the gradual, inexorable deterioration of our health care system that at the turn of this new century we are trying desperately to save.

St. Paul's, albeit an excellent hospital, was a far cry from the small institution I had left as an intern, and its politics seemed much more complicated than what I was used to. Headship and I, I came to realize, did each other no justice. I submitted my resignation in 1996, only three years after I had arrived, left my position in the ENT clinic, and moved across the road to a private office with two of my ENT contemporaries. Moving my practice from the clinic did not otherwise change my relationship with the hospital or the university, and I continued to be integrally involved with the training of both Residents and medical students.

Sinonasal surgery does not provide much leeway for error. One is operating between the eyes and below the brain which are an eggshell away. One needs little imagination to realize that the complications can be catastrophic. The training of Residents in this skill is necessarily a delicate issue. Therefore I often smile to myself when I think of explaining our teaching methods to lay people. How could they understand why someone would go to the morgue at seven in the morning to suck mucous from a cadaver's nose in order to dissect the intranasal anatomy? And while the latter part might be fascinating, the former, if you think about it (which one tried not to), is about as disgusting as it sounds.

If it had not been for Dr. Doyle, I would never have become head at Shaughnessy, since it was on his recommendation that I applied. Obtaining the position, which I suspect he also played a large part in, was the last thing I had expected. Similarly my early involvement with The Canadian Society of Otolaryngology, Head and Neck Surgery was also a result of Dr. Doyle's influence. In 1985, in the first year of my practice, he recommended me to the council as the B.C. provincial representative, a position that I took and held for two terms—ten years. By that time I was so familiar to everyone that I was elected as secretary where I spent another five years. After completing my term in 1999, I became second vice-president. Although it was not originally my intent to become intimately involved with our Canadian Society, I am glad that I did. It has been a valuable learning experience, a means of (trying to) contribute to our specialty, an opportunity to make a number of good friends, and lots of fun.

Similarly, had it not been for my involvement with the council, I might never have been appointed to the Examination Board of the Royal College of Physicians and Surgeons of Canada. I can't say it hasn't been hard work. However, I feel confident that the cause is a good one. The ENT Residents who become the examination candidates work very hard through their years of training, providing invaluable service. Ironically, volunteering as an examiner is one way of paying them back.

Medicine, like all of society, has changed a great deal during my years in practice. I guess I have, too. My medical career has not been glorious, exotic, or heroic. I have tried my best to bide by Osler to "First do no harm." I have taken great satisfaction in small therapeutic victories. When I first decided to become a physician it really was the social aspect and my desire to help that attracted me. I am not convinced in retrospect that ENT was the best choice. Just the same, I would like to believe that my patients for the most part would give me their stamp of approval.

To all those following behind, good luck.

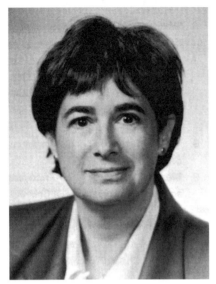

Dr. Vera Frinton, 1970

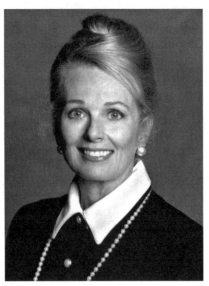

Dr. Linda Warren, 1970

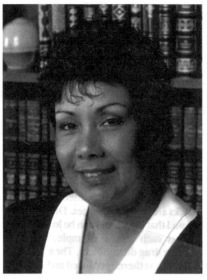

Dr. Hedy Fry, 1971

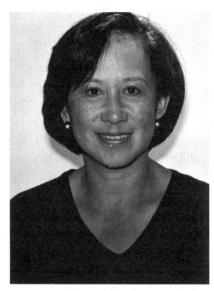

Dr. Lorna Sent, 1971

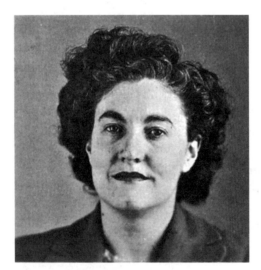

Dr. Mary Marshall Bailey, 1971

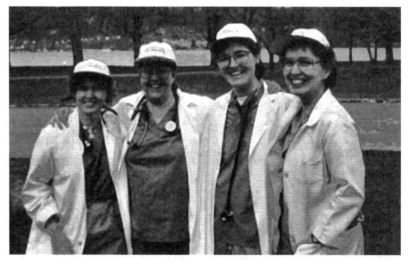

Dr. Rosalie Swart, Dr. Cathy Clelland, Dr. Sheila Fergusson, and Dr. Lianne Lacroix (1972) at the Elizabeth Fry Society Power Walk Relay '96

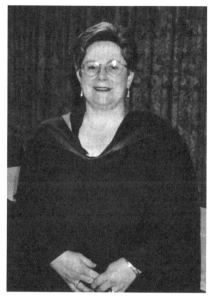

Dr. Shelley Ross, 1974

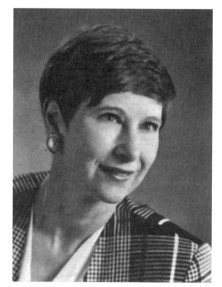

Dr. Jean Swenerton, 1975

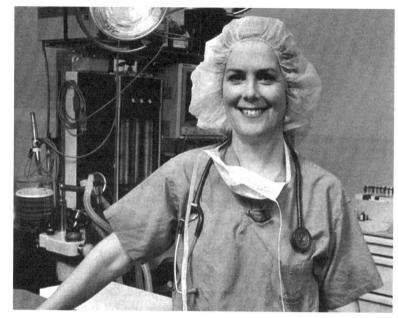

Dr. Lynn Doyle, 1978

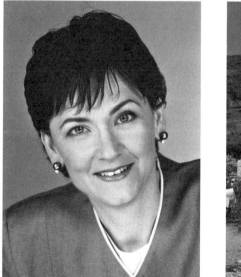

Dr. Maria Hugi, 1979

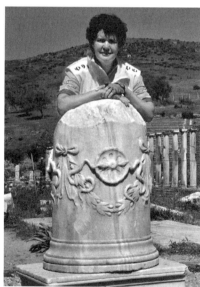

Dr. Valerie White, 1979

Notes from BC MEDICAL JOURNAL 1970 – 1979

January, 1970 Dr. Olive Sadler, West Vancouver, who has been a radio-therapist at the Cancer Clinic at Royal Columbian Hospital, New Westminster since 1951, retired on December 31st, 1969.

New members BCMA include: Dr. Eve Rotem, Vancouver; Dr. Jean McIlveen, Victoria; Dr. Libuse Tyhurst, Vancouver; Dr. Enid Pine, West Vancouver; and Dr. Katherine Mirhady, Vancouver.

Dr. Mary Campbell, a graduate of University of Toronto in 1906 and registered in B.C. in 1910, died January 2, 1970.

February, 1970 Dr. Violet Larsen has died. She graduated from the University of Alberta in 1940, and practised in Saskatchewan. She enrolled in the post-graduate course in anesthesia at UBC in 1954, following which she practised in B .C.

The B.C. Branch FMWC will hold two interesting panel discussions at the Academy of Medicine, Vancouver, March 5th on "Medical Women in Practice" and March 12th on "Frontier Medicine" with guest speaker, Dr. W.D. Watt, Hospital Superintendent, United Church of Canada.

In Creston, B.C. there is a plague of lice among school children. Over 100 people are acting as volunteers checking all school children.

Electoral Districts of BCMA have revised borders as approved at the 1969 Annual Meeting.

March, 1970 Dr. Richard L. Simmons and his wife, Dr. Sandra Simmons, have arrived from Middlesex, England to practise in Creston, B.C. UBC expects 600 applicants for Medicine for 60 places..

April, 1970 There are 2,883 members of BCMA; 274 doctors are not members, including probably half who are retired doctors.

In Oliver, B.C. Dr. Robert Rowed has taken over the practice of Dr. Glen Champion. He will be joined in practice by his wife, the former Dr. Roma Cessford.

St. Paul's Hospital Maternity delivered 1,700 babies last year.

Two Williams Lake doctors, the husband and wife team of Dr. Derek Cooper and Dr. Patricia Anne Cooper, left recently for volunteer service at the same hospital in Dominica, West Indies. The project of volunteer service is sponsored by Canadian Executive Service Overseas and the Canadian Medical Association. Another group, Canadian Overseas Medical Aid, has sent 14 physicians from British Columbia to Dominica since January this year. These volunteer groups were organized to relieve overworked Caribbean colleagues.

Infectious Hepatitis in B.C. increased by eight percent last year over 1968, to more than double the provincial rate of 1966. There were 2,160 cases, compared to 2,000 the year before. Gonorrhea cases increased from 4,200 to 4,800. Dr. W H. Sutherland delivered the 1970 VMA Osler Lecture. His topic: "The New Revolution."

May, 1970 Dr. W.D.S. Thomas of the Department of Obstetrics reports there were 44 maternal deaths from abortions during 14 years, 1955 to 1968. This represents 22.4% of 197 maternal deaths studied during this period. In Victoria the "Live Better" clinic has opened for advice on health issues "to live a little bit better."

The B.C. Branch FMWC elected officers: Dr. Yang-shu (Sue) Hsieh, President; Dr. Patricia Rebbeck, Vice-President; Dr. Joan Ford, Secretary; Dr. Beverley Tamboline, Treasurer; Dr. Beverley Barron, Social Convener; and Dr. Doris Mackay, Past President.

June, 1970 Article on "Extended Care in B.C." by D.G. Adams, BA, MD, CM, Medical Consultant, BCHIS, and Doris Mackay, MD, CRCPC, Medical Consultant BCHIS. There are eleven facilities now for extended care patients; there were none in 1965.

Victoria Medical Society marks the 75th Anniversary. When founded in 1895 there were 29 doctors in Victoria. The Society now represents 270 physicians. New members of BCMA include: Dr. Katherine Costley-White, Vancouver; Dr. Sophie Andriaschuk, Vancouver; and Dr. Ljerka Lisicar, Essondale.

July, 1970 Summer Externship in Kenya: student W.H. Barclay, Med. 4, was met in Nairobi, Kenya, by Dr. Marlene Hunter, formerly of B.C.

Barclay writes for the *Journal* about his experiences: "The Unspoiled Land." Dr. Marlene Hunter is one of two Canadian doctors at Tumutumu Hospital, 80 miles north of Nairobi.

August, 1970 Continuing Education UBC speaker Dr. Betty Poland will give lectures in October at the Royal Jubilee Hospital in Victoria on Obstetrics and Gynecology.

(In the August, 1970 *Journal*, there was a notice by the City of Vancouver advertising for an assistant Medical Health Officer for the Geriatric Program, indicating the requisites "for the man applying for the position"!)

September, 1970 BCMA reports included the report of the Maternal Welfare Committee whose members include Dr. Molly Towell and Dr. Herminia Salvador, with Dr. W.D.S. Thomas as Chairman.

October, 1970 Research Fellowships with grants approved by the Canadian Heart Foundation included three from UBC. Dr. Esther Anderson received one.

November, 1970 New members of BCMA include: Dr. Valerie Priest, Burnaby, and Dr. Elizabeth John, Vancouver.

In the Continuing Education Series Dr. Doris Kavanagh-Gray will give lectures in February, 1971 to the Burnaby doctors on "Acute Cardiac and Pulmonary Problems."

January, 1971 A new Revelstoke Hospital has been opened to replace the 37-bed institution built in 1914. The 60-bed hospital cost $300,000.

New BCMA members include the following women: Dr. Shirley Baker, West Vancouver; Dr. Ruth Gingrich, Bella Coola; Dr. Carol Herbert, Vancouver; Dr. Marjorie Papple, New Westminster; and Dr. Herminia Salvador, Vancouver.

In 1970 there were 1,226 physicians in British Columbia.

February, 1971 Meals on Wheels program in Vancouver and Richmond provided 22,839 meals to home-bound persons in 1970. Volunteers numbered 300 people.

March, 1971 A rubella outbreak occurred in 1970 and a second wave in 1971. Rubella vaccine is available for all children one to 12 years.

This year in Prince Rupert there is a great increase in the number of infectious hepatitis as expected. Peak of the last epidemic was in 1963. At least 400 cases are expected in 1971.

April, 1971 Dr. P.G. Ashmore was the VMA Osler lecturer this year and his title: "If Osler Were Alive Today." This had an amusing anecdote about Johns Hopkins Medical School where a wealthy Baltimore lady gave $500,000 for the medical school with strict qualifications beginning with: "1: That women be admitted to the school on the same basis as men. 2: That the building be designated: The Women's Memorial Fund Building. 3: That a lay committee of six women be appointed to supervise the extracurricular affairs of the women students." The trustees accepted this immediately—half a million bucks is half a million bucks and Osler and his associates found that they could live with it, too.

May, 1971 For the B.C. Centennial Anniversary July 20th babies born in the first 71 minutes of July 20th will be given $100 to commemorate the anniversary of British Columbia entering the Canadian Federation (1871–1971).

Dr. Patricia Rebbeck has been chosen President of the B.C. Branch Federation of Medical Women of Canada (FMWC) for 1971–72. Other officers are: Dr. Joan Ford, Vice-President; Dr. Beverley Tamboline, Secretary; Dr. Gwen Sandy, Treasurer; Dr. Herminia Salvador, Social Convener; and Dr. Yang-shu (Sue) Hsieh, Past President.

July, 1971 District #3 Vice-Delegate BCMA, Dr. Shirley Rushton, has completed her term. Dr. Betty Wood is an officer of the B.C. Radiological Society.

August, 1971 Statistics: Population of British Columbia in 1970 was 2,137,000, an increase of 70,000 over the year before. Birth rate was 17.1 per 1,000 population. Illegitimate births: 13.9%.

New members of BCMA include: Dr. Lynn Nash, Rutland; Dr. Tanya Wulff, Vancouver; and Dr. Marlene Hunter, West Vancouver.

Book Reviews: *Pulmonary Edema in Man and Animals* by Aldo A. Luisada, MD, St. Louis, reviewed by Dr. Doris Kavanagh-Gray. *Technique of Lymphography and Principles of Interpretation* by Hans Kuusk, Publisher: Warren and Green, reviewed by Dr. Vivien Basco.

September, 1971 BCMA Annual Reports: Dr. Molly Towell is a member of the Committee of the Foetus and Newborn; Dr. Herminia Salvador is a member of the Maternal Welfare Committee.

October, 1971 Dr. Margaret Anne Lees was director of the Clinic Day in Powell River, B.C. Dr. Patricia Johnston was elected to the Victoria Medical Society Library Committee.

December, 1971 The new hospital in Kaslo, B.C. opened in December.

January, 1972 BCMA President is Dr. David Bachop.

When it was stated in a previous *Journal* that Kelowna was the first to have a Co-ordinator of Family Life Education Program, Dr. Elizabeth Patriarche, Director of Family Life Education Program in Victoria, wrote to the *Journal* explaining that the Greater Victoria School Board had had a Family Life Education Program since 1964.

February, 1972 New members of BCMA include: Dr. Margaret Ormston, Fort St. John; Dr. Laverne McKinstry, Vancouver; Dr. Norma Calder, West Vancouver; Dr. Patricia Blackshaw, Surrey; Dr. Mary Lee, Vancouver; and Dr. Alvera Witt, Vancouver.

The Travel Clinic of the Children's Hospital reported that 1,768 patients were examined, sixty-five percent of those were for orthopedic consultations.

New Dean of Medicine at UBC is Dr. David Vincent Bates.

April, 1972 Dr. Mary Miller is a member of the Drug and Rehabilitation Committee.

Dr. F.S. Hobbs, MD, is Chairman, Editorial Board of *BCMJ*.

May, 1972 *Journal* article: "Skin Diseases of Indigent Youth in Vancouver" by Dr. Lynne Davies, Dr. Roberta Ongley, and Dr. J.C. Mitchell.

June, 1972 B.C. Branch FMWC elects new officers: President, Dr. Joan Ford; Vice President, Dr. Beverley Tamboline; Secretary, Dr. Frances Forrest-Richards; Treasurer, Dr. Gwen Sandy.

Noted in the *Journal* an advertisement for United Church Home for Girls, Sussex Ave., Burnaby.

August, 1972 "An Appreciation" by Dr. Olive Sadler on the death of Dr. Ethlyn Trapp: "News of her death will start a wave of sorrow among colleagues, friends, and patients which will encircle the earth, but this sorrow will soon give way to happy recollections of shared experiences and pleasant encounters."

Port Alberni, B.C.: Four physicians will take up practice in Port Alberni, including Dr. John Quirk and his wife Dr. Helen Currie, formerly of Woodstock, Ontario.

September, 1972 There is need for a Department of Family Medicine at UBC. Ten of the 16 medical schools have either an established or approved formal Department of Family Practice.

The new Medical will contain Billing Numbers of Doctors.

Dr. Patricia Baird, Department of Genetics, is requesting reports of cases of infant congenital gastroschisis for her studies.

B.C. Branch FMWC members are to meet at the home of Dr. Josephine Mallek, Oct.12th, to hear Dr. Erica Crichton speak on The Hastings Report.

October, 1972 *Journal* article: "Preventable Deaths due to Hemolytic Disease of Newborns in B.C. (September, 1965 to December, 1969)," by R. Elizabeth Manning, MD and A.F. Hardyment, MD, CRCPC.

December, 1972 Dr. Gladys Story Cunningham, BA, MD, MCOG, FRCOG, died on September 8, 1972.

January, 1973 Dr. Kenneth Hill is the President of BCMA.

Dennis Cocke is B.C.'s Health Minister. Telex has been installed in the Academy of Medicine and College Library.

February, 1973 Gonorrhea is now of epidemic proportions in Canada. The highest rate is in the Northwest Territories, the Yukon Territory, and the four western provinces.

New BCMA members include Dr. Mary Robb, Pot Hardy, B.C. and Dr. June Steinson, New Westminster.

March, 1973 The Age of Consent has been lowered from 19 to 16 years.

April, 1973 Dr. Richard Foulkes is giving sessions defending the Hastings Report during April and May, 1973.

Total Population in B.C. in 1972 was 2,247,000, an increase of 62,000.

May, 1973 Women MDs are trying to get the same Disability Insurance as men MDs. Dr. Joan Ford, the immediate Past President of the B.C. Branch FMWC, led the women doctors in requesting that their $600 per month be extended to equal that of the male doctors for both Plan I and Plan XI. The coverage at present for female members is limited to $600 per month as a benefit of Plan I (three years for sickness and lifetime for accident). The limit is extended for females who provide evidence that they are the sole support of themselves and their families. The B.C. Branch has recommended to the Insurance Company that coverage be extended for females on both Plan I and Plan XI, with payment of added premium to take into account the additional risk (actuarial tables show a higher rate of disability for females under 50 years of age than for males).

At the Annual Meeting of the B.C. Branch FMWC Dr. Beverley Tamboline was elected President. Other officers were: Dr. Frances Forrest-Richards, Vice President; Dr. Hedy Fry, Secretary; Dr. Roberta Ongley, Treasurer. Social Conveners were Dr. Laverne McKinstry and Dr. Anne Derks.

June, 1973 New BCMA members include Dr. Patricia Chipperfield, Burnaby; Dr. Judith Dowd, Vancouver; Dr. Wendy Fidgeon, Surrey; Dr. Catriona D. MacLean, Vancouver; Dr. Olive Sinclair, Essondale; Dr. Avelina Tuason, Essondale.

July, 1973 Dr. Molly Towell, Associate Professor of Obstetrics and Gynecology, gave a report from her UBC research on "Toward New Knowledge of Effects of Stress on Delivery of the Fetus."

New BCMA members include: Dr. Gerda Allison, Vancouver and Dr. Wendy Palmer, Victoria.

August, 1973 Dr. Doris Mackay was elected Chairman of the Section of Physical Medicine and Rehabilitation at the Annual Meeting of BCMA.

New BCMA members include: Dr. Anna Albrecht, Comox; Dr. Adele Evans, Vancouver; Dr. Ulana Farmer, Vancouver; Dr. Frances Galvon, Calgary; Dr. Jeanine Olsen, Essondale; Dr. Eleanor Payne, Vancouver; Dr. Connie Mei Sui, Vancouver; Dr. Edith Trachsel, Kamloops.

September, 1973 Outpatient Ambulatory Services begin at Vancouver General Hospital. New BCMA members in September include Dr. Lorena Kanke, Vancouver.

October, 1973 *Journal* article by Drs. Linda Warren and Walter Knickerbocker, Department of Radiology: "Polypoid Pyelitis Cystica."

There were 65 cases of Hansen's Leprosy in Canada on record, July 1973, with 63 from the Far East. In British Columbia there were nine cases.

November, 1973 New members of BCMA include: Dr. Marion Ferguson, Kamloops; Dr. Tonka Kamburoff, New Westminster; Dr. Linda Ottley, Vancouver; Dr. Adele Preto, Salmon Arm.

Winners of the 1973 Upjohn Post-Graduate Study Awards for British Columbia are Dr. Ilse Destrube, Victoria; Dr. W. Mitchell-Banks, Prince Rupert; Dr. D. M. Miller, Courtenay.

January, 1974 *Journal* article: "Whipple's Disease" by Mary Trott MD and Helen Emmons MD. Both doctors are from the Department of Diagnostic Radiology.

Dr. Wendy Fidgeon topped the polls in the recent school board elections in Surrey. There are 30 mental health centres located throughout

B.C., 20 of which were opened during the past four years. Boarding Home program has 1,450 patients in 200 boarding homes. The number of patients in Riverview have continued to decrease from 1966 to 1973.

Shaughnessy Hospital is now B.C. Medical Centre at the Shaughnessy Hospital Site as announced by Dennis Cocke, Minister of Health.

February, 1974 There have been 200 cases of diphtheria in B.C., 82 in Victoria. There have been six cases of polio since 1972. Gonorrhea has increased by fifteen percent from 1972 to 1973. Dr. Elspa Davies, anesthetist, died at age 39, on February 16th in Burnaby.

The February *Journal* discusses the summarized Foulkes report. The report came out three and a half months late and at a cost of one-half million dollars. It contains 1,100 pages, and is condensed for the public.

New members of BCMA include: Dr. Mary Davidson, Vancouver; Dr. Jean Lee, Essondale; Dr. Sharylee Barnes, Vancouver; Dr. Patricia Montano, Queen Charlotte Islands.

March, 1974 For more than 80 years the United Church of Canada (or its predecessors, the Methodists and Presbyterians) has been operating acute care hospitals in coastal and northern areas of British Columbia. In 1974 there are 11 full time physicians and final year medical students looking after several thousand people. Dr. Donald Watt is Superintendent of Hospitals and Medical Work, United Church of Canada.

April, 1974 The Greater Vancouver Mental Health Project West End at Harwood St. has psychiatrist, Dr. Ingrid Pacey in charge.

Fifteen percent of practising doctors in B.C. are graduates of UBC Medical School. Thirty-three percent are foreign medical graduates from the U.K., U.S.A, Eire, Australia, New Zealand, and South Africa. Eight percent are from other countries. The balance of forty-four percent are from the rest of Canada.

Over half the doctors in B.C. have Royal College Certification or Fellowship. As of September, 1973, there are 3,651 practising physicians in British Columbia.

New BCMA members include: Dr. Miriam Schaffrin, Vancouver; Dr.

Helen Penny, Victoria; Dr. Mary Norris, Langley; Dr. Molly Towell, Vancouver; Dr. Linda Warren, Vancouver.

May, 1974 The Health Budget this year is $548 million. CU&C and MSA health insurance companies are now transferred to Government coverage. Dr. Hector Gillespie is the President of BCMA 1974–1975. District #6 Vice-Delegate is Dr. Patricia Blackshaw.

June, 1974 The Vancouver General Hospital purchases an EMI Scanner for $350,000. BCMA dues rise to $40, beginning 1975. There were 9,000 legal abortions performed in British Columbia in 1972.

From January to March 1974, there were 163 persons in B.C. with toxigenic strains of corynebacterium diphtheria. Most of these were asymptomatic carriers.

July, 1974 Dr. Frances Forrest-Richards, Victoria, has been elected President of B.C. Branch FMWC. She succeeds Dr. Beverley Tamboline, Vancouver. Dr. Hedy Fry is Vice President, Dr. Roberta Ongley is Secretary, and Dr. Tanya Wulff is Treasurer. Fire destroys most of the top floor of the BCMA section of the Academy of Medicine building.

In Memorium: Dr. Lillian Fowler died June 23, 1974. She was the first woman anesthetist to be honoured by an appointment to the consulting staff of the Vancouver General hospital in 1920. She worked at VGH for 25 years.

August, 1974 Dr. Carolyn McGhee is Medical Director of the Child Development Centre in Prince George, B.C. Dr. Moira Chen-Yeung MB, FRCP(C) is one of the authors of the *Journal* article: "Rehabilitating Patients with Chronic Airway Obstruction."

Case Report by Dr. Betty Wood and Dr. T.O. Myolwin: "Nitrofurantoin Lung in a Child."

Rubella cases are on the increase, 140 in six months. Drs. Dale Stogryn and Joan Strogryn completed internship at the Royal Columbian Hospital and have a contract with the provincial government for a two-month service in Rivers Inlet and Port Renfrew. This is a summer medical service for 3,000 fishermen in coastal areas and 2,000 working out of Rivers Inlet.

Dr. Heather Watson, McBride, B.C., has been awarded a $2000 research fellowship at B.C. Cancer Institute. She will be studying effects of lymphography on the lungs. Dr. F.S. Hobbs retires from medical practice after 42 years service in Obstetrics and Gynecology.

September, 1974 B.C. women doctors entertain women medical students, interns, and residents September 19, 1974, at 8 p.m., at the home of Dr. Roberta Ongley, Secretary of the B.C. Branch FMWC.

New members of BCMA include: Dr. Diane Banikhin, Vancouver; Dr. Mavis Burrows, Calgary; Dr. Barbara Copping, Dr. Claire Hamilton, Dr. Hilary King-Lam Hui, Dr. Hilary Lee, Dr. Gillian Lockitch, Dr. Lea Manraj, Dr. Ingrid Pacey, all of Vancouver; Dr. Theresa Patterson, Salmon Arm; Dr. Joan Stogryn, New Westminister.

October, 1974: Dr. Josephine Mallek will be guest speaker at the Annual Dinner Meeting of the B.C. Medical-Legal Society, October 17, at the Marine Drive Golf Club.

November, 1974 The book *The Indomitable Lady Doctors* was reviewed by Dr. Frances Forrest-Richards. She notes that in early Canadian medical history many women graduates became medical missionaries in India and China, as there was the difficulty of licensure in Canada. Many hospitals in Canada would not offer internship to women graduates. Of the 200 women graduates in 1913, one quarter became medical missionaries. Dr. Maude Abbott, a Canadian who was world famous for her knowledge of congenital heart disease, was not allowed to present her first paper to the Medico-Chirurgical Society. It had to be read for her by a male member as women were not admitted to the Society in Montreal.

B.C. Medical Centre is one year old. Its purpose is to integrate and co-ordinate health care delivery of seven autonomous institutions in the Greater Vancouver Area: G.F. Strong, Vancouver General Hospital, UBC Health Sciences Centre, B.C. Cancer Treatment and Research Foundation, St. Paul's Hospital, Shaughnessy Hospital, and Children's Hospital.

Beds were reduced by ten percent from 1,700 to 970 at VGH. Shaughnessy Hospital is to expand its number of beds.

Diane Dahlman MD, a graduate of Memorial University, St. John's, who interned at VGH assumed duties with the Worker's Compensation Board as adviser to claims adjudication will be responsible for the medical care in the health unit.

Dr. Betty Poland, Associate Professor of Obstetrics and Gynecology, with the assistance of Dr. J. Miller's help, will conduct a study into the effects of contraceptives on later planned pregnancies. Sixty doctors will assist in the study.

All of the 80 students entering UBC Faculty of Medicine this fall are either Canadian citizens, or landed immigrants of several years duration.

The B.C. Branch FMWC is hosting the Annual Professional Women's Dinner at Hyatt Regency Hotel on November 14, 1974. The speaker is Judge Nancy Morrison.

December, 1974 Drs. Gillian A. Bowers and Leslie S. Bowers, British-trained practitioners, will set up offices in the ski patch First Aid huts.

There were 30 women doctors who became members of BCMA listed in the December *Journal*, a record number.

January, 1975 There are 10,910 doctors in general practice in Canada.

Vancouver physicians, Dr. Mel Shaw and Dr. Peter Allan, recently installed the first rechargeable heart pacemaker in Canada.

It was a great success when Drs. Dale and Joan Stogryn were sent as doctors to join the fishing fleet at Rivers Inlet and Port Renfrew following an appeal from the United Fisherman and Allied Workers' Union. The Drs. Stogryn have recommended the program be repeated next year.

February, 1975 Dr. Monica Shackleton has been named Medical Officer of Health, North Shore Union Board of Health.

March, 1975 In Memoriam: Dr. Eleanor May Pine of Vancouver died suddenly January 19, 1975.

Dr. Margaret Hutton of Victoria is a consultant with Dr. A.F. Hardyment's Prenatal Program of British Columbia.

April, 1975 Guest Editorial of *BCMJ* of April 17th by Dr. Frances Forrest-Richards MD, FRCP(C). She is the President of the B.C. Branch

Federation of Medical Women of Canada. She titles the editorial "A Prescription for Women." In 1967, the United Nations declared 1975 International Women's Year. "With that much time for planning, you'd think it would have begun with more of a splash, but the slow dribble of interest so far no doubt indicates the measure of low priority the status of women has. When all the rest of the world's problems are solved then and only then we'll look to the problems of women.

"Physicians know that women make up the majority of their practice. Do women get the priority of time and effort that these numbers merit? Are they being fobbed off with tranquilizers to dull the edge of frustration of doing equal (and often more) work for less pay, at being passed over for promotions, at coping with child-rearing, of living in a kitchen ghetto, at being 'put down' as stupid after putting hubbie through college?

"What do women want, you may say?

"Have you ever listened, really listened long enough to find out? It may not be a job, a career, a new house, a trip, another baby. It could be simply the freedom to be.

"Charity begins at home, they say. A good start for consciousness-raising in 1975 could be to look at (and listen to) the artificial lives of doctors' wives, the humiliation of the deserted wife, the low pay and high level of responsibility of the office receptionist, the ambiguity of the position of 'the other woman,' the pre-mastectomy patient abandoned to her fears.

"It is unlikely that the conservative medical profession will ever be a radical force for social change, but at least it could be less resistant to change in the perpetuation of the status quo.

"Try listening to yourself. Have you ever called a menopause patient 'girl' or 'honey'?

"Ever tell a young woman it's a 'waste of time and money' to stretch her brain at college or university because she'll 'only get married anyway'? Ever address your female colleagues in a letter as 'Gentlemen' instead of 'Doctor' or 'Colleague'? Ever tell a woman who is going to lose a breast that she's 'got another'? Ever oppose pregnancy leave and insurance because 'men don't get pregnant'? Ever say 'she thinks like a man'?

"Let's approach International Women's Year with something new in the way of prescription for women. Instead of pills to dull the mind and still the emotions arising out of social inequities, let's prescribe a listening ear, an open mind, a non-judgmental attitude mixed with a large amount of understanding."   —*Frances Forrest-Richards MD, FRCP(C), Victoria.*

In B.C. there are more Ontario-trained doctors than B.C.-trained doctors. Canadian-trained doctors in B.C. are 2,600, with 709 from Ontario Schools and 644 from UBC.

May, 1975   Dr. June E. Steinson of New Westminster died February 26, 1975. Maternal deaths drop about fifty percent over five years. Home deliveries to be considered "as a retrograde step in maternal care." There is no licensed midwife or flying squad available in B.C. as noted by Dr. Jon Schonblom, Chairman of the Maternal Welfare Committee.

Dr. J.M. Stephenson, Chairman of the Child Care Committee, states "Considerable difficulty has been reported in Vancouver in finding someone willing to accept reports of abuse."

May, 1975   Residents and interns are on strike in seven B.C. hospitals (300 residents). Ninety-four percent of PARI members voted for strike. Dr. Craig Beattie is President of PARI (Professional Association of Interns and Residents). The residents and interns are asking for parity with Ontario residents and interns.

July, 1975   Scoliosis referrals are requested by Dr. Judith Hornung who is doing a pilot study on students from Grade 5 through Grade 7.

More than 500 people attended an education forum in Prince George in May, 1975 to hear Dr. Adele Evans and Dr. Stewart Jackson of the B.C. Cancer Control Agency, Vancouver, and Dr. Tully Chambers of Prince George, discuss causes, prevention, and treatment of cancer.

August, 1975   BCMA fees are now $50 for members. In the 1975 medical class at McMaster University there are 52 women and 48 men.

September, 1975   Mr. J.E. Gilmore, BCMA Director of Communications, attends many meetings and he writes, "Something is missing. Where are all the women physicians? There are 300 of them in B.C. and not a single meeting where there was a woman physician sharing in the decision-making. It is 29 years since Dr. Ethlyn Trapp was President of BCMA. Are there no more Ethlyn Trapps out there?"

Dr. Marian Sherman, 84, Victoria, a gynecologist, who was one of the first women Fellows of the Royal College of Surgeons (England), has become the third person to win the Humanist Association of Canada Award. The award will be presented at the Association's convention in Ottawa in June.

October, 1975 *Journal* article by Frances Forrest-Richards MD, FRCPC on "Health Education for Women."

The B.C. Branch Federation of Medical Women of Canada has sponsored organized Medical Seminars for Women in B.C. The first one is in Vancouver at the Queen Elizabeth Theatre, October 18, 1975, and the second one is March, 1976. The program: "Physiology," Dr. Mirian Schaffrin; "Birth Control," Dr. Hedy Fry; "Venereal Disease," Dr. Elizabeth Whynot; "Abortion," Dr. Shirley Rushton; "Vaginitis," Dr. Lori Kanke; "Skin and Hair," Dr. Roberta Ongley; "Nutrition and Obesity," Dr. John A. Hunt; "Breast Cancer," Dr. Patricia Rebbeck; "Some Aspects of Psychiatric Illness," Dr. Libuse Tyhurst.

The Seminar in Victoria takes place October 19, 1975, with three panels on: "The Breast," "Food and Health," "Ages and Stages." In Courtney in November a seminar will be held with speakers Dr. Mary Wertheim and Dr. Pamela Aldis. A seminar will be held in Kamloops, February, 1976.

November, 1975 In reply to Mr. Gilmore's letter in the September, 1975 *Journal* Dr. Hedy Fry, President of B.C. Branch FMWC, writes, "Women doctors simply do not have the time to attend meetings. We are also housewives and mothers, serious 'feminine' women with no time for mundane activities like community involvement of BCMA."

Dr. Ruth Khim joined the staff of Worker's Compensation Board in September, 1975. She is a graduate of McGill University and has a Fellowship in Physical Medicine and Rehabilitation from the Royal College. Dr. Diane Dahlman left the WCB in March, 1975 to accompany her husband who has joined the staff of Imperial Oil in Toronto. Dr. Hedy Fry was elected Vice President of the Federation of Medical Women of Canada at the Annual Meeting in Calgary. Dr. Fry is President of the B.C. Branch

FMWC. The *BCMA Journal* has an excellent series of eight articles on current concepts in Medical Genetics.

December, 1975 Dr. Patricia Baird and Dr. Betty Poland are among the co-authors of the article "Genetics in Medicine in B.C."

There were 86 new members of BCMA in 1975; 37 were women who are working in Campbell River, Gillies Bay, Kamloops, Masset, Port McNeil, Powell River, Terrace, Trail, Victoria, as well as in the Lower Mainland.

January, 1976 The Free Pine Clinic is located on 1985 West 4th Ave. In charge of the clinic are Dr. Elizabeth Whynot and Dr. Art Hister.

Pharmacare was introduced by the NDP Government. Dr. Tanya Wulff, the Communications representative for the B.C. Branch FMWC, attended. In the first year class entering Medical School at UBC in 1976 there are twenty-four percent women. College of Physicians and Surgeons of British Columbia: In the college report of 1976 it was the first time doctors were documented as 'he or she' rather than all 'he' in most reports and speeches in the past. Postal codes introduced in January, 1976.

February, 1976 R. H. McLelland has been appointed Health Minister by the Social Credit Government of British Columbia.

March, 1976 873 candidates applied to UBC Faculty of Medicine 80 positions. Of those applying, 415 were from B.C.

April, 1976 Incorporation discussions begin for BCMA and doctors.

Project Scoliosis screening continues with Dr. Judith Hornung in charge. It has been announced that the controversial B.C. Medical Centre will not be built. The officers of the B.C. Chapter of the College of Family Physicians of Canada include Dr. Judy Hornung of Vancouver.

Provincial population is nearing two and a half million, (2,457,000) June 1, 1975. There was an increase of 64,000 over that of 1974. The province's population has doubled in the period since 1952.

Amendment re: landed immigrant physicians: They are now required to practise in an area of need for three years, or until Canadian citizenship is obtained, whichever comes first.

Human Rights Commission is to inquire into the propriety of the College requiring immigrant physicians to practise in areas of need.

June, 1976 Dr. Hedy Fry, President of B.C. Branch FMWC, reports that women doctors are available for part-time work and many would share offices.

August, 1976 The College of Physicians and Surgeons was ordered to cease and desist and to remove all geographic restrictions for immigrant doctors. The top two UBC medical graduates in 1976 were Jack Taunton and Susan Tha. Dr. Roberta Ongley of Vancouver is the newly elected President of the B.C. Branch FMWC. Vice President, Dr. Tanya Wulff; Secretary, Dr. Vera Frinton; Treasurer, Dr. Mirian Schaffrin.

September, 1976 Dr. Shirley Rushton of Vancouver worked at the Clinic sites during the Olympic Games in Montreal.

October, 1976 An article in the *Journal* by Dr. Moira Yeung for the Tuberculosis and Respiratory Disease Association on: "Survey of sawmill workers exposed to red cedar and other wood dusts."

Extended Care to open at UBC hospital. Dr. Doris Mackay is medical consultant for long-term care.

November, 1976 *Journal* articles with Dr. Gwen Ballantyne and Dr. Carol Miller among the authors on "Breast Cancer in B.C." including "Planning Rehabilitation" and "Negative Mammogram—What Does it Mean?"

December, 1976 Dr. Patricia Johnston is the Honorary Secretary of the Victoria Medical Society. Dr. Sarah (Sally) Hemming is now the Burnaby Health Officer. She was formerly assistant MHO with the Vancouver City Health Department. New members of BCMA include 56 women doctors.

January, 1977 The Epidemiological Oncology Unit is based in the Department of Health Care and Epidemiology at UBC. It is led by Dr. Brenda Morrison, biostatistician, and epidemiologists Drs. Mark Elwood and Michael Verner.

Dr. William Jory is President of BCMA.

There is an increase in Giardiasis in British Columbia. Doctors advise treatment with quinacrine, metronidazole, or furzolidine.

BCMA Section of Obstetrics and Gynecology has asked its Chairman, Dr. Lori Kanke, Vancouver, to write to department heads in hospitals throughout the province concerning home deliveries. She also will ask the department heads to meet with the hospital officials to try to find ways to make hospital stays more acceptable to the kinds of care now requested by the public.

Cervical cancer accounted for sixty-two percent of 1,144 uterine cancer deaths in the 1963–1974 period.

The BCMA officers for 1977, and its 28 affiliated societies, have only two women: Dr. Roberta Ongley, President of the B.C. Branch FMWC and Dr. Hedy Fry, Vice President of the Federation of Medical Women of Canada. (This confirms James Gilmour's observation in the September *Journal* "that there were no women physicians sharing in decision making.")

February, 1977 The Seat Belt law passed in British Columbia.

"Drugs used in the Treatment of Asthma" by Moira Yeung MB, FRCP(C) and Stefan Grzybowski MD, FRCP(C) was printed in the February *Journal*.

The Canadian Medical Association and the Australian Medical Association plan a combined meeting in September, 1980, in Vancouver.

March, 1977 Dr. Carol Miller, Radiologist and Ultrasound specialist, interviewed by the New Westminster newspaper *The Columbian* states, "Ultrasound is a good preliminary procedure because it eliminates use of dyes, enemas, and exposing of the body to radiation." Sixty percent of her patients are obstetrical.

April, 1977 *Journal* articles: "Cancer in Children; An Overview" by Dr. J. Mavis Teasdale MB, ChB, DCH, FRCP(C), Pediatric Oncologist and Dr. Vivien Basco MD, ChB, FRCR, FRCP(C), Radiation Oncologist; "Leukemia and lymphoma" by Drs. J. Mavis Teasdale, E. Barton, S. Israels, D.F. Smith, and Vivien Basco; "Solid Tumors in Childhood" by Drs. P.C. Rogers, Vivien Basco, P.G. Ashmore, and D.M. Chan.

Dr. David Boyce is the new head of Cancer Control Agency of British Columbia. Dr. Thelma Cook is St. Paul's Hospital Trustee to Vancouver Regional District's Hospital Advisory Committee.

Rubella article: "A clinical statement prepared by an expert subcommittee of the Perinatal Programme of British Columbia under the chairmanship of D.M. Kettyls MD, DPH, FRCPC. The membership: Dr. Molly Towell, Dr. Sydney Segal, Dr. Margaret Pendray, Dr. P.J. MacLeod, Dr. A.F. Hardyment, Dr. Herminia Salvador, and Dr. T.D. Stout."

The *BCMJ* Editorial Board for 1977: Dr. F.S. Hobbs, Chairman; Dr. A.F. Hardyment; Dr. W.A.H. Dodd; Dr. W.J. Mitchell; Dr. D.W. Jones; Dr. R. Pratt.

May, 1977 A Forum Panel on "Cancer" with Moderator, Dr. Graham Clay, a cancer surgeon at Vancouver General Hospital and Chairman of the BCMA Cancer Committee. The panel includes four specialists: Dr. Linda Warren, radiologist and instructor in radiology at UBC; Dr. Ann Worth, Director of Pathology at the Cancer Control Agency of B.C.; Dr. F.R.C. Johnstone, Professor of Surgery at UBC; and Dr. Ian Plenderleith, Head of Medical Oncology at CCABC. The forum was held at Queen Elizabeth Theatre, sponsored by the *Vancouver Sun* newspaper in co-operation with BCMA and Yukon Division of the Canadian Cancer Society. There were 2,100 in attendance.

Dr. Doris Kavanagh-Gray was chosen as the VMA Osler Orator for the 56th Annual Osler Dinner. Dr. Kavanagh-Gray is the Head of Cardiology Division at St. Paul's Hospital and Clinical Associate Professor, Faculty of Medicine UBC. She is the second woman to present the address in 56 years. (Dr. Ethlyn Trapp was the first). Her topic: "Health: The Reward for Individual Endeavor." The lecture is printed in the August *BCMJ*.

June, 1977 Six scholarships donated by Burroughs Welcome to medical students across Canada are $1,200 each. Medical student Cynthia E. Lauriente, UBC, was awarded one of them. The scholarships are designed to help medical students pursue supervised research projects during the summer.

A $25,000 grant for study of fetal movements in normal and abnormal pregnancies has been given to researchers Dr. Molly Towell and Dr. Bernard Wittman by the B.C. Christmas Seal Society to cover the capital cost of an ultrasonic scanner which monitors fetal movements in the womb.

Dr. Honor Mary Kidd died April 27, 1977, at age 70. Her medical interests centered on Pathology and Research investigations which she carried on for many years.

August, 1977 Dr. William Webber has been appointed Dean of Medicine at UBC. Dr. Patricia Johnston, Victoria, agrees with Dr. Peter Banks that the proposed split of Victoria General Hospital into a northern and southern division is an expensive and potentially dangerous mistake.

October, 1977 Dr. W. McClure, Registrar of the College of Physicians and Surgeons of British Columbia, is retiring at the end of 1977. Dr. Craig Arnold, Deputy Registrar, succeeds him as Registrar.

December, 1977 Vancouver surgeon, Dr. Patricia Rebbeck, has joined the Editorial Board of the *British Columbia Medical Journal*.

Dr. C.E. McDonnell writes articles on B.C. Medical History in the September, October, and November *Journal*, which are most interesting reading. Items include, "At the time of incorporation of the City of Vancouver in April, 1886, four physicians formed the basis of private practice in Vancouver," and "Medical care on Burrard Inlet in the years 1877 to 1882."

In 1977, new members of BCMA include the greatest number of women doctors—41 of the total of 308 new members.

January, 1978 Dr. F.S. Hobbs, Editor of the reports in 1977 there were 51 papers published by the *BCMJ*: 15 scientific, 23 general medical and 13 features. British Columbia Medical Association now has 5,500 members.

Journal article by Dr. Moira Yeung, Associate Professor of Medicine UBC, and Dr. Stefan Grzybowski, Professor, Department of Medicine, UBC: "Study into effects of grain dust exposure in B.C. grain elevators."

Facilities of WCB Rehabilitation Clinic have moved from Heather St., Vancouver to Richmond, and renamed Leslie R. Peterson Rehabilitation Centre.

February, 1978 There were 19 cases of tuberculous meningitis in British Columbia. Four were under five years of age.

March, 1978 In Memorium: Dr. Wan Ching Rebecca Woo died November 6, 1977. Dr. Helena Bozena died November 12, 1977.

April, 1978 The Prince George Regional Hospital development will cost four million dollars. A 48 bed Detoxification Centre opened in Vancouver.

In 1977, 46 B.C. doctors left B.C. for the U.S.A., nine specialists and 37 general practitioners. *Journal* article: "Emotional Sequelae of Elective Abortion" by Ian Kent MD, FRCPC, R.C. Greenwood MD, Janice Loeken MD, and W. Nicholl MA (Cantab).

May, 1978 A Public Forum took place in New Westminster on: "What's new in Cancer." Panelists were Dr. R.W. Dunn, Dr. Joan Ford, Dr. Gerald Coursley, Dr. James Glezos, and Dr. Michael Noble.

June, 1978 Dr. Patricia Rebbeck is on the Board of Directors, BCMA as a District #3 delegate. Dr. Hedy Fry and Dr. Beverley Tamboline are vice-delegates District #3.

B.C. Branch FMWC members giving radio talks and on panels: Drs. Tanya Wulff, Hedy Fry, Bev Tamboline, Shirley Rushton, Vera Frinton, Pat Blackshaw, Betty Poland, Dorothy McWatters, Elizabeth Whynot, Sue Stephenson, Frances Forrest-Richards, Betty Patriarche, Roberta Ongley, Pat Johnston, and Ellen Wiebe.

There are 500 women doctors now in B.C. and a growing number are participating in medical affairs.

June, 1978 Comment by James E. Gilmore, Director of Communications: "Comes the Revolution. First it was bumper stickers, and then it was t-shirts . . . and now it is a woman on the Board of Directors. Is nothing sacred anymore?

"You may have missed it in the election results—Dr. P.M. Rebbeck elected in District #3. Spelled out it reads Dr. Patricia Mary Rebbeck, who also happens to be B.C.'s lone woman general surgeon. Greybeards confirm that Dr. Rebbeck is only the second woman to gain entry to the Board

chambers although the first, the revered Dr. Ethlyn Trapp, went right to the top and was BCMA President in 1946.

"For B.C. watchers, and more particularly, for BCMA woman doctor watchers, the signs have been there for some time. Dr. Rebbeck's vote-getting was not an isolated breakthrough, for a growing number of women doctors have been speaking out—as all doctors should—on matters affecting their profession and the public.

"While the Federation of Medical Women has been the rallying point, by no means has it been the only platform for leaders of the 500 women MDs in B.C. Radio talk shows, television interviews, health forums, Society and District delegate elections, and Planned Parenthood are just some of their activities. And Dr. Rebbeck preceded her election by being appointed to the Editorial Board of the *Journal* last year, another trail-blazing first for female physicians.

"Out front with Pat Rebbeck are Tanya Wulff, Hedy Fry, Bev Tamboline, Pat Blackshaw, Betty Poland, Dorothy McWatters, Elizabeth Whynot, Sue Stevenson, Roberta Ongley, Pat Johnston, Ellen Wiebe, Frances Forrest-Richards, and Betty Patriarche. There are more, but you get the idea.

"While we do not wish to make too big a thing about a woman being elected to the Board of Directors, it is a good omen for the future."

In June, 1978, Dr. Bluma Tischler, Medical Director of Woodlands School, was awarded the 1978 Research Award of the American Association of Mental Deficiency, for her development of a new method of detecting and treating a rare disease, phenylketonuria. In the 102-year history of the award only one other Canadian has received it.

July, 1978 Dr. F.S. Hobbs, Editor and Board Chairman of the *B.C. Medical Journal* for the past 12 years has announced his decision to resign.

Journal article on "Lymphoma Diagnosis," with Dr. Ann Worth as co-author.

New executive of B.C. Branch FMWC: President, Dr. Vera Frinton; Past President, Dr. Tanya Wulff; Vice President, Dr. Shelley Ross; Secretary, Dr. Marion Akrigg; Treasurer, Dr. Lorena Kanke; Public Relations, Dr. Hedy Fry; Social Convener, Dr. Jean Carruthers.

President of Planned Parenthood of B.C., Dr. Dorothy McWatters, comments that it is ironic that three million dollars are spent on therapeutic abortions, but nowhere near that on preventive programs.

Penny Ballam of the 1978 graduating class in medicine at UBC is the winner of the Hamber Medal. She had the highest cumulative record of all the years of the medical program.

Dr. Margaret Buchanan Forster Sylling died in Vancouver on May 5, 1978, at age 79 years.

Dr. E.C. McCoy, former executive director of BCMA and now President, MD Management Ltd., has been awarded a Commemorative Medal in honour of the 25th anniversary of Her Majesty's reign.

Fort St. John: Working with Dr. Margaret Ormston of Fort St. John, B.C. this summer will be Janet Kusler, second year medical student at UBC, under a program to encourage medical students to practise in rural areas when they graduate. Supporting students in the program is the Provincial Government, while the Royal Canadian Legion is donating $40,000 a year to UBC Department of Family Practice, which is organizing the program. A fellow student, Kathleen Malloy, will be working with Dr. Anthony Kenyon in Fort Nelson.

Journal article: "Five year survey of lip cancer seen at BCCI 1960–1965" by Frances Lai-Wah Wong, BSc (third year medical student at UBC) and Stewart Jackson MD, FRCP.

August, 1978 The suggestion that patients sign their own insurance cards stirred the ire of several practitioners enough to write letters to the *Journal*, including one by Dr. Mary Murphy, Surrey.

Journal article: "Genetic Amniocentesis Program in B.C. (1971–1977)" by Betty Poland, MB, BS, FROG, and Lydia Suderman, RN.

There were 548 women over 38 years of age who had amniocentesis procedures performed at Vancouver General Hospital.

September, 1978 Dr. Elizabeth Kubler-Ross spoke at the Orpheum Theatre in a six-hour symposium on "Death and Dying."

In Memorium: Dr. Irene Mary Clearihue of Victoria died June 7, 1978.

WCB, new appointment: Dr. Lois Karabilgin has been appointed as a clinic physician.

Dr. Patricia Rebbeck, Vancouver surgeon, has been appointed Chairman of the National Service to Patients Committee of the Canadian Cancer Society for 1978–1979.

October, 1978 *Journal* article: "First Standard Perinatal Records Produced in B.C." by Dr. Molly Towell and Dr. Brian Dixon-Warren.

December, 1978 Dr. A. Milobar is BCMA President.

New BCMA members numbered 245, including 39 women doctors.

January, 1979 Dr. Patricia Johnston of Victoria was recently elected as both President and Communications Officer of the Victoria Medical Society.

March, 1979 Elizabeth Guy, first year medical student at UBC, was awarded a scholarship by the New York Life Insurance Company.

April, 1979 Article in the *Journal*: "Prognosis of Epilepsies" by Dr. Jean Arcide.

May, 1979 J.H. Tegenfeldt has been appointed Executive Director of the new Children's Hospital. Article in the May *Journal* by Dr. Katherine Mirhady: "Mainstreaming in Public Education (including handicapped among regular students)." Article by Roberta McQueen MD, FRCP(C): "Mental Health: What are our Priorities?" Dr. Josephine Mallek has been chosen as the VMA Osler Lecturer for 1979. Her topic is "Osler Takes a Wife." Dr. Molly Towell has been awarded the UBC Killam Senior Fellowship in recognition of her outstanding achievements in Perinatal Research.

BCMA Annual Reports include: Section of Dermatology report by Dr. Margaret Johnston. Health Planning Council had 14 committee reports, including: Dr. Shirley Rushton as a member of the Athletics and Recreation Committee. Dr. Patricia Rebbeck gave the Annual Report of the committee on Delivery of Health Care. Dr. Vera Frinton, President of the B.C. Branch FMWC, gave a report.

July, 1979 Newly elected executive of the B.C. Branch FMWC, 1979–1980: President, Dr. Shelley Ross; Past President, Dr. Vera Frinton;

Vice President, Dr. Lori Kanke; Treasurer, Dr. Marian Akrigg; Secretary, Dr. Sue Li Yong; Social Conveners, Dr. Dorothy Goresky and Dr. Thais Hall.

Women medical students at UBC received awards: Dianne Ripley, the Dean M.M. Weaver Medal; Patricia Pierce, the Dr. H.A. Henderson Memorial Award; Heather MacNaughton, the CIBA Prize in Psychiatry, and Elissa McMurtrie, the Max and Susie Dodek Memorial Prize.

August, 1979   At the Canadian Medical Association Annual Meeting Dr. William Thomas was elected by nomination from the floor to be CMA President.

Dr. Roberta Ongley is the new Chairman of the BCMA Section of Dermatology; Dr. Shirley Rushton is the Chairman of the Athletics and Recreation Committee of the Health Planning Council; and Dr. Hedy Fry is the Chairman of the Nutrition Committee.

UBC medical graduate Claire Wilson was the recipient of the 100,000th degree awarded at UBC. Claire will be interning in Nova Scotia.

Vancouver Medical Association: The first woman to become President of the 81-year-old Vancouver Medical Association is Dr. Patricia Rebbeck, member of the BCMA Board of Directors and a member of the Editorial Board of *B.C. Medical Association Journal.*

Dr. Beverley Tamboline is member at large of the VMA and Dr. Hedy Fry is Communications Officer of the VMA.

October, 1979   The main *Journal* articles were on Physiotherapy.

Dr. Eve Gulliford of Salmon Arm writes an Appreciation of Dr. Harold Pickup and his loyalty to the people of Alert Bay.

November, 1979   *Journal* article on "The Use and Abuse of Drugs in Sports" by Dr. Shirley Rushton.

December, 1979   Dr. Doris Kavanagh-Gray has been appointed Chairman of the Continuing Advisory Subcommittee (CASC) on Cardiac Care.

There were 308 new members of BCMA in 1979, 47 of them women.

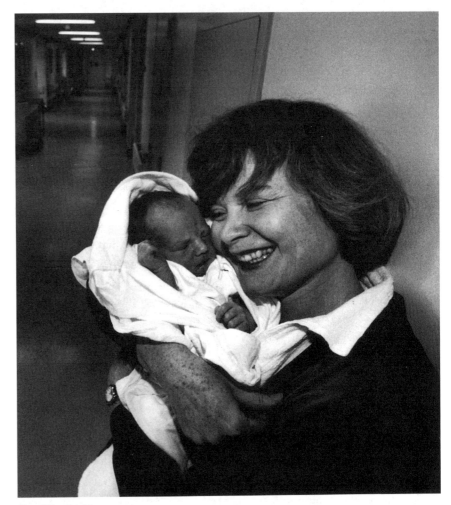

Dr. Kirsten Emmott, 1974

Stories from **1980 – 1989**

There were 975 new registered women doctors from 1980 to 1989.

1980
Dr. Vera Gellman
Dr. Maria Hugi
Dr. Theresa Isomura
Dr. Joan H. Scruton
Dr. Patricia Warshawski

1981
Dr. Elizabeth Barbour
Dr. Jean Hlady
Dr. Leslie LeHuquet
Dr. Kirstie Overhill
Dr. Peggy Ross

1982
Dr. Carol Katherine Dingee
Dr. Judith G. Hall

1983
Dr. Cicely Bryce
Dr. Sharon Lee

1984
Dr. Lynn Doyle
Dr. Frances Elaine Patterson

Dr. Caroline Penn
Dr. Doreen Tetz

1985
Dr. Sueda Akkor
Dr. Jean Louise Beck Jamieson
Dr. Rozmin F. Kamani
Dr. Caroline Ying-Mei Wang
Dr. Valerie White

1986
Dr. Heidi Oetter

1987
Dr. Christine Loock
Dr. Trine Larsen Soles
Dr. Lori Vogt

1988
Dr. Marjorie Docherty
Dr. Teresa Milia
Dr. Wendy V. Norman

1989
Dr. Alice Huang

DR. VERA GELLMAN

The story of my career goes back a long way, as far as my genes I suppose. Our children's ex-school principal recently told us that important to a successful career are high-quality genes and a stable happy home. I had the genes, but my stable happy family life was abruptly interrupted by the entirely sudden and unexpected death of my school teacher-father on Christmas Eve of 1937. I was twelve. My mother at thirty-five was left a widow with no pension, no life insurance to claim, no skills, the rent, and two pre-teenaged daughters, girls with ambitions. To make matters worse, World War II would break out eighteen months later.

We were living in a London suburb on a London County Council housing estate. At my own insistence I had started at the local grade school at the age of three-and-a-half. My sister, one-and-a-half years older, had been enrolled at the usual age of five. I wanted to go to school too and would hang my hat and coat next to hers in the school cloakroom and protest vehemently when made to put them on again to go home. Finally the teachers and mother succumbed. I could already read so was allowed to stay. By now my bright sister had been elevated to the next grade and we were never in the same class. Throughout the school we were the youngest in our respective classes. We were blatantly bribed by our mother to excel. She would give us two shillings and sixpence for coming top of the class and a lesser sum for second place. We made sure we always got the half-crown.

At eleven years I "sat for the Scholarship." On the basis of this exam I was awarded a Junior County Scholarship which entitled me to go to the grammar school of my choice. I chose the Mary Datchelor Girls' School in Camberwell Grove, S.E. London. It was a prestigious semi-private school sponsored by the Clothworkers' Company of London, and was situated at the bottom of Camberwell Grove where my grandparents lived. The building now houses the London headquarters of the Save the Children Fund. I had always admired the sophisticated Datchelor girls in their navy blue uni-

forms and "pudding-basin" hats. Moreover, the school was building a swimming pool which would soon be ready for use. I wrote an entrance exam, was interviewed by the school principal, and was accepted to start in September 1936.

My father's school was also in Camberwell and each morning we would set out proudly, me in my "pudding-basin" hat and music case in hand. We caught a bus and then a train, then we would have a short walk to our respective schools. My school consisted of "Scholarship girls" and "paid for" girls. The latter had been there since kindergarten and each was designated as "mother" to one of us. Despite our disparate backgrounds we very quickly melded and those of us with cockney accents soon acquired the "plum-in-mouth" accent of the middle-classes. The way you spoke was very important in those days. Friendships were formed which in some cases were to last a lifetime. My friend Mary and I still meet when I go back to London.

Academically I was now more challenged. I never did win the half-crown again, but the incentive to excel was firmly entrenched. I always ended up second or third in my class and every year received one, sometimes two, school prizes. The top place was invariably held by a very nice girl, Margaret Pitt, who was good at everything. Later during our evacuation to Wales, we were to become room-mates in one of our billets. From there we both went to Cambridge, she to read Geography and I to read Medicine. Margaret died a few years later from cancer. What a terrible waste of a brilliant intellect!

After the death of my father, the family went to stay with my grandparents in Camberwell. Their rented five-storey terrace house was just up the road from my school, so this was very convenient for me. My mother eventually found work in a London County Council food supply depot where she operated a small telephone switch-board for the princely sum of three pounds a week. She held this job for the next thirty years.

By now the threat of war was looming. Britain was totally unprepared and fully expected an imminent air attack on London. It was considered unsafe for the children to stay there. My school decided to evacuate to the country. We were each allowed one case and a carrier bag. Our list of essentials included a chocolate bar, a packet of biscuits, and a box of sanitary pads. I presume that our parents were advised to explain the use of the latter, as I remember my mother's embarassed "little talk" and her reassurance that "the Queen uses them too."

For three consecutive days we sat in the assembly hall at school with our hats, coats, and bags beside us ready to take off at a moment's notice. Meanwhile Neville Chamberlain was negotiating his famous "peace in our time" deal. Suddenly the crisis was over and school life returned to normal. The rest of the story is well-known. War broke out the following September and we waved goodbye to our tearful parents on Charing Cross Station. Our destination was unknown.

For me this was the start of a great adventure. I had always wanted to go to boarding school and this was the next best thing. From now on the school was to be my guardian, the teachers my surrogate parents. I was thirteen, just about to become fourteen, and I never lived at home again.

For the first ten months we were billeted in homes in little villages around Ashford in Kent. My first foster mother was Mrs. Woodcock, a simple country woman in an apron and shoes with turned-up toes. There were two children, Betty aged twelve and Billy aged nine. Billy was always in need of a handkerchief. I shared Betty's bed and we bathed once a week in the kitchen in a tin bath. Milk was delivered to the houses directly from the farms. One morning the milkman arrived with a beautiful "cauliflower ear" classically sustained when a cow flicked him on the ear with its tail while being milked.

After about three months of separation from their family, my friend Mary's parents decided to rent a small house in Ashford and I was invited to live with them. It was a very happy arrangement. Mary was the middle girl of three and older than me by only twelve days. We were all "Datchelor girls" and got along well. My mother was able to visit occasionally and was reassured as to my happiness.

The school shared the facilities of Ashford High School. We had lessons in the mornings and the Ashford students had theirs in the afternoons. We were given plenty of homework, but still found time to explore the countryside, help on the farms, roll bandages at the Vicarage, and knit socks for soldiers.

It was the period of the "phoney war." We had each been provided with a gas-mask which we had to carry at all times. Lessons were interrupted from time to time for air raid drills when we had to don our gas-masks. We quickly discovered that if we exhaled forcibly we could make a marvelous loud noise caused by the vibration of the rubber flaps on our cheeks. It was not long before this became absolutely forbidden.

There was an occasional air-raid warning in the middle of the night. Mary's parents had arranged with the pub across the road that we could shelter in their cellar. We would trundle across in our night attire with blankets, books, and gas-masks, and would read or chat, becoming gently and pleasantly intoxicated by the smell of beer. After an hour or so the "all clear" would sound and we would return to our beds.

After France fell Ashford came within the direct line of invasion by Hitler's forces. Once more we were uprooted and taken by train to an unknown destination. This time the journey was longer and the names of the stations on the way became more and more unpronounceable. We finally stopped at one called Llanelly. We were in South Wales. A few years ago among my mother's papers I found a postcard which I had sent her on June 24th, 1940 on arrival in Llanelly:

One morning the milkman arrived with a beautiful "cauliflower ear" classically sustained when a cow flicked him on the ear with its tail while being milked.

Dearest Mummie,

We arrived very safely at about 8:15. We are at Llanelly and I am billeted in a very nice place. My address is 31 New Rd. c/o Mrs. Rosser. It is very nice so far.

Mrs. Rosser is a fairly old lady and her husband is too. I think her daughter and her son live with her. I think I shall be very happy here, but that is all I will say because do you remember how marvelous I said Mrs. Woodcock was? We had a very long journey, but we enjoyed ourselves and we had a wonderful reception. All the children waved and cheered us.

Mary is in No. 13, New Rd., and Pat and Jean, the twins, are at 45. There is also one of our girls next door, but I don't know who. I have a lovely little room to myself and there is a dog here. I could tell you more but there is no room left, so do not write until you receive a letter.

Love Vera xxx

I was happy with the Rossers and stayed with them for three years until Mr. Rosser retired and they moved to Gloucester.

Meanwhile the war became more earnest. We were in steel-works country and the industrial town of Swansea was only twenty miles or so away. Air-raid warnings became a nightly routine. At first we would huddle in the cupboard under the stairs, but this became too uncomfortable for five of us and a dog. As we became more used to the raids we would stay in bed, cross our fingers, and shiver until the "all clear" sounded. We could hear bombs falling on Swansea, as its centre was systematically razed to the ground, but generally only received the odd spare bomb unloaded at random by the German planes on their way home.

My poor mother and my sister whose school had decided to return to London from Brighton after the fall of France were in the meantime suffering through the London Blitz. They had by now moved to Lewisham to share a small house with my aunt. The Anderson shelter in the garden became their permanent bedroom.

School life continued throughout the turmoil. We shared the Llaney Boys' School for lessons and used the church crypt for assembly and as a day-time air-raid shelter. Academically, life was also becoming earnest. Some time during my fourteenth year I had decided I wanted to become a doctor, and nothing would shake me. My reasons were the usual altruistic ones, but also I had read historical accounts of the early women pioneers in medicine and of Marie Curie and was incensed at the ridicule and discrimination they endured. I was already becoming a feminist. Women doctors were still rather unusual and this was a challenge I could not resist.

At fifteen we were preparing for the "School Certificate" exam. Our curriculum was still fairly general, but for those of us with university aspirations the inclusion of Latin was essential to gain exemption from writing the university matriculation exam, the first hurdle for university entrance.

We wrote the "School Certificate" exam in the church crypt and I satisfied the examiners that I was potential university material.

I had passed my first hurdle and next was to convince my mother to let me aim for a career in medicine. Her initial reluctance was purely financially based, and with good reason. But my school principal managed to convince her that we could face that problem when the time came. A firm decision was important at this stage because I would have to rearrange my curriculum with a bias toward the sciences. So it was settled. I would aim for a medical career.

In two years I would write the exam for the "Higher School Certificate" (today's "A" levels). My studies were devoted to Chemistry, Physics, Biology, Mathematics, and English Literature. I especially enjoyed Biology, dissecting worms, cockroaches, frogs, rabbits, and smelly dogfish. I became adept at cutting one-cell-thin sections of plant stems with a cut-throat razor and staining them in gorgeous colours to demonstrate the xylem and phloëm. I had always been good at art and loved to draw what I saw under the microscope.

There were only a half-dozen students in the Science sixth form and we considered ourselves elite. Our teachers were devoted to our success. We eventually wrote the Higher School exam, and on the basis of my results I was awarded a Senior County scholarship and exempted from having to sit the first MB exam (equivalent to pre-med). The scholarship would take care of my tuition fees but not my living expenses.

Meanwhile life was by no means all work and no play. Because of the bombing in London we were not allowed to go home for school holidays until we reached our final year. Instead teachers would take us in groups to farming camps where we joined other volunteers in fruit-picking and potato-picking to help the war effort. Also in term time Mary and I would work on a small local farm, cutting and stacking hay, bringing in the cows for milking, and searching the hedges for guinea-fowl eggs.

In the sixth form (Grade 12), we were recruited for fire-watching, sleeping overnight on camp beds in the school staff room. We learned how to extinguish incendiary bombs with a stirrup pump, but fortunately were never required to use our skills.

At sixteen I experienced my first autopsy. I was visiting my sister, by now a student at a teacher's training college evacuated to Cardiff. Her friend's boyfriend was a medical student at Cardiff University and smuggled me into the morgue on the grounds that I was a medical student. It was a case of silicosis, common among the miners in South Wales. I was most interested and fortunately was asked no questions.

In 1943 the Rosser family was preparing to move and I was transferred to my final foster home with the Alfords. Margaret Pitt was already living there and we became room-mates and good friends. The Alfords were a lovely childless middle-aged couple who took a great interest in our budding careers. Mrs. Alford was no great cook, and we ate Spam and chips (French fries) every day for our main meal. On Sundays we ate the week's meat ration. Convinced that she was anaemic, as well she may have been on that diet, Mrs. Alford supplemented her intake with "Dr. Pink's pink pills for pale people" which she offered round as after-dinner candies.

It was now my last year at school and this was devoted to securing a place at University and finding the extra funds to cover my living expenses there. In those days University was not open to all. One earned a place by writing an entrance exam and surviving interviews with various members of the faculty. Places in medicine were limited to ten in each of the two women's colleges at Cambridge. I applied to Girton College and was selected to take the college entrance exam. To my great delight I was offered a place. I had wanted to go to University, but Cambridge was beyond my wildest dreams.

I now had to find the additional funding to cover my expenses. There were at the time a number of organizations in London which awarded grants to impecunious students. Their great advantage was that they were gifts, not loans, and were pledged for a certain number of years. With the help of one of my teachers I applied to the Draper's Company, the Thomas Wall Fund, the Clothworkers Company (our own school sponsor), the Gilbert Foyle trust Company (of Foyle's Famous book shop in London), and the London Schoolteacher's Association. Each pledged a small grant which, together with my Senior County Scholarship, would take care of my expenses at the University for the next three years and the subsequent three years of hospital training.

There was still another hurdle to overcome. My place at Girton College, Cambridge was subject to my prior acceptance at a hospital. Cambridge Medical School had no specific hospital affiliation and most London teaching hospitals at that time were not taking women. The Royal Free and the West London Hospitals in Hammersmith were the only two all-women medical schools. After an interview with the Dean I was accepted at the West London. It was not until 1945 that, under threat from the government of withdrawal of funding, all teaching hospitals were forced to open their doors to women.

In July 1944 my happy school days ended. My return to London is a complete blank in my memory. All I know is that over the course of five years I had become an independent, adaptable, and mature nineteen-year-old. I had had a great experience and was ready for the next.

The following September I went up to Cambridge. You always go *up* when you go to Cambridge, even if you come from the north of England. When you leave Cambridge you go *down*, and if you leave in disgrace you are *sent down*.

Cambridge functions on the collegiate system. Students belong to and live in a college. Lectures and labs take place in University Departmental buildings in downtown Cambridge. Girton College is a mile or two outside the town and students bicycle in for lectures. Because of the wartime constraints, rooms in college were in short supply and new students were placed in approved accommodation in nearby homes. Once more I found myself living in someone else's home. This time it was the large and lovely house of Professor Lennard-Jones. My college was just across the road where I had my meals. Professor Lennard-Jones was Plummer Professor of Theoretical Science. He became famous in his field as creator of the "Lennard-Jones potential" and was knighted in 1946.

After my carefree years in friendly Wales, I was totally unprepared for the rigid Victorian atmosphere at Girton. I was now addressed as Miss Annett (my maiden name). Students were expected to dine in "Hall" a certain number of times a week, presided over by "High Table" where the mistress and dons ate. If we wished to leave the Hall before the meal formally ended we bowed to High Table. "Gentlemen" were not allowed in our rooms between the hours of 6 p.m. and 7 p.m. when we were supposed to be changing for dinner. There was of course a curfew and if we planned to spend an evening in town we signed out and in at the Porter's Lodge. This was called "signing an exeat." Dressing gowns could be worn at breakfast as long as pyjama trousers or nightgown did not show underneath. I found these restrictions oppressive and inhibiting. No wonder the male students called us "Blue-stockings"!

Cambridge offered an infinite number of alternatives to studying. I joined the Jesus College Choir, and was selected for the University women's netball team. I had always been very keen on netball and later was to play against Oxford, thus earning my "half-blue." Outnumbered ten to one by male medical students, "Blue-stocking" or no, there was no shortage of invitations for evenings out. Mrs. Lennard-Jones began to be concerned about the number of evenings I was spending not studying. She expressed her concern to my college supervisor and by the end of the Michaelmas term a room was found for me in the college. I now had to sign "exeats," which was just as well!

As each female student arrived she would be greeted by the stomping of two hundred pairs of male feet if she was homely and wolf-whistles if she was attractive.

Anatomy, Comparative Anatomy, Physiology, Inorganic Chemistry, Biochemistry—there was no end to the new knowledge we were expected to absorb. Together with the male medical students we attended lectures and labs in the various university departments.

Professor Harris, the Anatomy Professor, was a formidable character who did not tolerate whistling. If anyone whistled in the vicinity of the Dissecting Room he would burst from his office shouting, "Remember, you are in the presence of the dead!" He also hated women medical students. "Intimidate the students" was the name of his game and we all dreaded getting him as an examiner in the orals.

The lecture theatre in the Anatomy School was built along the usual lines with tiers of benches and entrances in the pit. As each female student arrived she would be greeted by the stomping of two hundred pairs of male feet if she was homely and wolf-whistles if she was attractive. These days this would be regarded as sexual harassment. We just laughed at them.

If the women's colleges exerted an unusual vigilance over their students, there was good reason. At that time women were not accepted as full members of Cambridge University. They attended lectures with the men, sat for the same exams in the same rooms, usually passing with better grades, yet they were denied full privileges, including a proper degree. The women's colleges were negotiating with the University authorities for full acceptance and we were therefore expected to behave with absolute decorum. It was not until 1947 that women were finally admitted as full members of Cambridge University.

World War II ended at the conclusion of my first academic year. V.E. Day occurred in May 1945, and provided that we had resided on campus for the requisite number of days, we were allowed to go down to be with our families. V.J. Day followed three months later during the long vacation.

In May 1947 I succeeded in passing the Tripos examination and went *down* for the last time. For us women there were no graduation exercises and no piece of paper signifying our achievement over the last three years.

I had enjoyed my university years, but was happy to shake off the feeling of excessive supervision. The West London Hospital Medical School was altogether different. We were treated as adults. It was a small school and for the first year consisted only of females. Later when London teaching hospitals were obliged to accept women, the West London accepted men. I lived in the students' hostel for one year, then shared an apartment on the Hammersmith Road with five other female students. Living close to the hospital gave us an advantage in that we could be called in quickly when interesting cases were admitted.

We worked in "firms" of about six students supervised by a Consultant and, together with the Ward Sister, would follow him on rounds examining and discussing his patients. The wards were large, each with about twenty beds. Patients would all be sitting in bed, newly scrubbed and freshly pyjama-ed, ready for examination, and there would be absolute silence.

In those days the mystique of healing was still carefully preserved. Patients were kept in ignorance of their illnesses, test results, and treatments. Certain dreaded words were never uttered in their presence. Cancer, tumour, and growth were referred to as "neoplasm." Tuberculosis was "phthisis" and syphilis was "lues." To be fair these terms were usually used in bedside discussions of differential diagnoses so as not to worry the patient unduly. But the extraordinary thing was that patients seldom asked questions. I remember being absolutely amazed when, a few years later as a resident in a Chicago hospital, I was approached in the corridor by a tiny black haemophiliac boy saying, "Hi! Do you want to see my haematoma?"

After ward rounds at the West London there would be refreshments for the Consultant in the Sister's office, dainty sandwiches, cakes, and coffee served from a silver pot. Inflated by the deference bestowed on them, many Consultants became prima donnas or the male equivalent. One gynecology Consultant, after himself examining the patient, would make us each in turn examine her vaginally while he sat down to write his notes. For the poor patient it must have been like gang-rape! The Consultant would then return and, slapping one of us heartily on the back, would say, "Well, what did you find? Bag of nuts? Bunch of keys? Statue of Napoleon?" A Cardiologist at the Middlesex, my husband's hospital, was known to have sent someone out into the street where men were working with hydraulic drills to ask them to stop drilling because he was trying to listen to a patient's heart murmur.

The West London Hospital had no maternity ward and since we were required to deliver twenty babies to complete our obstetrics course, we had to transfer to the West Middlesex Hospital in Isleworth for a few weeks. The West Mid. had an excellent training facility for midwives. Like them, we were required to wash the sheets after a delivery, no matter what time of night or day. But it was a great experience, and we shared the joy with our patients when their babies were born.

One of my deliveries was particularly startling. The mother was an unwed elderly primip. When the baby emerged it appeared at first to have two heads. There was in fact an enormous retinoblastoma pushing out of the infant's orbit. There was also a nodule on the skin and at autopsy a further metastasis was found in the intestine. I wrote up and published this exceedingly rare case.

Contagious diseases requiring admission to hospital were in those days confined to Fever hospitals. West London students would bus to the Fulham Fever Hospital to see the cases there. There were the usual cases of scarlet fever, measles, German measles, etc., but there was one, a seventy-year-old man, who had both herpes zoster and chicken pox simultaneously. He was isolated in a single ward. After ushering us into his ward, the Registrar asked, "By the way, has anyone here not had chicken pox?" I had not. Sure enough, sixteen days later I came down with chicken pox, then passed it on to one of my flat-mates.

My healthy childhood was to catch up on me once more a few years later when I was in practice. I caught mumps from a patient and passed it on to my husband, who was at the time my fiancé.

After my three years of clinical training I was eligible to return to Cambridge to write my final exams. I passed and in February 1951 attended a convocation (women were by now full university members) and received my MB, BChir (Cantab) degree. The following year I became eligible to receive an MA. There was no exam. It was a peculiarity of Cambridge that a Bachelor's degree could be automatically elevated to a Master's after five years. Since I was never aware of having received a BA, I wasn't going to bother, but in 1956 after we were married my husband persuaded me. We attended the convocation together and I became Dr. Vera Gellman MA, MB, BChir (Cantab).

After qualifying I did a series of house jobs to expand my experience. These were six-month appointments, and after each came the tedious business of application and if selected, attending an interview for the next job. A House appointment in one's teaching hospital was a valuable indication of one's worth and helped in securing subsequent positions.

In January 1951 I became House Physician to Dr. Geoffrey Konstam, Cardiologist at the West London Hospital. At the age of twenty-six I received a salary for the first time in my life. It was thirteen pounds per month plus board. We house staff were on call twenty-four hours a day and were off duty every other weekend. If, however, a Consultant chose to admit patients during a weekend off, we were expected to be there to write them up and organize their tests ready for ward-rounds on Monday morning. We took all blood samples ourselves, did lumbar punctures, catheterized for sterile urine samples, and out of hours did electrocardiograms on a portable machine. We were on call for Casualty (ER) one night a week, and whether we were up all night or not, were expected on ward rounds the following morning.

Other House jobs followed, each with its new experiences, demands, and rewards. At Lewisham Hospital as House Surgeon to Dr. A. Cavendish on the UG ward, I became adept at circumcisions and dilating strictures. "Thank you, Doctor, for your pains," murmured one poor old man. As House Physician to Dr. N. Coghill, gastroenterologist, of the West Middlesex Hospital, I would follow him, together with a Ward Sister, on bed-pan rounds each morning. He insisted that the stools be fresh. At Christmas time he was presented with a tiny doll-house stool freshly painted in glossy brown paint: "A fresh stool for you, Sir."

In 1953 I returned to the West London Hospital and worked for eight months as Casualty Officer dealing with an unlimited variety of emergencies. I

At the age of twenty-six I received a salary for the first time in my life. It was thirteen pounds per month plus board.

learned to take X-rays and develop them, reduce fractures and splint them, and stitched up countless lacerations sustained by drunks "fighting for the freedom of Ireland."

In June 1952, when I was House Physician to Dr. Leslie Cole at Addenbrooke's Hospital, Cambridge, something occurred which was to change the direction of my career and ultimately my life. An epidemic of Salmonella typhimurium broke out on the wards. Patients admitted for simple appendectomies were dying. The Public Health Officer was called in and the hospital was promptly closed. Every stool passed by everyone working in the hospital had to be submitted for bacteriological examination. This went on for about six weeks until the source of the infection was traced to the hospital's milk supply. A single farmer supplied the hospital with milk and his equipment was unsterile. Meanwhile the hospital staff had time on their hands. It was a beautiful summer. We sunbathed on the roof, played tennis, and fell in love. No fewer than six couples eventually married, including Derek and me.

When in 1954 we became engaged I decided that general practice would best fit in with a future family life. I became Trainee-Assistant in a well-established family practice in Woolwich, S.E. London. The government was at that time offering grants to encourage practitioners to employ young assistants for one year. There were two female partners in the practice, Dr. Eileen Wise whose father "old Dr. Wise" had started the practice

at the turn of the century, and Dr. Eileen Gorman (Helen), her protegee. Helen was a few years older than me. They used the government money to provide me with a car, so the first thing I had to do was learn to drive. My maiden voyage was to visit Derek who was working at Aldershot, about thirty miles away. It took me three hours!

The two Eileens lived in a multi-storey terraced house on Burage Road and the surgery was in the basement. I had a room in the attic. We would see patients in the surgery in the mornings and evenings, and house calls, which were the rule rather than the exception, were fitted in between. As well as working in the practice I had a part-time appointment with the Department of Public Health. I examined and gave shots to school children and held pre-natal clinics.

It was a true family practice with a large component of obstetrics and pediatrics. Many of the pregnant women had themselves been delivered as babies by "old Dr. Wise" or his daughter. All uncomplicated deliveries were conducted in the home by nurses trained in midwifery. They were skillful, competent, and very experienced. Things rarely went wrong, but if they did we were called in.

Derek and I were married in 1955, and we spent one more year in England living in an apartment in Eltham while I continued with my Public Health clinics and he worked as Registrar at the Middlesex Hospital. The more senior positions were becoming very hard to acquire. People had been languishing in Senior Registrarships for years while waiting for Consultant positions to be freed up. There was certainly no hope for Derek of climbing the next rung of the ladder without a further qualification, a B.A. (Been to America). The United States was considered at the time to be the ultimate in medical research and training, and scores of young physicians were leaving England for this reason.

In September 1956 we crossed the Atlantic, Derek with a one-year Fellowship from the Middlesex and I with a Fulbright Scholarship. We travelled on the Queen Mary, a five-day stormy sea journey. There were no jet planes in those days. Safety ropes were in place in the dining rooms, but we hardly saw any fellow travellers at meal times. On the last day of the crossing we woke early and went up on deck to see if we could sight land. There was a row of matchboxes on the horizon which, in the course of the day, gradually enlarged into skyscrapers. We passed the Statue of Liberty and finally entered the harbour in Manhattan. We were greeted by the usual flotilla of little boats sirening their welcome. It was a truly unforgettable experience.

We spent one night in New York and the following morning caught the train from Grand Central Station to Chicago. Derek had arranged to spend his Fellowship working in the Renal Unit at the Research and Education Hospital (R & E) in Chicago, and I had an appointment as Resident in Pediatrics at nearby Presbyterian and St. Lukes's Hospitals. Both were teaching hospitals in the University of Illinois. I wanted more experience in pediatrics in preparation for returning to practise in London after a year.

We were about to experience a series of culture shocks which these days do not seem very remarkable, but after the rather formal and penurious atmosphere of post-war England, made a great impression on us. In the railway dining car, for example, we were amazed at the size of the steaks which people were eating. Only four years away from the food rationing at home we remembered that each of these steaks would have represented a week's meat ration for a whole family.

On arriving in Chicago I met the Head of the Department of Pediatrics, Dr. Heyworth Sanford. He greeted me by my first name, which I found nice and friendly after the formal "Dr. Annett" of London days.

At Presbyterian St. Luke's Hospital I was responsible for the patients of several pediatric practitioners. Each thought that he was more deserving of my time and attention than the others. Catering to them all was exhausting, and so I jumped at the opportunity when after three months Dr. Sanford offered me a Residency in the Research and Education Hospital where there were eight Residents to share the responsibilities and the teaching was excellent.

The wards at R & E were a veritable museum of pediatric conditions. At any one time on the ward there would be a half-dozen adrenogenital syndromes, a Kleinfelter's Syndrome, a progeria, several Wilm's tumours, a case of phenylketonuria, several congenital hearts and so on, not to mention a few F.L.K. (Funny-Looking Kids) awaiting diagnosis. I had at one time under my care a pair of monovular twins with congenital hydrocephalus. I published a paper on them in the *Archives of Diseases of Children*. I was also co-author with I. M. Rosenthal *et al* of a paper on "The effect of stress on patients with congenital virilizing adrenocortical hyperplasia," which was published in *Paediatrics* in 1960.

One of the most unusual cases was that of a four-year-old black boy whose mother had noticed a swelling on his hard palate which had been there for a week or more. It was pale, smooth, and hard, and did not seem to be tender. There was much speculation as to what this could be. He was presented at grand rounds and all manner of specialists were called in for consultation. It was thought to be a bony tumour and biopsy was recommended. On the morning that he was slated for surgery I met the Resident who was caring for the child and enquired how the procedure had gone. He smiled and produced from his pocket a test tube containing the "tumour." It was a half pistachio nut shell and it had fallen out as my colleague was examining the swelling prior to surgery.

We were enjoying Chicago. Determined to make the most of our year in the U.S.A., we attended meetings in the east and in the west, seeing as much of the country as we could on the way. Then we were persuaded to stay on for a further year.

After the second year, plans were underway for our return to England, but as the time approached we discovered that neither of us was anxious to return to the competition for jobs that would surely await us. Our career opportunities were much greater on this continent and so we decided to stay. However, our Exchange-Visitor visas were nearing expiry and we would have to leave the U.S. for at least two years.

In August 1958 we crossed the border into Canada and, starting in Victoria, travelled by bus to Winnipeg, stopping off to visit every medical centre on the way. We were greatly impressed by the Winnipeg Clinic, a well-organized group of about thirty specialists with their own laboratory, X-ray facilities, dieticians, etc. They were looking for a well-qualified Internist and had been advised by colleagues in the west that they were

At any one time on the ward there would be a half-dozen adrenogenital syndromes, a Kleinfelter's Syndrome, a progeria, several Wilm's tumours, a case of phenylketonuria, several congenital hearts and so on, not to mention a few F.L.K. (Funny-Looking Kids) awaiting diagnosis.

about to receive a visit from us. Within weeks of returning to Chicago, Derek received an invitation to join the Winnipeg Clinic.

In October 1958 we left Chicago with all our personal possessions strapped to the roof of our 1952 Chevy which we had purchased for $600 two years previously. We rented a brand new apartment in Winnipeg, then flew back to England to take leave of our families and collect the rest of our worldly goods which had been in storage. They occupied two large wooden containers. We returned with them on the Empress of France. It was November by now, and as we entered the St. Lawrence Seaway, it began to snow. By the time we reached Quebec City, the snow had turned to a blizzard and the visibility was nil. We were stranded in the middle of the Seaway, fog-horns sounding, for fourteen hours.

We eventually arrived in Montreal and disembarked, fully expecting a long and tedious confrontation with customs since we were importing a long list of household items. However, it happened to be Grey Cup day and the game was about to begin. At the sound of a whistle all the customs officials suddenly disappeared and we were whisked through in minutes. We continued our journey by rail to Winnipeg. They had had a blizzard too and were digging themselves out when we arrived. Banks of snow six feet high surrounded us. We had never seen so much snow in our lives!

To help with the family coffers I used to read electrocardiograms for Dr. Frank Matheson's Farnham Study in my spare time.

By now we had been married for three years. With the prospect of at least one steady income it was time to think about starting a family. I also wanted to write the exam for Certification in Pediatrics while my newly-acquired knowledge was still fresh in my mind. It would be expedient to do this before assuming the responsibilities of motherhood. Despite my years in practice and as a Pediatric Resident, the College insisted on further clinical experience. I worked in the Outpatients Department at the Winnipeg Children's Hospital and in the Allergy Department at the Winnipeg Clinic and studied in my spare time.

In November 1959, seven months pregnant, I wrote the exam, then accompanied by my husband, flew to Toronto for the orals and passed.

Shortly after that Dr. Harry Medovy, Pediatric Department Head, University of Manitoba, offered me a position as Director of the Poison Control Program and University Lecturer based in the Children's Hospital. I would be provided with a part-time secretary and an honorarium of $100 a month.

In January 1960 our son was born. The Directorship of the Poison Control Program offered an ideal way of combining my career with that of mother and homemaker. It would also provide me with a *pied à terre* in the hospital so that I could attend rounds and keep up with new pediatric trends. My office was a desk in the corridor outside the Emergency Room which I shared with my secretary. I was to hold this position for the next thirteen years, by which time I had graduated to a proper office and Assistant Professorship and my honorarium was doubled. To help with the family coffers I used to read electrocardiograms for Dr. Frank Matheson's Farnham Study in my spare time.

Our daughter was born February 1961, and with the help of a devoted nanny I was gradually able to increase the time spent on my work, which I found intellectually rewarding. However, until the children started school, my afternoons were always with them.

Canada's Poison Control Program was the brainchild of Dr. Harry Medovy. The centre in the Winnipeg Children's Hospital had been set up a year or two previously, but it needed nurturing and developing. In essence I was responsible for the establishment and administration of nine daughter centres across the province. The principal centre maintained a twenty-four hour information service for physicians, the public, and other hospitals on the toxicity of household products, plants, etc. I consulted on clinical matters, instructed nurses, Residents, and students, and worked with government departments and voluntary agencies to educate the public on the prevention of poisoning. I gave talks to school children and service clubs and interviews on television and radio. To extend the reach of my educational program I organized teams of lay people to give lectures and slide presentations which I prepared.

In the early years, Canada had no legislation requiring warning labels on toxic household products. In my lectures and media interviews I took every opportunity to point out this fact. The local branch of the Consumer's Association of Canada contacted me and adopted the issue. Using Poison

Centre statistics, prepared statements, and letters from me to the Minister of Consumer and Corporate Affairs, they lobbied successfully for a Hazardous Products Act which finally passed in 1968–1969.

In the early sixties glue sniffing became a popular pastime among Winnipeg school children. Experimentation with other drugs soon followed. The Poison Control Centre became the information source on these issues for concerned parents and teachers. I answered numerous requests for lectures and seminars on the subject. My paper "Glue Sniffing Among Winnipeg School Children," published in *The Canadian Medical Association Journal* in 1968 was, I believe, the first in Canada on that subject. Later in 1977, after I had left Winnipeg, I was invited to make a presentation on "Solvent Inhalation Legislative Controls" at a seminar jointly sponsored by the Ministry of Tourism and the Addiction Research Foundation of Ontario. The proceedings were published in a booklet titled *Solvents, Adhesives, and Aerosols.*

For the three years from 1961 to 1964 I contributed a monthly column to *The Manitoba Medical Review* on various aspects of poisoning, and in 1971 the Winnipeg Horticultural Society asked me to write an article on "Poisonous Plants in Our Environment" which they published in their magazine *Prairie Gardens.*

I worked for several years with the St. John Ambulance Society, giving lectures and demonstrations and acting as a consultant. I was asked to contribute a chapter on Poisoning to the third edition of their First Aid handbook. In 1970 I was honoured at a special ceremony by the Priory of Canada of the Most Venerable Order of the Hospital of St. John of Jerusalem, with a resolution that "the special thanks of His Excellency the Prior and the Priory Chapter be conveyed to Vera Gellman MA, MB, BChir, (Cantab) for valuable assistance rendered in the furtherance of the work of the Order in Connection with the Priory of Canada." It was signed by His Excellency the Govenor General Roland Michener.

Throughout the years 1962 to 1977 I was a member of the Safety Promotion Committee of the Canadian Pediatric Society and served as Chairperson from 1964 to 1967.

In 1972 we left Winnipeg for Ottawa. I was presented with a plaque by Mayor Juba "in recognition of the outstanding contribution to the young citizens of Manitoba in the prevention and relief of suffering, involving poison control and close association with the operation of '999,' the City of Winnipeg Emergency System."

The Board of Directors of the Children's Hospital of Winnipeg also honoured me with a citation "in recognition of her devoted service as Director of the Poison Control Centre and as a testimony of the high regard in which she is held by her colleagues."

My husband had been appointed to a position with the Federal Government in Health and Welfare at Ottawa. Finding work for me was going to be a problem. I had become highly specialised, too highly, in fact. Only one person with my expertise was needed in a city and Ottawa already had a Poison Control Director. The Federal Poison Control Unit, which was responsible for distributing information to the centres across Canada, was looking for a Toxicologist to review this information and suggest treatments in cases of ingestion. The work was within my sphere of expertise. I applied for the position and was accepted. But it was boring and my chauvinistic immediate superior gave me no scope for initiative.

After a year, I decided to approach the Director of the Product Safety Branch, at that time in the Department of Consumer and Corporate Affairs. Jim Black supervised the research and development of regulations to the Hazardous Products Act and was responsible for teams of field inspectors and enforcement officers. We had met several times at interdepartmental conferences and I was impressed by his intelligence and dynamic approach. To my great delight he said he was planning to ask me if I would be interested in joining his group. He needed the prestige and credibility of a physician to add weight to the department's debates with industry on the safety of their products. I was offered the position of Chief of Research and Development. Unfortunately, although my prestige as a physician was the reason behind the offer, I could not be paid as a physician because Health and Welfare was the only government department with physicians on their payroll. As an employee of Consumer and Corporate Affairs I would come under the category of Scientist, which belonged to a lower pay-scale than physician. (The story of my life!) The work sounded interesting, so I accepted anyway.

It was the Trudeau era and my first requirement was to become bilingual. Like many others I had taken French at school and knew how to conjugate a verb in French, but could not converse. I attended one of the government's total-immersion French schools in Hull and spent seven months thinking, writing, speaking, and dreaming in French. What is more, I was being paid to do so (thank you, taxpayers). At the end I was quite fluent, but alas, did not have to speak French once during my next five years with the Federal Government.

As Chief of Research and Development in the Product Safety Branch I supervised a group comprising two engineers, a chemist, and a textile chemist, and worked in liaison with departmental lawyers. I researched the causes of accidents, especially but not exclusively in children, due to household chemical and other products: toys, equipment, clothing, etc.

I was particularly interested in children's equipment and toys. There had been a few instances of strangulation of infants whose clothing buttons had caught in the wide holes in the mesh surrounding their playpens. Regulations were introduced to define the maximum allowable dimensions of the mesh holes. Several babies had died, their heads trapped between crib bars. These tragedies resulted in amendments to the Cribs Regulations in the Hazardous Products Act. Death in infants with tiny baby rattles impacted in their throats led to the promulgation of regulations regarding the size of rattles and other toys and so on.

The variety of work was unlimited. We dealt with the electric kettle problem. Lead solder was in use inside electric kettles in those days, giving rise to lead levels in boiled water beyond the limits of potability, a situation particularly dangerous to formula-fed infants. Silver-tin solder is now used. My colleagues and I researched dimensions for safe car seats, construction of hockey and bicycle helmets, the flammability of children's clothing and toys, labelling of hazardous household chemicals, and of course, child-proof safety caps. Whenever I struggle with and curse the safety-cap on my medication, my husband laughs and says, "You have only yourself to blame!"

All of this work required frequent discussions with industry, which necessitated travel to other Canadian cities. I worked closely with my counterpart in the U.S.A., often travelling to Washington to do so. I made presentations as a representative of my department at scientific meetings, gave radio and television interviews, participated in the TV program "Marketplace," acted as an expert witness in litigation suits, and attended briefing sessions for the Minister Herb Grey, then later Andre Ouellet.

The work was extremely interesting and intellectually satisfying, but social life in Ottawa left much to be desired. Our children were by now embarking on their own careers at University and it was time to move on. In 1979 my husband was offered the position of Vice-President, Medicine, at the Vancouver General Hospital. Who could resist? He would have about ten working years ahead of him and I could now retire in a balmy climate and make jam.

We moved to Vancouver in 1979 and found a nice house in the British Properties. But our successive moves in Canada had been to increasingly expensive cities from the property point of view. Here we were in our mid-fifties with a large mortgage to pay. There was nothing for it but for me to find work. I needed a part-time position, preferably less demanding than my last. I talked to Dr. Rob Hill who was at that time Acting Head of the Department of Pediatrics at U.B.C. He later became Head. Rob needed help with some of his administration chores, and with my experience in a government department I might fit the bill. We agreed to try each other out for six months in the first instance. I became Assistant Professor and part-time Assistant to the Department Head for the next eight years. This time I was paid according to the scale for physicians.

It has been a motley career and a far cry from the family physician once envisioned. But it has been interesting and rewarding intellectually if not always financially. To me the most remarkable thing is that my career in medicine ever got off the ground, and for that I must thank my resourceful school teachers, the various institutions which supported me, and my mother who made sacrifices. My most heartfelt thanks belong to my husband who encouraged me throughout, at times even paying for the privilege of having a wife with a career.

DR. MARIA HUGI

Born: 1953.
Graduated: UBC Medical School, 1979.

I must say that I felt flattered and privileged when Eileen Cambon asked me to contribute to this book. When it came to writing my story, however, I struggled long and hard with the content. What was my bailiwick, I mused, as I scratched at the healing scars on my ever-ravaged chest wall? Befitting of my long struggle with breast cancer, I am currently recovering from a prophylactic mastectomy and reconstructive surgery. I decided it was better to write about the most profound influence on my life, which is having to endure a major life-threatening illness at a young age while juggling children, marriage, early menopause, a career, and volunteer work.

I will put other influences of my life on the back burner. I will not belabour you with the fact that I am a Swiss immigrant whose family, like thousands of other Europeans, fled a decimated post-World War II Europe for a brighter future in Canada; that my father was a skilled labourer and a fundamentalist Christian; that my mother and two sisters were homemakers; and that I grew up in Terrace. I will not dwell on the fact (well, maybe a little) that my elementary and high school education in Terrace left a lot to be desired; that less than five percent of my high school graduating class went to university. In hindsight, it is hard to believe I used to envy First Nations children as they were shipped off to residential schools every September. In elementary school, I can remember class sizes of fifty-five students, with one teacher riding herd over us. The class bully in my Grade 6 class was fifteen years old. In Grade 7, one of my classmates became pregnant, allegedly by her father. Along with all too many girls in my high school, I grew tired of being "hit on" by more than the occasional male teacher, so much so that my favorite teacher was the overtly gay French instructor. I could relax in his class and concentrate on my studies.

I will also not bore you with the fact that, although I am armed with a wonderful and powerful degree, I found medical school to be an intimidating, grueling, and character-crushing experience. I always thought I was the only one having a rough time because, after all, most of my classmates had well-educated parents, better schooling, better support systems, straighter teeth, and more money than I had. Imagine my surprise then, when at a recent impromptu gathering of nine women from medical school, I discovered that, despite their privileged upbringings and my perception of how self-assured they seemed to be, these women had all struggled in medical school.

After medical school, I completed an Emergency Medicine residency in New Orleans and was finally able to apply what I had learned. I then worked for years as an emergency department physician in southern Louisiana, almost exclusively in teaching hospitals designated to care for the poor and uninsured. I was appointed, and still am, a board examiner for the Emergency Medicine specialty exams. From my time in the U.S., I became permanently infected with the American spirit where all that matters is "life, liberty, and the pursuit of happiness." I developed a tremendous, lasting respect for the sanctity of individual freedom and responsibility. The "don't mess with me or I will reach for my guns and lawyers" attitude rubbed off on me.

I married a fellow Canadian, an Emergency department physician, whom I had met as a medical student while he was an intern at St. Paul's on his way to New Orleans for further training. We bought a house in the suburbs, beach property in Florida, and worked hard at our careers. I gave birth to two sons. Then, at age thirty-six, when my second son was four months old, I diagnosed breast cancer in my left breast after interpreting a vicious-looking mammogram.

I had a Stage III poorly differentiated invasive cancer, a T3-N1-M0 cancer rank and serial number with a thirty- to sixty-percent five-year survival and a pathological description I had thought was reserved only for medical textbooks.

I had a Stage III poorly differentiated invasive cancer, a T3-N1-M0 cancer rank and serial number with a thirty- to sixty-percent five-year survival and a pathological description I had thought was reserved only for medical textbooks. My treatment included a mastectomy, oophorectomy, chemotherapy, radiation to the chest wall and axilla, tamoxifen, and psychiatric therapy. I also had my bone marrow harvested in Omaha, Nebraska, for future use and research purposes. I felt like Job during treatment. I had several episodes of cellulitis, abscessed teeth, mouth ulcers, anal fissures, and conjunctivitis, not to mention a bout of pneumonia that rendered me septic and in isolation in hospital.

My stormy course with chemotherapy was partly my fault. I kept hounding my oncologist to give me more chemotherapy despite my low white count and kept berating her that my hair was not falling out fast enough. Not that my oncologist was not aggressive; she pulled out all the stops, broke into clinical trials, and came at me with guns blazing in true American style, all the while insisting, "I want you to be around for those kids," as I clung to her for dear life.

Several episodes occurred during treatment. My infant son had to have neurosurgery at the age of six months for a prematurely fused lambdoid suture which, due to my illness, my husband and I failed to notice in a timely fashion. He lost a lot of blood and required a blood transfusion. Because of the cancer, I could not give him my blood. As a mother and a physician, this shook me deeply. He has become my Wednesday's child, full of woe. Was it because I could not bond properly with him or was I subconsciously blaming him for my cancer? Was it because my husband had difficulty adjusting to my second pregnancy and it was to be that pregnancy that almost killed me? I must say that, during my illness, my husband showed his true colours, which had often been hidden by the stresses of marriage. He said the magic words that made all the difference: "I wish this was happening to me instead of to you."

During treatment, I tried to stay in some sort of shape by swimming and had an embarrassing moment when my breast prosthesis floated away from me only to be scooped up by a young male doing a vigorous front crawl. He was heard to say, "What the f . . . ?" when he abruptly stopped swimming to compose himself.

I mentioned psychiatric therapy in my list of treatments, and found great comfort in my sessions with my elderly and wise Freudian psychiatrist (though I knew that I was getting better when he started snoring loudly during one of my tales of woe). It took me a long time to realize that the diagnosis of cancer does not stop at the neck, and I give him as much credit for my survival as I do my other physicians.

Friends were a great support to me. One of my dear friends, Theresa Isomura, understood my fears and flew down to New Orleans to see me through a crucial time, the weekend before the start of chemotherapy. Leaving behind a busy work schedule and three children under six years old, she moved in and took over the household, looking after my kids and my husband and holding my hand.

One time, a most bizarre episode occurred when an elderly gentleman in a big white Lincoln pulled up beside me, gazed at me through rheumy eyes, and proceeded to tell me how good I looked. There I was, looking like the wrath of God, with a hat perched haphazardly on my bald head, no make-up, not even lipstick (why bother? I was going to die anyway) and some guy makes a pass at me! I was thunderstruck that anyone could see me as attractive and immediately suggested to my admirer that he should get his cataracts checked!

After treatment, my fight with breast cancer was far from over. What faced me now was its aftermath. I developed severe lymphedema in my mastectomy arm, rendering it twice the size of the other arm. For nine years, I ran the gamut of therapies—compression sleeves and pumps, manual lymphatic drainage—with minimal effect. In my desperation to relieve the lymphedema, I even ended up smuggling in a drug not approved by the Health Protection Branch (HPB) / Food and Drug Administration (FDA). Touted by a *New England Journal of Medicine* article as being effective against lymphedema, it was called benzopyrone and I got it from Australia. After taking it for six months, I was alarmed to find out through the grapevine that it was pulled off the market in Australia for causing severe liver damage and deaths. Needless to say, my respect went up considerably for the HPB and U.S. FDA.

I have also been plagued by numerous episodes of virulent erysipelas-like cellulitis in the arm, caused by trivial injuries such as a hangnail or a paper cut, always streptococcal in nature and exquisitely sensitive to penicillin. When I get these infections, I try to avoid the hospital and treat myself with intravenous penicillin at home. For the past two years, I have stopped all lymphedema therapy and my arm has behaved. In fact, the infection rate has gone down.

Another result of the treatment was the onset of early menopause. After six years, I could no longer stand its ravages. I felt like a dried up prune with no lust for life. I would chafe and bleed in the vaginal area after skiing or vigorous walking. Having sex was horrid and out of the question. My bone density studies was falling by three percent every two years. I started wolfing down calcium only to develop a kidney stone. I gained weight, lost my figure, could not get a decent night's sleep, and was not thinking as sharply as before. Despite my high risk for breast cancer, I started taking estrogen and progesterone and have concluded that indicting menopausal women with a history of breast cancer to a life without hormonal support is exacting a cruel cure.

Seven years after my treatment, probably because of the estrogen surging through my veins, I had reconstructive surgery with a saline implant. As part of my pre-operative workup, I insisted on having my mastectomy site scanned with ultrasound for any signs of metastasis. Much to my alarm, a filling defect was found between the lung and the chest wall. When it was needled to show lymph fluid, I developed a fifteen percent pneumothorax.

In view of my poor prognosis, my husband moved us back to Canada to be closer to family. It was a difficult move for me; I felt I was coming back here to die. Returning to work was also difficult. After working a few shifts, it became painfully obvious to me that I had become extremely rusty as an Emergency physician. Fortunately, my colleagues assigned me to areas where I could wreak little damage and urged me to take some continuing medical education.

In true Job-like fashion, my list of medical curses related to breast cancer mounted. Due to the radiation damage to the tissues of my chest wall, my saline implant hardened and developed a capsular contracture. My kids could literally bounce a ball off my implanted breast. I decided in 2000 to have a prophylactic mastectomy because I could not stand the mounting yearly risk for breast cancer in the allegedly healthy breast. I had to wait, however, until Health Canada came to its senses and released silicone gel breast implants for women with breast cancer. Perhaps my endless badgering e-mails to Health Canada and my very public stance on the safety of silicone implants paid off. I had the hardened saline implant removed and now have two soft silicone implants, which will slowly be expanded with saline over the next few months.

Although I do not believe in fate, I could imagine its cruel finger pointing at me when an Aboriginal woman arrived at Emergency during my shift, short of breath and reeking of rotting flesh. My worst fears were confirmed when I removed her clothing and saw her cancerous breast. I saw that finger pointing my way again when a middle-aged woman with an old mastectomy scar arrived in shock and died because the breast cancer had metastasized to her pericardium.

Unfortunately, working has also contributed to my stormy medical history. After resuscitating a Burmese refugee who turned out to have full-blown AIDS and active TB, my PPD skin test converted. I had to take INH for one year, despite the risk of liver toxicity at my age. What irked me was the fact that this poor man had been languishing in Canada for eight months with no medical care, all the while potentially infecting those around him. Two weeks of TB medications would have rendered him non-infectious, and triple therapy for his AIDS would have given him some quality of life. I contacted the government repeatedly, urging them to medically screen refugees more diligently, but got nowhere. I then went to the media and was immediately branded a racist and, unbeknownst to me, became a poster girl for a white supremacist web-site. The irony is that my Jewish husband urged me not to go public with the story and predicted that I would be branded a racist.

But, as much as I try, I cannot restrain myself from speaking up. I am quite vocal about breast cancer issues and have joined virtually every organization that involves breast cancer. Since 1994, I have helped run a breast cancer support group in my neighbourhood, called "Treasure Chests." I have participated in numerous federal government forums and workshops on breast cancer, and felt privileged to be a survivor representative to Health Canada's committee for the development of national clinical practice guidelines on how to treat breast cancer. I have been called upon to speak at public forums in British Columbia and Ontario and have been interviewed extensively by the media. My Cassandra-like attitude to breast cancer has sometimes given me less than rave reviews, but I was thrilled to receive the Canadian Cancer Society's "Medal of Courage" in 1998 for my cancer advocacy work.

I have written articles for medical journals, books, and magazines, and am forever writing newspaper items which have landed me in hot water several times. When I wrote an article pointing out that AIDS gets more federal funding than breast cancer, I was branded a homophobe. When I argued, in another article, that there was no link between silicone implants and disease, I received an anonymous death threat in the mail. But the *coup de grace* occurred when I wrote an article based on sound epidemiological data for the *Journal of Clinical Oncology*, that cancer survival rates are better in the United States than in Canada for all socioeconomic classes except the poor. The hate mail generated by the article was staggering. Again my long-suffering husband cautioned me not to go public with the article as I was setting myself up for malicious attacks and character assassination. "Oh no," I brayed, "people need to know the truth."

Unfortunately, a reporter came gunning for me and alerted not only me but also my employers of my presence on a white supremacist web-site. He then threatened to do a hatchet job on me in an article for the weekend paper. It was time to "reach for my lawyers." I chose the attorney who made legal history by successfully suing the U.S. government. He was able to keep my name out of the paper. It was a sobering lesson in civil rights for me. When freedom of speech and freedom of press collide, freedom of press always wins. As my lawyer keeps reminding me, newspapers buy ink by the barrel and can always print the last word.

All this activism has taken its toll on my husband and kids; on many occasions, they call me Donna Quixote rather than Mom, especially when I get that crazed look in my eye. My greatest source of joy and hope is my family, particularly my two sons. I treasure each moment with them (except the homework and hockey ones) and am thrilled to watch them grow. I call my second son my "tumour-marker" and revel in the passing of his birthdays. My sons are now eleven and thirteen and know I fully expect them to become doctors. They will have to have a degree in medicine to take care of themselves if, heaven forbid, they inherit my medical history. But above all, I will want them to look out for me and take care of me in my old age. And that is a prospect I truly want to enjoy!

DR. THERESA ISOMURA

My grandmother was a nurse in Nagoya General Hospital in Japan. She came to Vancouver in 1920 after crossing the Pacific Ocean for twenty sea-sick days. She was a picture bride and her spouse-to-be, my grandfather, had come to Vancouver in 1905 at age eighteen. He had been adopted by a couple who had no sons and inherited six houses and half of Kerrisdale, which was forest and bush land at the time.

He had lost most of his properties by 1922 when he went bankrupt. My grandmother borrowed twenty dollars and an iron, and started a dressmaking business. She rented a store on Commercial Drive, 'Isomura Dressmaking Store.' She had quite a flourishing business and had up to three ladies working for her. My grandparents had three sons—the eldest was later to be my father.

In May 1942, my grandparents suddenly lost everything and were forced by the Canadian Government to evacuate with their family to Greenwood, British Columbia. After the war ended, the family went to eastern Canada, and spent some years in Kingston, Ontario, where my father studied physics and mathematics at Queen's University. He went on to complete his undergraduate degree at McGill University. After he was accepted into McGill Medical School in August 1951, my parents decided to marry. I was born in December 1952, and my sister Mary Ann in 1955, the year my father graduated from medical school.

My father interned, then spent four years studying surgery at St. Mary's Hospital in Montreal after which he decided to work in Point St. Charles near Montreal. Point St. Charles was where the Irish settled after the potato famine in Ireland, many of whom worked on the St. Lawrence Bridge. My father was one of three English-speaking doctors who worked for an Anglophone population of 13,000 (sixty percent of whom were of Irish descent). My father had a busy practice and enjoyed his work. The office was in our house. After he spent much of the day at the hospital and in his office, I remember many evenings when my mother would accompany my father on house calls late at night.

Medicine was my father's life. He also became involved in social issues in the Point, trying to organize support for the poor. My sister and I remember him returning from a house call on Christmas day and packing our toys and going back to the house he had visited because the children had not received anything for Christmas. I made many good friends in Point St. Charles. I had a glimpse of poverty, learned to value friendships, and had great times playing baseball in the back lane, skating on an outdoor rink, or walking to Expo '67 with friends. I attended the St. Gabriel's School, a public Catholic girls' school taught by nuns. The sisters were strict but kind-hearted and dedicated to teaching. They took great pains in preparing us for our first Communion and Confirmation. We attended Mass with the boys, the first Friday of every month. They also prepared us each year for the St. Patrick's Day concert. Since he was an Irish saint, March 17 was a school holiday, but we all had to attend the concert.

I think my sister and I were the only Japanese Canadians with shamrocks, but on St. Patrick's Day everyone is Irish. I completed high school at James Lyng and then attended two years of CEGEP at McGill University.

It was a very interesting time, with the FLQ and the October Crisis in the province of Quebec occuring while I was attending an Anglophone university. During this time, my career interests were uncertain and I was considering teaching, since a career in medicine appeared too consuming. In 1970, my father was concerned about the politics in Quebec and decided to move west to Richmond, British Columbia, to start a general practice. He packed the maroon Chevrolet family car and headed west. My sister flew to B.C. several months later, and after I completed my second year of CEGEP I also flew to B.C. My good childhood friend, Joanne, had also decided to move to Richmond, and this made my transition to the other side of Canada easier.

My father's practice became very busy; he saw primarily Japanese-speaking patients who were appreciative in having him as their family doctor. I guess the genetic pull to the sciences and medicine was pretty strong for me. I attended the University of British Columbia and completed a Bachelor of Science degree in biochemistry. I became curious about the biochemical cause of illnesses, applied and was accepted into medical school at UBC. I met my future husband Greg in an anatomy class. We were grouped alphabetically in anatomy and histology classes. What attracted me to him was his great sense of humour, which has continued to be an important part of our relationship. We made many good friends during medical school and shared many hardships as a group. We lost one of our classmates to suicide in our second year and another to lymphoma our third year. Shortly after our graduation, a classmate died in an avalanche. To date, we have had two reunions, both great get-togethers.

After completing UBC Medical School in 1979, Greg and I did our internship at the Royal Columbian Hospital in New Westminster. Since we wanted our holidays at the same time, the intern director arranged for us to work as partners during our internship year. This meant we were doing one in two calls for twenty-four hours. It was an interesting year. One evening after I had dinner at my mother's house I brought some dinner to Greg, who was in the OR assisting Dr. Allan, an obstetrician. The next day Dr. Allan commented to one of my intern colleagues, Martha McCarthy, "I think there is something going on between Isomura and Harrington." Her reply was, "I hope so. They are getting married next week."

Greg and I married in November of our internship year. The wedding was fun; all twenty interns from the Hospital attended. We were sad to see the year end. We learned a lot and had great memories.

After our wedding, Greg went on to a Urology Residency Program at UBC. I did general practice locums for a year before applying for the Psychiatry Program at UBC. During my locums, patients with anxiety and depression triggered my interest in psychiatry as I was trying to find ways to help them. My father-in-law, who was a psychiatrist, appeared to be such a normal person that this also helped me to decide that psychiatry might be a specialty I could enjoy.

Dr. Allan commented to one of my intern colleagues, Martha McCarthy, "I think there is something going on between Isomura and Harrington." Her reply was, "I hope so. They are getting married next week."

After completing my studies in psychiatry at UBC, I was four months pregnant when I went to my oral exams in Edmonton in June 1985. Greg had started work at Maple Ridge Hospital, and I worked at the Burnaby Psychiatric Services doing Community Psychiatry, and also at Shaughnessy Hospital in the Sleep Disorder Clinic.

Sleep was not something I was doing much of. I had returned to work after two-and-a-half months of maternity leave, and Angela had colic for a few months, crying most nights. I can remember feeling more tired than most of the patients I saw in the Sleep Clinic. We had our second child Naomi in 1988, and shortly after I wrote my specialty exams in Sleep Disorders. We started Angela in Montessori preschool when she was three-and-a-half years old. Although we had a live-in nanny, Tessie, she did not drive, so Greg and I would take turns driving Angela to and from school. I was usually late because of work duties and she would be the last one to be picked up, looking very unhappy. We had Megan in 1990, which was the same year Tessie left and found Rose for us.

Rose initially worked full-time and over the last three years has continued to work part-time for us. She has been invaluable helping with child care, driving, doing housework, and taking care of us. Greg and I have made it a priority to attend the special school events as we realize how important it is for the children.

The Sleep Disorder Clinic had moved to UBC, and after working in this field for ten years I decided to leave and devote my time to my work in Burnaby and to my family. During this time, I was asked to teach Residents and provide a psychiatry rotation at Burnaby. I enjoyed imparting knowledge about psychiatry and helping people understand how it feels to make someone better. In the meantime, the girls became involved in a few more activities, playing sports and piano and attending a French Immersion School program in Coquitlam. We have met so many wonderful parents and made so many friends through the girls' activities. Although this makes our lives busier, we are trying to enjoy every moment.

To deal with stress from work and get into shape, I started walking during my lunch hour with my friend Daniella. I belong to a running group, and was encouraged to do the Kelowna Marathon in October 1999 and in October 2000, and I completed the Victoria Marathon. Training and marathons have given me another perspective on life.

My work has changed again over the last year and a half. I have been involved in a Shared Care Pilot Project working more closely with family physicians in their offices with a mental health nurse. I have also been involved with the redevelopment of a Psychiatry Department at the Royal Columbian Hospital. This has been a real challenge, but an honour to come back as a full-fledged specialist to the hospital where I interned. I will still be continuing my work at the Burnaby Psychiatry Services.

I enjoyed the many aspects of psychiatry, and was privileged to have my family and children who have given me a better understanding of my work. My work has also given me a better appreciation of my family, children, and husband. I cherish my family and the many good friends I have made along this path: Joanne Teraguchi, Maria Hugi, Martha McCarthy, Margaret Duke, Heidi Oetter, Sherry Fulton, Danielle Derrick, and Gindy Bir, to name a few. The support of my family and friends has given me the courage and energy to do what I have done and to take on the challenges which lie ahead.

DR. JOAN H. SCRUTON

I graduated from Sheffield University, United Kingdom, where I also did my house-jobs. I did emergency medicine and general medicine (cardiology and internal medicine). David, my husband, then got into the internal medicine rotation in Aberdeen, Scotland. I had hoped to do pediatrics, but at that time there were no places. My next choice was cardiology, and I had great experiences there working on the Coronary Care Unit, putting in temporary pacemakers, doing cardiac cauterizations, and even Coronary Angiograms. It is difficult now to believe that I actually did that. I took part in a Double-Blind Trial comparing Nifedine with B-blockers in controlling hypertension. I missed out on a trip to Rio de Janeiro and Spain which was paid for by the drug company. My consultant would not take me because I was pregnant! One hair-raising trip was escorting a patient with a nurse on the sleeper (night train) from Aberdeen to London. He had a Hb. of three grams because his aortic valve replacement was haemolysing his red cells and he was going to London for a new valve. We had an oxygen tank under the bed on the train and some other resuscitation equipment. Fortunately nothing untoward happened. Another man I escorted from Aberdeen to Edinburgh for surgery had oedema up to his armpits due to a VSD secondary to his myocardial infarction. Another palpitating experience was helping a man with the heart-lung machine during cardiac surgery. In Aberdeen we did not have theatre technicians, just the consultant and I; and he used to go off for coffee, leaving me alone. I was petrified I would get the three-way valve directing the wrong way. I never was very good with three-way taps.

We came to Canada twenty-one years ago and realized a dream of my husband. I was very unsure whether I wanted to be here for quite some time. In November, 1978, I was despatched to Toronto to get an Enabling

Certificate. I had to discontinue breast-feeding my second son in order to do this. My husband had booked me a room for one night, and I was quite in awe of its size, the number of towels, and the dining room with white table-cloths and pink napkins folded in a fan shape. I enjoyed a few hours of shopping in downtown Toronto and took some exciting Lego back home for the children's Christmas. I was impressed with the cleanliness of the underground system in Toronto. So that was my introduction to Canada. I have not been to Toronto since we were destined to go to Prince Rupert. One of the carrots, as far as my husband David thought, was that I could have a horse (a dream since age ten); the only problem was that it was not possible in Prince Rupert. That dream had to wait for another twelve years to come true.

David came out to Canada in January, 1979. I remained to finish selling our house and came to Canada in March, 1979. My father-in-law came with me to help with looking after Colin, aged three, and Andrew, aged fourteen months. During our first five days in Prince Rupert it rained non-stop! I was unable to work for the first five months in British Columbia because I had not done the six-week post-grad obstetrics even though I had done lots as an undergrad. This I found frustrating, almost hurtful, but in order to get a temporary licence I had to go to Lions Gate Hospital in North Vancouver to fulfil this requisite. I was lucky to have support from my sister-in-law and my mother-in-law who came for three weeks to look after my kids and husband while I was away. Then of course we had to study again and sit the LMCC exams—not easy with two small boys to look after at the same time. Sitting the exams, which involved hours of answering multiple choices and questions, was taxing—a type of exam we were not used to. Anyway, we did succeed.

I did locums at first, and then worked part-time in the Greene Clinic, the same clinic as David. I gradually increased the work-load as the kids became more independent at school. It was difficult juggling clinic time and getting away in time to pick up the children from nursery school (you were not allowed to be late). Like any working mothers there was always the problem of finding baby-sitters. On more than one occasion I had to rush to Maternity to deliver a baby and leave one of my children at the nursing station. On one Sunday morning while we were enjoying a rare cup of tea in bed, I was called to go out by helicopter to one of the Native villages where I had to assess a girl with premature rupture of her membranes and

escort her back to Prince Rupert. It turned out that the concern was that it was her fourth baby, and the possibility that she might deliver before we returned. In fact the opposite happened, and we had to induce labour the next day.

One of my fortés which I had developed was reducing shoulders. I just seemed to develop a knack of quietly talking to the unfortunate patient while doing the necessary manoeuvres at the same time. Our Clinic's duties included having one of the doctors fly via float plane to Port Simpson for a day-long clinic. If you have ever seen the movie "Never Cry Wolf," you will understand what the plane journey is like. It was often so windy that it left you with a dry mouth.

I was the only female physician for eight of the twelve years of our stay in Prince Rupert, so naturally I attracted a lot of gynecology. At one Christmas party I was given a holster with a speculum on one side and a Pap-smear stick and swabs on the other, because for many days I was continually trotting up and down the hall with speculums.

It was actually quite tiring working in Prince Rupert. We were always on call and did shifts in Emergency on a regular basis. I often did my husband's night calls because he worked full-time. I worked part-time and was a much lighter sleeper, conditioned by work and kids to be up and down every night. We had a skeleton of specialists. After the first four years we had no obstetrician, and I got used to that after about six months. My worst shift was on a New Year's Eve. With people fighting and knifing each other and car accidents, there was blood everywhere. The situation became so bad that I had to call Dr. Greene in to help. He was the surgeon on call; he has long since retired but is apparently alive and well at age eighty-six.

We had a third child, a daughter, in 1981, whose arrival completed the family. I took eight months off, but on resuming work I would be up twice in the night with the baby and in and out to Emergency at different times.

So finally came the decision to relocate. We moved to the Comox Valley in 1991. David stayed on in Prince Rupert, leaving me with three kids in our new house on four-and-a-half acres. I was the guinea-pig, so it seemed, left to find locum work. This happened fairly quickly. I worked half-time with a girl returning from maternity leave, and the rest of the time filled in with bits for several other people. Then I worked for two years full-time.

David came down in April, 1992, but for the first six months I was oscillating between work, home, and children's activities. Emergency again was compulsory. I shared hospital privileges with the girl whom I shared a practice with, but did not get my own for five years. This was very political, as others who came after me received privileges before I did!

Here in the Comox Valley we have a Hobby Farm. So, as before, my time was divided between medicine, family, and animals. I have a strong maternal instinct, which is why I could never work full-time and leave the care of my children to anyone else.

We are contemplating moving to Denman Island. We'll stop work at our current clinics but continue working with Dr. Doreen Tetz, a single-handed general practitioner who is somewhat isolated and on call twenty-four hours a day throughout the year. So again we are putting ourselves into a more isolated area where specialized help is much nearer.

DR. PATRICIA WARSHAWSKI

Curriculum Vitae

Born: February 14, 1953 in Vancouver, B.C.
Marital status: Married with two children.
Education: Sir Winston Churchill High School, Vancouver, B.C.,
  1968–1971; Undergraduate Studies, Faculty of Science, UBC, 1971–1974;
  Faculty of Medicine, University of British Columbia, 1974–1978; First
  Year Resident, Department of Pediatrics, UBC, 1978–1979; Rotating
  Intern, Royal Columbian Hospital, New Westminster, B.C., 1979–1980;
  General Practice, Surrey, B.C., 1981–present.
Activities: Federation of Medical Women of Canada. Member at Large,
  B.C. Branch, 1986–1987; Member at Large, B.C. Branch, 1987–1988;
  Treasurer, B.C. Branch, 1988–1990; Member at Large, Vancouver
  Area Branch Federation of Medical Women of Canada (FMWC);
  Secretary, National FMWC, 1990–1991; Member at Large,
  Vancouver Area Branch FMWC, Childcare Committee, National
  FMWC, 1991-1992; President, Vancouver Area Branch FMWC,

Childcare Committee, National FMWC, 1992–1993; Past President
  Vancouver Area Branch FMWC, 1993–1994; Member at Large
  Vancouver Branch FMWC, 1994–1998; Treasurer Vancouver Branch
  FMWC; FMWC National Honorary Secretary, 1998–1999; FMWC
  National Awards Committee Member, 1999–2000.
Other Activities: Chair off and on, Library and Education Committee
  Surrey Memorial Hospital, 1991–ongoing.
Other Organizations: British Columbia Medical Association; has worked
  for Planned Parenthood for years starting in the early 1980s.

1981

DR. ELIZABETH BARBOUR

I enjoy living in the country—the beautiful fresh air, the clean water, and the lovely silence that urban people probably never experience. I also like the sense of community found in smaller areas as people tend to help each other in times of trouble. Although this closeness often comes at the expense of privacy and anonymity, it is nice to walk down the street of your town and feel bonded with the people you meet on your way.

My practice is about forty-five minutes away from the town of Nelson, in the unincorporated village of Slocan Park, located in the Slocan Valley and with a population estimated between 2,000 to 4,000 people. One of the main industries is logging, but there are also lots of folks who do business via the computer. There are self-employed people, small farmers, and a large underground marijuana industry here as well. A number of people in the Valley came in the 1960s with ideals of alternative lifestyles. Their arrival subsequently led to a polarization between loggers and environmentalists. Life is never dull because of the diversity of people coming from different backgrounds.

I did my undergraduate degree in Arts with majors in Religious Studies and English at the University of British Columbia. After graduation I spent some time in the work force before returning to UBC to do undergraduate science courses required for my application to medical school. My arts background and the time spent working in a non-medical area have helped to give me a better feel for the human side of medicine. I am particularly interested in how people's personalities and life histories affect their physiology. Each disease takes place within the frame of a personality, and often the type of response can really affect the outcome of the illness. Having done a fair bit of reading in comparative religions has also been helpful for looking after people who are facing death and who may or may not have the spiritual resources to handle palliative issues. I feel that it is important to give these patients genuine support and care by drawing upon my own spiritual resources.

After finishing my internship at St. Paul's Hospital, I came to Nelson to begin general practice, as I yearned for the rural lifestyle and was aware of Nelson as a particularly beautiful and clean country setting. The hospital here has an excellent medical staff with the advantage of having Internal Medicine, Pediatrics, Gynecology, Neurology, and Surgical specialists for backup. We also have a very fine ICU. At the regional centre in Trail, specialists, CT scanning, and Nuclear Medicine are also available. From 1982 until 1996, I had a very busy practice in Nelson itself, which also included Obstetrics. From 1989 until 1991, I was the Chief of Staff at the local hospital and also chair of the steering committee for regionalisation. We were one of the earliest regions to achieve a cohesive agreement. While much ill has been done in the name of regionalisation, I still feel proud of the consensus-building we achieved in Nelson.

In 1995, I developed rheumatoid arthritis and it was clear that it would be necessary for me to withdraw from some of my many activities. I dropped my political involvement and began planning to move my practice out to the Slocan Valley, where I have been living since I came to the area. In doing so, I eliminated a half-day that I otherwise would have spent on the road. I also ceased to practise Obstetrics, so that the late night mad dash for town was no longer an added stress. At this time, there was no medical doctor practising in this end of the Valley, and no dentist or other medical services were easily available. About an hour farther north in New Denver, there were two fine practising physicians who were also associated with the small hospital there. However, patients from my part of the Valley would typically drive the forty-five minutes to Nelson for any medical needs.

After leaving my practice in Nelson, I was able to interest a local entrepreneur in becoming the owner/landlord of a clinic facility developed in Slocan Park. This is the site of my practice. The other tenants include a dentist, a massage therapist, a chiropractor, a doctor of traditional Chinese medicine, and a holistic health practitioner. (I might add that this is the classic spectrum of health services offered in the Slocan Valley region.) We are hoping to add services for lab work in the near future. My practice has grown and is generally welcomed as a very useful service for the area, particularly for the seniors who live at the new development home at Passmore, approximately five minutes from my office. Since I pass their door twice a day on the way to and from my office, I can easily stop in for house calls for any medical needs there. I would say that my involvement in initiating the development of the clinic and bringing these services to the local folks are something I am particularly proud of. I am very happy to think that the more vulnerable members of our community, such as the elderly, are now able to get medical attention more easily. Now that I am based here, it is easier for me to make house calls.

I really enjoy my small hobby farm, my horses and organic vegetable garden, and feel a real sense of belonging and privilege in being connected with this community in such a positive way.

DR. JEAN HLADY

Although I never planned to be a doctor, I was exposed to the medical field at a young age as my mother was Head Nurse in Pediatrics at St. Paul's Hospital. I remember being taken up to the ward at Christmas time to visit the staff and patients. Occasionally I would hear about certain patients, but I remember in particular one story about a poor child whose head was stepped on by a horse.

Initially I was in the field of psychology at the University of British Columbia, but I was not too keen on running rats through mazes, so I switched to genetics soon afterwards. I was not planning on going into medicine, but I got a summer job one year as a nurse's aid at Vancouver General Hospital. I met an orderly there who was a medical student, and he told me that I should apply to medical school since I had all the qualifications. I decided to apply, and then did not quite know what to do when I got accepted! I never thought I was smart enough for entering into this field. But I decided to give it a try.

Overall I enjoyed my years in medical school, in spite of our heavy workload. I made some good friends whom I have kept in touch with for twenty-five years. We got along well with everyone in our class, and continue to have wonderful reunions every five years.

I ended up receiving the Gold Medal in my class, which was quite a surprise. The headline in the *Vancouver Sun* at the time read: "Sex No Bar to Prize Winner." The interviewer asked if I had ever felt discriminated against because of my sex, and I had to honestly say, no, I had never experienced such discrimination, but that I had taken lots of teasing—all in fun.

On my first day I was on my own treating a farmer who had lost both his arms in a machine. The farmer came in first, followed by the arms. Needless to say, the arms could not be saved.

I headed off to intern in San Diego, California. It was an eye-opener to attend the weekly clinics in Tijuana, with a particular focus on early detection of cervical cancer. Sometimes I heard about how women in labour sneaked across the border in trunks of cars, in hope of having their babies born in the U.S. so that the whole family could immigrate to the country. It was also interesting to experience first hand the U.S. Health Care System. There were several people who had to mortgage their homes in order to pay the hospital bills. We were told to stop ordering bilirubin tests for the babies whose families could not afford them. This was something I had not been used to. It was here where I also saw my first child abuse case. I still remember the child's name (incidentally, I missed the diagnosis at first). Never did I expect that I would later spend most of my professional life in the child abuse field.

After the internship, I answered an ad and ended up in Lloydminster, Alberta, as a GP for two years. I really learned to stand on my own feet medically—with a little backup from specialists—after managing a bus crash with close to a hundred victims (many minors), a head-on crash with twelve serious victims, and a six-year-old child with seventy percent burns all in the first few months. On my first day I was on my own treating a farmer who had lost both his arms in a machine. The farmer came in first, followed by the arms. Needless to say, the arms could not be saved. The people in the community were wonderful, and I came very close to staying permanently. My life would have been very different had I made that choice.

But I met a physician who had emigrated from York, England, and he encouraged me to work there in pediatrics as a house officer. I did this and, again, it was a wonderful experience. It could be quite hair-raising at times, such as managing an obstructed epiglottitis patient on your own. I met many wonderful people there too. It was fascinating to compare the U.S. and the British Health Care Systems.

By this time I had decided to pursue a career in pediatrics. It was very gratifying to see children recovering rapidly even though they tend to fall ill very rapidly. It was usually more difficult to handle the parents of these sick children.

I applied to the Hospital for Sick Children for my residency. During the interview I was asked why I thought I was good enough for their hospital. I was rather surprised by that question, but I must have handled the interview all right because I was accepted. The years there were very difficult, but I saw many interesting children, and fortunately was able to pass my fellowship exams.

My heart was out west, so I returned to Vancouver in 1980 as a teaching fellow in pediatrics. I really enjoyed teaching the students and eventually ended up directing the second and third-year Pediatric Teaching Program for five years each. In 1996, I received the Excellence in Teaching Award in Pediatrics for the Undergraduate Program.

I was also working regular shifts in the Emergency Department of the new Children's Hospital at the time. In fact, I started working in the Emergency Department when the hospital first opened. For the first little while we were able to cover the ER from home. Things are certainly different now! I found emergency very exciting and challenging; one never knew what would come through the doors next. One time we had a film crew filming a day in the life of emergency while a young child was being brought in with her arm caught in an industrial meat grinder (they brought the whole grinder in). The film crew, who were all large men, went three shades of green and nearly fainted while I had to take charge.

As an emergency physician I was asked if I would see a few of the child abuse cases, as many of them came through the ER. Well, things evolved from there and before I knew it, I was the local expert on abuse issues. Eventually I became more interested in this area and felt that this work was vitally important.

I was able to secure funding to significantly expand the Child Protection Team at the Children's Hospital. When I took over the director's position from Dr. Jim Carter, the staff of the unit consisted of several part-time physicians and a social worker. Now our unit has a staff of fourteen, some full-time and some part-time. The most complex cases from B.C. come to us. The work is, of course, very stressful, but I have a wonderful staff to work with, which is why I have lasted so long in the field. We all try to keep a sense of humour, although things can be difficult at times.

Besides working in the Child Protection Team, I have been working in the General Pediatric Clinic since the hospital opened. I feel strongly that it is important to keep a balance between General Peds and Child Protection. In the General Peds Clinic, however, many of our patients are in foster care or are underprivileged. Over the years I have seen a lot of intriguing pediatric problems, and I have learned many things, especially the importance of always listening to the nurses; they may make the diagnosis when you have missed it.

I have been offered university academic positions (I am a clinical professor now), but I have no real interest in the academic tenure track. Hands-on patient care was what I enjoyed the most, although I was an examiner in pediatrics for the Royal College for five years. That was a great experience. I still enjoy teaching, but now it is mostly restricted to the Child Protection field. I now teach other professionals about child abuse: lawyers, social workers, police, and dentists, to name a few. I have taken on more of a provincial role in the protection field now, consulting with the Ministry for Children and Families and sitting on an advisory committee to the Children's Commission.

I have no desire to advance "up the ladder" anymore. My only ambition now is to work in an underdeveloped country for a period of time. Many of my medical school colleagues have entered 'glamorous' sub-specialties, such as plastic surgery, orthopedic surgery, anesthesia, and so on. My daily work is anything but glamorous, treating children who have been subjected to the most horrendous forms of physical and sexual abuse. Many of these children have been raised in grinding poverty and the future seems bleak to them. I consider it a privilege to have been able to work with these children, to have, perhaps, improved their lives in some small way. Looking back, I would not change a thing for the experiences I have gained throughout my career.

DR. LESLIE LeHUQUET

It is of value to record the experiences of ordinary women as their contributions are rarely thought noteworthy. Still, it is somewhat intimidating to have to look back on one's life and judge whether any portion of it might be thought to rise above the banal and be worthy of interest to others.

I was born in Halifax and raised around the same area, although most of my memories are of the rural areas of Lawrencetown, Mineville, and Preston where I spent the summers roaming on my own. These communities have all grown up now and acquired considerable respectability, but when I was young they were very sparsely populated and quite poor.

Mineville and Lawrencetown are small habitations joined by the Mineville River that flows into the Atlantic at Lawrencetown beach. My ancestors built and maintained the dykes that kept the seawater from the fields near the Mineville Bridge, but by the time I was old enough to explore, these areas had returned to marshlands. I spent many summer days poling through these marshes and canoeing miles up and down this river to Lawrencetown Beach.

Lawrencetown Beach is one of a series of extensive sand bars that stretches along the eastern shore of Nova Scotia. I have visited beaches all over the world, including the famous Long Beach of Tofino and North Beach of Graham Island, Queen Charlotte Islands. I would rate the coast of Nova Scotia as one of the most impressive. The waters off Nova Scotia can be exceptionally cold, and learning to swim in such temperatures has allowed me to enjoy afternoon dips in glacial run-offs to this day.

Mineville itself was an unusual place for an adventuresome child as the woods were filled with disused mine shafts and collapsed tunnels that we were taught to recognize by the shallow overgrown depressions. An unwary step might very well have meant a trip to the underworld.

My family owned the area known as the Shanghai Mines. Although the holdings were extensive, it was a meager remnant of the land granted by Cornwallis to my seafaring ancestor for piloting the ships of General Wolfe up the St. Lawrence River to the Battle of the Plains of Abraham. I enjoyed exploring the ancient gravesites and finding familiar names on headstones dating from the 18th century. Even as a teenager I was fascinated by the clustering of deaths that suggested disease outbreaks.

In my time the public school system of Nova Scotia was flexible enough to include students of varying degrees of ability, and there was money to hire the best teachers. It allowed me the luxury of progressing as quickly as I wished. The major problem with the system was gender bias, especially towards academically ambitious female students, an attitude that started in homes where physical abuse for many women was a daily fact of life. It was the fear of being trapped in such a cycle that accelerated my learning, driving me to start in the Honours Biochemistry Program at Dalhousie University by the time I was sixteen.

There was very little money left for rent and food, and for a time I lived on cabbage and stale bread mixed with mustard. If I was lucky I was able to find leftover food at the hospital, but there was always a line-up for these treats.

The scholarship applications had to pass through the hands of the school counsellors for pre-approval and authentication, and I remember vividly being told that despite having the highest grade point average, I would not be permitted to apply for university financial assistance. The rationale was that I would be unfairly competing with males who would be supporting families and putting their education to better use. I was not eligible for any academic awards at my grade level either as I was "jumping the queue" by leaving high school a year early.

In contrast, Dalhousie University was very supportive of any student with ability and ambition regardless of gender, and allowed selected applicants to choose their own course of study, provided an academic standard was maintained.

I was very fortunate to have found the academic challenges enjoyable, and I was able to graduate *cum laude* with a BSc in Chemistry and Math by the time I was nineteen. I was immediately accepted into Dalhousie Medical School after graduation and completed those studies by the time I was twenty-three.

Even with student loans and bursaries I remember working three jobs at a time to afford the books and other expenses of post-graduate education. I envied students from wealthier families who were able to focus solely on their studies. With courses running all year round there was very little money left for rent and food, and for a time I lived on cabbage and stale bread mixed with mustard. If I was lucky I was able to find leftover food at the hospital, but there was always a line-up for these treats. The training system was extremely hierarchical at Dalhousie, and the senior resident or house officer had first dibs on any leftover food on the patients' trays. The next in line was the junior resident, then the intern and clinical clerk, and the final turn came only to the medical student when the floor matron released the meals instead of sending them back to the kitchen. If we were on call, the hospitals sometimes would provide us meals, and I remember that the dieticians used to give us special Maritime treats for breakfast. The specialty of the house at VGH was kippers and strawberry jam, while the Provincial Lab was famous for its Mulligatawny soup.

The Halifax Infirmary was a very spooky place to work. The on-call rooms were reached by a series of underground tunnels. The nuns ran the hospital, and we were never even provided clean sheets for our on-call beds. The sleeping accommodations were so unkempt that many of us preferred to sleep on any free couch or chair on the wards. If I remember correctly many of the facilities in the Halifax area were connected underground, but few of us would travel these alone and rarely at night.

I lived in a single-room apartment with one other girl, but there usually seemed to be one or more boys also sleeping on the floor or curled up in our chair. There was no impropriety; it was just a dry roof and a warm spot. They just seemed to be there when I got up in the morning, having arrived long after I was asleep. I never had time to wonder about introductions as, being the only medical student in the group, I was up and out hours before any of the rest awakened.

Medical school at Dalhousie was, for me, a revelation. Women were accepted, not just tolerated. Every student willing to work was encouraged and supported. I especially enjoyed surgery and entered a surgical internship with the endorsement of the Halifax surgical group. The surgeons were all male, and while the humour may not always have been politically correct, their hearts definitely were in the right place. I spent most of the time in the surgical suites in stitches from the teasing that was usually directed at me, the most junior person. Outside of Halifax, though, others were not as enlightened, and in some of the smaller hospitals the going could be pretty rough for females. The attitude towards women was considerably less enlightened when I worked in Saint John, New Brunswick.

I met my husband while fulfilling my obligations as junior house officer at Camp Hill Hospital in Halifax. John was the senior house officer during my tenure, a UBC graduate and Dalhousie Family Practice Resident who had moved from an Internal Medicine Residency. We met while attending a very ill gentleman whom we believed had a treatable condition. Unfortunately, the Head of Service, convinced that this patient was not salvageable, overruled us and the man died without any diagnostic investigations. On autopsy he was found to have a benign perforated duodenal ulcer and not pancreatic cancer. It was this case and its complicated ethical issues that brought us together.

We have now been married for twenty years and look forward to another twenty. During my internship we chose to leave Halifax and acquire a more rural experience in New Brunswick. The living conditions and attitudes were considerably different than those in Halifax. All the interns in Saint John were housed in a two-storey lodge next to the railway tracks. It was so cold that we often had to huddle in groups under blankets in the common room to stay warm in the evenings. The men on the second floor had the worst of it as there was often ice layered on the inside of the windows. We had a single kitchen which we rarely used; as our salaries barely covered transportation and books, we had little money left for food. I remember being given a large zucchini and some onions that we sliced and layered with a little cheese that someone else had acquired. It was a wonderful feast for twenty of us. Imagine a gourd that could feed such a large group of hungry, young people, and one harkens back to the story of the loaves and the fishes.

Initially I was not allowed to live with my husband in Saint John. It was not considered proper that there be any fraternization between ranks of staff. As my husband was a year ahead we were not supposed to be housed together, and the administration refused to allow us to even stay in the same building. It was not until we threatened to write to the Office of the Dean in Halifax that we were assigned married accommodations.

Ours was a basement apartment with a living room so wet that one of my texts actually splashed when it slipped off of the table. There was one-quarter inch of ice on the inside of all of the windows for the entire winter, but at least we were able to spend some time together. At Christmas we decided to pool our resources and invite a number of our colleagues to a Christmas dinner. Knowing that medical students ate lots whenever the food was free, I planned on serving both ham and a large turkey with all of the fixings.

Unfortunately, the ham was fatter than we thought, and some of the drippings pooled onto the base of the oven. Subsequently, when we cooked the turkey the stove caught on fire. This was the first of many of the cooking conflagrations that seemed to have marked the goal posts of our marriage. It seemed a simple matter for us to shut the stove down and open the door periodically to throw in baking soda and then flour; the problem arose when we tried to relieve ourselves of the choking smoke. The windows were frozen and solidly shut, and we were unable to chip away enough of the ice inside the room to free the sashes. We resorted to opening the door, unaware that this apartment building had a fully functional and monitored smoke alarm right outside our door. A klaxon crowed, cries of alarm were heard, and many feet clattered. Someone shouted to another to grab warm clothes, as there was five feet of snow outside and ten feet of drift. The fire department fortunately arrived with amazing dispatch and cancelled the siren before everyone figured out that we were the culprits. The dinner was a success anyway because we were not to let a simple fire prevent us from cleaning out the oven and starting over with the turkey. The neighbours were relieved when we finally left.

Saint John was very cold and the winter conditions were often severe enough to shut the city down. I remember trekking through waist-high snow to reach a cleared thoroughfare so that the police could pick us up to man the Emergency department. Saint John had a busy emergency and it was not unusual for me to see 120 people on a shift. Some of the cases were particularly gruesome as it was not unheard of to have a semi-conscious alcoholic brought in to have the maggots cleaned out of his or her multiple pressure sores. The police also brought in those whom they felt were at risk on the street for being set on fire by the local rowdies.

Saint John Hospital had a psychiatric crisis unit, and the experiences that I lived through there would probably fill at least another page. It was at the Infirmary in Halifax where I came face to face with the real tragedy of mental illness. One case lingers with me still. My preceptor assigned me the duty of interviewing a special case, the nineteen-year-old son of a personal friend, a successful student and athlete, who had been having some depression problems for several years but had not been adequately treated. He had been referred to the unit for specialized assessment, as no one had been able or perhaps willing to make a diagnosis. He was a well-built and very handsome young man almost my age who spoke well but seemed somehow distant. It was subtle, but there was something suspiciously wrong with his attitude and the content of his speech. His writings confirmed the disordered thought of the frightened early schizophrenic who sensed the barrier being raised

We watched as eagerly as other residents for the barges during the winter, as sometimes transport through the treacherous waters of Hecate Strait of such essentials as fresh vegetables and fruit, baby formula and milk, was impossible.

between life around him and his own diseased reality. It was my first contact with an early schizophrenic before complete decompensation, and it was saddening for the whole department to confirm the diagnosis. I followed his treatment for some time, and when I last saw him he was wandering the sunny corridors of the secure psychiatric unit in Dartmouth. It was hard to imagine anyone looking so lost. It was difficult to accept the loss of a personality that had begun with so much potential, and I have never again been able to approach a family struck by schizophrenia without compassion and a sense of shared loss.

The Infirmary was a major referral centre for psychiatry, serving not only the Maritimes but also the French islands of St. Pierre and Miquelon. Earlier in my medical school training I was instrumental in setting up a French medical terminology reference for non-francophone medical students. I was therefore assigned the patients from the islands, most of whom were candidates for electroconvulsive therapy (ECT) as they were already dangerously depressed by the time it was deemed necessary to fly them out to Halifax. Almost all of these patients were male. It was not always easy communicating with these francophones, as their accents were entirely different from each other and from the Acadian twang and Quebecois gutturals that I was used to.

On my graduation John and I were approached to fill two vacancies in the Queen Charlotte Islands. John had been to the area before, but it was entirely unknown to me. We spent almost all of our money buying a van and camping gear, including a red pup tent to camp our way cross-country. We had just enough cash to pay for the B.C. registration and licensing fees. Our trip began in September when there was already frost in the Maritimes, and we greatly appreciated the Hudson Bay blankets we had been given as wedding presents to provide much needed insulation against the early morning chill.

We survived rush hour in Montreal, driving our van and towing my Gremlin; then became entrenched in a sand pile in Kenora, blown down in a biting sub-zero gale on the flats of Manitoba; and experienced the surreal while celebrating our wedding anniversary in a high-rise restaurant in Calgary during a hot air balloon festival. The sunset sky was filled with the gaudily-coloured floating behemoths, and it was almost as if we could reach out and pass their passengers a basket of hot fresh rolls from our table. The trip was a life experience that I would not have missed despite some physically uncomfortable moments.

The van and Gremlin travelled to the Islands by Seaspan barge, a name that we would soon recognize as an essential link to southern coasts and supplies. We later learned to watch as eagerly as other residents for the barges during the winter, as sometimes transport through the treacherous waters of Hecate Strait of such essentials as fresh vegetables and fruit, baby formula and milk, was impossible. While all our possessions made the sea voyage, we travelled by plane from Victoria to Prince Rupert and then by floatplane to Masset. It was my first experience travelling in a plane with a manually-operated landing gear, and I will never forget watching the pilot madly pumping on a long lever to his right side as the plane was taking off. I remember wondering whether this strenuous activity was a form of cranking that the operator would have to periodically perform throughout the flight to keep us airborne. I hoped that his shoulder stayed healthy at least for the duration of our trip.

Masset, for me, was not much different from the Maritimes. I was used to the fishing camps and the sometimes primitive conditions. Despite the warnings from the local Health and Human Resources clinic, it was necessary to choose an allegiance for one of the groups (Haida, townspeople, or military personnel), and we had no problems getting along famously with everyone except the health unit managers who seemed to resent our easy social acceptance.

Masset and Old Masset, or Haida, were the most northern settlements on the most northern island of the Queen Charlotte Island archipelago. We provided a full spectrum of medical care except for surgery which required general anaesthesia. Complicated medical emergencies were shipped out by helicopter to Prince Rupert or sent by ambulance and ferry to Sandspit, and then by Lear Jet ambulance to Vancouver.

Medical air evacuations were always fraught with risks. Although we lost no one during our tenure, there have been fatal crashes while trying to fly in or out in the treacherous conditions.

Masset was a military "listening station" to monitor Soviet radio traffic. We were fortunate to share the facilities and staff of the CFB hospital, yet we sometimes found ourselves tied up by the secrecy surrounding the visiting spooks.

I remember one very frantic holiday weekend. The last flight to escape the weather had gone out of Sandspit more than twenty-four hours before carrying my husband, who was the only other doctor on the Island at the time, and an emergency case to the Vancouver General Hospital. The MPs brought in a lost-looking older man with a history of chest pain. He had been found wandering on the beach, and would not give anyone his name or background. After a most frustrating and unrewarding interview I was informed that this was an American intelligence specialist and that his own medical team was prepared to fly in from the States to take care of him.

It was nice of the Americans to offer to take care one of their own, and I certainly did not need the extra work, but they did not understand that we were locked in by winter weather conditions. I remember vividly that this was also the same weekend that I had a diphtheria case. Military feathers were ruffled when I overruled protocol and bumped the spymaster so that the infectious disease case could have the only private room.

The idiot savant code-breaker fortunately turned out to have nothing seriously wrong with him, but it was several days before his team could come and collect him. In the meantime my seventy-two-hour shift was an almost continuous stream of emergencies ranging from drug overdoses to obstetrical malpresentations. I remember falling asleep on the X-ray table and being awakened by one of the nurses to attend to a stabbing. I also remember having to handle a psychotic crisis not my own.

Psychiatric disease takes up a major portion of general practice, especially in isolated communities, as it seems that the more borderline and fragile personalities gravitate away from "civilization." While in the Charlottes we had at least three homicidal psychotics, and it was very nerve-wracking to have to deal with them alone at night. I do not remember eating during that hectic weekend. I was only able to grab a cookie and a glass of juice from the tray that we kept for our walking blood bank which had also been called out in full force.

The walking blood bank was what we called the group of volunteers who were on call to attend the lab when we needed blood. Since we were too isolated to get the blood products shipped in and were too ill-equipped to maintain stores of product ourselves, we simply tried to find a match in the local population whenever we needed blood. The service was amazingly efficient, and we were able to stabilize more than one GI bleed while being locked down by adverse weather conditions.

We were given accommodation overlooking the Delkatla Slough. This complex was affectionately known as the Slough View Apartments. The walls were paper-thin, and it was not unusual for us to know what problems we may have to deal with in the morning after overhearing the ruckus the night before. My office appointments often began over morning coffee, as patients from the surrounding apartments would show up at the door before breakfast.

I vividly remember being awakened in the middle of the night by snow landing on my face. One member of the couple upstairs had been locked out after staying too long at a party and was throwing snowballs at the windows to attract the attention of the other more sensible and less inebriated member. Unfortunately, the trajectory of the projectiles was somewhat low and they were whistling through my open window instead. The discussion that ensued between the partners was *sotto voce*, but I was still able to hear enough of it that I set my alarm clock earlier, knowing that I would probably be hearing from one or the other before I left for the office in the morning.

It was in Masset that I was awakened for the first time by an earthquake. I had often felt minor tremors while visiting Victoria, but this violent shake and coincident explosive crack was different. It was a five on the Richter scale, and we were almost over the epicentre. A new hot springs appeared as a geyser visible at low tide just off shore.

My favourite memories of the Charlottes are always coloured green. It was there that I first experienced the temperate rain forest of the Pacific Northwest. The forests of the Maritimes were mainly hardwood, with some softwood conifers. The forest floor was usually dry and covered with needles or low transition bushes. In the Charlottes everything was deep green with long draperies of lichens and moss. The forest floor was a series of lumps and ridges created by fallen and rotting nurse trees whose shapes were distorted by the thick living verdant carpeting.

I travelled in my squat red Gremlin daily to Juskatla to manage the small clinic that served the logging camp of the same name. One day I was shocked to have an eagle blocking the entire view of my windshield. The young eagle was even more startled and kept looking over its shoulder as it attempted to gain enough height to avoid ending up in my front seat. This silly bird had been stuffing itself on a road kill just on the shoulder as I was passing. Unfortunately, it chose to lift off right in front of my car, and it was so gorged that it misjudged the effort necessary to out-fly the vehicle. Although I am sure it ended up with indigestion, I was relieved to arrive at

work with my car intact. The Delkatla Slough was a major stop-over for the large migratory birds, so we often did not have to go very far from our front door to get front row seats of the action.

The same area, though, also attracted a different and far less welcome migration—mushroom pickers who travelled from Ontario and Quebec to harvest psilocybin, the 'magic mushroom,' for its hallucinogenic affects. Mushroom intoxication was a nasty thing to have to deal with in the emergency, especially if alcohol was also a factor. I remember a twelve-year-old boy who required six large men to subdue him in order for us to treat. These visitors were a scourge, and caused considerable damage to the local environment and morale. They encouraged truancy among young teenagers who were recruited as mushroom gatherers for this lucrative and illegal industry.

We might have had the smallest kitchen on the Island, but we did develop a reputation for entertaining and good food. Our fresh beer-battered fried red snapper and halibut were popular, and guests were caught licking out the serving bowls of our Amaretto mousse. We created this exotic dish from the boxed chocolate Whip and Chill, and we used Amaretto liqueur instead of water. Shortly after our introduction of this delicacy to Masset, the Co-op had a rush on chocolate Whip and Chill and had difficulties keeping it in stock.

We were invited out in turn to experience traditional Haida customs and cuisine. Salmon, fresh caught in gill nets stretched across the Yacoun River, were wrapped in skunk cabbage leaves and roasted between preheated rocks. The numerous riverside smoke houses were a source of wonderful cured fish. We always ensured that the fish was thinly sliced before smoking a sufficient length of time as botulism was and still is a very real risk with partially smoked fish.

We even had a short time homesteading when one of the other doctors, a long term Masset resident, asked us to move in and care for his small farm in his absence. I was no stranger to this kind of living, and I had no qualms about pinning down the gander nesting near the henhouse with a wire rake while I collected the eggs.

We enjoyed the time, but found the demands of one in two call combined with the poor remuneration finally too much. It was exceedingly difficult and expensive to arrange continuing medical education from such an isolated area, and both of us decided that enough was enough. After we left there was considerable difficulty finding replacements.

We still were not prepared to move into the city, so we moved to Gold River, a pulp mill and logging town at the head of Nootka inlet on the west coast of Vancouver Island. The isolated towns always preferred to get a medical couple, thinking that they could hire two doctors for the price of one. Although well-meaning, they often did not realize that the night work was twice as demanding for a married couple as for two unrelated physicians because there was no relief. If one was called out, the other was up as well.

We had one weekend off in every four weeks, and were expected to be available twenty-four hours daily, seven days a week all year round including all holidays. Even then there was always someone who complained that the doctor was never around! Still it seemed a vacation compared to what we were used to in the Charlottes.

We did see and do a great deal of interesting medicine while in Gold River. We often had serious and unusual industrial accidents to attend to. If there was no surgeon available in Campbell River, one had to transport serious cases for two hours to Comox. One of the most memorable incidents occurred to a mill worker who was servicing a huge hog fuel press when it suddenly closed down. The lock-down system had not been followed correctly, and the machine was started up while he was inside. He walked away alive only because there was just enough sawdust left in the bin to prevent the vise from closing down on him. An imprint of his body was clearly left in the debris after he was pulled free. He was seen in the clinic with a case of shakes, and needed to get a medical pass so he could go home to think about the meaning of life.

Like many small towns, Gold River provided housing for a doctor, as there was no rental accommodation generally available. The doctor's house in Gold River was much better than many of the accommodations we had been assigned before, but we still suffered dreadfully from draughts. I remember watching my long nightgown billowing around my feet as I nursed the baby in the early hours of the morning. For this reason we started intermittently using the wood-burning fireplace in the living room.

Our entire record collection was stored on plank and brick shelves next to the fireplace, and some of the records were stacked at floor level. I would often play records while nursing my new daughter, and I was appalled one day to select a disc from those on the floor which folded like soft toffee around my hand as I pulled it from its cover. The floor beneath the records proved to be hot, and a call to the fire department brought speedy rescue in the form of the fire chief with his pisspot (the endearment used by those in the know to describe the hand-held and hand-pumped extinguishers). The chief took great delight in taking his fire axe to the ceiling of the carport, creating an access to the smouldering danger lurking between the walls.

We loved Gold River and we enjoyed the support of the Health Clinic Board who was appreciative of the long hours and the physician's workload. The on-call demands were not a problem if the population base did not abuse the system, but many rural physicians noticed a change in expectations during the early 1980s. Before this time the town doctor was only called for life-threatening emergencies, and people respected the physician's off hours. Unfortunately, people started to think of the town doctor as a twenty-four-hour drop-in service similar to the local twenty-four-hour gas station or coffee shop. It was this type of increasingly common discourtesy that convinced us that isolated practice was incompatible with having a family life. It was the impossibility of raising our infant daughter, Ariel, and working non-stop for twenty-four hours a day that finally drove us farther south.

Drug addicts from Vancouver travelled a route hitting every emergency clinic up the Island to obtain drugs for fabricated medical conditions. You only had to give in once and the word went out that you were a soft touch.

We still could not see ourselves working in a major centre and stopped in Parksville, joining a well-established clinic of three other physicians. The call obligations were still horrendous as we covered weekends from 5 p.m. Friday evening to 8 a.m. Monday morning. John and I could spell each other off, but even with the two of us working it was not unusual to see sixty to seventy emergencies a day. We were the ambulance stop for patient stabilization before continuing on to Nanaimo, so the cases ranged from major trauma and cardiac arrests to ear infections. These weekends were usually one out of every five to seven and were in addition to the evening call rota.

One trick to handling the busy emergency call was to never prescribe narcotics to patients you did not know personally. I had learned this while in Gold River, as the drug addicts from Vancouver travelled a route hitting every emergency clinic up the Island to obtain drugs for fabricated medical conditions. You only had to give in once and the word went out that you were a soft touch. You would soon have a constant stream of transients appearing in your clinic demanding a controlled substance. The situation was never safe, as doctors were known to travel alone and carry drugs with them. The most senior of our group warned me that he never attended the clinic at night without driving by and checking out the person waiting for him first. If there was any doubt he called the RCMP and they would come by in case he needed assistance.

There has always been an element of risk in handling emergencies alone. It was not a big problem in the Charlottes as almost everyone was seen through the hospital emergency department. In Gold River we used to carry radios whenever we had to be in the clinic after office hours. On one occasion I had a particularly bad fright while I was in the clinic alone at night reading X-rays. I heard heavy footsteps coming down the hall. There was no phone in the X-ray lab and the radio could not transmit because of all the equipment and shielding. There was only one door that led right to the person making the noise. I was rapidly thinking about my options when a deep voice called out, "Eh, Les. How're things?" My luck was holding out again, as it was the local RCMP popping around to check on me. Never say that there is not a cop around when you need one, as I have been in several very tight and potentially very dangerous situations when either an RCMP or local police constable happened to drop by.

Unfortunately, the RCMP was not around when my husband was followed home one night in Parksville. We lived on a rural acreage with a long driveway. John came home to pick me up for a medical meeting. Our two young children were to stay at home with our teenaged babysitter. We were about ten minutes absent from the vehicle, but it was long enough for

someone to break into the car and steal our emergency medical supplies out of the trunk. Considering that there had been several torture-murders of physicians in their homes by drug-seeking addicts within the preceding several months, we were badly frightened for the safety of our children and ourselves. The RCMP were sympathetic, but warned us that a security system was useless in our area, as the officer who alone covered the huge area from Nanoose to Bowser at night could not be counted on to respond in a hurry. We took their advice and obtained a large Airedale, and I started sleeping with a 12-gauge shotgun and a supply of shells.

Eventually John decided he had had enough of the wear and tear of general practice, and entered a Pathology residency in Vancouver. We sold both of our practices and the house. Unfortunately, the timing was not as perfect as we had hoped, and my replacement was not able to take over the practice until three to four months after we had to move out of our house. The transition time was an interesting one for all of us, as the only accommodation I could find was a one-bedroom condo on Rathtrevor Beach. Our family of four, the nanny, and my sister, who was visiting for the summer, all took up residence in June. It was cozy, but the family spent all of their time on the beach during the day and the evening, coming in only to do laundry, eat, and sleep. The children learned to swim and John sailed his Laser in the bay. It seemed like a vacation even though I continued to work.

Our move to Vancouver began another time of change. I was unwilling to send the children to daycare, having visited all the local facilities and found them seriously wanting. I decided to take time off instead of reinventing myself as a locum. I did volunteer work with the St. John's Ambulance and took on the responsibility of joining the boards of both the Delta Hospital and the Delta Home Support Agency.

We became financially lean and had to give up our car. The rhythm of our lives changed, but both John and I had time for fun with our growing family. We staged elaborate parties for the children, with home-made costumes and themes set both indoors and out. One party was particularly memorable as John and I, at the request of our daughter, created a medieval theme complete with painted cardboard swords, hand-sewn black capes, and a flying dragon piñata that swooped down on the clothesline over a huge refrigerator carton castle in the backyard. We created the most wonderful cake sculptures for every birthday. Our daughters still make special requests for these elaborate confections even though they are now teenagers.

John's completion of his training meant that we were able to move back to the Island in 1992 as there was a place waiting for him at Nanaimo Regional General Hospital. I moved back into general practice in Parksville, and decided to branch into palliative care. Palliative Care has become my field of interest as the complicated disease processes found in this group of patients require a physician to use all of his or her expertise in pathology, pharmacology, and medicine. Palliative Care is a branch of medicine where physician interest can make such a difference to a patient and family.

I now run the Symptom Control clinic through the Nanaimo Cancer clinic, and act as the palliative care physician liaison with Home Nursing as well as maintaining a general practice in Parksville. It is almost as if our lives have come full circle; John's training in pathology and my experience and training in palliative care dovetail. Once again, we find ourselves working together on difficult cases as patients advocate for the best care.

Nowadays it is common for women to practise medicine, although many work shorter hours to afford time with their families. I believe this change of attitude probably makes them better doctors. As our daughters are getting ready to move on to their careers and both are considering medicine, John and I look forward to more freedom to advance our own education.

As I look back on our time and adventures shared together, I realize that it really has been a good time. I would do it all again.

Curriculum Vitae

Employment: Queen Charlotte Islands, B.C., Family Practice, Obstetrics and Emergency Medicine, Haida Medical Clinic, Masset Health and Human Resources Centre, Juskatla Family Clinic and Emergency Centre, 1981–1983; Gold River, B.C. Family Practice, Occupational Health and Emergency Medicine Gold River Health Clinic, 1983–1984; Parksville, B.C. Family Practice and Medicine, Parksville Medical Clinic, 1984–1988; Vancouver, B.C. Family Practice and Health Education Locum Tenens, St. John's Ambulance Centre, 1988–1992; Parksville, B.C. Family Practice Locum Tenens, 1992–1993; Parksville, B.C. Family Practice, Heritage Centre Medical Clinic, 1993; Nanaimo, B.C. Palliative Care, Nanaimo General Regional Hospital, 1994 ; Nanaimo, B.C. Palliative Care, Outpatient Palliative Care and Symptom Control Clinic, 1997.

Education: Dalhousie University associated hospital in Saint John, New Brunswick, Rotating Internship, distinctions in Surgery and Obstetrics and Gynaecology, elective training in Anaesthesia, Neonatology Intensive Care, and Surgical Intensive Care, 1980–1981; Dalhousie University Halifax, N.S. Doctor of Medicine, 1976–1980; Dalhousie University Halifax, N.S. Bachelor of Science with Distinction, major in Chemistry, minors in Mathematics and Languages, 1973–1976.

Family: b. 1957 Leslie Ann Crook to parents Capt. Wm. H. Crook and Lt. Ethel Mae Laing rtd. in Halifax, N.S.; m. 1980 Dr. John Blais Le Huquet, Halifax, N.S.; b. 1983 daughter Ariel Lauren LeHuquet, Campbell River, B.C.; b. 1986 daughter Katherine Elise LeHuquet, Victoria, B.C.

Appointments: Active Staff Halifax Infirmary, Active Staff Grace Hospital, Active Staff Victoria General Hospital; Active Staff Sir Issac Walton Killam Hospital, Halifax, N.S., 1980; Active Staff Saint John Regional Hospital, Active Staff St. Joseph's Hospital, Saint John, N.B., 1981; Active Staff Masset Hospital Masset, QCI, B.C., 1981–1983; Associate Staff Campbell River Hospital, Campbell River, B.C., 1983–1984; Active Staff Nanaimo Regional General Hospital, Nanaimo, B.C., 1984–1988; Medical Facilitator Healthy Aging Program, Vancouver, B.C., 1988; Board Member Delta Home Support Services, Ladner, B.C., 1988–1989; Chairman Board Delta Home Support Services, Ladner, B.C., 1989–1992; Board Member Delta Hospital, Delta, B.C., 1990–1992; Member Quality Assurance Committee Delta Hospital, Delta, B.C., 1991–1992; Active Staff Nanaimo Regional General Hospital, Nanaimo, B.C., 1992–2000; Member Palliative Care Team Nanaimo Regional General Hospital, Nanaimo, B.C., 1995; Co-ordinator Palliative Care and Symptom Control Clinic Nanaimo Regional General Hospital, Nanaimo, B.C., 1997; Vice-President

Medical Staff, Nanaimo General Hospital, Nanaimo, B.C., 1997-1999; Palliative Care Physician Liaison to Community Care, Nanaimo, B.C., 2001–.

Memberships: College of Family Physicians of B.C.; Upper Island Hospice; Mid-Island Hospice; National Cancer Institute of Canada, Clinical Trials Group, Symptom Control Committee; Canadian Pain Society; Phi Rho Sigma Alpha Eta.

DR. KIRSTIE OVERHILL

Stories From the Country

I was born in Montreal in 1956 and grew up in Ottawa. I did not have a rural upbringing, except when I visited my grandparents in the Laurentians and in Revelstoke, B.C. I did, however, suffer adolescence in the suburbs of Ottawa, and the intense boredom of that experience has inspired me to seek other choices in my own life. I rebelled in high school and disliked the courses, with the exception of biology, which was interesting. I left school early and completed Grade 13 at Ottawa University where I obtained an entrance scholarship to continue with a science degree. After two years of biology I applied to medical school, in part because everyone else was doing that, and I was pleased to receive early acceptance.

I thought I was very grown up at the mature age of nineteen, but now realize I was completely naïve. I only applied to one medical school because each application cost $20! Part way into first year I was shocked to find out about the meaning of on call, which started in third year! I certainly consider myself fortunate to have been so happy with a career which I entered with so little foresight.

Nevertheless, my time at medical school from 1975 to 1979 was a difficult experience for me. The work was very hard and unremitting, and I did not necessarily have the maturity to cope with it well and pace myself properly. My health began to break down in second year and by third year I had lost thirty pounds and developed asthma, the treatment for which was adrenalin shots and theophylline which made me sicker. Even worse, I was not given lung function tests and was routinely underdiagnosed because I seldom wheezed. I remember begging to be admitted to Emergency and being turned away, and after that just coping at home even when I was cyanosed. I do not remember any of the professors commenting on my obvious illness, but then I did not ask for advice either as we were all caught up in the stoicism needed for 100-hour work weeks and studying. I kept going mostly because it did not occur to me to quit. Needless to say, when graduation came around, it was the happiest day of my life.

Besides my illness, however, I found there was also a fair bit of harassment at medical school, more of a general intimidation on the part of men rather than sexual. The women students liked to complain it was hard to get dates since we were surrounded by young nurses who were better rested by far, more attractive, and less cranky!

After medical school, I went on to a Residency in Family Medicine at McGill University (Montreal General Hospital) where I had a good experience. There were some very committed and inspirational professors (some of them specialists) who had a genuine enthusiasm for primary care. I also had tons of fun exploring Montreal's night life and burning the candle at both ends. I was chief resident for half of my final year and had my first experience with administration.

Immediately upon graduation in 1981, I moved to British Columbia with the intention of getting my feet wet, medically speaking. I wanted the challenge of a small-town practice if I could find a small town I wanted to live in. My first job was a summer locum in Ashcroft, B.C. "Boy are we glad to see you," said the doctor who greeted me, one of the two in town. Everyone asked the new receptionist, "What's the new doctor like?" I had some of the most exciting challenges of my career in Ashcroft, especially when I was the lone physician in Emergency with no one else available. I intubated a newborn baby successfully to treat a mucous plug, when my only previous experience had been on the ACLS plastic dummy. The first patient I ever injected with IVP dye went into anaphylactic shock. I saved a cardiac arrest, diagnosed strange diseases, and left a little less green.

After Ashcroft, I worked in Okanagan, Vancouver, and Queen Charlotte City where I met my present husband. In 1982 I moved on to Gibsons, B.C., and found the place I wanted to be. At that time, Gibsons was a community of

3-4,000 people where they used to film the Beachcomber's TV show. The town is close to Vancouver on the mainland, but separated by Howe Sound and only accessible by ferry during the day. In the early 'eighties, there was no shortage of doctors in general, but few women had made the move to the small towns, and this was to my advantage in finding work. In a period of six months I bought a house in lovely Roberts Creek just up the coast, joined the local practice, and had my husband-to-be moved in with his two small boys aged five and six. I was twenty-six, and very anxious about having to learn how to cook. I guess I was still completely naïve.

The work in Gibsons was interesting and demanding. At that time the hospital was largely run by the GPs, with only one sturdy country surgeon. I shared hospital duties (including the ICU), helped cover the busy ER, and started an obstetrical practice. My role models were the highly-skilled, busy GPs who also took on anaesthesia in some cases. The older ones in particular were from what is now a dying breed—the rural GPs prior to the days of helicopter evacuation. I still remember fondly their stories of daring-do such as high forceps deliveries on the kitchen table, solo C-Sections, endless work, and practical jokes played on each other. Sometimes there would be stories of daring-don't, too, like, "the time I delivered a ten-pound breech at home in bed and took the pledge never to do another home birth."

One of these fine old-timers was a man that we young doctors referred to as Father because he was known for his endless skill and aplomb in emergencies as well as being renowned for being very lucky. Many evenings when I was sweating it out, hovering over a sick patient, I would call him for advice in hope of sharing a little dose of his luck. "Kirstie, if I'm not worried," he would say expansively, "then you don't have to be," and my anxiety would magically abate.

Another veteran was known for his judgement of human character and empathy for patients. Among other jewels of information he passed on to us, he recognized what came to be known as the Swan Syndrome, the condition in which unfaithful husbands are the ones most likely to criticize the quality of their wives' care.

As time went by I developed my own tales of crises, critical care, and cases won and lost. In my memory, it seems the most urgent problems always happened at night when bright lights failed to dispel the gloom as I struggled to save accident cases or stabilize the critically ill. Vancouver was very far away on those nights when the weather was bad and flights were not available; colleagues who would come and share the risk were a blessing.

The most terrifying experiences were always obstetrical in the days before we had an obstetrician. I once delivered thirty-three-week twins (the second one with a high MityVac extraction of the undescending head); and on other occasions had to do sudden forceps deliveries for distress of babies. The most stressful event of my career developed from a Primip delivery on a night when our surgeon was away. Although there was no concrete signs to alarm me, the labour was dragging on in an unsatisfactory way and I was beginning to get a prickly feeling that all was not going to go well. Considering the long delay in obtaining help, I phoned Vancouver and after consultation they chose one of their senior residents to do a Caesarean in our hospital.

The epidural test dose was in when the resident arrived and there were early signs of fetal distress. He performed an examination and the fetal heart rate promptly dropped to sixty and stayed! The resident called for an immediate C-Section under general anaesthetic to save the baby.

The women students liked to complain it was hard to get dates since we were surrounded by young nurses who were better rested by far, more attractive, and less cranky!

The anaesthetist hesitated briefly then complied, but was not able to intubate her. The mother was now in grave danger of aspirating, and her life took precedence over the baby's distress, so the anaesthetist elected to wake the mother and proceed with the epidural, but she had a pseudo-cholinesterase deficiency and the paralysis could not be reversed. At this point the anaethetist turned to the resident and said, "Can you do a tracheotomy?" and the resident said, "I don't know how." I really thought we would lose both mother and child. It took thirty minutes for two anaesthetists to finally get an intubation tube in and then the baby was delivered, thankfully in good condition. It was days later, after transfer to Vancouver, that the mother was finally given a clean bill of health. This particular case was a terrible experience for me, being responsible for arranging the situation, but helpless to fix it.

Another time, I delivered a baby who was unexpectedly distressed at birth and began having a seizure. I spent a week full of guilt as to whether I had done something wrong before a CT scan revealed that the baby suffered from a congenital brain abnormality.

Emergency always had its surprises, of course. There was one little boy who had completely dislocated his elbow, as an X-ray showed. I was waiting for the surgeon while the child wandered in the hallway. The tired mother told her older son to "go bring your brother back in here." This was followed by a loud scream which echoed down the hall. I arrived on the scene to find the mother berating the older boy, saying "don't grab his sore arm!" and the boy protesting that he "didn't know it was that one!" and meanwhile the small patient was experimentally moving his elbow again, finding the dislocation nicely reduced. I wished I had seen how it was done and wondered if I could bill for the reduction.

Some of the greatest successes in primary care are lives saved in the most quiet, undramatic way, like when you detect an early illness because you know your patient does not seem to look right.

Overall, it was a wonderful experience to deliver babies and watch them grow, and I loved the challenge of hospital work and using my skills to the fullest. Some of the greatest successes in primary care are lives saved in the most quiet, undramatic way, like when you detect an early illness because you know your patient does not seem to look right. Once, in the middle of an outbreak of viral gastroenteritis, I correctly diagnosed a toddler with bowel obstruction. Over fifteen years I saved two lives by diagnosing cancers on driver's medical exams, and a couple more by noticing black spots (early melanomas) during the course of other examinations.

I spent my first five years in practice feeling hopelessly green, and the next five picking up confidence before my knowledge started to become out of date. After the 'eighties, I started to notice that Gibsons was not as far as it used to be from the city. This was partly due to my improved confidence, but part of it was also a change in atmosphere among the medical community. I felt less of an obligation to handle everything by myself and more willingness to send patients to the specialists in town.

During my seventeen years in Gibsons, I ended up with a sideline career in administration. The origins of this were humble enough. It was the tradition at St. Mary's Hospital to elect those doctors who missed the November Medical Staff meeting to various positions. And I was elected as Secretary of the Medical Staff for six months before I knew it, followed in annual order by Vice-President, President, and then three years as Chief of Staff. I remember receiving a questionnaire at that time asking what barriers I had encountered as a woman in holding these various positions. In fact then, as with later positions, I was merely susceptible to the plea that there was no one else who would agree to take the job.

I worked hard in administration, but came away with the feeling that, if you hope to see changes extend beyond your term of office, you are probably going to be disappointed. I did get a reputation for being rather verbal and was often called upon by my colleagues to come to various meetings and educate various people, in a very polite way of course! Later on I enjoyed committee work with the BCMA and the College of Family Physicians where I ended up as Chapter President and briefly on the National Communications Committee.

I do not want to neglect the story of my family completely. I met my husband in March 1981 on Jungle Beach in the Queen Charlotte Islands. Our first date was a boat ride to the west coast of the Charlottes, and I attracted his interest by not getting sea-sick. While I worked in Gibsons my husband completed his PhD in Geography and taught at Simon Fraser University; we raised two sons and added a daughter in 1991. My husband had to be a patient man, of course, to put up with my schedule. I shall never forget the look he gave me when I invited eight three-year-olds to a party, and then promptly left for a delivery at the hospital! I learned early that talking about my work at the dinner table was not allowed because it was considered far too gory.

In the early days in Gibsons I did have days off after call, and we took advantage of the sabbatical system to take four months off and cruise in our sailboat up to Prince Rupert and back. The real crunch came after my daughter was born and I was approaching my forties. Our sons did not seem to mind my hours and absences, but my little girl sure did. From the time she was born until she was six, I did not even have an afternoon to spend alone with her. (Finally I had nasal surgery which brought me a blissful week at home by myself.) Even so, what my daughter mostly remembers of her early childhood is me leaving her.

As the 1990s wore on, taxes went up, income went down, raising the kids became more expensive, and overhead climbed. Our group tried to make adjustments by bringing in part-time practice for the female doctors, but it was always a struggle to accommodate the different needs of the minority female partners. For years, people would say to me, "How do you do it?" and I would answer, "Simple, no hobbies and no social life." This line began to wear thin as the years passed, and I finally made a move in 1999 to an even more rural life on Cortes Island to work as a solo physician in a salaried position three days a week. Now I can look back with nostalgia at those exciting years while enjoying my new, more balanced life.

In 2000, the general agreement is that the new physicians do not want to work in rural areas. I see this trend, perhaps an unfortunate one, of new graduates working in walk-in clinics and then spending their high salaries on eco-adventure holidays. Why not have an adventure job and an eco-life instead? Medicine was not a calling to me when I was younger, but over the years it has been a whispering in my ear. I am learning to listen to what it has to tell me.

DR. PEGGY ROSS

I graduated from the University of British Columbia Medical school in 1958 and did a rotating internship at the Vancouver General Hospital. After marrying Jock Ross, a businessman, I moved to Toronto to do a specialty in Anaesthesia. Our four children were born while I was training and working in Anaesthesia. In fact, I was the first female on the Anaesthesia staff at the Toronto Western Hospital. Needless to say there were the usual problems relating to child care, but fortunately my nonphysician husband had more regular hours than I did and hence we managed. The year I wrote my Fellowship exams we had three children under the age of five. The only quiet time I had to study was between 4 and 6 a.m. Sleep deprivation was a way of life.

One rather amusing incident during my residency was one evening when there was a serious accident on the Gardner Expressway. We were running eight operating rooms treating the injured. I was very pregnant at the time, and unfortunately my membranes ruptured while I was doing one of these cases. I asked the circulating nurse to please get me some relief or I would be having my baby in the middle of the OR floor. She explained that all the available Anaesthetists were already in the ORs. The only one who wasn't in hospital was the department head—and he didn't take calls. This particular man did not really want to have women in the Anaesthesia residency program. He was not amused to have to come in and relieve me in the middle of the night. I quickly departed from the OR and my daughter was born some two hours later. I really did believe in working until I went into labour! In those days there was no such thing as maternity leave. I took two weeks of my holidays off when my children were born and then went back to work—trying to make the point to the mostly male staff that women really were reliable employees.

On completion of my training, I spoke to the head of the department of Anaesthesia in Toronto to ask about employment. He offered me a job at $5,000 less than the male applicants as he said, "You have a husband to support you."

It was always a balancing act to run a household, be a good parent and wife, and work full time as an anaesthetist.

My husband and I moved back to Vancouver, and I decided to take some time out from Anaesthesia as the move was a difficult adjustment for my four children. I had planned to be a full-time wife and mother for one to two years. That became fourteen years.

When I decided to return to practising Anaesthesia, I did a Fellowship at the Vancouver General Hospital to update and upgrade my clinical skills. The staff and department head were most supportive of my desire to re-enter the work force. I was somewhat of a novelty as I had been away from clinical work for a significant period of time.

When the new B.C. Women's Hospital opened in Vancouver, I joined the staff to work there full time.

My youngest daughter entered medicine at the University of British Columbia and I was appalled at the harassment and discrimination that she encountered—similar to what I had endured some thirty years earlier. I then decided to try to improve the work and study environment of the UBC

Faculty of Medicine. Dr. Judith Hall and I started a committee to deal with harassment and intimidation in the Faculty of Medicine. One of the recommendations of this committee was to have an Associate Dean of Equity. I applied for the position and was appointed in December, 1993. This was the first such position in any medical school in North America. In this position I started a course for first year medical and dental students called Peggy's ABCs—Attitude, Boundaries, and Communication. I also started workshops to teach medical students how to recognize and deal with harassment and intimidation.

I am now fully retired as an Emeritus Associate Dean Equity and Associate Professor Anaesthesiology. My daughter works full time as a General and Hepatobiliary surgeon in Victoria.

1982

DR. CAROL KATHERINE DINGEE

I was born in New Brunswick. After graduating from high school as valedictorian and Governor General's Medal recipient I attended the University of New Brunswick in Fredericton majoring in geology. I graduated with a BSci Honours in Geology, was on the Dean's List, and maintained a four year General Motor's Canadian College Scholarship. I also enjoyed joining the sport parachuting club.

As a geologist I worked in New Brunswick, Ontario, and British Columbia. Field work was never dull. On one solo excursion in a remote clear-cut area I was mapping down a steep bank. The trees had fallen across the stream four to six feet above the stream base making it very difficult to walk. I was crawling backwards on my stomach over the trees and thistles trying to negotiate the fall to the riverbed as gently as possible. I got a foothold on what appeared to be a large black rock, but it turned out to be a beaver that didn't want to be disturbed—I don't know which of us was more alarmed! Later that day I sank up to my hips in a bog. A quiet career in medicine looked good at that point and I felt it was time for a change.

I attended Medical School at Memorial University of Newfoundland, 1977 through 1981, and received my BMedSci and MD there. An elective in Internal Medicine in London, England was a good clinical experience and provided an opportunity to travel in Europe.

I did the Family Practice Residency in Vancouver starting in 1981 and sandwiched a year of locums in northern British Columbia between the two years of the program. Consequently, I have great respect for rural doctors and their working conditions, experience, and responsibilities. The Family Practice Residency Program in Vancouver was excellent and rotations through Cardiology and Psychiatry at Shaughnessy Hospital were highlights. One of my rotations was in Internal Medicine and Emergency at St. Vincent's Hospital. Dr. Gord Robertson supervised the residents, all of whom benefited from his mentoring.

Working in the north stimulated my interest in procedure-oriented medicine, and I was encouraged by Dr. Ron Hancock at Shaughnessy Hospital to apply to General Surgery. Just before I started my surgical residency I was introduced to the general surgeon of a family member. After I enthusiastically outlined my plans for entering General Surgery, he was silent for a moment and then thoughtfully said, "Is there anything I can say or do to make you change your mind?"

Undeterred, I entered the General Surgery residency in 1984. Dr. Patricia Rebbeck was one of the few female clinical surgeons, but many of the surgical residents were female. The residents' interest in patient care and the ability to "get the job done" was more important to most staff surgeons than gender issues. Patients were largely supportive and even enthusiastic about having a female resident on the case—except one patient who "didn't think girls were allowed to be doctors."

The five year residency was an intense, often exhausting but usually enjoyable learning and working experience. We were fortunate to work at Shaughnessy Hospital. The volume and variety of the work there provided a great clinical opportunity to rapidly advance the degree of patient care responsibility. An unexpected benefit was that if your birthday fell during the rotation you would be serenaded by Dr. Ron Hancock with an operatic "Happy Birthday to You!"

I remember especially the mentoring of Drs. Ian Cleator, Ron Hancock,

Pat Rebbeck, and Trevor Sandy. I also worked with these surgeons on research projects and received the Residents' Research Day second prize in 1987 and the first place senior prize in 1988.

I received my FRCS(C) in 1988 and started my practice in General Surgery at St. Vincent's and Mount St. Joseph's Hospitals in 1989. I am also currently consulting staff at the British Columbia Cancer Agency, Vancouver Hospital, St. Paul's Hospital, and am the Acting Associate Head of Surgery at Providence Health Care. My professional interests are in breast disease and I am co-investigator in the NSABP trials.

I met my husband during my surgical residency, so he appreciated from the start what the lifestyle of a general surgeon was like—working long and unpredictable hours, worrying over sick patients, spending lots of time on call for emergencies. Cutbacks in hospital beds and fee schedules in recent years have made practising more difficult and there never seems to be enough time to spend with family. Presently I am taking violin lessons with my daughter and struggling to keep up with her!

DR. JUDITH G. HALL

After high school in Washington and college at Wellesley, Judith came back to Seattle to study medicine. By the time she graduated in 1966, she had already taken an extra year for a master's degree in genetics, with a thesis on fetal haemoglobin. She says, "The labs were very busy at that time and the only way I could do research was to come in at night!"

She went to Baltimore for internship, followed by a fellowship in clinical genetics. At Johns Hopkins, she then went through pediatric residency and a year of pediatric endocrinilogy where she furthered her particular interest in children with short stature. She returned to Seattle in 1972 to start a clinical genetics service, based at Children's Orthopedic Hospital. This spread to clinics in medicine and prenatal diagnosis at the University, and then to outreach clinics throughout the WAMI (Washington, Alaska, Montana, Idaho) program. "This was an exciting time," she says, "for putting clinical genetics into practice."

After a few years, she was in search of more financial stability (like many academics in the U.S.A., she had been dependent on soft funds), and considered several possible situations, including Toronto. When Pat Baird heard that Judith was interested in a move, she immediately asked her to Vancouver, where she was attracted by the challenge of building a provincial service and pleased at the opportunity of staying in the Pacific Northwest; she came to UBC in 1981. The next eight years were taken up with the development of the Clinical Genetics Unit which provided service ranging from prenatal diagnosis to adult disease. After a sabbatical year at Oxford, her return coincided with the day of Don Hill's funeral. She was urged to consider the headship in pediatrics. This brought about considerable soul searching as to her future career; she had thought of applying for the headship in medical genetics, soon to become vacant, but felt that pediatrics presented the greater challenge; she also hoped she could support genetics from the outside. There were possibilities in the States, but she knew she wanted to stay in Canada.

Judith took over (the headship) in the fall of 1990 and attacked her new responsibilities with enormous energy, identifying the residency program and departmental organization as targets for immediate attention. Genuine clinical teaching units were formed.

(The above information is from the book Paediatrics in B.C. A History, with Particular Emphasis on the UBC Academic Department, *written by Dr. Robert Hill; he has kindly given permission to include it for Dr. Hall's biography.)*

Curriculum Vitae

Appointments: Intern, Mixed Med/Ped, Baltimore City Hospital, Baltimore, M.D., 1966–1967; Fellow, Medical Genetics, Dept. of Medicine, Johns Hopkins Hospital, Baltimore, M.D., 1967–1969; Assistant Resident, Harriet Lane Home, Pediatrics, Johns Hopkins Hospital, 1969–1971; Fellow, Pediatric Endocrinology, Dept. of Pediatrics, Johns Hopkins Hospital, 1971–72; State of Washington Licensure to Practice, 1972; American board of Pediatrics Diplomate Certificate, 1973; American Academy of Pediatrics, Fellow 1973; British Columbia College of Physicians and Surgeons, 1981; Royal College of Physicians and Surgeons of Canada, Fellow (Pediatrics), 1981; Canadian

College of Medical Genetics, 1984; American Board of Medical Genetics, 1984; Royal College of Physicians and Surgeons of Canada, Fellow (Medical Genetics), 1992; American College of Medical Genetics, 1993; Royal College Physicians of London, Fellow, 1997.

Employment Record: Assistant Professor Medicine and Pediatrics, Division of Medical Genetics, University of Washington School of Medicine, 1972–1976; Associate Professor Medicine and Pediatrics, Division of Medical Genetics, University of Washington School of Medicine, 1976–1980; Professor Medicine and Pediatrics, Division of Medical Genetics, University of Washington School of Medicine, 1980–1981; Clinical Professor Voluntary Faculty, Department of Pediatrics, University of Washington School of Medicine, 1981; Professor, Department of Medical Genetics, University of British Columbia, 1981; Professor, Joint Appointment Departments of Medicine and Pediatrics, University of British Columbia, 1981; Professor and Head Department of Pediatrics, University of British Columbia, 1990–2000.

Leave of Absence: a sabbatical study leave at Genetics Laboratory, Department of Biochemistry, Oxford University, Oxford, England with Professor John Edwards, July 1, 1988 to June 30, 1989; received the Senior Killam Fellowship Award, 1988–1989, and the Detweiler Travel Fellowship 1988–1989.

Teaching: Lecturer, Medical Genetics 440, 1981–1990; Small Group Leader, Medical Genetics 440, 1981–1990; Supervisor of Medical Students and Residents on Clinical Rotations in Medical Genetics, 1981–1990; Director, Medical Genetics Fellowship Program, 1981–1990; Numerous Grand Rounds and Continuing Education Courses, 1981–present; Moderator Grand Rounds, Department of Pediatrics, 1990–1996; Medical Genetic Fellows lectures, 1994–1998; Genetic Counsellor program lectures, 1996–1998; Oversaw Education in Department of Pediatrics at undergraduate, resident, sub-specialty resident, and CME levels, 1990–2000; Pediatric Undergraduate Course Introduction, 1991–2000; Professor Rounds for Pediatric Residents, 1993–2000.

Dr. Hall was Visiting Lecturer to forty-five Universities and Hospitals around the World, 1979-2000, and received over thirteen Research Grants as the Principal Investigator from 1980–1993. She has written seven books, over 245 refereed publication in journals, over 240 abstracts, edited over 100 Pediatric and Genetic works, served on dozens of committees of the University of British Columbia, Children's Hospital, and scholarly societies, as well as societies concerned with the welfare of children.

Dr. Hall has received over thirty awards for scholarship, Service Awards, and teaching including the UBC Senior Killam Fellowship 1988–1989, Science Council of British Columbia 1996 Gold Medal-New Frontiers in Research Award, B.C. Science World Hall of Fame 1993, YWCA 1994 Woman of Distinction (Health, Science, and Technology), was awarded the Oxford University Press Award of Excellence for the Best Book in Clinical Medicine in 1993, for *Human Malformation and Related Anomalies* by R. Stevenson and J.G. Hall 1994, and the Order of Canada Officer in October 1998.

As Dr. Robert Hill wrote after Dr. Hall became Head of Pediatrics for the first of two terms, "She attacked her new responsibilities with enormous energy." She continued with this energy to edit, review, and write many scientific articles, serve on numerous committees, teach, and lecture all over the world.

1983

DR. CICELY BRYCE

Dr. Cicely Ford Bryce was born in Vancouver and attended Queen Mary Elementary School and Lord Byng High School. Here is her story:

I was accepted by Cambridge University to become an undergraduate medical student in the spring of 1976. In 1979 I became a second year transfer medical student at the University of British Columbia and completed my MD in 1982. Graham Bryce and I had established a serious interest in each other in 1976 after being admiring friends during high school. He pursued his medical training in Toronto. We were granted two internship places at the Royal Columbian Hospital in New Westminster, British Columbia, and we committed to staying in the same place together and were married.

We alternated our post-graduate training where necessary, focusing first on my sub-specialty in Medical Oncology, and then on Graham's in Neurotology. Our trek for locum dollars and knowledge included northern British Columbia, Honolulu, and Oklahoma City. Wherever we went, Graham made me a comfortable nest, often out of thrift shops and similar outlets, and at the end of our specialty training we had no debt and some cash for a house.

We settled in Vancouver, had a third little girl, and I became a staff oncologist at the B.C. Cancer Agency. Graham became head of the Division of Ear, Nose and Throat at St. Paul's Hospital. We both worked hard in our interesting specialties. I am proud of my role at the BCCA as chair of the professional staff and tumour groups.

For holidays the whole family travelled the B.C. coast in our boat, one memorable trip to old coastal native Indian village sites on remote islands. For variety we all travelled to Nepal in 1997 with Aunt Joan Ford who has worked as a locum for years in Nepal, and my parents and brother accompanied us. Our youngest was only five, but with five doctors in the family on the trip, we all felt safe! We continue to enjoy our Bowen Island retreat.

Our lives have changed, however. On December 18, 2000 Graham dissected his right internal carotid artery from severe coughing, and an embolus was thrown to the right middle cerebral artery with resulting massive brain injury. How I value what was done for Graham by the practitioners of medicine and nursing. Graham had stabilized by Christmas and soon began rehabilitation.

As a family we are thoroughly launched into our new disabled lifestyle. In the process we have collected three different electric wheelchairs (including a portable one), two vehicles with electric lifts, and a tennis chair. We have a wonderful extended family on both sides who help us with chauffering Graham to St. Paul's for work and meetings, to Richmond for tennis for the disabled, to entertainments, and even to skiing for the disabled. I have been trying, in the domestic, recreational, social, career, and extended family spheres, to do as much as always to ensure that the losses for each, of Graham, myself, and now eight-year-old Marguerite, twelve-year-old Nessa, and thirteen-year-old Sydney, are kept to a minimum.

By February, 2001 Graham re-started meetings to raise funds for the Elks Hearing Resource Centre, which is a communication program for Deaf and Hard of Hearing Children aged zero to six years. He had been a member of the Board for eight years, and under his leadership had embarked on a major fund-raising campaign.

Along with Graham's dream of having a Resource Centre for Children, my project was to have in this Centre a special place dedicated to Graham for all his efforts, called "The Graham Bryce Room." I organized a surprise celebration party for Graham in July, 2002 and invited the 167 people who had donated $97,000 to the Centre on Graham's behalf. (One-hundred and fifteen were able to attend.) It was a great success, and I spoke on that wonderful day with thanks to all of them.

DR. SHARON LEE

I am originally from Nelson, British Columbia. I graduated from the University of British Columbia Medical School (along with my twin sister) in 1983, interned in London, Ontario and have been practising in Terrace, B.C. since 1985.

My areas of particular interest are psychiatry, obstetrics, and occupational medicine. I was also involved in the formation of the Terrace Hospice Society.

1984

DR. LYNN DOYLE

I have been very fortunate; I was born into a family where we were encouraged to reach for the stars. I am the eldest of three girls and at no time in my family was I discouraged from attempting things because I was a girl. In high school I did encounter a few teachers, mostly women, who thought my abilities at pie crust 101 were much more important than math and science. Fortunately by then I had been taught to stand up for myself, and home economics took a back seat to math and science.

I did my undergraduate training at Simon Fraser University. The University of British Columbia seemed far too large and impersonal for a little girl from Lynn Valley. During my undergraduate years at Simon Fraser, working towards a Bachelor's degree in biochemistry I continued to do well. In typical Lynn style I continued to believe that it was the older and smart students who went into medicine. About halfway through my third year at Simon Fraser I realized that maybe I was one of those students. I had always been interested in medicine and always believed that I should find a career where I added something to society rather than just took from it. I applied to medicine as a third year science student and was the first alternate to not be selected that year. This was the time when only eighty students were accepted from nearly 800 applicants. I finished the fourth year of my undergraduate training, got a degree in biochemistry from Simon Fraser University, and reapplied to medical school and was accepted outright. In those days we fortunately did not have to decide what style of medicine we wanted to practise until at least partly through our third year. I wonder what kind of medicine I would be doing now if I had to do what the modern students have to do—decide what kind of medicine they want to practise practically the first week in medical school.

Once again, in typical Lynn style, I had decided that I liked surgery; there was something about the operations that I loved, but I did not think I had what it took to be a surgeon. I was sure I was not tough enough to be a surgical resident. I nonetheless loved surgery and decided the best way to get it out of my system once and for all was to do one year straight surgical internship. This way I would never be able to look back and wonder. Part way through my first year I began to think that maybe I really was tough enough to be a surgeon. I sure loved the operations, and I therefore applied for a surgical residency. I guess the rest is history. I have been told that I was the first woman in Canada to obtain my certificate of special competence in vascular surgery. I have to say that I really do not feel like a pioneer. I was lucky enough to be born at a time when women were just starting to be accepted into surgery training. Along the way I have experienced some anti-female discrimination, but mostly I have been welcomed and encouraged. Most of my mentors have been men, and I feel grateful and thankful for their help, encouragement, and the faith they have shown in me.

My forays into medical politics has again been typical Lynn. I had been very unhappy and dissatisfied with my life as a physician. Like many physicians I have been frustrated by the effects of the continuing spiral of health-care cutbacks and restraints. I found the more I grumbled and complained the more unhappy I was. Some wise friends and mentors basically told me that I was going to put up or shut up. Those who know me well know that I do not shut up well. With the help of women physicians, who refer to themselves as grandmothers, I gained some political experience and knowledge by becoming involved with the Vancouver Branch of the Federation of Medical Women of Canada. Colleagues and mentors recognized my potential, helped me hone my skills, and encouraged me to become involved with the British Columbia Medical Association.

In 1996 I ran and was elected to be a district delegate from Vancouver to the BCMA. When I arrived at the BCMA I was like a deer in the headlights. I was welcomed and encouraged. Several experienced physicians helped me and served as mentors. As it happens all these mentors were men. I am grateful to every one of them. I arrived at the BCMA in some turbulent times, and I nonetheless found a group of people who welcomed and encouraged me and listened to what I had to say. My affiliation with BCMA continues. In 1999 I was elected to the executive as the honorary secretary-treasurer, then was elected to the "next rung in the ladder" in early July, 2000, becoming the chair of the general assembly. Dr. Heidi Oetter was President-elect in July 2000 and will be the third woman to become president of BCMA. The work at BCMA can be time-consuming and frustrating, but it also can be very rewarding. I personally find it much less frustrating to participate to try to improve the health-care system and physician conditions than to sit on the sidelines and complain.

I somehow manage to scrape together enough time to tend and expand my Galiano Island garden, knit, and learn how to quilt. Even though home economics took a back seat to science, I am told that when I do really cook, I am a good cook. My meals always get compliments. I have a very understanding and supportive husband and have been exceedingly lucky in many ways. Lest you think my life has been totally charmed, I do have a sister who has been chronically and severely ill for several years. Her illness has totally altered her life and significantly affected the lives of me and the rest of the family.

(Dr. Lynn Doyle became the President of BCMA in 2002 when the turmoil with the B.C. Government was at its worst. She has managed to calm the storm somewhat and has made some good recommendations.)

DR. FRANCES ELAINE PATTERSON

My parents met and married in Britannia Beach, British Columbia, in 1940. My mother was of English extraction predominantly and my father was Ukrainian. (He changed his name to Patterson, as he could not get work with a Ukrainian name!) My mother was the homemaker and my father an electrician. I am the youngest of five children. My parents had a hard life, having lost their first child as an infant, and the next eldest who drowned in young adulthood. One sister is estranged, but I have another dear sister who has lived with me for ten years in Nelson. In retrospect, my childhood was not too bad, although there were problems, especially with my father; they were certainly less than most of the families I see today.

Never having had anyone in a remotely professional capacity in their families, my parents were pleased but astounded when I commenced training in Medicine. My father was somewhat of the "why-don't-you-just-be-a-secretary-then-get-married-and-have-children" sort, but never to the extent of interfering with my education, which I paid for myself anyway. I applied for medical school with the encouragement of a boyfriend who had just been accepted into medicine.

I had graduated first in my high school class of 500 students. The completely different level of competition at the University of British Columbia was a shock, but I settled in and worked hard. It is hard to believe I spent eight years of my life there—no traipsing around the world with a backpack, for I worked for a year before university and every summer to pay for my education. I was in debt when I finished, but not nearly as much as the students are now.

I could not wait to get out of Vancouver, so I spent an interesting and hard-working two years doing my CCFP in Newfoundland. My home base has been the West Kootenays ever since then, and I enjoy small-town life. I have never married and have no children. Most of the time this is fine, but every once in a while, it feels hard.

I have been fortunate with my health apart from kidney surgery while in fourth year of medical school (the worst year of my life), bouts of depression, and most recently osteoarthritis and vitreous detachment. Being single allows you to set whatever goals you can for yourself. Recently, I have become more concerned about saving money for retirement due to my arthritis. I have spent thirteen of sixteen years doing locums, only three years in a steady practice in Nelson. For ease of retirement, I am grateful not to be tied to a practice, especially in today's medical political climate.

In all honesty, if I had it all to do over again I would not go into medicine. No sour grapes—I am grateful for the many satisfying experiences, and I know I have been of help to many people, and even saved a life or two. But most of my more wonderful moments in life have been connected with performing in theatre and music. I am a reasonably good singer and a better actress. The best moments ever were when I got standing ovations from forty to 800 people for my performances of "Shirley Valentine," a one-woman play which consisted essentially of two hours of monologue. Most years, for more than twelve years, I have done two to three plays per year, at the amateur and more recently professional level. I also took the two-year Selkirk College Professional Music Program in Nelson from 1994 to 1996, but sadly I have not continued much with music since then. My last performance of any sort was as the witch in the opera *Hansel and Gretel*. I dislike it when I am just working and not rehearsing for something, as has been the case this year.

Originally I had planned to retire from medicine at age fifty, but I strongly suspect I will be shifting gears into something else in a couple of years. The trick is to stay out of debt, and to keep your material wants and needs relatively simple.

Curriculum Vitae

Born: September 22, 1956.

Education: BSc, University of British Columbia, 1978; MD, University of British Columbia, 1982; CCFP, (Certification of the College of Family Practice), Memorial University of Newfoundland; Licensure in the College of Physicians and Surgeons of British Columbia, 1984; Completion of ACLS, most recent 1998; Completion of Pediatric Life Support course, most recent 1992; Completion of Neonatal Advanced Life Support course, most recent 1990.

Experience: General Practice locums in various areas of British Columbia. All the usual General Practice duties, including Emergency Room, Surgical assists, Obstetrics, 1984–1989; General Practice in Nelson, B.C., 1989–1992; Medical Director at Willowhaven Private Hospital (Long-Term Care), Nelson. Frequent locum physician at Mt. St. Francis Hospital (LTC), Nelson, 1989–1995; 1988–1998: Medical Officer at Canadian International College (for overseas students); 1992–present; resumed G.P. locums, mainly in Nelson area. Privileges at Kootenay Lake District Hospital (active staff). Not practising Obstetrics since 1982.

DR. CAROLINE PENN

My interest in medicine goes back a long way, probably to about age fourteen. My father, Michael Penn, was a family physician who trained at Cambridge University and then at St. Bartholomew's Hospital in London before joining my mother in Victoria, British Columbia. Through exposure to his work and various jobs as a medical receptionist and physiotherapy aid, I continued this interest through high school and university. However, I elected to study biology at the University of Victoria, and for a time entertained the idea of becoming a marine or wildlife biologist. On graduating from UVic in 1974 and having no firm plans, I applied to CUSO and set off to Europe. While travelling that summer I heard that I had been accepted for a teaching position in rural Ghana, West Africa. I

had three days at home before leaving again, this time to Africa. En route I attended CUSO's cultural orientation program at the University of Western Ontario in London, Ontario, and cultural, teaching, and language training sessions once on site in Ghana. I spent a year teaching biology in Ghana in a small town called Offinso, which was north of Kumasi in the Ashanti region. It was one of the memorable times of my life, though it had frustrating moments and certainly gave me lots of reasons to look critically at the way foreign aid is offered. I taught forms one to four biology to 300 young African students in a rural school within a secondary rain forest clearing. My first "gift" from my students was a dead black cobra, just one of the many deadly snakes which lived in that area, not to mention an array of outsized insects such as centipedes and scorpions, which lived in and around our little house. Travelling to Abidjan, Ivory Coast, for the New Year 1974, sleeping on the ramparts of old slave forts of the Ghanaian Coast in Dixcove, and navigating the markets of African villages for our plantain, ground nuts, and yams, are just a few of the many memories which constitute a story in itself.

On returning from Africa in the summer of 1975, I felt quite useless and so joined my brother, Andrew, who was studying medicine at Cambridge. I sat in on his lectures and worked in the town before taking a job as an *au pair* for the ski school director of Zermatt, Switzerland. I had always dreamed of working in Africa and spending time in the Alps, so this seemed to conclude these aspirations. The job in Zermatt was mainly housework as my boss applied his seven-day-a-week work ethic, but I believe that my resolve to make something more of my degree was strengthened by scrubbing innumerable floors in their chalet. The rewards of this job were the few hours of freedom that I had to ski the many beautiful slopes within sight of the famous Matterhorn.

Returning home to Victoria in 1976, I began to apply in earnest for medical school, and also worked as a substitute teacher. In 1977–78, while completing my final semester in the PDP teaching program at Simon Fraser University, I received word of my acceptance to the University of British Columbia and so began a new phase of my life. I found medicine a lot of hard work, but enjoyed it more and more as I reached its clinical phase. In my fourth year I spent three months in Christchurch, New Zealand, doing an elective in psychiatry and medicine. My psychiatric placement was in a chronic psychiatric hospital and had a fascinating array of characters for whom I provided general medical care. I found a few extra weeks to explore the South Island's fabulous West Coast (by motorbike) and the rolling sheep country near Mount Cook.

My first year of internship was in Edmonton, Alberta. It was a good year and very hard work with long hours. I recall doing CCU and obstetrics and being on call for twenty hours at a time with eight hours off before starting all over again. When possible I went with Alpine Club friends (winter and summer) to hike and ski in the Rockies near Jasper and Banff. I stayed on another year in Alberta, transferring into the second year of the Family Practice program. This program had an appeal as it offered electives in obstetrics in Red Deer, Alberta, as well as an elective in an arctic nursing station. In May and June of 1984 I flew to Cambridge Bay on Victoria Island in the high arctic to do a two-month elective in a nursing station. At sixty-nine degrees latitude North, there was probably no other physician between me and the north pole. It was a very wonderful two months in which I had the experience of practising with a team of nurse practitioners in a setting with few lab facilities or other props. We did our own gram stains, dispensed our own medication, and an Inuit woman had been trained to do X-rays. Any serious injuries had to be evacuated to Yellowknife or Edmonton, as did all maternity cases at that time. We made rounds to the homes of older Inuit and to small settlements such as Pelly Bay (near Hudson Bay) and Bay Chimo on Bathurst Inlet. I had some exciting medivacs—one to the arctic mainland (Hope Bay) to medivac an Inuit with a broken femur, and one to Pelly Bay. I met the intrepid northern pilots and flew in single Otters above the sea ice, landing on frozen lakes and bays. I met a celebrity, "Zachary," the Inuit who was the star in the movie of Farley Mowat's "Never Cry Wolf," and I experienced the coming of summer to the tundra with its thousands of migratory nesting birds and rivers with arctic char. I had the opportunity to work with a wonderful doctor, Dr. Brian Finnemore, who came to the arctic to do a locum and who was a great mentor.

On completing my Family Practice residency, I left Alberta to return to British Columbia and spent the summer and winter doing locums in the Kootenays. Although I do not consider myself adept enough at the surgical skills required for remote locums, I found the other challenges and rural personalities appealing and interesting. After a summer in Nelson, I spent four months doing a solo locum in New Denver, a beautiful setting on the Slocan Lake, surrounded by mountain ranges such as the Valhallas. Once a week I would drive to Slocan City and do a clinic there, which was set up in a local motel unit. I recall an American couple, newly arrived in town, asking if I was the resident cardiologist!

Around this time I first met my husband who was a bush pilot, flying Beavers on floats. His family had gone "back to the land" in the Slocan Valley during the early 1970s. He was in transition, having decided to go back to school, so we returned to Vancouver and began twelve years of school which took him through his BA, MA, and ultimately his PhD in psychology from UBC in 1995. During this time I did locums, first on the north shore and then in Burnaby. In the fall of 1985 we bought round-the-world airline tickets and embarked on a short but memorable trip which took us to many wonderful places—India (the Taj Mahal, Varanasi on the river Ganges), Nepal (trekking near Annapurna), Thailand and Burma (Rangoon, Mandalay and the mystical Pagan on the Irrawaddy river), and then Singapore, Australia, New Zealand, and home.

Practising travel medicine enabled me to learn more about public health, vaccines, and prevention of tropical illness and has been something I have done part-time ever since.

From 1987 to 1988 I did a one-year locum at Reach Clinic on Commercial Drive in Vancouver. It was an enjoyable year, working as part of a team in a clinic that had a varied population. The clinic started years ago as a youth street clinic and evolved into a community health centre with physicians, nurse practitioners, a pharmacist, a dentist, and allied social services. We did a lot of case conferencing, house calls in East Vancouver, and deliveries at St. Paul's Hospital. I worked with physicians such as Sandy Witherspoon, another fine mentor. Towards the end of the year I was expecting my first child and so made a decision to stop doing locum work and take a more predictable job. I was approached by Dr. Janice

Kirkpatrick, who worked in Ladner, to share her practice with her. In January 1989 when my daughter was five months old, I began part-time practice there and remained for almost ten years. Janice proved to be a fine associate with a wonderful sense of humour. We managed to juggle having two children each, alternating our maternal leaves, and working out hours that enabled us to see our office and hospital patients each day and cross over for each other on days off. We worked in Ladner, with the Delta Hospital across the road. It was ideal as we could walk to the hospital to do rounds, and the Emergency Department could handle our urgent cases. With no pediatrician or psychiatrist in the community, we did a lot of this ourselves and developed a good rapport with our available specialists. During this time I also worked with Planned Parenthood, doing a weekly evening clinic.

From 1995 to 1997, I was Head of Family Practice at Delta Hospital. Despite some reluctance to take on this responsibility (with a four- and a six-year-old at home), I surprised myself by tackling it and enjoying being part of a medical advisory committee. I can't say it was always easy. Our children were daycare kids, my daughter starting at nine months at the Simon Fraser University daycare, and then later both children attending the UBC daycare system. For the four years that my husband spent at UBC doing his PhD we lived in a townhouse in student housing and I commuted two to three days a week to Ladner to work. I remember some days when I would work a full nine-to-five day, chair a Family Practice meeting, attend a general staff meeting, and then attend a Medical Advisory Committee meeting consecutively, getting home at 11 p.m.

Around 1994, on a whim, I submitted a resumé to Dr. Rusung Tan, asking him if he needed any physicians to work in a newly-established travel clinic. He hired me, amazingly, sight unseen. Since my days in biology and living in West Africa, I had never lost interest in tropical medicine and this type of work fulfilled, vicariously, my continuing interest. I began doing weekly clinics in the downtown office of the Travel Medicine and Vaccination Centre (TMVC), often a morning travel clinic, and then commuting to Ladner to do family practice all afternoon. Practising travel medicine enabled me to learn more about public health, vaccines, and prevention of tropical illness and has been something I have done part-time ever since,

along with my family practice. Around 1998, I was asked to act as an associate director of this travel clinic and took on the job in addition to my weekly clinics. The extra responsibilities included scheduling doctors, writing monthly memos (about malaria or recent disease outbreaks, etc.), answering questions from nurses, doctors, and patients, and dealing with complicated cases.

I continued to work in family practice in Ladner and greatly enjoyed the experience of getting to know patients and their families and providing care to all age groups. Although I did not do obstetrics, we did some prenatal care, and did a bit of pediatrics. We provided surgical assists at the local hospitals and could admit and treat patients in hospital. After undergoing an office practice assessment in the 1990s by the College of Physicians and Surgeons of B.C., I was asked to be a peer assessor, and I have done several assessments annually since then. I also participated annually as a Medical Council of Canada examiner for the MCC Qualifying Examinations Part Two.

By 1995 my husband had finished his PhD and several years of post-doc positions and finally obtained a tenure-track position at SFU. I saw an opportunity to make a transition and so applied to SFU Health Services and took leave from my practice in the fall of 1998. I have worked part-time three days a week at SFU Health Services since then and we are finally able to buy a home (my first at age forty-five) in Port Moody. My present job involves primary care to the student population and responding to emergencies on campus, as well as travel counselling and various outreach programs. The latter has included advising and participating in orientation programs for students travelling overseas for field schools each year. I was acting as Medical Practice Leader while Dr. Gultaj Somani took maternity leave in 2000. I continued my second career in travel medicine, working one to two clinics per week for the Travel Medicine and Vaccination Centre. I also work from home with the aid of a computer, one to two days per week, accompanied by our nine-year-old son who has elected a non-traditional route to his schooling.

I have enjoyed a fulfilling, busy career and must extend much credit to my husband, Jeremy, who has been tirelessly supportive of my career (as I hope I have in small measure been to his) and as a parent through my long hours of work.

DR. DOREEN TETZ

Mine was not a conventional route to medical school. I suspect this is true of many women doctors. I was working in Chilliwack at a medical clinic, a job I was very pleased to have after waitressing and chambermaiding. My marriage was failing due to the impetuousness of youth. The future was not bright. A single mom without a high-school diploma doesn't have many doors open to her. Concurrently Germaine Greer was telling me I could open any doors I pleased. It was one of my employers, Dr. Tony Borschneck, who was the catalyst. When he found out that I would really like to become a doctor, he quipped "Just do it," decades before Nike had even thought it. Tony, an ex-policeman who approached medical school from a Grade 9 education with a wife and three kids, was a study in possibilities. I tossed my hat into the ring. From 1972–1976 I worked days and studied nights. I was able to get my first year university equivalent at our local night school and save enough money to enroll at the University of British Columbia in the fall of 1976. Three days before registration Wade (my son, age seven), and I moved into our hut in the Family Housing area at UBC. Neither of us had really ever been out of Chilliwack. Definitely wet behind our ears.

Feeling pretty full of myself at getting this far, I was abruptly humbled by my first midterm marks. Lesson number one, community college does not equal university. I had to learn to study! In the spring of 1979 I received my first acceptance letter to Queens University. Ecstatic is an understatement of my reaction. It was about a week later that my acceptance letter from UBC arrived. That was to be my choice. While I remember my pre-med years as a transition time of neurotic preoccupation with marks, my medical school years were a treasure.

One day I met Vona who would become a true friend. We came to medical school with very similar pasts and formed a bond that would sustain us both through the years to come. We studied endlessly on the phone each night, we exchanged clothes, we laughed and cried together. We both ended up in skimpy danskins at one of our infamous skit nights. These were good years—challenging, stimulating, and uproarious. They were also flexible enough years to accommodate a growing teenager.

Med school is demanding, parenting is demanding, and while my friendship with Vona eased the load, it was my mom who selflessly gave time and care to Wade to fill in for my gaps. Wade, who was ten to fourteen during my medical school years, became the most self-sufficient independent teenager. He deserves an honorary degree. We have great pictures of Wade and Vona and me on graduation day.

I interned at St Paul's Hospital. I think it is safe to say that I started to run out of energy this year. I have a strong allegiance to St Paul's, but many memories are blurred, with what I now know all too well as sleep deprivation. I elected to do another year after internship to get my Certification in Family Practice. Suffice it to say this was a limp to the end. I was exhausted!

During my intern year I met Dr. Art VanWart who was piloting a project combining St.Paul's internship with the two year Family Practice rotation. His associate was looking for a locum for one year just at the time I was completing my Family Practice residency. I signed up for one year and stayed for seven. During these—my Kerrisdale years—I also was part of a group of family doctors teaching interviewing skills to first year medical students. Also I sat on the UBC medical school admissions committee (1988). I remember thinking back to the time when I dropped out of high school. My home economics teacher, Mrs. Pucher, was so distraught. She enfolded me in a big hug with tears running down her cheeks. It was while I was sitting with the admissions committee in those very formal offices at UBC that I thought of Mrs. Pucher and how pleased she would be.

On the very last day of the very last year of this marathon I met my partner, Peter. Fortified with champagne sipped elegantly from a large old bedpan, I went with some friends and neighbours to a Doug and the Slugs dance at the Vancouver Commodore. It was loud, raucous, and dark. When people ask how we ever got together (Peter and I), we both just say: it was dark and we were drunk. Peter owned property on Denman Island. It became our yearly ritual to spend August on Denman developing this five-acre alder forest. We moved a fourteen-foot travel trailer on to the site and started what appears to be a life-long project. Denman did not have a resident doctor, so when the word got out that we were there, I would start to see a few of the accident-prone tourists. These visits watered a little seed of a thought about starting a practice on Denman Island. In my heart I knew I would be happier living back in a rural environment. We committed ourselves to this idea in 1987 and on December 1, 1991, I worked my first day in a clinic that Peter built on the road edge of our property. When I was transferring my banking to the Comox Valley, the then bank manager asked me how busy I thought I would be. I told him I planned to see five to six patients per day in my small one-person (no staff) clinic. This truly was my intention. Twelve people came on the first day and within a week I was as busy as I was in Vancouver. Time to hire some staff!

Rural medicine in one-doctor communities takes a unique mind-set and a very understanding partner. You are never OFF. It took a while to come to terms with this, but surprisingly it works for me. I can only think it has to do with growing up on a farm where there is work to do every day—sometimes there are emergencies and sometimes it's quiet. To those people who say, "But you don't have a life," I answer, "This is my life and it is extraordinarily rich."

Rural medicine in one-doctor communities takes a unique mind-set and a very understanding partner. You are never OFF.

People get sick in ways that are universal and in that way city medicine and country medicine don't differ. There are, however, stories to tell that are uniquely rural. In 1998/99 we had two high cliff rescues of seriously injured patients. Our first happened at 9 p.m. in the spring (and therefore dark) when a man was found barely conscious halfway down a 100-foot cliff. The fire department, our emergency service allies, set up a series of pulleys and ropes, and with Peter behind me, I was lowered down the cliff to the patient. This is not a pleasant thing to do to one's perineum. We ultimately stabilized the patient and lowered him to the beach for a Coast Guard Rescue. He made an amazing recovery from serious injuries, and we dined out on the adrenalin from that call for some time afterwards. Several months later an MVA patient went over another cliff. Feeling both experienced and comforted by the new harness that the fire department purchased, I made another ropes and pulleys descent. But it gets better! The Labrador Helicopter was called in from Comox and hovered over the beach to pick up our patient. His condition was fluctuating and the paramedics asked for a physician escort. It is probably important to stop here and explain that I don't like heights and I'm not fond of cold water. Nevertheless, it took about a nano-second for me to agree with this, and in what I can truthfully say was one of the most exciting moments of my life, I was hoisted in a "Velcro hold" by a not-unattractive SARTEC into the Labrador Helicopter. The patient did well and I was thrilled beyond belief.

My other "rural story" is a quiet reflection of the life that I love here. It is a life that is filled with critters. Deer, geese, beaver, racoons, muskrats, eagles—the list is endless and I have a soft spot for them all. I was working one Friday afternoon when Doris (my receptionist) and I were getting ready to wrap up the day at 5 p.m. A last patient came to the door. She was a young woebegone frail woman, who as it turns out was just passing through. She had some vague abdominal complaints. As I took her history it became clear that this woman needed much help. She was impoverished, had no place that was home, and was travelling with an abusive man. She suffered anxiety and was unable to eat. My examination revealed no acute organic problems to be fixed, and as I led her back to my desk to talk, I was struggling to find some small pearl of wisdom I could bring to this ephemeral meeting. A few minutes into our talk a startling transformation took place. Janey (not her real name) was looking over my shoulder out the window that sits beside my desk. It is a low window, only sixteen inches from the floor. She was smiling. I turned around and there was Beatrice, our clinic beaver that had been visiting us every day in the late afternoon for the previous few weeks. Earlier that week she had dropped a small fir tree in the clinic garden, much to the delight of the waiting room patients, and much to the chagrin of Peter the landscaper. She was particularly alluring that day with her front teeth on the low windowsill and her bright orange-toothed smile. Janey was enchanted, and this led to talks of her childhood in rural Quebec where she had last seen beavers. We talked of her parents and family and she became visibly stronger and confident. She started to see new possibilities for herself and left the office that day full of hope. I gave full credit to Beatrice. About one year later I received a card with a beaver on the front. Inside was written: "I'm doing well, Janey."

There are many more stories to tell and it is true the load is very heavy for rural doctors, but the rewards are commensurate, and with colleagues like Beatrice, you are never alone.

1985

DR. SUEDA AKKOR

I was born in a small town in rural Turkey. We moved to the capital, Ankara, where I attended Grades 1 and 2. Shortly afterwards, we emigrated to Canada. My parents were very hardworking and ambitious even though they did not have a post-secondary education; at a very early age, they instilled in me, my sister, and brother the principle of "first work, then play." I remember studying constantly during those early years in Canada, and it always seemed that I would never finish all the work that needed to be done. Nevertheless, I graduated from Grade 13 with a ninety-eight percent average and won the school's science award and a three-year scholarship to the University of Toronto.

At the age of nine, I made the decision to study medicine. This decision stayed with me. After studying first year sciences at the University of Toronto, personal circumstances took me back to Turkey for a year. Prior to going, I had completed several university entrance type examinations. My marks offered me two opportunities in Turkey: studying medicine or studying engineering. I chose medicine and studied for one year. I then made the decision (after long contemplation) to stay on in Turkey. I completed the six-year medical program at Istanbul University.

These six years were challenging times for me. There were many riots and demonstrations at the university because of the political circumstances in Turkey. The rest of my family was still back in Canada and I was alone. I did not really fit into the culture and after I was married at age twenty-one, all my medical studies were done while living in a two-bedroom apartment with my mother-in-law. Often there was no water or heating, and I studied in the bedroom with gloves on and wrapped in a blanket. My mother-in-law had manic-depressive disorder which had not been previously diagnosed; I diagnosed her as I studied psychiatry. Unfortunately, she ended up committing suicide during my final year.

It was a difficult year while studying and supporting my then husband. I managed to graduate from medical school in the top five percent of the class, and returned to Canada shortly after my graduation. I worked as a medical technician while waiting to take the examinations required for all "foreign medical graduates." I passed the exams and was qualified to do my internship in 1983 at McMaster Medical School in Hamilton, Ontario. I also published an article in a medical journal during this time.

After my internship, I decided to do further speciality training in Internal Medicine in Vancouver, but I could not afford to travel there for the interview! Fortunately I was able to do the interview by telephone. I was offered a position and travelled across the country in a van a with few pieces of furniture. After two years of intensive training in Internal Medicine, I decided to apply to Ophthalmology and was accepted. As I began my residency training, I was faced with another personal challenge—my then husband of nine years attempted suicide. After a very difficult time our marriage ended and he returned to Turkey.

I continued my training in Ophthalmology and passed my fellowship exams in 1989. I was offered a position at the Ophthalmology Department of the University of British Columbia, which I accepted. I first joined a busy private practice in East Vancouver and later a solo practice downtown. During my first five years of practice, I travelled up to Kitimat and Fort Nelson, B.C., to do visiting consultant clinics in those areas—an experience which I enjoyed very much. At UBC, I lectured to medical students and was the undergraduate program director for several years. I have given talks on ophthamological topics to general practitioners and other medical colleagues as well as the public. I also wrote a chapter on "The Red Eye" for a general medical therapeutics book, of which the third edition has just come out.

In more recent years, I was a co-founder and owner of a refractive laser centre where I performed laser refractive surgery during the early stages of this exciting field. After a second marriage and a child, I made the decision to let go of the refractive aspect of my practice. Presently, I have a solo practice in downtown Vancouver, which is highly satisfying, and am clinical assistant professor in the UBC Department of Ophthalmology. I also conduct visiting clinics at a nearby nursing home to provide eye care to elderly patients who are unable to visit an outside office and am on a geriatrics committee, where our goal is to provide optimal care to the elderly population.

DR. JEAN LOUISE BECK JAMIESON

Jean Louise is the second daughter of Drs. Dick and Jean Beck, and was born in 1960 in Vancouver, B.C. She graduated from Queen's University with a BA in 1980 and from the University of British Columbia with an MD in 1984. She interned at Memorial University Hospital of Newfoundland and went into General Practice in Fort St. John, B.C. where she had earlier done an elective in the final year of medical school. After a year and a half, she left to travel, doing a Diploma in Tropical Medicine in London, England, and some further training in New Zealand.

Jean Louise went back to Fort St. John in 1990 and joined the Ministry of Health Program to retrain in Public Health. She took the exam for MHSc in Health Care and Epidemiology and worked for the Ministry of Health and then for the newly-founded Community Health Council.

She is now married with two children, John (b. 1992) and Margaret (b. 1995), and lives in semi-retirement in Squamish.

DR. ROZMIN F. KAMANI

Many major milestones are due to the very people we elect—our politicians. In my life I have Ayatollah Khomeni and a premier of British Columbia.

I arrived in Canada in 1979 after having lived on two other continents—Africa where I spent my early youth, and Iran where I commenced my medical training. Due to the political unrest in Iran, I completed medicine and Family Practice Residency in Winnipeg. I felt I was adept as a chameleon. I had lived through tropical weather, desert storms, and winter blizzards, all in the span of twenty-four years.

In 1985, when we arrived in Vancouver, my husband and I with our two children felt we had "earned" B.C. (and its milder west coast influence). However, I had not been prepared for the storm created by Premier Bill VanderZalm. In denying me a billing number, my freedom to practice was taken away—as was the case for many other graduates.

Some wise person once told me that when one door closes look for the open window. One such window opened for me as I sat in desperation in the Vancouver airport. I was temporarily fleeing to Ontario when I spied a front-page headline in *The Vancouver Sun*. The Socreds had called the Ombudsman's recommendation on WCB "stupid." Intrigued by the word "Ombudsman," I decided to pay him a visit. He arranged to have my case investigated, and later that summer I was granted an unrestricted MSP billing number.

During these years of turmoil I found quiet support from the Federation of Medical Women of Canada. My husband and I attended a "Dual Doctor Marriage" panel discussion organized by the FMWC's B.C. Branch. I was quickly seized to help out with registration as the attendance flowed out into the hallway. It was standing room only. In 1989, the membership of the B.C. Branch of FMWC voted me in as President. I had a large executive and a membership of nearly 400. Women physicians addressed issues of childcare, patterns of practice, and women's health. Later that year the B.C. Government proposed to restrict abortions. I was hurtled into the realm of media and news releases. This crescendo culminated with a very successful private meeting with the then Justice Minister, Kim Campbell. Today, abortion remains in this country as a medical service.

At my first Board meeting as the national Honorary Secretary of FMWC, I found myself becoming the editor of the FMWC newsletter. A couple of years later I became the national President of FMWC. The experience gave me the opportunity to not only have opinions, but to actually express them and influence others. The Federation of Medical Women of Canada provided a springboard for many a woman physician in future leadership.

(Dr. Rozmin F. Kamani wrote her story for the BCMA News *of Nov/Dec 1995 and has given permission to include it in this book.)*

DR. CAROLINE YING-MEI WANG

The earliest notion I had about a career in medicine was introduced to me, quite casually, at a young age. A family friend had asked me, "What do you want to do when you grow up?" which startled me since career planning was the farthest thing from my simple mind at the time. However, being the obliging little girl I was and feeling that I was expected to produce an answer, I quickly searched my mind for a limited list of "girl" careers of that era and answered, "a nurse." Afterwards, when my parents suggested why don't I become a doctor instead, I realized that it was okay for a girl to think about being a doctor, too. That my father was a physician, of course, might have been a factor. It would be many years before I actually thought seriously about what I would do for a career. However, I am always grateful to my parents for signaling to me from early on that anything is possible to achieve.

I was an only child, which was unusual in those days for a Chinese family. I was blessed with the most loving, devoted parents and to them I was the centre of the universe. My father and mother were, like many others of their generation, forced by historical events and twists of fate to leave their families in Northern China to go to Taiwan during the revolution when Mao Ze-Dong and the Communist Party took over the rule of China. My father was studying medicine at the National Defense Medical Centre in Shanghai when his school was abruptly transferred to Taiwan. Cut off from their relatives and denied any form of communication due to political circumstances, it would be over two decades before they were to establish contact with their families. Thus I was born in Taiwan, where I lived for seven years before coming to Canada.

My father was one of the earliest physicians to emigrate to Canada from Taiwan. Upon completion of his medical training and serving several years in the army, he was determined that he would one day return to see his parents and relatives in China. This was not possible as long as we lived in Taiwan, so my father wrote and passed the necessary examinations to go to Canada. It was again by fate that we settled in British Columbia. After my father had originally applied and was accepted by a hospital in the United States for residency training, the U.S. immigration denied him entry, stating as the reason that he would likely not return to Taiwan in the future. My father then applied to Canada and was accepted to begin a rotating internship at the Royal Columbian Hospital in New Westminster, B.C. Expecting to see a land of snow and wilderness, he never imagined what a beautiful country awaited him.

My mother and I arrived in Canada in 1965, exactly three months after my father had landed. Our family was considered fortunate, since reunification of families had been frequently denied for several years due to immigration hurdles. When my parents came to Canada, they had no savings and their plane ticket was purchased with a friend's loan, but what they did bring was priceless—their knowledge, skills, determination, strong work ethic, and a fierce pride typical of most Chinese immigrants of that time. I can only wonder at the courage and determination it took for them to adjust to living in a foreign country. However, self-reliance was the norm and my parents, like most other immigrants, held high hopes and worked hard to seek a better life and future for their family.

When I arrived in Canada at the age of seven, I did not know a word of English. I had not quite completed Grade 1 in Taiwan, gaining only the most rudimentary basis of the Chinese written language. In the fall I was registered in Grade 1 at the neighbourhood elementary school. There was no ESL in those days, so I was put into a regular class, with total immersion in English. At that age, learning a language seemed natural and effortless. My teacher was very kind and initially worried that I did not comprehend my English, as for a long time I did not utter a single word. One day, desperate and unable to contain myself any longer, I broke the silence with my first words to the teacher, "May I go to the washroom?" Seeing her delighted reaction, I turned chatty after that. Towards the end of that year, I was allowed to advance early to Grade 2 to catch up with my grade level, which was merciful considering that I was already tall for my age.

Because of frequent moves, I actually attended seven different schools during seven years of elementary school. Despite this, I did well in school. I was very shy in grade school and was constantly dismayed by the considerable attention I received, particularly for excelling in art. By the intermediate grades I had fully caught up in English and from then remained at the top of my class. Being an only child of immigrant parents, the expectation to excel in school was inescapable.

We eventually settled in Kelowna, where my father set up in solo practice. It was an idyllic place to grow up, a friendly community in the beautiful Okanagan valley with a small town closeness. Life seemed uncomplicated and carefree. I became an avid hockey fan, and my worst nightmare was to have my favorite team and idol, Bobby Orr and the Boston Bruins, lose in the Stanley Cup playoffs. There was little academic pressure as most of my classmates did not plan to go on to university and were content to find a job upon graduation from high school. While lamenting the lack of competition in school, I was fortunate to have some excellent teachers who stimulated my curiosity and were an inspiring influence. Developing a wide range of interests forms an important aspect of one's personal growth, and my participation in various activities, including the school band, student council, editor of the annual club, and co-editor of the newspaper club, all became invaluable experiences. However, what I found most exciting was the school debating team which was excellent training not only in public speaking, but more importantly, on developing both sides of an argument. Discovering my passion, I went on to win several debating tournaments in B.C. and represented our province in the Western Canada Debating Tournament in Winnipeg. Debating is an important skill that trains critical thinking and objective analysis of an issue, and proved to be of enormous value in future years.

I was the top student in my school throughout the high school years, but was kept humble with frequent reminders from my father not to limit my sights to my own school and to seek understanding in learning. Humility is an important virtue for the Chinese, but it is all too often misunderstood by the Western culture which by contrast is boastful and frequently preoccupied by image. I recall an amusing incident when an acquaintance asked my father about how his daughter was doing and when my father replied jokingly, "She's a little dull," the woman promptly looked upon me with great pity and responded, "Oh, that's too bad." I don't think my parents would go so far now to show humility at my expense. However, most Chinese people, even the highly accomplished, tend to appear relatively low key.

My parents were strict and overprotective by Canadian standards, but rather typical of many traditional Chinese parents. I was not allowed to go out and never dated in high school. However, I accepted that the rules of my family were different and therefore I was not subject to the usual peer pressure during my teens. Since filial respect was a strongly engrained value, disobeying one's parents was simply unfathomable. Most of all, I had enormous admiration and respect for my mother and father, who are principled, caring, models of truth and integrity. Being the only Chinese in my

school, although fortunate not to have experienced discrimination while growing up, I remained conscious of my distinct ethnic background. I was taught to be proud of my Chinese culture and heritage, to be an independent thinker and resist pressures to conform to "the crowd" for acceptance.

While in high school I had already decided that I wanted to become a doctor. It was not an easy decision because I was interested in so many things. The greatest influence for me to become a doctor was undoubtedly my father, who devoted his life as a physician to helping others. To him medicine is a calling and he was proud to be in this noble profession. He genuinely loved the practice of medicine and was a meticulous and skilled diagnostician. I marvelled at his gift for communicating with people as well as his empathy for others. He worked long hours, was on call for his patients day and night seven days a week, and went to extraordinary lengths to help people. My father taught by example, living a simple and virtuous life, and showed how caring and giving can bring unparalleled joy and satisfaction.

Entering the University of British Columbia in Vancouver marked a major transition, since it meant leaving my sheltered home in Kelowna and moving into the student dormitories on campus. While it was exhilarating to have a taste of independence, it was also the beginning of an entirely new experience in developing responsible study habits, time management skills, and social interactions. Certainly I didn't know what burnout was, as up to then studying had occurred sporadically, usually on the night before examinations, and I had the energy and exuberance of a young colt just released from the corral. Suddenly at UBC I found myself in large lecture halls along with several hundred other first-year students in the Faculty of Science, squinting to see the professor and his notes flying by on the overhead projector. In contrast to my lighthearted mirth, most of the other students wore the serious look of "pre-med" students in which every step was calculated on how to get into medical school. Now that I found myself surrounded by the competition I always craved, I felt very small and understood what my father was talking about.

Living in the student residences formed an important part of my university experience, and soon I more than made up for my previous social isolation with hordes of new friends. Studying time was compressed between long chats in the cafeteria and library, and friends knocking on my door to go for nighttime snacks. I was terribly naïve socially, and the first time a boy attempted a friendly kiss it so terrified me that I fled into my room and hid under the desk. Organizing parties took a toll on my marks by my third year, which was particularly demanding with a heavy course load. When I failed to gain admission on my first application to medicine at UBC, I was disappointed but not surprised. During my fourth year I chose Honors Physiology as my major, which gave me a valuable glimpse on what it was like to do research as well as writing a graduation thesis.

When I was accepted by the first of several medical schools upon graduating with a Bachelor's Degree in Honors Physiology, I thought that it was the happiest day of my life. The next four grueling years in UBC medical school was to transform an innocent schoolgirl into a young physician ready to face the world. I was struck by the quality and brilliance of my medical school classmates who were obviously all highly accomplished and talented young men and women willing to dedicate their futures to medicine. Entering the world of medicine was fascinating, challenging, but also extremely demanding. Faced with a tidal wave of knowledge to be absorbed, it was also training in scientific thinking, organization, and prioritization of information.

Clinical training showed how the art and science of medicine are combined in the practice of medicine, in which a sound basis of knowledge in differential diagnosis and the ability to communicate with the patient are both indispensable tools. I began to appreciate medicine as a discipline that not only demands hard work and personal sacrifice, but also ethics, sound judgement, maturity, compassion, and even physical endurance. During clerkship, the initial excitement of carrying a pager and being awakened in the middle of the night quickly settled into the sober reality of chronic sleep deprivation and cycles of mind-numbing fatigue after thirty-eight hours on call. I graduated from UBC in the Class of 1984, proud to have finally earned an MD, but realizing this was only the beginning of a long journey and uncertain of the road that lies ahead. Curiously, my graduating medical school yearbook, which characterized me as "carefree" also wondered " . . . after she becomes a real doctor, will she manage to come back down to earth to pick up her paychecks?"

I began a rotating internship at St. Joseph's Hospital in London, Ontario, finally fulfilling my wish to get out of British Columbia to see and experience another part of Canada. It didn't take long for me to feel homesick, and although I enjoyed my year in Ontario, I suddenly appreciated the beauty of my home province which I had previously taken for granted. It was also during my internship year when I started to feel my biological clock ticking, and decided it was time to get married. I met my husband, Anthony, when he was doing his cardiology fellowship training in Vancouver, and we became better acquainted during my year in London while he trained in Ann Arbor, Michigan, a few hours drive across the border.

Four grueling years in UBC medical school were to transform an innocent schoolgirl into a young physician ready to face the world.

After marrying, Anthony and I settled in Vancouver where I worked doing locums in the Lower Mainland and Okanagan and discovered, to my surprise, that I enjoyed general practice very much. It was immensely rewarding to be able to apply one's knowledge in helping large numbers of people and families over time through a trusted doctor-patient relationship. From practising Family Medicine, one gained a unique and wide perspective on life, the human condition, and an intimate understanding of people of all ages. I joined a group of physicians at the Island Clinic in Richmond in 1986, buying a practice from one of their associates. Practices were selling for exorbitant sums, thanks to restrictions on physician billing numbers just imposed by the provincial government as a part of a scheme to limit the number of doctors in B.C. This was the first taste of how politics and economics would affect physicians, their professional practices and lives.

Medical school and internship provided no preparation on how to run a medical practice, and young physicians had to quickly learn how to run an office practice and a business, in addition to practising good medicine. This would become a formidable challenge, as I was to discover, particularly as doctors' fees are fixed by the government and do not reflect the actual quality of service provided, while physicians were forced to absorb increasing office overhead expenses in the face of lack of fee increases. Having gone into medicine for altruistic reasons but expecting that a medical doctor would not have to worry about earning a living, I would learn like most other physicians that this assumption would no longer hold true in the new era of health care cutbacks and politics. The astounding reality of more and more doctors who cannot afford to retire after dedicating their lives to a difficult profession to save the lives of others is a sad reflection of the values as well as devaluation of the medical profession by society today.

A unique challenge for women in medicine is balancing the demands of their career with that of their family. When both spouses are physicians it also presents an added challenge, especially for families with children. After having four children in six years, two boys and two girls, I now salute all mothers I encounter and especially those with young children. Parenthood is a gift that has given us the ultimate joy, and perhaps the most important challenge for us as physicians is finding the time and energy to nurture our children while shouldering heavy responsibilities to our patients and towards our society.

My involvement with community organizations began with my desire to improve the health care of the growing but underserved Chinese population by organizing Health Fairs on disease prevention and health promotion. My enthusiasm and passion for helping the Chinese-Canadian community and my physician colleagues began with my involvement as a Board member of the Chinese Canadian Medical Society (CCMS) from 1990 and led to serving as its President in 1996–97. This became the training ground for learning to run meetings and organize events, and ultimately was the unintended foray into organizational politics. Our work for the community also led to building bridges with other professionals, community leaders, and organizations, including the Vancouver Medical Association and the Federation of Chinese Medical Societies in North America (FCMS), both organizations of which I would later serve as President.

Interestingly, reactions to my involvement in leadership positions were varied, with many assuming that I must possess personal motives and/or ambitions. It was the perceptive few who understood my passion and zeal to realize a certain vision, its pursuit of which had serendipitously led me down this road. I was also to learn a lesson on the personal price that one sometimes pays when standing up for principles within certain organizations in defying the politics of self-interest. When I discovered that voicing my opinions about policy decisions and arguing for the necessity for informed debate led to personal attacks, I left the organization that I had poured numerous hours and years in serving to start a new organization, the Association of Chinese Canadian Professionals (B.C.) in 1999. Creating a new organization with its mission to unite professionals to serve the community as responsible leaders of society has been enormously rewarding and successful. Besides meeting and working with terrific people, it has allowed us to extend our reach to a diverse group of professionals who share this common interest and vision, and to take an active part in contributing to the future of Canada through advocacy, public education, youth mentoring, and nurturing of tomorrow's leaders.

My venture into medical politics began in 1998 when I became a Board member of the British Columbia Medical Association (BCMA). I was excited to be a part of this excellent organization with a proud history, led by fine and dedicated physician leaders deeply committed to improving health care for patients in B.C. Through BCMA and the Vancouver Medical Association, I feel honoured to have the opportunity to advocate not only for my physician colleagues who play such a valuable and indispensable role in providing our B.C. citizens with high quality health care, but also for necessary changes to save our Medicare system from inevitable future collapse.

Our challenges continue and the future path remains uncertain, yet guided by principle, compassion, strength, and perseverance, I remain optimistic about the future. For me, medicine has meant so much more than just a career; it has indeed been a calling. I feel very grateful to be in this noble and challenging profession that benefits all mankind, while allowing me the opportunity to help improve other people's lives and to make meaningful contributions to the future of our society as a whole.

DR. VALERIE WHITE

I received my medical degree from Memorial University of Newfoundland. Wanting to leave Newfoundland as soon as I was old enough, I did my internship at Mount Sinai Hospital in Toronto and then kept coming west to do internal medicine in Vancouver the following year. Upon deciding that the internal medicine specialty was not for me, I was accepted into the pathology residency at the University of British Columbia in 1981. In about my third year, I realized that I had seen specimens from all the parts of the body except the eye, and so I did an elective with Dr. Jack Rootman, who subsequently convinced me to do ophthalmic pathology as a sub-specialty. Following residency, I did a one-year fellowship with Drs. Alec Garner and Ian Grierson at the Institute of Ophthalmology at Moorfield's Eye Hospital in London, England, and a second year with Dr. Dan Albert at the Massachusetts Eye and Ear Infirmary in Boston. I then took up my current position in Vancouver.

My sub-specialty of Ophthalmic pathology is unique in British Columbia and unusual in Canada. It provides me with an opportunity to liaise with clinicians who are often used to being neglected by their pathology colleagues. My primary aim is to provide a timely and accurate histopathology service to the ophthalmologists of B.C. and to provide consultation for other pathologists throughout the province. I see approximately 1,200 ophthalmic pathology specimens per year, most from Vancouver, but several from different regions of the province. With Dr. Rootman, I have also provided consultative services worldwide. I have written numerous clinico-pathologic correlative papers (frequently with other members of the ophthalmology department) pertaining to different areas of ophthalmology, and several textbook chapters.

My main research interest has been in the area of the genetic changes in intraocular (uveal) melanoma for which I have collaborated with Dr. Doug Horsman at the B.C. Cancer Agency. I began by collecting fresh samples of these rare tumours for cytogenic analysis, and we were one of the first groups to show the recurrent findings of monosomy 3 and trisomy 8. In a further project, we used molecular biological techniques to show that a few more tumours with two chromosomes 3 cytogenetically had only one effective chromosome 3. We have reported that these cytogenetic changes are predictive of outcome in patients with ocular melanoma.

Another area of endeavour is a collaboration with Dr. Susan Lewallen, a tropical ophthalmologist, in an attempt to correlate the histopathology of the eyes in children dying of cerebral malaria in Malawi, Africa with the antemortem clinical findings. This is part of a larger postmortem study on the pathogenesis of cerebral malaria funded by the NIH under Dr. Terrie Taylor of Michigan State University. In March 1998 and 1999, I went to Blantyre, Malawi to work as the pathologist on this project.

I am an avid cyclist and have cycle-toured in many areas of the world, including Europe, Hawaii, Mexico, Alaska, Yukon, Newfoundland, Alberta, and of course B.C. Some of my hobbies include trying to learn to play the guitar and speak Spanish. My husband Alex and I have purchased a sailboat, and we hope to improve our sailing skills. Beginning in October, 2000 I go on a one-year's leave of absence to travel, cycle and sail. (June, 2000.)

Curriculum Vitae

Education: Memorial University of Newfoundland, BSc Program 1973–1975; Memorial University of Newfoundland, MD 1975–1979; Rotating Internship, Mount Sinai Hospital, Toronto, Ontario, 1979–1980; Resident, Internal Medicine, University of British Columbia, Vancouver, B.C., 1980–1981; Resident, General and Anatomic Pathology, University of British Columbia, Vancouver, B.C., 1981–1985; Fellowship, Royal College of Physicians (Canada), General and Anatomic Pathology, 1985; Diplomate, American Board of Pathology, 1985; Clinical Fellow in Pathology, Vancouver General Hospital, Vancouver, B.C., 1985; Research Fellow, Ophthalmic Pathology, Institute of Ophthalmology, University of London, London, England, 1986–1987; Research Fellow, Ophthalmic Pathology, Massachusetts Eye and Ear Infirmary, Harvard University, Boston, Massachusetts, U.S.A., 1987–1988.

Employment Record at University of British Columbia: Clinical Fellow, July–Dec. 1985; Assistant Professor, 1988–1999; Associate Professor, July 1999–present.

Other Employment: Assistant Pathologist 111, Vancouver General Hospital (VGH), Sept. 1988–Sept. 1989; Associate Pathologist 1, VGH, Sept. 1989–Sept. 1990; Associate Pathologist 11, VGH, Sept.

1990–Sept. 1991; Pathologist, VGH, Sept. 1991–Sept. 1993; Consultant Pathologist, Vancouver Hospital & Health Sciences Centre, Sept. 1993– ; Consultant Pathologist, British Columbia Cancer Agency, 1989– ; Consultant Pathologist, British Columbia Children's Hospital, Vancouver, 1991– ; Consultant Pathologist, St. Paul's Hospital, Vancouver, 1993– .

Teaching: includes pathology to medical students, and supervision of graduate students and Fellows as well as course co-ordinator. She gives numerous presentations at Rounds for the Pathology, Ophthalmology, and Neurosurgical Departments.

Other: Dr. White is a Journal Reviewer, Consultant on more than 300 ophthalmic pathology cases from local, national, and international sources, has published over sixty journal articles, and written several textbook chapters. From the time she was awarded the Gold Medal in Medicine at Memorial University in 1979 she has received Fellowship Awards, Research Grants, and the Residents' Award for Ophthalmology Teaching Excellence, UBC, 1992.

1986

DR. HEIDI OETTER

Dr. Heidi Oetter graduated in 1985 from UBC Medical School and registered with the College of Physicians and Surgeons of British Columbia in 1986. Her general practice was a busy one in Coquitlam, B.C., and being a member of both the Department of Family Practice and the Department of Psychiatry at the Royal Columbian Hospital, New Westminster, B.C. added to her workload.

She became active in the B.C. Medical Association, and was Chair of the General Assembly from 1999–2000 and a Board Officer from 2000–2001. In June 2001, she became President of BCMA, the third female doctor to take on the task. (Dr. Ethlyn Trapp was the first, from 1947–48, and Dr. Hedy Fry was the second, from 1990–91.) It was quite a task for the President at a time when negotiations and conflicts were most difficult between doctors and the B.C. Government.

Geraldine Vance, Director of Communications and Public Affairs at BCMA, describes the leadership skills and communication expertise of Dr. Heidi Oetter after she was inaugurated as the President of BCMA and soon became the most media-assaulted Head of the Association in anyone's memory. Vance writes:

"The contract negotiations that started in 2000 ended in a place that no one would have predicted. Following an orderly process of arbitration sessions before Former Chief Justice Allan McEachern, the general assumption was [that] the government would implement the agreement awarded by him. On March 5, 2002, the Provincial Liberal government made history by overturning the arbitrated agreement and imposing a settlement on B.C. physicians. Just as physicians had not expected the actions of the government, it is fair to say [that] the government in no way anticipated the fire it ignited when passing this legislation. The reasons for B.C. doctors' anger and subsequent response were complex and not solely tied to the overturning of the arbitration, but it was the 'straw' that broke the very large camel's back.

"In the period immediately following the government's overturning of [the] legislation, physicians from across the province did the only thing they could: they took job action to get a fair deal. Dr. Oetter, therefore, was put in the midst of a protracted and escalating public defence that would have tried the skills of the most experienced media spokesperson.

"In a month period, Dr. Oetter did over 200 interviews on the service withdrawals. I well remember her first press conference. We walked into the Wallace Wilson room at the BCMA to find at least twenty reporters with TV cameras, multiple radios, and the hungry looks of dogs who had been denied their dinner waiting to pounce at the assembled media people. This was one of the most difficult media conferences I had seen and I have seen some tough stuff in my time. Questions flew at her from all directions, reporters talked over one another, and the quest was relentless to get her to call off the service withdrawals.

"I remain amazed and impressed at how well Heidi handled herself and the hundreds of media interviews that followed. She was calm, articulate, compassionate, and never once lost sight of the fact that she was the voice for all B.C. doctors and that it was her job to tell their story. The only sign she was ever under stress in these situations was that when she had had enough her head would shake ever so slightly and the hair on the crown of her head would flutter a bit. That was the sign to call the press briefing or interview to an end.

"Aside from the media work, Heidi also did the behind-the-scenes work with the BCMA Board and staff to find resolution to the situation while running a busy family practice. I can only assume her stamina came from the training at medical school. In spite of dark circles emerging under her eyes and her clothes getting looser from burning up so much nervous energy, Dr. Oetter maintained her cool and delivered her care under great pressure.

"During the period we came to dub as 'our troubles,' Heidi Oetter was one of the most recognized faces in B.C. When she took trips to Costco to stock up on groceries, she was greeted by fellow shoppers who had seen her on the evening news, and she became a regular fixture at media outlets in the city.

"There is a saying around the BCMA that the President-of-the-day is always the President that was needed. This is most certainly true for Dr. Heidi Oetter. She did her job with grace and courage and distinguished herself as a great advocate for B.C. doctors. My working relationship with her remains one of the best I have enjoyed with any leader."

Dr. Oetter continued to be active in the BCMA and was invited to join the Editorial Board, eventually becoming editor of the *B.C. Medical Journal*. She later became a Deputy Registrar for the College of Physicians and Surgeons of British Columbia.

1987

DR. CHRISTINE LOOCK

Dr. Christine Loock was born and raised in Texas, and was beckoned to come north of the border to reclaim her birthright through her strong family connections to Canada. Her mother, a second generation Canadian, completed nurses' training at St. Boniface, Manitoba. After receiving a *summa cum laude* BA (Chemistry) from Southern Methodist University (SMU), Dallas, Christine attended Harvard Medical School, graduating in 1981. She responded first to the call of the west and was chosen for a prestigious residency spot in Pediatrics at the University of Washington. Then a call from the north brought her to Canada, where she married, began a family, and subsequently completed her Pediatric Fellowship at UBC, receiving her FRCPC in 1985. She was a Fellow in Genetics at UBC from 1985–86 and a Fellow in Medical Education at the Harvard Macy Institute, Harvard Medical School, in 1996.

Dr. Loock is an Associate Professor in the Department of Pediatrics at UBC, and is a Developmental Pediatrician at B.C. Children's Hospital and Sunny Hill Health Centre for Children. Her clinical work and research focus on children with neurodevelopmental disorders and birth defects, including Fetal Alcohol Syndrome (FAS) and craniofacial conditions. She is recognized as an expert in the field of FAS in Canada. She is also a medical consultant for the Vancouver Coastal Health Authority, where from 1991–1993 she helped conceptualize, design, and implement Sheway, a child health program for pregnant substance-using women and their children in the Downtown Eastside. She continues to provide pediatric outreach consultation there through a partnership with the YWCA Crabtree Corner and the inner city schools.

In 1999, Dr. Loock was appointed by the Federal Minister of Health to the Board of the Canadian Centre on Substance Abuse (CSA). In 2000 she was invited to sit on Health Canada's National FAS Advisory Committee, and was subsequently appointed to its sub-committee on Diagnosis and

Screening in October 2001. She is the co-author of the Canadian Medical Association's 2005 publication "Fetal Alcohol Spectrum Disorder: Canadian Guidelines for Diagnosis."

As well as clinical and research work, Chris is very involved with teaching both students and residents, and with undergraduate curriculum design and development. She organized, developed, and for five years directed the "Doctor and Patient in Society" (DPAS) course, has authored/co-authored four problem-based learning (PBL) cases, and designed and implemented the Phase VI theme based on the Medical Council of Canada objectives on "Considerations for Ethics, Law and the Organization of Health Care" (CLEO). All four graduating classes that have participated in CLEO have ranked this the top theme.

Dr. Loock serves on numerous committees within the Faculty of Medicine and other medical organizations, including the BCMA, Health Canada, and pediatrics associations. Her publications are many, including journal articles, book chapters, and videos. She has been a visiting lecturer in the United States and United Kingdom, and many times an invited presenter provincially, nationally, and internationally.

Chris has received many awards for her teaching, academic, and athletic achievements. One of the first awards she received in high school was the "Betty Crocker Future Homemaker Award" (in addition to being the graduating Valedictorian)! She was the first woman to earn a varsity letter from SMU (on the men's team). In 1996, she earned the Southern Methodist University's Distinguished Alumni Award. The most recent award is the SMU Lettermen's Association 2004 Silver Anniversary Mustang (SAM) Award for her twenty-five-year distinguished service after graduation, presented on February 12, 2005. She is the first woman to receive the award which is presented to a former student-athlete who lettered at least twenty-five years ago and who has made significant contributions to his or her community after graduation. Another significant award was that of Outstanding Canadian Immigrant of the Year Award from the Canadian Bar Association, Immigration Lawyers Section, in April 2002. She is also an Honorary Alumna of the UBC Medical Alumni Association.

Chris has also had an outstanding athletic career in springboard and platform diving. She was a five-time U.S. National Diving Champion, and won a bronze medal at the World Championships in 1975. At age twenty-one she was ranked the top female diver by the international aquatics federation (FINA), and competed in the 1971 Pan Am Games. In 1979–80 she took a year off from her medical studies to train for the Olympics (combining this with research), but a number of countries including the United States boycotted the 1980 Olympic Games in Moscow. She was the first woman in the U.S. to receive a National Collegiate Athletic Association post-graduate scholarship to study medicine.

At the Pan Am Games in South America Chris met a Canadian Olympic diver, and a decade later, while she was doing her Pediatric residency at the University of Washington, this young man was studying law at the University of Victoria. He fortunately persuaded Chris to join him in Canada. She works collaboratively and consults with her husband, Ronald G. Friesen, who is Director of Education of the Continuing Legal Education Society of B.C. They are the proud parents of three children, two girls who are competitive national age group divers, and a son who is now an undergraduate at UBC.

DR. TRINE LARSEN SOLES

I was born in Vancouver in 1957, but did not live in B.C. for any length of time until I returned in 1979 to attend graduate school. My childhood was spent in Quebec City, followed by a move to California in 1962. My family returned to B.C. every summer like homing pigeons. I remember the small towns where my various cousins and grandparents lived, and how I enjoyed the times I spent there. Perhaps that was why I ended up practising in rural B.C. I always thought it was the most beautiful place in the world.

I graduated from Menlo Atherton High School in 1974, Menlo Park, California. I went on to UC Berkeley and majored in Zoology, with an interest in Genetics. I graduated with a BA in 1978 and worked for a year for International Health Services in East Palo Alto. This organization was the brainchild of Dr. Charles Beale, an American physician who had a long history of humanitarian work. His career included serving as a medical missionary on the Ivory Coast. He started IHS to develop medical devices and programs that would improve delivery of health care in the third world, and in poor areas of the U.S. Projects during my time there included development of a rapid home test for Group A strep and an educational nutritional program for pregnant teens to be used in the local school system. He was an inspiring man to work for, and helped further my medical aspirations.

Following that year, I returned to Vancouver to pursue a MSc in Genetics. I worked for Dr. Robert Miller in the Department of Microbiology, but divided my research between Microbiology, Biology, and Biochemistry. At that time Genetics was an interdisciplinary degree. I finished my Masters in 1982, and entered the UBC Faculty of Medicine that fall.

I enjoyed my time in medical school. After my first year I returned to the Microbiology Department for a summer research project. It involved making monoclonal antibodies, and my major memory is of trying to cannulate the tail veins of mice as part of the process! Eventually, the mice were sacrificed, and their spleens dissected out. I consoled myself with the thought that the experience would probably enhance my procedural skills for the following years. Second year saw the introduction of clinical sessions. A strict dress code for the times was enforced; men were required to wear a tie and women skirts or dress pants. One of my classmates obeyed the letter of the law with a leather string tie, black jeans, etc. In retrospect, I wonder at our compliance.

That summer, we were given the option of participating in the Summer Rural Placement Program. This was (and still is) a popular elective, and students participated in a lottery to pick a spot. I drew number 112 out of a possible 120, and thus wound up arranging my own elective. I went to Osoyoos, where I had relatives who were happy to give me free room and board for the summer. This community of 2,700 provided an excellent exposure to small town medicine. I gave my first injections, sutured wounds, put on casts, assisted in the OR, and helped with deliveries; in short, a medical student's dream. However, Osoyoos is a retirement community, and social opportunities were limited. By the end of the summer, I decided that rural medicine was great, but would be very difficult as a single person.

UBC had the typical curriculum which concentrated clinical exposure in third and fourth year. I enjoyed this portion much more than the first two years, and flirted with the idea of specializing in pediatrics. However, in fourth year I made some personal choices which returned my focus to rural medicine. Actually at that time it was not nearly as well-publicized or as trendy as it is becoming. All I told people was that I intended to practise in a small town. Most of them thought I was crazy. My husband-to-be and I became engaged in February of the fourth year. He was working as a forest technician in Golden, B.C., so that was where I hoped to practise. I had applied to a variety of internship programs selected due to their proximity to Golden, and was matched to the Family Medicine Residency at the Royal Alexandra Hospital in Edmonton.

At that time the Alex did not have a reputation for treating interns well. However, I found it to be a tremendous place to train, with a heavy emphasis on procedural skills. Because I intended to pursue small town practice, my preceptors made sure I had lots of hands-on experience, especially in the ER, OR, and obstetrical suite. The high patient volume provided a good opportunity to see a lot of pathology and the associated diagnosis and treatment.

I served as the Professional Association of Residents & Interns (PARI) rep for my year in Edmonton. These associations were still sort of a novel idea, as was the idea that interns should be well paid and the frequency of on call limited. One in two was still pretty common, and one in one not unheard of. Certain Plastics residents had been known to spend six weeks straight in the hospital. Our contract read one in three, and most of the rotations did go along with that.

I had intended to complete the second year of the Family Program, but Golden was advertising for a locum and I was not looking forward to a commuter marriage. Dan and I got married in November of my internship year and he spent the winter in Edmonton with me. He returned to Golden in May. The second year of Family Medicine consisted of taking turns filling in deficiencies in the call rota, and the thought of eight weeks covering call for the detox ward in Internal Medicine just did not seem like it would further my medical education. I was worried that someone else would snap up the job in Golden (I was rather naïve about rural physician supply in those days). I did not need the second year to get a B.C. licence, so in June of 1987 I finished my internship and moved back to B.C. One week later I was working at the Golden Medical Clinic. I was initially hired for three months to replace a partner doing a locum overseas. My billing number was a "locum number" and I could only work to replace someone else. At the end of the three months I had to apply for a permanent number to work in Golden. I did get one, but it was geographically restricted. Eventually, the legislation restricting billing numbers was turned down in the courts, and I became the proud possessor of an unrestricted B.C. billing number!

During my first year in Golden I lived in terror of the major trauma off the highway. Holiday weekends were particularly stressful. Many Calgarians head for the Okanagan Valley every long weekend, and this was before the mandatory seatbelt legislation in Alberta. The treacherous curves of the Kicking Horse Canyon generated a fair amount of business for us. One such Friday I was assisting a colleague with two patients who had a head-on collision in the Canyon. After appropriate stabilization it was decided that I should accompany the patients to Calgary via the local air service. We loaded both patients—an ambulance attendant and myself—into the plane and took off. It was the first time I had ever been in a small plane, and I was surprised how bumpy it was. Then the patient on the spine board began vomiting. I had to flip the board sideward and suction her while the plane bounced around. The ambulance attendant retired to the rear of the plane with a bag about this time, and the pilot was quite amused. Finally, we landed—to find out we had been flying on the edge of a tornado. The airport was closed; hence, I spent the night at the home of a friend of the pilot. I shared a sofa with the ambulance attendant, and the friend bought us pizza (I had taken off without any money). The next morning we finally got back to Golden and the return flight was much less traumatic.

During my first year in Golden I lived in terror of the major trauma off the highway. Holiday weekends were particularly stressful.

I was the third woman doctor to come to Golden. The first one predated me by four years, and stayed for two. She left to be married. The second one came as a summer locum and stayed part of that year. When I arrived, there had been a ten-month gap, and I spent the first few weeks in the office catching up on everyone's Pap smears. Eventually, the group decided that since I married a local boy the odds were better on my staying around. I became an associate in the clinic in 1988, and have practised in Golden ever since. One important factor in my decision to stay was the support of the other physicians in town. From the moment I arrived I knew I could call on them for back-up at any time. The learning curve of all the things you do not really know until you have been in practice for a few years was made much easier because of their help. Services in town include an acute care hospital, intermediate care facility, and extended care beds. Our OR services include Caesarean section, appendectomy, D&C, hernia repairs, etc., which have already been provided by GPs with extra training. Finding people with skills to continue the service has proved more challenging as the years go by. Our last two recruits have come from South Africa, as did the physician just before me.

In the summer of 1988, I became pregnant with my first child. As the only female physician in the group I was determined not to slack off just because of my condition. I worked full-time until December when I developed a nagging cough. I felt miserable, actually, but did not get anyone to examine me until I developed a persistent fever. Unfortunately, I had developed pneumonia, and was admitted to hospital on Christmas Eve for IV antibiotics and ventolin. I felt horribly guilty because I was supposed to be on call on Boxing Day and several of my partners wound up covering for me. On the 28th I developed these peculiar cramps and then went into pre-term labour at thirty-one weeks. I had a series of tocolytics, but laboured most of that night. There were no neonatal beds in Calgary, so initially they would not accept me. Plans were made to transfer me to Vancouver or Edmonton—but first there was a blizzard and then it got dark (you can only get a plane in here during daylight hours). My labour did stop overnight and in the morning I went by ground to Calgary. Travelling in the ambulance as a patient was an experience I could have done without. I spent three weeks in Foothills Hospital, the first on complete bedrest. Interestingly, despite the fact I was on IV antibiotics for pneumonia, only one physician listened to my chest during my entire stay. That was the admitting resident, on the day I was admitted. On an Obstetrics floor, they seemed only to worry about the obstetric problems.

At thirty-four weeks, I was permitted to go home, and went on to deliver at term in Golden. I took two months off after Hester was born. When I returned to work I began an ongoing struggle to find adequate child care. The first babysitter had no understanding of the demands of my job, and would cancel at a moment's notice. One call day my sitter cancelled and I had my baby at three different places over ten hours. Add in trying to breastfeed, and it is perhaps no surprise that I developed more medical problems five months postpartum. I eventually had surgery to drain a persistent sinus infection and after that cut back my practice to three office days per week (my partners all work four). I have continued that schedule to the present, although there have been a number of periods when I worked more, due to staffing shortages at the clinic. Over the next three years I had two more children. With my second pregnancy I stopped doing call at thirty-two weeks and worked until two days before my son was born without any difficulties. With the third I went into labour at thirty-six weeks, winding up with inpatients and a fully-booked office. I did rounds after I delivered, but cancelled the office!

The day after Paige was born I was in my hospital room early in the morning. My roommate was a nurse at our hospital. She came down the hall, running back to tell me that a lady had just walked in at term and was crowning. So I got out of bed, put on my bathrobe, and went down to the labour room. Sure enough, the baby's head was visible. I turned to the nurse, asked for a pair of gloves, and delivered the baby. The baby required resuscitation, and I was waiting for the placenta when my colleague showed up. Afterwards, the new father wanted to know why some woman in a bathrobe had delivered his baby! The mother had recognized me so was not at all perturbed. She was so amused by the story that she approached the newspaper, and now my daughter has a nice little article in her baby book. Unfortunately, Paige had group strep infection and had to stay in hospital for nine days and have antibiotics and phototherapy. We were unable to find a locum for my maternity leave or for the summer. I went back to work at the clinic two weeks after we were finally out of the hospital. I just did occasional half days, but even that helped.

Paige was an easygoing baby except for one thing. She absolutely refused to take a bottle. This resulted in me taking her along on call, for deliveries, and even on a transfer to Calgary. I had to accompany a girl who had her head stepped on by a horse, a depressed skull fracture with persistent vomiting. I could not leave the baby for the required eight hours for a round trip, so she came along. I left her asleep in the ambulance when we took the patient to the ICU. When I got back to Emergency I found her sitting on the counter, with a row of accusing faces. "Someone left this baby in the ambulance!" "Oh, she's mine," I replied. They looked at me in confusion. "Well, I'm breastfeeding," I explained. They all shrugged, thinking I was just another peculiar rural doctor.

That summer was one of my most difficult times. My husband's work required him to be out of town from Monday to Friday. The three kids were forty months, twenty-two months, and four months. They were in an excellent family daycare, but I was alone at night and we lived nine miles out of town. I had a busy maternity practice, and either scrambled for overnight babysitters or took all three in with me. My son had a difficult summer, with a bout of viral meningitis followed by a broken collarbone and sprained neck. Eventually, my daycare provider started spending nights at my house, which she did off and on for two years. She literally saved my sanity during that period of my life. Later my husband started his own business with an office in our basement. It gave him somewhat more flexibility and then we broke down and hired a live-in nanny for a few years. Somehow we got through all that. Now my children are old enough to be left alone for brief periods and my husband works out of home. Life is suddenly so much more flexible.

I somehow was elected Chief of Staff during one of my brief maternity leaves. My tenure coincided with the implantation of "Regionalization" in B.C. I think it was a big part of the eventual deterioration of Medicare as we

When I got back to Emergency I found her sitting on the counter, with a row of accusing faces. "Someone left this baby in the ambulance!" "Oh, she's mine," I replied. They looked at me in confusion. "Well, I'm breastfeeding," I explained.

know it, and it was my first exposure to political manoeuvring and cost-cutting strategies disguised as improved access to care for rural patients. My cynicism about the motives of politicians and the Ministry of Health started developing then. I was involved in numerous meetings in my area to develop a regional plan for the East Kootenays. The eventual outcome was that no consensus was reached, and we lost the previously approved funding for an ER renovation in Golden. Seven years later our hospital has fewer beds, fewer nurses, and the same inadequate ER we had when I started in Golden.

I stumbled across the Society of Rural Physicians (SRP-B.C.) in 1997 by virtue of attending an educational meeting in Banff. I did not realize until later that the organization was only four years old. I ran into a few old friends and was amazed to find I had more in common professionally with doctors from rural Quebec and Newfoundland than with most of the doctors in B.C. The Society was born out of a group of rebels in Mount Forrest, Ontario, who were the first to publicize the issues of rural working conditions and remuneration for on-call services. The first meeting involved forty people in the basement of some hotel in Montreal in 1994. From there it grew. In 1997, political action came to B.C. when a group of doctors in the north decided to pursue the issue of on-call remuneration for after-hours work. Their approaches to government met with little response, so in January of 1998, they began a job action which dragged on until June and eventually involved eighty physicians in twenty-two communities. My community was the most involved in southern B.C., which sort of took me by surprise since we were well-staffed at the time. One of my partners suggested we needed to support our colleagues, and we wound up participating because we really thought they had a point. During the eleven years I had been in Golden we had repeatedly struggled to replace doctors who left and were having increasing difficulty finding locums. We knew it was only a matter of time until we were in that position again, and incentives would certainly help us recruit.

It was a long and stressful confrontation, made more difficult by our political naïveté. We were lucky to have a united group of local physicians and a very supportive community. We met with Lucy Dobbin, the Ministry consultant who was hired to find a solution. Her report was accepted in June, and it took another three months of fighting with the Ministry to get the contracts implemented. During all this, I became more involved with the SRP-B.C. We felt it was necessary to have a separate rural group from the BCMA to ensure that our special problems had a voice. I organized a drive that resulted in a significant increase in our B.C. membership. From there, the B.C. group went on to have a provincial rural e-mail discussion group, an annual educational conference, and annual meetings of the SRP-B.C. We have a separate executive, and I have acted as treasurer in the past two years. On a national level we are part of the Northwestern Committee of the SRP-B.C., and I am currently the Chair of that committee. In conjunction with the BCMA we have been involved in establishing the Rural Issues Committee, which approached the Ministry of Health with a view to negotiating a formal agreement based on the Dobbin deal. We had actual negotiations from March of 1999 through March of 2000. I was also on the negotiating committee, and we did reach an agreement with government on March 28, 2000. That deal is in the process of being implemented now, and another set of negotiations are scheduled to begin in October.

I never had any particular interest in politics. My goal in going into medicine was to make a difference in people's lives in a positive way. As a physician I think I have accomplished that, and I have felt privileged to share in momentous events with my patients. However, there comes a time when the day-to-day achievements are not enough. We are living in a time when our system is in trouble. There are not enough of us to do the job required in rural medicine. And so I have added another aspect to my job description. Perhaps healing on a broader level is required for our medical system to survive. Whether we can fix things remains to be seen. Right now I am not sure I would encourage my children to pursue a medical career. I hope things will evolve so that I could do so with a clear conscience!

DR. LORI VOGT

I graduated as a specialist in child psychiatry from the University of Manitoba in 1986, and as part of a resident payment contract, I was placed fresh out of residency into the Chief of Psychiatry for a 1,200 bed mental hospital 200 kilometres from my hometown of Winnipeg. The Brandon Mental Health Centre had been the pride of its day when it opened . . . but its day had been more than half a century earlier. Now it was a chronic backwoods hospital complete with full cage beds, antique insulin therapy, and hydrotherapy rooms still fully equipped but cobwebbed in the attics. The facility and patients were all in various states of decline. Some had been condemned for years and were said to be haunted. That was true of both buildings and people.

Despite having spent the extra time to do a fellowship in Child Psychiatry, the Province of Manitoba saw fit to completely overwhelm me by placing me as the only certified psychiatrist in this old-style madhouse where ninety-nine percent of my patients were adults, the majority over fifty. Some had been there since lobotomies were popular in the 1950s and wandered, vacant-eyed, about the grounds accompanied by staff. Some were murderous lunatics who were kept "at the Lieutenant-Governor's pleasure" after having shot up their families or their schools in some long-ago drama. It was quite the challenge for a greenhorn doc fresh out of university. I was fortunate to have a competent team of psychiatric nurses, social workers, and psychologists, with a handful of generally competent family physicians visiting the place on a daily basis. They were all so happy to have a real psychiatrist about the place and I was treated with respect and made to feel welcome.

There were some who balked at the idea of a lady psychiatrist leading the place, but the Chief Nurse ruled with an iron hand, and he liked me. We worked very hard there. It was the time of the great "de-institutionalization" movement, so I headed a team of professionals whose job it was to review every patient in the place and arrange for community placement. For most, this meant specially created geriatric wards in existing government-run care homes, but our team tried in every case to discharge to family or group home type resources who could help these deeply institutionalized patients have a new life after decades in "The Hill." By the time I left there, we had managed to place nearly 800 patients in the community in less than eighteen months. Each one of these patients was personally examined by me and had their medications adjusted as necessary. Some had not seen a psychiatrist in five years. As well we had about sixty acute, emergent, and short-stay beds which I consulted to. I lived on the grounds in a splendid old house with wonderful views of the Assiniboine River Valley. A consequence of this perk was that I was often called to certify a death in the geriatric ward in the middle of the night, or to see acute psychiatric emergencies sent from "down the hill" at the general hos-

pital. By the time eighteen months of my twenty-four month contract had passed I was very near stir crazy with stress from constant unofficial on call and the myriad other duties that came with the job of Chief.

I sought the advice of my accountant, my lawyer, and my colleagues. The political scene in Manitoba was very unfavourable to doctors at the time—the NDP were waxing in power and we remained among the lowest paid psychiatrists in the country, with no end in site. Manitoba charged the highest marginal tax rate in the country in the NDP years. I had had about twenty-five too many of the harsh prairie winters. I began to set my sights west, to the beautiful city of Victoria, where I had vacationed since I was a child. The tax rate in B.C. was favourable: if I moved, I would save more than $5,000 that year in income taxes alone. My lawyer had advised me that the Province of Manitoba would not be happy about my leaving with six months left on my contract, but we thought we could cover the costs of successfully fighting that off for less than my tax refund for the year. Little did I know just how unhappy the province would be.

My (then) husband and I began to scheme as to how to leave with the least disruption. We found an old school bus at a rural municipality auction. It had been in service until that year, and was perfectly roadworthy. At $1,000, it was a bargain and would move us, our pets, and our belongings easily. I painted the windows with scenes of the West Coast—whales, big trees, flowers, and rainbows—in the style of the hippies of a decade earlier. No one could look in. By night we gradually packed all our belongings in it. We told everyone we were converting it to a camper and planned to travel the following summer. By the time it was fully packed and ready to go in late September, it bore a distinct resemblance to a Mexican tour bus, with motorcycles hanging off the front and back, loaded to the rafters and beyond. A couple of pet cats who got loose inside completed our little version of travelling mayhem. The plan was that my husband would drive the bus to Victoria with a friend for company and locate a rental house. I would follow a month later, as soon as I could give notice, and drive my little black TR8 convertible alone through the mountains to join him. It was dicey planning to leave in late October as there could easily be a blizzard, and I wanted to leave Manitoba before the snow came and my tiny two-seater car turned into a frisbee on skis.

Just before I was to announce my departure to my boss in Winnipeg, a final insult was dealt to me. It was bad enough that they had never employed me as they had agreed to, as a child psychiatrist. Suddenly, despite my competence in their assigned role as head of a chronic mental hospital, they decided that a classmate who had not even passed his specialty exams should be named as my "supervisor" and travel out twice a week from Winnipeg at nearly double my rate of pay! I could only think it was because he was an older male, and I a fresh-faced twenty-eight-year-old woman. My husband had already left for the coast with the bus. Feeling rather miffed and angry about this latest turn of affairs, I wrote a terse letter of resignation, which I kept in my pocket awaiting the right moment. The day I planned to give it to my new "supervisor," he called me into his office and began berating me for various aspects of work that certainly could have had better psychiatric coverage—if I had chosen to abandon sleep entirely. After he finished his rather long list of my supposed deficiencies, I stood silent for a moment.

He asked if I had anything to say. I smiled and handed him my resignation letter. "Just this," I told him. "I had thought to give you a month's notice, but I'm leaving tomorrow. I quit."

He asked if I had anything to say. I smiled and handed him my resignation letter. "Just this," I told him. "I had thought to give you a month's notice, but I'm leaving tomorrow. I quit." I turned on my highheels and with a flourish of my skirt, walked out the door. My "supervisor" had done me the supreme favour of erasing any left over pangs of guilt I felt leaving the many fine people I had worked with at "the Mental." As I cleared the elaborate wooden carved doorway, I heard him ask behind me, "Was it something I said?"

There were only a few things left to pack, and I worked through the evening. I could leave at sunrise. Everything went smoothly and with the weather forecast that Halloween calling for a large snowfall, I felt it was now or never. It dawned a brilliantly sunny day, and although it was crisp, I put the top down, put on my sunglasses, and fired up the powerful V-8 motor. I rumbled slowly down the hospital's long winding driveway and watched in my mirror as the grand old ruin faded from my view. Then I headed west onto the TransCanada Highway and opened the throttle. Not a moment too soon. I could see to the east in my rearview mirror huge storm clouds which were already dumping feet of snow over Portage la Prairie. A few flakes flew across my windshield, but within an hour I had crossed the border into Saskatchewan, and from there on the sun shone clear and brightly all the way to Vancouver. I felt free and empowered and with no stress for the first time since I had entered medical school.

Years later, a colleague who had been my dear friend and helped me through the experience in Brandon, told me that day I handed in my resignation, my bosses in Winnipeg had gone to a judge and got an injunction to physically hold me in the province should I attempt to leave. A Sheriff had been dispatched before the sun rose that morning, trying to catch me before I left Brandon, but he had been turned back at Portage la Prairie because the RCMP closed the highway due to snow. He arrived later that day, but I was two provinces away by then. Like I said, I had no idea how steamed the province would be when I left. They attempted to sue me for all by wages for the previous four years that I had been in their employ. I had to fly back once to attend a hearing for discovery, after which they made a hasty settlement. A good lawyer is a wonderful asset for any doctor, and mine was true to his word. In the end, the lawsuit cost me less than my tax refund that year.

My troubles were not completely over. It was good I had budgeted to take a month off to get settled in my new hometown of Victoria. Although I had a guaranteed job in the Queen Alexandra Centre and my arrival coincided with the opening of the new Jack Ledger Psychiatric Hospital for Children and even though there was a shortage of child psychiatrists to staff the place, and when I arrived I was the only female child psychiatrist in Victoria, the government in its wisdom would not grant me a billing number. British Columbia felt it had too many doctors in general and had declared a moratorium on all billing numbers, even for specialties that were in a shortage like mine. Without a billing number, I was free to work but I could not be paid. I spoke with the Professional Association of Residents and Interns in B.C. and joined their legal challenge to the legislation, and settled in for a wait. Being a practical person, and having recently been on salary, I applied for Unemployment Insurance benefits, which I had paid for in all my occupations for over fourteen years and never needed before. The lady at the office couldn't believe a doctor was applying. She suggested I obtain employment in a related field, like child minding! I had another suggestion for her which should probably not be printed. Basically I made the point that I had no other job training except my twelve years learning to become a doctor, and running a mental hospital. I had paid the insurance according to the rules and was eligible for over six months in support benefits. That would buy me some time. The PARI-B.C. suit was settled less than a year later and billing numbers were once again granted more freely, but I did not have to wait that long.

Victorians made me feel very welcome despite my unemployed status and kindly invited me to all sorts of gatherings so I could meet people. I had lunches and dinners with the who's who of Victorian society. Many were interested in my situation and did their best to influence the powers that were to grant me a billing number as a special exception to the rules. After six weeks collecting unemployment, making contacts, writing letters, and speaking to PARI-B.C., I was getting nowhere fast, and even at the highest rate UIC still meant living like a student again. I was truly tired of Kraft dinner, however much I still like it as a treat now. It was time for desperate measures.

The Ministry of Health seemed like a good place to start. I thought of camping out at the legislature, but it was November, with cold, dreary weather, and the office on Blanshard was in a 1960s style building with wide corridors and open foyers. And dry heat. One could sit comfortably a long time, watch everything, and see the world of Health go by. I took to sitting there for an afternoon, or a whole day, on several occasions. I recognized people from their news shots and gradually got up the nerve to confront the deputy minister as he stepped onto an elevator. I told my story—a doctor unable to work when their new health showplace had agreed to hire me. The elevator didn't go all the way to the top floor before the DM got out. I'm not sure he cared. I had been civil and hoped to have been heard. A few days later I was able to do something similar to the actual Minister in the foyer, but he pushed past me without acknowledging me. I felt discouraged.

I had heard that the Province of British Columbia was hiring salaried foreign graduates on temporary restricted billing numbers to work in the B.C. counterpart of Brandon Mental Health, Riverview. I phoned the Chief Psychiatrist one day to see if I could at least stay afloat working there. We chatted pleasantly while I explained my plight, and afterword, he said, "You don't want to work here, believe me. Don't come here." I was somewhat shocked, but did not call back. I heard many stories about Riverview in later years that made me glad I had heeded him.

Next I called the College of Physicians and Surgeons of British Columbia in Vancouver, thinking they might be of assistance. Their attitude was one of why had I bothered to move to B.C. at such an awful time, how could I be so stupid? It was not the welcome I expected from the registrar and supposed defender of the right of the medical profession. All of these events conspired with the increasing length of time without work to make me quite depressed. After the social buzz of Christmas and New Year wore off, and the rainy dull winter caused mildew to grow in every corner of the house we were renting, I kept house, went to medical meetings and education events, but basically just moped around. Maybe moving to B.C. hadn't been such the great idea I thought it was on that day when I flourished my resignation. In January, I had to fly back to Manitoba briefly to answer the lawsuit the Province of Manitoba had launched against me. I dressed nicely, ready for court—I was, after all, a young blonde back then. Behind me at the departure gate, was the Premier of B.C. He was talking and laughing and I turned around to see who it was. Congenially, he said hello, introduced himself as the Premier, and asked how I was. Life presented me with another satisfying opportunity. All the frustration of the previous two months leaked into a broad sarcastic smile. I shook his hand warmly and introduced myself as "one of those doctors you won't let work even though your hospitals need us." I'm sure that didn't help my cause, but it certainly made me feel better. The Premier was speechless and much subdued as we cleared security and boarded the plane.

It seems people who work in high places in government often have children. And sometimes those children are in dire need of a psychiatrist. One such person phoned all of my psychiatry colleagues and got the same

When I applied for Unemployment Insurance benefits, the lady at the office couldn't believe a doctor was applying. She suggested I obtain employment in a related field, like child minding!

answer—long waiting lists due to the general shortage of child psychiatrists, and oh, did they know Dr. Vogt was available and just needed a billing number? One of my colleagues, Ric Arnot, took the time to phone me at home and let me know that there was an acute situation and how quickly could I be in business?

Lo and behold the next week I was opening my new office in a space below Phil Ney, next to the Eric Martin Institute, complete with unrestricted billing number. Patients were booked for a month solid as I helped clean up the long waiting lists held by other doctors. Sometimes it is a good thing that there can be a personal touch in politics. In my case it was a win-win situation for everyone concerned, and all caused by a little child's distress. The child recovered and I was launched into my new career in my new home. There was the input of literally dozens of concerned people in Victoria who helped me in so many different ways in that first year. I was so fortunate to have landed here when I did, despite the initial struggle. When I was finishing my residency, my supervisor told me that if I planned to make a move, I had to do it early in my career or it would not happen until my retirement. I have seen that play out with so many of my classmates. At the time of my move west, I felt like I was completing a migration begun a century ago by my ancestors. They had come to Canada from Russia in 1875, just in time to build sod houses on the prairie, and never made it further for four generations. In this generation, many of my prairie family have moved to the west coast.

Life has changed much since that time, but I never regretted making the bold move, a move which outlasted the marriage that brought me to B.C. Every time I drive over the Royal Oak Overpass and catch the view of the mountains, every sunny trip on the Swartz Bay Ferry, every winter when I don't have to shovel anything but cherry petals, I am thankful for living here.

DR. MARJORIE DOCHERTY

I was born in Bannockburn in Scotland of Braveheart fame on the 28th of February, 1958. Byburn is a small mining village which was the site of the famous battle of 1314 when the Scots finally managed to pull off a victory against the English. It was quite an important battle because it meant that Scotland then remained independent for the next 300 or more years and allowed us to maintain our identity as a country. So I grew up in the background of that fearsome and proud history. I think every child in Bannochburn can probably recount the battle details to you before they even get to school.

I spent some of my pre-school time in the Shetland Islands to the northeast of Scotland and continued to spend my summer holidays and most of my Easter holidays there until I went to high school. My mother was born and raised in the Shetland Islands and all of her family were there, so my background is a mixture of Lowland and Highland Scotland. My mother was a nurse and later on became a dressmaking teacher; my father was a Headmaster with a mixed background as a mathematician and a physical education instructor as well as being a physical education Sergeant during the War.

I think I always, always wanted to be a physician except for one brief year when I considered being a vet or a nun, and my father curtly informed me that I could never be a nun because I could not keep the vow of silence. He thought obedience might be a problem, too. So probably from the age of eight onwards I wanted to be a doctor.

I realized that the competition for going to Med school was very stiff. I probably did quite well in school without much effort until I hit my higher examinations, pre-entrance exams which we had in Scotland at that time. In that year the teachers had a strike and I ended up being on a two-day school week for most of the year, which was really quite a catastrophe when you were about to sit for your final exams, so I did not get into medicine that year.

I went for career counselling, and when I went to the Career Fair and spoke to a young male physician who was there to advise about medicine, he said, "Oh, women don't do medicine apart from obstetrics, that's about babies, and old women do that stuff." So it was not very encouraging, but I refused to give up.

I had to do most of my hunting down and investigating the qualifications required to get into medical school on my own. I went as far as to phone Dublin Medical School in Ireland and tried to find out if I could get in there, much to my parents' horror because the "troubles," as they call them, of the Protestant-Catholic conflict were very high at that time.

I finally secured a conditional acceptance from Aberdeen University in the northeast of Scotland, and I was incredibly delighted. Scottish parents are very good at bringing you down to earth. When I was jumping up and down in ecstasy that I had this conditional acceptance, my dad looked me in the eye and said, "I'll congratulate you when you qualify." I was certainly brought down to earth at that point.

I spent five years in Aberdeen University and graduated in 1981. I thoroughly enjoyed Aberdeen. I found the first eighteen months of the pre-clinical science quite tough, especially medical physics. When I got into the clinical portion of the training, I just revelled in it and thoroughly enjoyed every part of it.

Probably some of my early experiences in medicine started to form who I was as a physician. I realized that in clinical hospital medicine people did not pay much attention to what people were feeling, and if in presenting your case history you brought in emotional elements of the patient's anxiety or sexual difficulty or relationship difficulty, you got a kind of a raised eyebrow from the consultant in internal medicine who might consider this entirely irrelevant to the condition of Lupus or whatever you happened to be dealing with at that point in time.

I worked very hard in Med School and because I had struggled to get in, I think I always felt that at any point in time I might fail, so I probably over-compensated and over-worked, ending up graduating in 1981 with a Commendation Degree in Medicine in the top ten in the class and also the top woman. Our class was about fifty percent women and fifty percent men, about 135 of us. As the top woman, I got the Louise Tomory prize, and I also got the Matthews Duncan Medal in Obstetrics and a couple of Distinctions, so as I said I guess I overdid it somewhat in my anxiety about passing.

As a young, impressionable, and newly-graduated physician, I thought that medicine had all the answers. I certainly thought senior physicians were somewhere near to approaching God.

I graduated as Dr. Marjorie A. Hooks, which was my maiden name, and got married a week later to Dr. Henry Docherty who came from Bishop Briggs in Glasgow. Aberdeen University had a long history of graduating more physicians than it could accommodate in its own hospitals and so routinely supplied physicians to Inverness in the North of Scotland, the Shetland and Orkney Islands, and to the borders of Scotland, Dumfries. Although I could find a job in Aberdeen, unfortunately my new husband could not, so I moved down to Glasgow to work with him. Because I thought I might go on to a career in internal medicine, I had chosen two rather tough internships, with six months in Professor A.C. Kennedy's Department of Medicine and Endocrinology, and six months in Professor Carter's Department of Surgery. Both these rotations were rather grueling, involving mainly one and two on call and on one occasion a two and three on call.

As a young, impressionable, and newly-graduated physician, I thought that medicine had all the answers. I certainly thought senior physicians were somewhere near to approaching God.

As I rotated through the different aspects of medicine and surgery, it was a truly exhausting year. I have to admit the amount of pathology I saw and the amount of experience I got probably could not be rivalled in ten years of a forty-hour week. It was not hard, however, to see what sort of stress it put on your relationship and marriage, and this was compounded when one day one of my husband's co-workers came up to me and asked if I knew my husband was ill with the flu; I did not, and asked him to send my husband my best wishes. I realized at that point that I had not really seen him for about two weeks, even though we tried to communicate on the phone most days. The hospital switchboards were very much against personal phone calls. If they realized you were on a personal call they would cut you off, or worse, listen in. So we had to devise all sorts of reasons that he would want to talk to me about patients and have these metaphors or coded conversations about who was going to bring home milk for supper.

At the end of that year I wondered what a qualification in internal medicine would do to my thoughts about marriage and family, and realized that Britain at that point was only interested in dedicated career women. Therefore I applied to quite a few rotations in family medicine, which in Britain was a three-year rotation, and found great difficulty in finding one that I could do. It was not that I was not well-qualified to apply, but in Britain it was quite difficult to find six-month obstetrics that did not involve doing terminations of pregnancy. I was somewhat of a conscientious objector to performing terminations, but was quite happy to counsel them and look after them if there were any complications. Also at that time in Britain you could not be a principal of a practice or sit your MRCGP without having done six months' obstetrics, so I was in somewhat of a bind. I eventually got a job in Falkirk Royal Infirmary, thanks to a lady obstetrician who had known me as a Med student and who kept tactfully steering conversations away from abortions in my interview. They hired me without ever knowing that I would not do that for them, although she certainly did, and she was one of the women in medicine I looked up to because she was such an advocate for patient care and so kind and so well-grounded as a physician. She had never married, had no children, and had virtually no personal life outside her obstetrics. I also noted that her male colleagues sometimes treated her with little smirks or innuendoes and did not seem to give her the esteem that she was probably due.

So I did my year of obstetrics and pediatrics in Falkirk Royal Infirmary, Scotland, and got some tremendous experience there, especially in obstetrics. We were just a general hospital and most of our senior staff were immigrant physicians trying to get their membership in Britain prior to going back home. This gave rise to some difficulties in understanding different cultures and different training backgrounds. But on the whole we all got on quite well.

One experience during that year probably shaped me as a physician. One of the seniors I met in this hospital came from a large obstetrics teaching hospital, and she was receiving further training in obstetrics in order to achieve consultancy. I should pause here to say that the system in Britain is very different. When you get your membership it is really just permission

to carry on to further training, and it is often nine or ten years post-graduate before people achieve consultancy in the National Health System. The lady who worked with me was a Registrar and had probably graduated five or six years earlier and had her membership. She was a great obstetrician and a good teacher, kind and funny. Yet sometimes her behaviour was very erratic. You would call her some nights and she would swear at you and be unpleasant and not come when asked to. So finally one night came when I had to deliver a breech on my own, and as I was inexperienced, I did not feel terribly comfortable doing a C-section on someone who was fully dilated and had lots of other complications. My friend and senior obstetrician passed out during the surgery, leaving me with an abdomen full of blood and other complications. I coped with the situation until my senior colleague got there and talked to the other senior house officers in my training grade, and the next day we all had to come to the sad conclusion that although we really enjoyed this lady and felt very loyal to her, we had all known for quite some time that she had an alcohol and drug problem. I and two of the other female house officers screwed up our courage and met with our senior consultant and talked to her about our concerns for this lady, at the same time urging him to help her because she was so good. We were absolutely devastated to realize that all of the senior staff had known that she had a drug and alcohol problem. It was the reason why she had been sent to a small district general hospital, although she would have in fact had more supervision and help in a teaching hospital.

However, none of them had told us, and nobody had helped her. It was almost like they were farming her out to a smaller hospital where they thought taking on more responsibilities may help to sober her up and take care of her problems. She never came back to work; I do not know what happened to her. She just vanished from the area, and in subsequent years, I tried to find her in the medical directory but could not, so I cannot finish her story for you. But I took her story with me; since then I have made caring for my colleagues' well-being as part of my mantra for the rest of my medical life.

During that year in Falkirk the government made a one and two rotation or on-call rotation illegal, and so one and three or one and four was the maximum you could do. Rather than hiring more staff, the District General

Hospital decided that they could use Senior House Officers, which would have included me working with the interns on a one and three basis. After being on call so much for so long, I just could not philosophically deal with that and felt that it was a very obvious waste of time and training. I decided therefore to try to go back into internal medicine, because I felt somewhat, I guess, under-stimulated in the Family Practice program in an academic sense. Family Practice programs at that time were not quite as streamlined as they are now. Much to everyone's amusement I managed to secure a place in a Glasgow infirmary. I guess it was quite unusual for a married woman coming from community practice to go back into a teaching program. It was interesting that at my interview they asked me all sorts of questions about what my husband thought of me working and studying there and asked very little about what I thought of medicine and what I wanted to be.

I thought of becoming an endocrinologist. A couple of things happened that changed that direction for me. My husband was in a Family Practice program and he thought he might like to spend a year in Canada. I had spent three months in Canada as a fifth-year medical student and had done an elective in Alberta, and had thoroughly enjoyed Canada, the people, and the way of life.

Another thing that happened was that one of the registrars who worked in respiratory medicine in Glasgow Royal appeared to be getting passed over for promotion and had decided to go to Canada and become a GP Internist. He chose to go to Alberta and came to talk to me about life in Canada. To make a long story short, once he became established there, he met a lady from Slave Lake, Alberta, at a rural practice meeting. They talked about their urgent need for physicians. He then called me and asked me if my husband Henry and I would consider coming out to Canada. We had no intentions of doing that, but we did come out on holiday and visited the Rockies. We went up to Slave Lake and visited the practice there. We sensed that there was a dire need for physicians and certainly a dire need for physicians who could do some surgery, obstetrics, and emergency work. I went home to think about it. I could visualize my career in endocrinology, but at the same time I realized that I would need to sacrifice a lot of my relationship time as well as the option of having children, because once you finished climbing up the ladder, you may be too old to have children. So we

finally came to Slave Lake, Alberta, my husband in 1984 and me in January 1985, to see what it was like for a year, and we just never went home.

Northeast of Edmonton, Slave Lake was a small community of about 5,000 people, but serviced a much larger area of about 13,000 by the time you took in all the outlying districts and Native reserves. I think what struck me mainly was how friendly people were and how much they depended on each other's skills. Everyone in the community was treated with equal respect. If you are a physician in a small community, it does not necessarily mean that you are more important.

You are somewhere up there with the guy who keeps the roads clear, the RCMP officer, the teacher, and perhaps the telephone engineer, because all these people are links in the community. Then there are the pharmacist and the people who brave the bad weather to bring in supplies and the pilots who fly out sick patients when the road conditions are too bad or you do not have the time to send them down. All in all the community integrated very well and I really enjoyed my time there.

At my interview they asked me all sorts of questions about what my husband thought of me working and studying there and asked very little about what I thought of medicine and what I wanted to be.

When I was bemoaning the fact to one of my friends who had emigrated to Canada many years before me that Slave Lake did not have a blood gas machine or the ability to do liver function tests, he said to me with a twinkle in his eye, "I don't know if Slave Lake needs you, but you need Slave Lake." What he really meant was that it was time for me to learn how to use my hands and eyes again rather than to depend on investigational techniques, because when you are in a small town, it comes down to a very adequate history, a thorough exam, and then using your head to do what you can in the situation you're in.

When we were expecting our first child I really wanted to have him in Slave Lake so that I could prove to people there that I believed in our medical system and our medical team. However, my colleagues, who were also my close friends, were quick to point out that they did not want to be the ones having to do a C-section on their close friend. Hence I ended up going to Edmonton to deliver and subsequently ended up having a rather complex labour and delivery befitting that of a female physician and the wife of a physician, with almost every complication in the book. Nevertheless, our son was born in 1986, and having given birth to a Canadian I began to realize that there was a likelihood that we may end up staying forever.

Almost all small town practices have inter-dynamic problems and medical politics problems in isolated communities. Our town was one of those that had some difficulties, and after four years we decided that perhaps it would be best if we could find our future in Canada elsewhere. With many mixed feelings and much regret, we left our practices, our patients and friends, and we started to look around western Canada to see where we would like to be. We almost ended up in Lethbridge because I had a good university friend whom I would have loved to be close to. Ultimately, through a series of twists of fate we ended up buying a practice in Kelowna, B.C. We moved there in 1988, approximately ten days before my daughter was born. Those were the days of billing restrictions and I could not obtain a billing number. Since my husband had bought a practice, he was able to practise immediately, but it was some eight months before I was allowed a billing number.

Although there were less than ten female physicians in Kelowna at that time, I was told that on application for medical privileges at the hospital, there was no shortage of female physicians, and I also did not fit their manpower plan. Eventually towards the end of 1988 I began to practise part-time, increasing in hours and diversity as the years went on. Our third child was born in 1990.

I continued to be more involved with teaching and eventually became a director of the Pediatric program and subsequently the Obstetric program for Family Practice residents in Kelowna General. I served as Head of Family Practice for two years and on the Family Practice executive for a further two years. I was involved in a community research project to promote the awareness of fetal alcohol syndrome and to identify those who were at high risk for it. I have been heavily involved in preventative health education, particularly in women's health issues. Over the last six years I have done many menopausal and women's health-related forums throughout the Okanagan Valley and down as far as Osoyoos teaching about preventative health in the pre-menopause and menopause, as well as sexuality and mood

disorders. I think our record was that Dr. Lianne Lacroix and I, also from Kelowna, had 750 women attending one of our forums.

Along with education, my other passion over the last twelve years in Kelowna has been physician wellness, a concern which has developed since I graduated from medical school. In my first and third years post-grad I became associated with two physicians whose mental health were seriously in question. One of them later committed suicide and the other developed chemical dependency. Through them I gained insight into how unsupportive and insensitive we have been in the past in regards to problems with physicians. In the last few years I have been sitting on the Physicians' Support Program (PSP) Committee of the British Columbia Medical Association (BCMA). I most recently took up the position of Chair of the PSP Committee in June of this year. It is my aim to increase preventative education among physicians and their families so that the program can offer more immediate support for physicians in difficulty, and also more work can go into preventing difficulties with physicians and their families.

At the time I graduated, like many other young doctors, I wanted to do something wonderful and become famous. I wanted to, perhaps, discover the cure to some important disease, or become a Professor of Endocrinology and manage some very important outpatient clinic. Over the years I have gone from an aspiring internist to part-time family physician, and in that time I evolved from a family physician to an educator. I spent a short while dabbling in medical politics. It is quite ironic that I am not allowed to disclose my work in physician support in intricate details. So I went from somebody who wanted to do something famous who was in the limelight to someone whose passion and important work must remain hidden and quiet.

When I was a medical student in Aberdeen University, my pediatric professor once said to me, "It's important to be a family doctor," and I replied, "Oh, I don't want to do that, I want to do something much more than that." He said, "Well, when you're a family doctor you help the ninety-nine people that everybody else doesn't see and they see the one you send on. They comment on your ability and care in terms of the one you sent on, but they never see the other ninety-nine who are kept well and are listened to and supported and guided through your care, and it's the ability to do that that makes a good family doctor and also a good teacher."

I think by the end of my career, I would have made a good family doctor and a good teacher. But now I am more inspired to become a good mother and mentor to my children. If they grow up well, whole, and happy, I will have felt that I have carried out my greatest task in life to the best of my ability.

Curriculum Vitae

Present Position: Active staff, Department of Family Practice, Kelowna General Hospital; Assistant Clinical Professor, Department of Family Practice, University of British Columbia.

Born: February 28, 1958, Bannockburn, Scotland.

Marital Status: Married, three children.

Education: University of Aberdeen, Scotland, 1975–1981; Graduated MBCHB with commendation from University of Aberdeen Medical School, Scotland, July 1981.

Awards: Mathews Duncan Medal in Obstetrics, 1981; Louise Tomory Prize for most distinguished female medical graduate, 1981; John Hunter Bursary, 1981, 1980, 1979; Distinction in Obstetrics, 1981; Distinction in Psychiatry, 1980; Distinction in Medical Microbiology, 1979; 2nd Class Distinction Anatomy, 1976; 2nd Class Distinction Physiology, 1976.

Employment: Internal Medicine Rotation, Professor A.C. Kennedy, University Department of Medicine, Glasgow Royal Infirmary, Glasgow, 1981–82; Surgical Rotation, Professor David Carter, University Department of Surgery, Glasgow Royal Infirmary, Glasgow, 1981–1982; Obstetrics and Gynecology, Falkirk Royal Infirmary, Falkirk, Scotland. This obstetric department dealt with over 2,000 deliveries per year, involving high-risk and primary care obstetrics, 1982–1982; Pediatrics, including Out-Patient Pediatrics and Pediatrics Intensive Care, Falkirk Royal Infirmary, Falkirk, Scotland, 1982–1983; Internal Medicine Rotation, University Department of Medicine, Glasgow Royal Infirmary, Glasgow, Scotland, 1983–1985, 1st year Medical Senior House Officer, 2nd year Senior House Office/Registrar position. This included clinic work in all areas of internal medicine and acute on call as Medical Registrar on 1 in 4 basis for east end of Glasgow. Also on call for one year to Hemophilia Unit of Glasgow Infirmary. This internal Medicine Rotation included extensive Out-Patient work, especially in the areas of respiratory medicine, gastroenterology, and endocrinology. Teaching involvement was on a weekly basis with medical Junior House Officers, dental students, and nursing staff, 1982.

Certifications: DRCOG exam, Diploma of The Royal college of Obstetrics and Gynecology, London, England; College of General Practitioners Family Planning Certificate (U.K.); DCH, Diploma of Pediatrics, Royal College of Medicine, Glasgow, Scotland, 1983; 1st Part MRCP examination, Glasgow, Scotland, 1984; LMCC exam, 1985; CCFP exam, Calgary, Alberta, 1989.

Employment and Continued Education: Emigrated to Slave Lake, Alberta, Canada as a Family Practitioner, 1985; Completed LMCC examination, May 1985; Slave Lake, Alberta. Family Physician, co-ordinator of Continuing Medical Education for Slave Lake General Hospital, 1985–1988, audit of medical charts 1986–1988; Preceptor for University of Calgary Family Practice Residents and Medical Students 1985–1988; ACLS Instructor in Alberta and British Columbia, teaching an average two courses per year during that period of time and also being responsible for helping put together a course involving certification of thirty of the nursing staff in Slave Lake. Organized weekly and monthly education events in Slave Lake. Involved in community education in schools and community college on all aspects of preventive medicine, family planning, and women's health issues, 1986–1994; Member of the Department of Family Practice, Kelowna General Hospital, Kelowna, B.C. Private practice involving a large volume of obstetrics and pediatrics and considerable involvement in mood disorders and counselling. Teaching in my practice has been since arrival in Kelowna, and over the years, have taught medical students, nurses, ambulance staff, family practice residents, and small group education sessions for family physicians, 1988–present.

Professional Activities: Membership Canadian Medical Association; Canadian College of Family Practitioners; British Columbia Medical Association; BCMA Section of General Practitioners; Federation of

Medical Women of Canada; College of Physicians and Surgeons, B.C.; Member of Drug and Alcohol Committee, Kelowna General Hospital, 1991; Head of Family Practice, Kelowna General Hospital, responsible for building strategic plan for the Department of Family Practice, and reconstructing credentialing process of Department of Family practice, 1992–1994; Preparation of review documents of the Principles and Procedures of the Department of Family Practice for Accreditation, 1992–1994; Member of Strategic Planning and Budget Priorities of Kelowna General Hospital, 1993; Involved in the development, initiation, and ongoing assessment of the Early Maternity Discharge Program of the Kelowna General Hospital in conjunction with Continuing Care in Kelowna and Kelowna Health Unit, 1993–1996; Involved in Development of Home IV Program of Kelowna General Hospital, 1994; Member of the Family Practice Executive, Kelowna General Hospital, 1994–March 1997; Member of Physicians Support Committee, Kelowna General Hospital, 1993–present; Member of Regional Mental Health Advisory Group, 1995–1996; Member of ASTAT Committee at Mental Health, 1995–1999; Member of Physicians Support Committee of the BCMA, 1996–present; Pediatric Reconfigurations Committee, Kelowna General Hospital, 1996; Teaching residents in my office one-half day per week, medical students on an average of one to two weeks per year, and in-servicing staff on request. Also considerable informal teaching at deliveries and in the case room, 1989–1994; Co-ordinator of UBC Family Practice/Obstetric Residency Program at Kelowna General Hospital and am Clinical Assistant Professor. This involves organization of residents, teaching rotations within the hospital and private practitioners' offices, and tutorials with residents on a weekly basis along with a final evaluation of residents at the end of each rotation. Development of manual for pedatrics residency program in Kelowna in 1994 and a manual for obstetric residency program in 1999, 1994–present.

Presentations and Workshops: From 1992 to 1996 presentations in Kelowna included the topics of Diabetes, Adoption Issues, Fetal Alcohol Syndrome, Menopause, Hormone Replacement and Osteoporosis,

lectures to the nursing and ambulance staff on Survivors of Sexual Abuse, Mood Disorders, Obstetrics; Stress and Female Physicians to the Kelowna Branch of FMWC; From 1997 presentations increased to two or three per month, in Kelowna and in Penticton, Vernon, Oliver, Kamloops, Salmon Arm, and Rossland. By 2000 the topic of Stress became a popular presentation, and at the BCMA Millennium Annual Meeting Dr. Docherty spoke about "Physician Family Stress."

Research:

Comparative study of General Practice office practice techniques in Shetland Islands, Scotland vs. Westlock, Alberta, 1981

Glasgow Royal Infirmary, "Retrospective Study of Outcome of Abdominal Pain in Hemophiliacs," 1984

Fetal Alcohol "At Risk Drinking in Pregnancy." This research was performed in conjunction with the Health Unit, Drug and Alcohol Services, Kelowna and Okanagan Neurological Association. The results were correlated over the period of 1994–1995 and published in May 1996 as a public education document reviewing the risks in lifestyle associated with pregnancy outcome. This research was multidisciplinary and performed on a voluntary basis with donated community funding. The documentation and publication has been developed with the hope of diminishing the frequency of at-risk drinking in pregnancy and the outcome of FAE and FAS (Fetal Alcohol Effect and Fetal Alcohol Syndrome), 1992–1996

Investigator in the "EQUOL" trial (Evista Quality of Life), 1999

Investigator in "RISC" trial (Coronary Intervention Study in Canada), 1999

Professional Aims: To promote Canadian medical education, to improve understanding and treatment of women's health issues, and to improve health and support for physicians and their families

DR. TERESA MILIA

I was born in Squamish, British Columbia on July 18, 1960. My parents were immigrants from Italy, coming over to Canada in 1952. As the third of seven children in the rural community of Squamish, I often took care of my siblings and I was well on my way to being prepared for a medical career in a small town. This was mentioned by the younger of my two brothers on the day of my wedding July 18, 1989, when he stated during the toast to the bride that I was always there for him, "fixing his booboos." And I had the drive to become a doctor, despite being in a coma for three days when I was two-and-a-half, after being struck by a car.

By 1978 I graduated top of my high school class, having led all grades since Grade 4. My mother encouraged us to study. I worried about the cost of university, but my mother assured me she would get another job in addition to running the family restaurant, helping my father run a trailer park, and taking care of my four younger siblings. It wasn't necessary as I received enough through scholarships, summer jobs, student loans, and an out-of-court settlement from my accident of years ago that I hadn't been told about until I reached nineteen years of age.

First year sciences at the University of British Columbia was difficult as I missed home and there were so many other good students. I remember phoning my older sister from the residence after exams in December, despondent that I didn't do well. Having survived first term, I improved enough to realize that I could still accomplish my dream. I made use of all the tutorials, old exams, and masses at St. Mark's on campus. I was pleasantly shocked to get 100% on the Calculus 101 midterm exam. Because of my first term, though, my marks were not high enough to get accepted into medical school after third year. Microbiology and my MCAT scores could have been better, too.

By fourth year I was doing "fun things" in Microbiology, like isolating bacteria from store-bought chicken that we had left on the counter overnight. I isolated campylobacteria and was so impressed, but I couldn't bring myself to throw away the chicken. Being the poor student that I was I baked it and served it to my unsuspecting older brother. He ate it, but I gingerly picked at it. Yes, he got food poisoning, and I was able to tell him the organism. We still laugh about it!

I reapplied to medical school after fourth year with no success. Being very determined I completed my credits for Botany in fifth year and applied again. I also applied to graduate school in Oceanography. I heard back from the Department of Medicine first—I was on the waiting list! Because of the expansion of the class to 130, there was a position for me in the September class of 1983.

Three of us rented an apartment with our brother. The next four years were a blur of studying, classes, and then as an MSI night call. For the last two years I continued to have family support, as I lived with my two younger sisters near the Vancouver General Hospital which was closer to classes than our previous residence on Fraser and 70th.

I graduated in 1987. I was the first student from Squamish to graduate from any Medical School. I was also the fittest female and the second fittest of the whole class in first year. I had trained for the marathon in the summer. Edmonton General Hospital selected me for their out-of-province intern position. I met my future husband, Ting, who was then and continues to be the most cheerful person I know. We had a lot in common—medicine, coming from a large family (ten), and most importantly, he was Catholic. The intern year passed quickly.

During the Obstetrics and Gynecology rotation, I assessed a pregnant woman with abdominal pain and thought she had appendicitis. The obstetrician on call was reached by phone and I told her of my suspicion. She put me on the spot by asking, "Well, does she or doesn't she?" I stood my ground and she sent a surgeon to see the patient. I was right and the surgeon was impressed, and more importantly, the patient did well. Needless to say, I thought about a residency in Obstetrics, but knew that the lifestyle was not for me. I really enjoyed my Surgery rotation and must have done well because I was offered a letter of reference from my preceptor, who encouraged me to apply for Surgery residency.

Most of my free time was spent with my boyfriend, Ting. We became engaged on February 1, 1988. During my internship I experienced the tornado which struck Edmonton. The casualties went to the Royal Alexandra Hospital, and we were on standby for any overflow, which didn't happen.

We interns were involved with the transfer of patients to the new Grey Nuns Hospital, and I felt privileged to be one of the first people to work in the new hospital and therefore involved with 'working out some of the bugs.'

Having finished the internship, Ting and I headed to Hodgson, Manitoba, for our first locum. Ting's brother, Kiong, met us in Manitoba to stay with us for a year as their mother wanted him to leave his questionable friends back east. After a month I was able to get locums in British Columbia. The first was in Salmo, a town of about 800, where our family had lived for six months in 1972. My mother accompanied me. I stayed with family friends of my parents. For two weeks I was the only doctor there and was on call every night. I was amazed that there was not one call! During the day, though, I remember having to make a house call because someone was having chest pain. The ambulance was already there and the patient was stable enough to get transferred to the nearest hospital in Nelson, twenty minutes away. It was inconvenient having to see patients in the clinic X-ray department and blood-letting office with neither lab facilities nor ECG. It was frustrating to send patients to Nelson for tests and not being able to get results quickly (no fax then). By giving over care to the ER physician in Nelson, I couldn't admit anyone because I couldn't do rounds on them in Nelson as I was the only MD in Salmo.

I really enjoyed my Surgery rotation and must have done well because I was offered a letter of reference from my preceptor, who encouraged me to apply for Surgery residency.

Hodgson, Manitoba had a self-contained facility that included a lab, X-ray, pharmacy, and hospital along with the clinic. It also provided accommodations and multiple benefits, but it wasn't British Columbia. Ting had a position for six months and was asked to stay. I also was offered a position giving care for the more isolated populations in the north that were accessible only by plane.

The third locum and a better job prospect was in Clearwater, B.C. This time my father helped me move. I enjoyed the people there, including the office staff, the doctors, and their families, but I missed my fiancé who was still in Manitoba. Ting decided to visit and be interviewed for a locum position in Clearwater. The interview went well, but there was only a need for one-and-a-half positions. To help them out, though, Ting worked in my place for the month of December while I did my fourth locum in my hometown of Squamish.

Before completing my locum at Clearwater I picked up an aortic aneurysm in a woman with upper back pain. She had complaints of muscle pains all over and had been to physiotherapists. I fortunately ordered an X-ray of her back and the aneurysm was seen on the X-ray. I give credit to the radiology technician, who called me from the hospital when the patient was still at the radiology department. The patient was transferred to Kamloops and then to Vancouver where she had surgery. She did well.

Squamish was busier than the other locums. It was a far larger community and night call was similar to internship. During one night in the Emergency, I was dealing with a patient with pulmonary edema when I got a call from Ting in Clearwater. He was shaken up as he had been in a motor vehicle accident earlier. He had rolled down a steep embankment called "donor hill." No one has ever survived an accident on that hill. Fortunately he was driving my sturdy '79 Ford LTD and his guardian angel was looking after him. He managed to get out of the vehicle, wade through the snow, and get to his office in time for the afternoon clinic!

When the one-month locum in Squamish was over, Ting, his brother, and I headed for Castlegar. I didn't consider settling in Squamish as I felt uncomfortable working in my hometown. While there, a classmate from elementary school days saw me as a patient and begged me for narcotics, which I refused.

The job offer in Castlegar was a locum position with the view to buying the retiring physician's practice. There were three other physicians in an association. They worked as a three-person practice with someone always off. (This required that each person take three months off per year). I liked the working conditions. There had been some controversy from the other clinic in town over giving me a job as they wanted someone with more skills in the community. After all, they had just lost one of the three GP surgeons in town. There had only been one female doctor in the past and none at the time I started there. I decided to give it a try, making the GP population eleven once again in a town of about 8,000.

Ting got a locum position in nearby Trail, twenty minutes away. The position became permanent and he now has one of the busiest practices in town. Ting's brother, who called me "Princess Diana," left just before our wedding in Squamish as he was to help arrange our second wedding reception in Malaysia where we would have our honeymoon.

We finally made our decision to call Castlegar home in January, 1990. I bought the practice and Ting had already joined the clinic in Trail. He didn't cover obstetrics, so we thought I should be closer to my hospital for obstetrics and night call. In May my father visited us and helped us select our future house. It turned out that four other doctors and three nurses lived within one or two blocks of our new house. I learned to keep in phone contact and not rely on a pager long ago when I was visited by police as my pager wasn't functioning while I was on call! Another time one of our OR nurses found the GP anesthetist she had been trying to reach standing in front of her in the checkout counter of one of Castlegar's four grocery stores. His cell phone batteries were dead!

I worked until three weeks before the birth of our son Christopher on December 2, 1990. I had a locum for my four-month maternity leave. When I went back I worked part-time with another female physician, whose husband had also been given a locum position for one of my partners who had left.

My son was a poor sleeper and I breastfed. I was constantly exhausted. By the time Chris was one year old we decided we should show our first-born to Ting's family in Malaysia. My mother-in-law returned with us to visit and to help look after Chris, and stayed from February to September when her daughter came from Malaysia to visit and accompany her home. My next pregnancies were complicated and I was transferred by medi-vac to Grace Hospital in Vancouver where Michael was born in 1993. In January, 1998, Christina was born in Trail, B.C. after a stormy pregnancy and another medi-vac trip to Vancouver in October to the Women's Hospital. (The medi-vac team recognized me from last time!) I was finally allowed to stay in my parents' second home in New Westminster where I was under the close monitoring of the nurses in the new home care program, and then back to Castlegar just before Christmas. I was back to work full time in July.

Our office practice had become a partnership somewhere along the way to allow a person to work as much or as little as they wanted. The volume had increased long ago, so we needed four doctors working weekly. We did get a surgeon in our practice who did GP work.

Around May is the time for our annual Enema Open, a fun golf and dinner for our office staff, doctors, and spouses. One of our two RNs, Ginny, and "the glue that keeps our office running," Chris, were the founders of this social event about twelve or thirteen years ago. In a recent event I was feted with an early fortieth birthday party. There were black balloons and streamers everywhere, as well as pictures of me from infancy on, including one of me doing the "catwalk" during the Miss Squamish Pageant when I was nineteen. Yes, I was embarrassed. My mother had secretly sent the pictures to our nanny who delivered them to Ginny at the clinic. All this work to surprise me! I was overwhelmed.

So far I have found the practice of medicine in the "country" very rewarding, despite the tedious paper work and occasional bad call. I delivered some of my older son's classmates and was the family doctor to others, so he would come home and ask me if I delivered a certain classmate or was I someone's doctor. I have become close to some of my patients, having known them for eleven to twelve years. I see quite a few in the town's five fast food drive thrus, banks, grocery stores, gas stations, and at the neighbourhood church. I recall once when I had three very sick patients in hospital. I worried about them and prayed for them that night. I was exhilarated to find them better the next morning. Practising medicine in a small town can be very rewarding.

DR. WENDY V. NORMAN

Curriculum Vitae

Education: Master of Health Science, student of University of British Columbia, Vancouver, B.C., 1999–present; Diploma in Tropical Medicine and Hygiene, U of Liverpool, United Kingdom, 1993; Anesthesia, UBC, Vancouver, B.C.; 1 year residency for GP-Anaesthetists, 1988; CCFP Family Practice Residency, University of Alberta, Edmonton, Alberta, 1985–87; MD, Queen's University, Kingston, Ontario, 1981–85; 2 years of Life Sciences, Undergraduate, Queen's University, Kingston, Ontario, 1979–81; 3 months of Science–withdrawn without penalty–University of Western London, Ontario secondary to 8-month illness (full recovery), Ontario, 1977; Grade 13 with Honours, Aldershot H.S. Burlington, Ontario, 1977.

Courses: ACLS Advanced Cardiac Life Support, Sechelt, 1997;

Ultrasound Training for Pregnancy Dating, Toronto, 1996; NRP Update of Neonatal Resuscitation, Sechelt, 1996; Obstetrical Emergencies Course, Sechelt, 1995; Airway Emergencies Course, Sechelt, 1995; NAF Risk Management Seminar, Philadelphia, 1994; HEP Health Emergencies Preparation, MSF Amsterdam, the Netherlands, 1993; NALS Neonatal Advanced Life Support, Lion's Gate Hospital, Vancouver, 1990.

Instructor & Provider Course: ATLS Advanced Trauma Life Support VGH, Vancouver, 1988; ACLS Advanced Cardiac Life Support, University of Alberta, Edmonton; updated every 3-5 years, 1985.

Work Experience: Medical Program Director, Breast Health Program Vancouver, B.C. Women's Health Center (WHC) of Children's and Women's Health Centre of B.C. (C&W)—A broad-based mandate to increase the provision and quality of breast diagnostic and assessment services throughout the province, as well as to supervise the provision of tertiary care diagnostic and assessment services and teaching in our multidisciplinary clinic; Medical Advisor to the Aboriginal Health Program, WHC; Relief work in CARE program, WHC; 1997–1998; Clinic Physician, Elizabeth Bagshaw Women's Clinic, Vancouver, B.C., 1997–present; Rural GP–Anaesthetist in B.C. Coastal community of Sechelt, B.C., 20,000 population, accessible by water or air only. Varied Family Practice (as only one specialist available locally–a general surgeon), included office and hospital care: ER & trauma, Obstetrics, Anaesthesia, ICU, house calls, 1989–1997; Branch Medical Director & Clinic Physician, Sechelt, B.C., Planned Parenthood Association–Sunshine Coast Branch Weekly Birth Control Clinic providing medical care, public information, and low cost accessible contraception. Associated community and school lectures in support 1989–1997; Clinic Physician Everywoman's Health Clinic, Vancouver, B.C., 1991–present; *Medecins Sans Frontiers*–Physician volunteer working in a Ler, S. Sudan, a primitive African village (few buildings, no running water, no electricity) in a war zone treating TB, Visceral Leishmaniasis (Kala Azar), malnutrition, malaria, obstetrics, and providing general medical care for a semi-nomadic community of approx. 50,000. (See also 'Teaching Experience.') Participation in clinical trials for TB and Kala Azar treatment regimens, Dec. '93–June '94; 6 months locum covering rural Yukon practice with Whitehorse, Yukon clinic work at outpost nursing stations, ER and trauma care in Whitehorse and helicopter evacuating of injured/ill persons from remote mountain areas, 1987.

Organizational and Teaching Experience: Clinical Instructor, Department of Family Practice, Faculty of Medicine, UBC, 1999–Present; Chair of Conference Planning committee, "Breast Health Centres—The Team Approach," an international interdisciplinary conference for professionals working in Breast Diagnosis and Assessment, Vancouver, B.C., 1999; Workshop Moderator: "Integrated Breast Assessment," and Conference Planning; Committee member, "Breast Cancer: Myths and Realities," Regional Conference, Vancouver, B.C., 1999; Conception, design and implementation of a 2-week intensive course in Breast Health for Rural Family Physicians jointly given at B.C. Cancer Agency and at Children's and Women's Health Centre, intended to enhance their locally available breast care expertise, and involving a mandatory series of public and professional lectures to be given by the participants in their home areas upon course completion. Accredited by the College of Family Physicians of Canada for 70 hours of CME, Vancouver, B.C., 1998; Oral Examiner for Family Physician Certificate candidate; Vancouver, B.C., 1998–present; presentation to B.C. College of Family Physicians and the Federation of Medical Women: "Breast Health—the Difficult Diagnosis." Vancouver, B.C., 1998; Lecturer, School of Rehabilitation Science, UBC, Women's Health Lecture in Medical Sciences Course, Vancouver, B.C., 1997; President, Provincial Board of Directors, Planned Parenthood Association of B.C., a provincial non-profit health care organization providing quality education and clinic services aiming to reduce the incidence of unplanned pregnancies and to improve related areas of reproductive health and behaviour for all British Columbians. Currently we run 39 branches throughout B.C., 1997–present; Vice President, Board of Directors, Planned Parenthood Association,

Vancouver, B.C., 1997; President of Sunshine Coast Branch, Planned Parenthood, Gibsons, B.C., 1996; Medical Director and sole physician running a TB inpatient program for over 100 patients, and a similar sized Kala Azar treatment program, overseeing work and design and delivery of nursing course for approximately 55 nursing and aid staff and ensuring ongoing research data collection. Taught English lessons in the evenings, Ler, S. Sudan, Africa, 1993–94; "Tuberculosis Treatment and Control using the Manyatta Cincinnati, U.S.A. regimen in a conflict zone in Southern Sudan." Presentation of research findings at a concurrent session at The American Society of Tropical Medicine Annual Meeting, 1994; President of Medical Staff, St. Mary's Hospital, Sechelt, B.C., 1992; Chairman of Utilization Management Committee, St. Mary's Hospital, Sechelt, B.C., 1990–91; Founding Branch Board Member and Branch Medical Director, Sunshine Coast Branch Planned Parenthood, Gibsons, B.C., 1989–97; Instructor, Neonatal Advanced Life Support Course, St. Mary's Hospital, Sechelt, B.C., 1991–95; Lecturer, Obstetric Nursing Course, St. Mary's Hospital, Sechelt, B.C.; Clinical Instructor/Preceptor, Family Medicine Residency, Rural Experience program, UBC, Gibsons, B.C., 1989–90; Director & Volunteer, Telephone Aid Kingston, a volunteer-run organization to provide a telephone distress line, Kingston, Ontario, 1979–82.

Awards: John Snow Prize in Epidemiology Awarded to the Graduate Student with the highest standing in the Health Care and Epidemiology Course "Measuring the Health of Populations" HCEP 502, UBC, 2000; Fellow of the College of Family Physicians of Canada, an honour recognising outstanding contributions to Family Medicine in Teaching, Research, and Community or College Leadership, and limited to no more than ten percent of Certificants of the College, 1999; Dr. Jeffery Dolph Memorial Award for compassion and caring in relations with patients and co-workers, conferred by the Planned Parenthood Association of B.C., 1997; Warrington Yorke Medal in International Community Health for top standing in the International Community Health course of the Diploma in Tropical Medicine and Hygiene, Liverpool School of Tropical Medicine, University of Liverpool, United Kingdom.

1989

DR. ALICE HUANG

The dandelion seed. That is how I began my last autobiography, which happened to be part of my medical school application in 1983! Back in those days, I viewed the dandelion seed as a metaphor for life; now, I view the weed as a nuisance in the garden. How life has changed!

I am the third child, and first generation Canadian, of Chinese physician parents. I was born in Kingston, Ontario, August 20, 1964, and grew up in Montreal where life revolved around ballet classes, piano, French Immersion at school, perfecting the cartwheel, and picking weeds from the lawn. In the first grade I wanted to be a doctor, but like any kid, my career aspirations evolved to fireman in Grade 3, astronomer in Grade 9, engineer in first year Memorial University of Newfoundland, then eventually back to medicine during undergraduate studies at Queen's University. My application to medical school, dandelion and all, must have either amazed or amused someone on the admissions committee. I was accepted at the University of Toronto Medical School in 1984.

There were 250 students in my class. Lectures took place in a huge, sloped lecture hall with three projector screens often running simultaneously. To this day, there are still people in my class whom I don't recognize! I devoted half of my time to studying, and the remainder to dancing and choreographing for "Daffydil," the annual medical school production. I managed to earn the Walter F. Watkins scholarship and the Canadian Foundation for Ileitis and Colitis Book Award over the four years. I graduated in 1988.

My rotating internship was at St. Paul's Hospital in Vancouver, British Columbia. I spent an amazing year exploring the west coast and learning how to be a real doctor. One of my funniest and most embarrassing anecdotes involved a night on call for the vascular surgery ward. One of the male nurses phoned me about 11 p.m. to say there was a seventy-year-old male patient who had been unable to void over the past two hours because of a persistent erection. Immediately I ran down to assess the patient, my mind frantically reviewing the possible causes of this gentleman's priapism. The patient and the three other gentlemen in the room were asleep. I had a difficult time awakening the patient because he was hard of hearing. I shouted my questions in order to obtain a proper history, and I performed my physical exam by flashlight! I concluded that this patient had priapism, but I was puzzled as to why he was not experiencing any pain. Since the books say that priapism is a medical emergency, I decided to wake up the urologist on call at home. He suggested that I go ahead and catheterize the patient, and he would see the patient in the morning. Well, there was a lot of chuckling on the ward the next morning! It turns out that the patient had had a penile prosthesis implanted, but never bothered to mention it to anyone. Luckily, the urology consult did not go to waste since he had an enlarged prostate which required surgery.

The helicopter pilot, Charlie, was located at the local pub, and once he dragged the chopper out of a barn, we flew to the site of the crash.

After internship, I headed off to Wanganui, New Zealand—a city with a population of 40,000 humans and 80,000 sheep! My plan was to work as a second year house surgeon, then travel New Zealand and Australia. I lived in the nurses' residence at the hospital, and loved picking fresh lemons from the trees on the hospital grounds. Wanganui Base Hospital was staffed by a mix of New Zealand, British, South African, Sri Lankan, and Canadian physicians. I was constantly encountering different styles of medical therapeutics and seeing a very different range of diseases. My most exciting medical experience there involved a helicopter transfer at a trauma scene.

There had been a head-on collision on the "desert highway," which runs alongside the three volcanoes of the North Island. The call from the ambulance at the scene came in at 10:30 p.m., requesting a helicopter transfer of two seriously injured patients. I loaded my coat pockets with gloves, syringes, and narcotics. The helicopter pilot, Charlie, was located at the local pub, and once he dragged the chopper out of a barn, we flew to the site of the crash. The view of the volcanoes by moonlight was eerie. I could see cars lined up for miles on either side of the accident scene. Landing the chopper in a tiny area was very tricky and scary. It required a series of tight turns to circle the chopper down. One patient had a pneumothorax, and the other had major head lacerations and a respiratory arrest. I managed to intubate the patient in respiratory arrest, and gave analgesics to the patient with the pneumothorax. The patients' stretchers were secured like shelving, one on top of the other, and I was squished in beside them in the chopper. I kept hoping nothing would happen en route, since I was manually bagging one patient, and there was no room to manoeuvre in the event of an arrest. The flight ended on the front lawn of the hospital, and lots of help had materialized in the emergency room.

Despite the stimulating work, I was very lonely and decided to quit after six months. I spent the following three months backpacking around New Zealand and Australia. I returned to Canada in May, 1990, realizing how much I had missed my family and my country.

After a year of general practice locums in the Vancouver area and the Northwest Territories, I enrolled in the one year GP-Anaethesia program at the University of British Columbia. The most important spin-off of this year was my meeting my wonderful husband-to-be in the operating room! Gerry was a fourth year medical student, doing his general surgery rotation. We used to chat while I finished off the anaesthetic, and he was left to suture the patient. He was very slow in suturing, so we had lots of time to talk! I used to purposely check all the operating rooms in the morning to see if he was there. Our romance blossomed from the operating room to the wards, then eventually down the wedding aisle when we were married in 1993.

I returned to working as a general practitioner in the Vancouver area, giving up the anaesthetics after six months, while my husband pursued his residency training in pathology.

My beautiful son, Christopher, was born May 11, 1996. Life has never been the same since! I returned to work after six months of maternity leave, and learned to juggle the stresses of daycare, commuting, breast feeding, daily household chores, and working weekend travel clinics. No wonder I was tired all the time! Gerry passed his pathology exams and landed his first job in Kamloops, British Columbia. We moved to the B.C. interior in August, 1998 when I was thirty-two weeks pregnant. Packing and moving with a big pregnant belly was challenging! Our beautiful daughter, Cynthia, was born October 13, 1998. I returned to work part-time when Cynthia was seven months. We bought our first home complete with fruit trees, dandelions, and visiting bears. The commute to work and daycare is only fifteen minutes, and there is never any traffic. This is life in a small city!

My children love to dash around the garden to collect the bright yellow dandelion flowers. I love to watch the innocent wonder in their eyes as they gaze at nature's creation. I can't help wondering if one day, they too may be inspired by something as simple as a dandelion seed?

Notes From BC MEDICAL JOURNAL 1980–1989

January, 1980 The Government of British Columbia is giving $400,000 over a four-month period, to provide additional medical examinations for Vietnamese refugees coming to B.C. Two thousand have already arrived and 8,000 more are expected by the end of 1980.

Dr. M.C. Petreman is President of BCMA 1979–1980. Hon. Rafe Mair is the new Health Minister. There were 4,912 physicians in British Columbia as of September, 1979.

In Memorium: Dr. Kathleen Stewart Graham, a well-known family practitioner in Vancouver, died on November 27, 1979. She was born in 1917 and graduated from the University of Alberta in 1943. Dr. Isabella K.A. MacDonald died at age 79. She graduated in Scotland in 1928 and came to B.C. in 1956.

Victoria: Dr. Patricia Johnston is the first woman to serve as President of the Victoria Medical Society in its 84-year history. She was honoured recently and presented with an engraved brooch.

March, 1980 In 1977 there were 37,000 live births in British Columbia. Ten percent or 3,934 were delivered by women 19 years and younger, 47 to girls less than 15 years of age. Of the 3,934, 52% were born to unwed mothers. Of 189 pregnancies occurring in girls under age 15 years, 142 were aborted. There were 11,285 therapeutic abortions in 1977, 35% on females age 19 and younger. There is a 33% higher perinatal mortality in very young mothers than the average, and 70% higher infant mortality. Statistics are from an article in the *Journal* on "Teen-age Pregnancy" by pediatricians Dr. Roger Tonkin and Dr. A.F. Hardyment.

Journal article by Moira Chan-Yeung, MB, FRCP(C) and Stephan Grzybowski, MD, FRCP, UBC Department of Medicine, Vancouver General Hospital, describes the work of the Occupational Lung Disease Unit, i.e., Occupational Asthma due to western red cedar exposure. The chemical (plicatic acid) has been identified, but the mechanism of this type of asthma is still unknown. The unit has conducted health surveys in six sawmills and five terminal grain elevators on workers in the Pulp and Paper Mill in Powell River, and is embarking on a study of Alcan chemicals and smelters in Kitimat to investigate the effects of fluoride exposure on lungs and the skeletal system.

A book by Dr. Louise Jilek-Aall, *Call Mama Doctor—African Notes of a Young Woman Doctor* was reviewed by Dr. Chunilal Roy, FRCP(C), FRCPsych(E).

Dr. Lynn Beattie has been appointed Acting Head of the Department of Geriatrics and Continuing Care at Shaughnessy Hospital and Acting Head Division of Geriatrics, Faculty of Medicine, UBC, effective February 15, 1980. Previously she had been the Director of the Geriatric Unit at Toronto Western Hospital, and Assistant Professor of Medicine, University of Toronto. She will continue as Head of Geriatric Medicine, Health Sciences Centre Hospital, UBC.

Dr. Virginia Wright, pediatric Pathologist, is Chairman CASC on Perinatal Care of the Perinatal Program of B.C.

April, 1980 *Journal* article: "Screening for Congenital Hypothyroidism," by Margaret Norman MD, FRCP(C) and Lorne Kirby PhD. The new screening program to prevent mental retardation is now established by the Provincial Government.

In Memoriam: Dr. Teresa Elizabeth Rush (Mrs. B.J. Trecice) died at home in Crescent Beach, August 12, 1979 at the age of 53.

May, 1980 The Honour Roll of the Council of College of Physicians and Surgeons of B.C. for those registered for 50 years or more has 46 members, including only one woman, Dr. Kathleen Woods Langston.

Dr. A.F. Mandeville is the new President of BCMA 1980–1981.

BCMA Annual Reports include those of the Health Planning Committee. Dr. Shirley Rushton, Dr. Judith Hornung, Dr. Kay Costley-White, and Dr. Wendy Fidgeon are members. Dr. Hedy Fry is Chairman of the Nutrition Committee. Consultant to the Committee is Dr. Doris Kavanagh-Gray.

July, 1980 Medical student Judy Chow, on graduation received the Dean M. M. Weaver Medal, the Hamber Scholarship in Medicine, the Frank Porter Patterson Memorial Prize, and the Peter Spohn Memorial Prize.

Debbie Holberg was awarded the Dr. A.M. Agnew Memorial Prize, and Diane Miller was awarded the Dr. A.B. Schinbein Prize and the Elizabeth Tong Ng Memorial Prize. Gail Stirling received the Ingram and Bell Limited Prize and the Max and Susie Dodek Medical Prize.

Journal article: "An Overview of Obstetrical Ultra Sound" by Mary Graham MD, FRCP(C).

August, 1980 Dr. Ellen Wiebe is the secretary-treasurer of the B.C. Chapter, College of Family Physicians of Canada.

September, 1980 Conjoint meeting of Australian Medical Association and the Canadian Medical Association is held in Vancouver, B.C.

November, 1980 *Journal* article: "Genetic Prenatal Diagnosis in British Columbia: An Update," by authors Barbara McGillivray MD, FRCP(C), FCCMG; Dorothy Shaw MB, ChB, FRCS(C), and Lydia Suderman, RN. Based on the experience of some 1,000 amniocenteses at University of B.C.'s program for genetic prenatal diagnosis of genetic disorders, the authors review the present indications for amniocentesis, ultrasound, and fetoscopy.

December, 1980 Facts from the Bulletin Forum produced by the Association of Canadian Medical Colleges in 1980: There were 1,746 graduates from Canadian Medical Schools in 1980. A record 32% or 560 graduates were women. In 1960 women were 7% of the graduates and in 1970 they were 12%.

January, 1981 Clinical Hypnosis Courses, March 21–22, 1981 with seven doctors lecturing, including Dr. Marlene Hunter and Dr. Tanya Wulff.

Health Minister Rafe Mair resigned from the Cabinet on January 6, 1981, and Richmond MLA Jim Nielson was appointed Health Minister. Mr. Mair is moving to radio station CJOR in Vancouver as an open-line host.

Worker's Compensation Board has given a grant of $149,000 to Dr. Moira Yeung and Dr. Stefan Grzybowski for a major health survey of pulp and paper workers in British Columbia to be conducted at MacMillan Bloedel's Powell River complex. Dr. Yeung has been doing research in Occupational Lung Diseases in areas such as Woodfibre on the Sunshine Coast and Alcan Co. at Kitimat.

February, 1981 Dr. Dorothy Shaw and Dr. T. Martin will give a one-day course in Obstetrics and Gynecology on March 5, 1981 in Burnaby, sponsored by the Division of Continuing Medical Education, UBC.

Medical School Admissions Update: In September, 1950, the Faculty of Medicine at the University of British Columbia admitted the first class of medical students composed of 57 men and three women. In September, 1980 the Faculty of Medicine admitted 73 men and 47 women for a total of 120. In 30 years the medical school has doubled its class size, and the male/female ratio has changed considerably.

The Surrey Medical Society has organized a tour of China for March 7–26, 1981, including three hospital visits, in Peking, Shijiazhuang, where Dr. Norman Bethune worked and is buried, and in Shanghai.

March, 1981 The last tuberculosis patients to be treated at Pearson Hospital in Vancouver were transferred in January, 1981 to the Ministry of Health's Willow Chest Centre at 2647 Willow St. Pearson Hospital will be used for long-term care patients.

A Tuberculosis Program has been set up for Indo-Chinese refugees. Over 7,000 have now arrived in B.C. from Southeast Asia, and 2,500 more are expected by the end of 1981.

Dr. Shirley Rushton, Chairman, Athletic and Recreation Committee, writes in her report that her committee has been lobbying the Ministers of Health and Education to make a statement endorsing one hour of daily physical education for all school children in B.C.

April, 1981 Balance billing has become illegal in British Columbia. Bill 16, The Medical Service Plan Act, designed to abolish balance billing and to put an arbitration procedure in place, is still on the legislature's order paper. A speedy passage deleted the arbitration section.

Canada West Medical Congress takes place May 30–June 5, 1981. Chairman of the Organizing committee is Dr. Hedy Fry. There will be 32 guest speakers (22 Americans, two from England, and eight Canadians) other than speakers from B.C.

May, 1981 Article: "The Social and Economic Needs of the Community Elders" by Dr. Elizabeth Luke, MB, FRCP(C), MRCP(Psy), DPM, MSc, of Victoria. Dr. Bill Jory is President-elect of BCMA. He was BCMA President in 1976, and is the first person in Canadian medical politics to be elected to the same position twice.

June, 1981 Dr. Raymond March is President of BCMA, the 81st President. The Health Minister is Jim Nielson.

In Memorium: Dr. Kathleen Belton has died.

Dr. Josephine Mallek received honorary Senior Membership in the Canadian Medical Association at the BCMA Annual Meeting.

July, 1981 Article by Betty Wood MD, FRCPC and Donald Newman MD, FRCPC: "Radiological Findings in Fetal Alcohol Syndrome."

New medical microbiologist on the staff of the Provincial Health Laboratory is Dr. Judith Issac-Renton, formerly Assistant Professor in the Division of Microbiology, University of British Columbia and assistant microbiologist with the Division of Medical Microbiology, Department of Pathology at Vancouver General Hospital.

August, 1981 *BCMJ* notes that "The UBC economist, Robert Evans, rejected the Canadian Medical Association's claim that the Canadian Health Care System is starved for cash. He said the system is overstacked with high-priced help. He said the system could easily get along with significantly fewer physicians and by making greater use of less expensive personnel such as nurses."

Medicare premiums have increased to $11.50 per month from $8.50 for individuals, and to $28.75 from $21.25 per month for families.

Daily hospital charge for in-patients will be raised to $6.50 from $5.50. Day-care surgery will rise to $6.00 from $5.00

Graduate medical students receiving awards include Catheryne Mecham-McConnell who won the Dr. H. Henderson Memorial Award, Penny Osborne the Dr. A.M. Agnew Memorial Prize, Sylvia Henderson the Dr.

W.A. Whitelaw Prize, Barbara Roper the Mead Johnson of Canada Prize in Pediatrics, Elaine Nabata the Lange Medical Publications Prize, and Ruth Campling, the Jack Foulks Memorial Prize.

September, 1981 Article: "Optimizing Pregnancy Outcome" by Dorothy Shaw MB, ChB, FRCS(C).

Dr. A. F. Hardyment praises his Board members and welcomes Dr. Patricia Rebbeck to the Editorial Board. He comments: "She has several distinct differences to bring to our Board. First, she is our only 'foreigner,' having qualified at Edinburgh in 1959. Second, she is a General Surgeon. Third, she is female. Dare I say she is probably the toughest reviewer in the group."

November, 1981 BCMA Committees Chairmen for 1980 to 1981 include: Health Care Delivery, Dr. Patricia Rebbeck, Athletics and Recreation, Dr. Shirley Rushton, and Nutrition Committee, Dr. Hedy Fry.

Dr. Ellen Wiebe is President-elect of the B.C. Chapter, College of Family Physicians of Canada.

Obituaries: Dr. Anna Farewell died in 1980.

January, 1982 There are many more advertisements in the *B.C. Medical Journal* from 1982 on, some full page. The Chairman of the Nutrition Committee, Dr. Hedy Fry, warns physicians of the growing problem in B.C. of clinics that promote weight-loss diets of 600 calories or less.

February, 1982 Article by D.V. Bates MD, FRCPC and Martha Grymalowski MD, FRCPC: "A Case of Silicosis."

The B.C. Chapter of the Physicians for Social Responsibility (PSR) began in the fall of 1981, and B.C. is the largest of five Canadian chapters. Dr. Dorothy Goresky is the President of the B.C. Chapter PSR.

March, 1982 The new Vancouver Detoxification Centre operated by the Ministry of Health opens at 377 East 2nd Ave. It will be used for cases now handled by the City of Vancouver "drunk tank."

The Ministry of Health advocates immunization against rubella for all children.

April, 1982 Article by Patricia Baird MD, CM, FRCPC, FCCMG and Adele Sadovnick, PhD: "A Cost-benefit Analysis of Prenatal Diagnosis for Down's Syndrome and Neural Tube Defects in British Columbia." Dr. Baird is Head, Department of Medical Genetics, UBC. Dr. Sadovnick is a research assistant, Department of Genetics, UBC.

Letter from Dr. Dorothy Goresky re: Physicians for Social Responsibility states that "Nuclear war is the most imperative issue of our time."

At the Sports Injuries Review at the Whistler Seminar, Dr. Jerilynn Prior, Endocrinologist in the UBC Faculty of Medicine, spoke on "Menstrual Changes in Sports." Up to 50% of female runners may report oligomenorrhea or amenorrhea due to changes in the hypothalamic-pituitary-ovarian axis which are physiological and reversible.

May, 1982 Health Minister Jim Neilson announced that Medicare Premiums are raised: $15 per month for a single person, compared to $11.50. For a couple there is an increase to $25 from $23, and for a family an increase to $32 from $28.75.

B.C. Health Research Projects: Since 1978 when lottery funds were first used for this purpose, $11.3 million has been awarded to support research in B.C. Dr. Joanne Weinberg of UBC received the largest award, $27,000 for studies on the effects of maternal alcoholism.

June, 1982 Dr. Roberta Ongley, a newcomer to the Board in 1981, was elected Honorary Secretary-Treasurer. Of the 5,000 members, only 50% participated in the vote. Dr. Bill Jory became BCMA President for the second time in five years.

There are 475 registered for the Canada West Congress in Vancouver.

July, 1982 HandyDart transport is now available in the Greater Vancouver Regional District for 12,000 disabled.

BCMA Fitness Fun-fest: The team Body Mechanics, headed by Dr. Shirley Rushton, participated in the Corporate Cup on May 30th. The 15-person team included Drs. Joanna Blaxland, Anne Gagne, Jerilynn Prior, and Nona Rowat.

August, 1982 Dr. Ellie B. Brisco, North Vancouver family physician, spearheaded the production of a film showing the experiences an expectant parent can anticipate in the Health System. The film is tentatively titled, "The Journey: You and Your Baby."

September, 1982 The article "Clinical Management of Malignant Melanoma in British Columbia" included authors Dr. Patricia Rebbeck and Dr. Ann Worth.

The Ministry of Health has donated numerous awards for health research, including $20,000 to Dr. Shirley Gillam, UBC Biochemistry Department, in order "to identify and separate cells and antibodies against rubella virus by recombinant DNA techniques."

Dr. Dorothy Goresky reports that Physicians for Social Responsibility, B.C. Chapter, has over 200 members of whom 75% are physicians.

October, 1982 Article by Dr. Tanya Wulff BSc, MSc, MD, CCFP: "Behavioural Treatment of Dysmenorrhea." Dr. Wulff is a family practitioner on staff at St. Paul's Hospital.

Another article, by Marlene Hunter BA, MD, CCFP: "Behavioural Treatment of Tension and Migraine Headaches." Dr. Hunter is a Vancouver family physician and a member of the teaching staff of the Department of Family Practice UBC, and a member of the Board of the B.C. Division of the College of Family Physicians of Canada.

An article: "Occult Breast Cancer Localization" by Donald Longley MD, FRCPC, Maureen Leia-Stephen MD, and Trevor Sandy MD, FRCSC.

December, 1982 The age limit has been lowered for amniocenteses to 35 years. The procedure can detect 40 genetic conditions that can lead to abnormalities at birth.

BCMA has established an ad hoc committee to examine the question of midwifery training and to report its recommendations to the Board in January. The committee consists of Dr. John Anderson, Dr. Charles Carpenter, Dr. Vera Frinton, Dr. Brad Fritz, and Dr. Hedy Fry.

Article: "Geriatric Challenge, Assessment and Rehabilitation" by

Bernice Wylie MD, FRCPC, Clinical Assistant Professor UBC and Consultant, Department of Geriatrics and Continuing Care at Shaughnessy Hospital and G.F. Strong Rehabilitation Centre.

January, 1983 Article in the *Journal*: "Sexual Abuse of Children: Questions and Answers," by William Maurice MD, FRCPC, Kate Parfitt MB, BS, FRCPC, and Lillian Maurice BA, RN, LLB.

Drs. Hedy Fry and Beverley Tamboline are BCMA delegates for District #3 (Vancouver).

February, 1983 Article by Margaret Norman MD, Director of C.H. Wills Newborn Screening Laboratory, Children's Hospital: "Problems in Screening for Congenital Hypothyroidism."

March, 1983 Guest Editorial by Patricia Baird MD, CM, FRCPC, FCCMG: "Mental Retardation in British Columbia. The scope of the Problem."

An article by Margaret Neave MD, DCH (London), former superintendent of Tranquille School: "Community Services and Programs for the Mentally Retarded."

Queen Elizabeth visited the Patient Activity area of the Health Sciences Centre Hospital, UBC.

May, 1983 Dr. Beverley Tamboline, President of Vancouver Medical Association, confers Prince of Good Fellows degree on three VMA members at the Osler Dinner, one of the these being Dr. Patricia Baird.

Dr. Ludmila Zeldowicz, a well-known neurologist, has given the library a copy of a unique book: *In the Warsaw Ghetto 1940-43: An Account of a Witness, the Memoirs of Stanislau Adler*. Adler and Dr. Zeldowicz escaped together from the ghetto. Dr. Zeldowicz brought his manuscript to Vancouver in 1946 and has been instrumental in overseeing its printing in Jerusalem.

BCMA officers for 1983–1984: Duncan MacPherson, President; Gerald Stewart MD, President-elect; and Roberta Ongley MD, Chairman of the General Assembly.

In Memorium: Dr. Emily Sterbak died. The Medical Staff of Woodlands School especially mourn her passing.

June, 1983 *Journal* article: "Chromosome Abnormalities and Advanced Maternal Age." Authors Judith Allanson MB, ChB, MRCP, (UK), Clinical Fellow in Clinical Genetics, and Judith Hall MD, MS, FAAP, FRCPC, FCCMG, Professor, Department of Medical Genetics, UBC, and Director of Clinical Genetics Services, Grace Hospital.

Dr. Dorothy Goresky is President of Physicians for Social Responsibility.

According to the BCMA Child Care Committee there is a rising incidence of teenage pregnancy with the related social problems. Mothers aged 15–19 gave birth to 29,000 babies in 1981 in Canada.

July, 1983 The recent decision to have the UBC medical class expand from 60 to 120 students has been challenged on a number of grounds, not the least of which is need. On the national scene there were at least 60 graduate doctors unable to find internship positions in the recent Match.

The BCMA Body Mechanics Team wins the Sun Life Corporate Cup for 1983. Among its 13 members are Dr. Joanna Blaxland and Dr. Connie Lebrun.

August, 1983 Bill 24 to ration billing numbers is not acceptable to BCMA. It is the 25th anniversary of Health Insurance coming into effect in July, 1958.

Dr. Ernest Bowmer gave the VMA Osler Oration in August, 1983. His title was "Communicable Disease Influences History."

September, 1983 After a decade of controversy over the site and services, the new $58 million, 496-bed Victoria General Hospital opened on April 17, 1983.

In 1980, over the previous seven years, the rate of pregnancies of girls 14 and under had increased 33% in British Columbia.

President, B.C. Chapter, Physicians for Social Responsibility, Dr. Dorothy Goresky, was one of four Canadians in attendance at the third Congress of International Physicians for the Prevention of Nuclear War, held in the Netherlands in June.

October, 1983 Dr. Ellen Wiebe is the 1983–84 Past President of the College of Family Practice. Dr. Marlene Hunter, West Vancouver is the Secretary-treasurer and Dr. Evelyn Shukin, West Vancouver is member at large.

Dr. Elaine Kennedy, Port Coquitlam, writes in the *Journal* to draw attention to a recently published Amnesty International report on Chile: "Evidence of Torture." She states that the role played by doctors and paramedical staff in the torture of prisoners is in direct contravention of the World Medical Association's Declaration of Tokyo, and the recently adopted United Nations Principles of Medical Ethics.

The first adolescent psychiatric unit in the province is in operation in the Department of Psychiatry, Vancouver General Hospital.

Dr. Patricia Rebbeck writes: "Woman on the Editorial Board" describing her first Board meeting and her anxiety being in company of the Editor, Dr. A.F. Hardyment, and other learned members. She need not have worried as it ended happily!

November, 1983 Article for the *Journal*: "Maturation Index, A Cytological Technique for Hormonal Evaluation." Authors: George Robinson, MB, BS, FRCPC, Jean LeRiche, MB, BS, FRCPC, Jasenka Malisic MD, FRCPC, and Kenneth Suen, MD, FRCPC.

December, 1983 "Galactosemia Screening Introduced for All British Columbia Newborns," an article written by Dr. Margaret Norman, Director of C.H. Wills Newborn Screening Laboratory, Children's Hospital.

January, 1984 *Journal* article: "Botulism Exotoxin in Treatment of Strabismus and Blepharospasm," by Jean Carruthers MD, FRCSC, FRCS (London). Dr. Carruthers is a specialist in pediatric ophthalmology and ophthalmic genetics, an Associate Professor, Department of Genetics, and Clinical Associate Professor, Department of Ophthalmology, UBC.

February, 1984 *Journal* article: "Embolization of Post-traumatic Carotid-cavernous Fistulae" by authors Jocelyne Lapointe MD, FRCPC, Douglas Graeb MD, FRCPC, William Robertson MD, FRCPC, and Robert Nugent MD, FRCPC.

Dr. Jocelyne Lapointe is a diagnostic neurologist and Assistant Professor of Radiology at UBC.

Victoria Medical Society membership has increased from 80 in 1948 to 350 in 1984.

Journal article: "Percutaneous Transluminal Coronary Angioplasty: Initial Experience." Authors are Arthur Dodek MD, FRCPC, FRCP (Cardiology), CACC, Doris Kavanagh-Gray MD, FACC, FRCPC, Richard Hooper MD, FRCPC. Dr. Kavanagh-Gray is a cardiologist, St. Paul's Hospital and Clinical Professor, UBC.

March, 1984 Dr. Barbara McGillivray, MD, FCCMG, FRCPC writes an article for the *Journal*: "Medical Genetics and Adoption." Dr. McGillivray is a pediatrician and Clinical Professor, Department of Medical Genetics, UBC.

There are 5,500 physicians in British Columbia caring for 2.7 million people. There are 1,700 children in B.C. legally adopted.

Dr. Ellie Bertha Brisco, North Vancouver, was the catalyst behind the production of the film "The Journey," an antenatal film produced by the Department of Biomedical Communications at UBC, in association with the Perinatal Film Society of B.C. This film is a half-hour colour documentary, suitable for pre-natal classes, senior high school students, medical students, midwifery, and associated professionals. Dr. Brisco is on the staff at Lion's Gate Hospital.

April, 1984 The *Journal* gives praise to the Family Practice Department: "In Vancouver we rely heavily on support from the various hospital Family Practice Department heads: Alex Cherkezoff, VGH; Art Van Wart, St. Paul's Hospital; Gary Feinstadt, Grace Hospital; Ivor Mickleson, Shaughnessy Hospital; Adam Waldie, UBC-Health Sciences Hospital; and Gordon Robertson and Sylvia Henderson, co-ordinators of residency education, St. Vincent's Hospital. Other hospitals (Burnaby General, Lion's Gate, Richmond) provide sites where our residents obtain specialty rotations in medicine, surgery, psychiatry, and emergency. Dr. Clyde Slade, who retires in July, 1984, was the founder and developer of the Department of Family Practice at UBC in 1977."

An editorial by Dr. Patricia Rebbeck: "Time to Practise Good Medicine" stresses it is time to explain treatment and alternatives for treatment to the patient.

Dr. Carol Herbert at the Campus Unit at UBC and Dr. Sylvia Henderson with Dr. Gordon Robertson are active in teaching academic Family Medicine in the Family Practice Department at UBC.

The BCMA Annual Reports at the General Assembly included the Nutrition Committee report by representative, Dr. Hedy Fry, who also presented the report of the Convention subcommittee. Dr. Mary Burgess presented the report of the Federation of Medical Women, B.C. Branch; and Dr. Estelle Stevens reported for the Section of Psychiatry. Dr. Dorothy Shaw is on the Medical Advisory Committee of Planned Parenthood of British Columbia, and Dr. Anne (Patty) Vogel is on the Committee of Athletics and Recreation.

June, 1984 BCMA is lobbying the Government of British Columbia to accept the need to use restraints for children under six years of age when in automobiles.

Dr. Connie Lebrun as team captain of North Shore Narcoleptics won over eight other teams at the BCMA Annual Meet in Stanley Park.

Dr. Gerry Stewart is the BCMA President for 1984–1985.

July, 1984 Guest Editorial by Dr. Georgia Immega: "The Language of Childhood Sexual Abuse."

"Review of the Vancouver Sexual Assault Assessment Project," an article by Carol Herbert MD, Elizabeth Whynot MD, and Georgia Immega MD. Dr. Carol Herbert is an Assistant Professor, Department of Family Practice UBC and co-founder of Vancouver Sexual Assault Assessment Project. Dr. Elizabeth Whynot, a Medical Health Officer for the City of Vancouver, is a General Practitioner, a co-founder of the Sexual Assault Assessment Project, and a Clinical Instructor in the Department of Family Practice UBC. Dr. Georgia Immega is a General Practitioner in Vancouver, a member of the Sexual Assault Assessment Project, and a Clinical Instructor in the Department of Family Practice UBC.

The July *Journal* includes three more articles on child sexual abuse: "The Role of Primary Physicians in the Investigation of Child Sexual Abuse," by Georgia Immega MD; "Sexual Abuse in Children: a review of the first year's experience at Children's Hospital," by authors Jean Hlady MD, J.E. Carter MB, and D.F. Smith MD, "Behavioural Indicators of Sexual Abuse in Children and Adolescents," by Teresa Cope MD.

Canadian Medical Association Honorary Senior Membership was given to six doctors from British Columbia, including Dr. Margaret Elizabeth Patriarche of Victoria,

August, 1984 Bill 26, the Hospital Amalgamation Act, was introduced in May, 1984 by Health Minister Jim Nielson and was given final approval on the last day of the Spring session, May 16.

September, 1984 Cancer Control Agency of British Columbia's new 44-bed clinical facility, the A. Maxwell Evans Clinic, was officially opened in Vancouver on September 26th.

Dr. Lynn Beattie, Clinical Director of Geriatric Medicine at the Health Sciences Centre Hospital UBC, is the President-Elect of the American Geriatric Association.

The authors of the article "Nutrition and Cancer" include Ann Worth MD, FRCPC. Dr. Jocelyne Lapointe is a co-author of two articles on "Digital Subtraction Angiography." Dr. Hedy Fry is a delegate for BCMA, District #3 Vancouver.

October, 1984 An editorial by Dr. Patricia Rebbeck "A Bigger Share" states: "Women doctors in British Columbia are not pulling their weight. I do not mean that they are not doing enough medical practice. I mean that they are not doing their fair share in the medical organizations. Only a handful stand for office in BCMA, they are not represented on enough BCMA committees, and most important they are not represented in the College of Physicians and Surgeons of British Columbia." She writes, "I consider the absence of women doctors in office in the College to be the most serious omission because the College is the organization that deals directly with complaints from the public, and because a proportion of these complaints are of sexual abuse of female patients. The presence of another woman would give some comfort for the female complainant. The process of facing the court-like College hearing must be daunting for a female complainant."

A *Journal* article: "Acute Asthma," by Stephen Lam MD, FRCPC, and Moira Yeung MB, FRCPC. Dr. Yeung is an internist, Head, Respiratory Division, Vancouver General Hospital, and Professor UBC.

November, 1984 *Journal* article by Vera Frinton MD, FRCSC: "Cervical Cancer Screening: Pap Smear Positive: Next steps in Investigation." Dr. Frinton is an Obstetrician and Gynecologist practising in Vancouver.

An article: "The Physician and Palliative Care" by Jacqueline Fraser MB, ChB. Dr. Fraser is a Palliative Care physician at St. Paul's Hospital, Palliative Care Unit.

Dr. Carol Herbert writes on: "Behavioural Prescription in Family Medicine." Dr. Herbert is Director, Division of Behavioural Medicine, in addition to being Assistant Professor in the Department of Family Practice UBC.

December, 1984 The editorial by W.A. Dodd MD, titled "Too Many Groups" questioned the need for a separate organization for women, the Federation of Medical Women of Canada. (There were several responses later in the Personal View column of the March, 1985 *Journal*.)

January, 1985 Dr. Gerald Stewart is President of the British Columbia Medical Association.

In the January *Journal*: Statistics on Abortion in British Columbia: With Hospital Abortion Committee approval, before twelve weeks of gestation in the year 1983 to 1984, there were 9,147 abortions paid for by MSP at a cost of $942,000. After twelve weeks of gestation, with Hospital Abortion Committee approval, there were 1,948 procedures, paid by MSP at a cost of $333,000.

Dr. Hedy Fry is the only female BCMA Board member this year.

The *Journal* writes that the British Columbia's renal treatment program is one of the best in the world and B.C. has for many years been a pioneering area in the treatment of renal disease. Dr. John Price, Head, Division of Nephrology, Vancouver General Hospital and Professor of Medicine and Research, University of British Columbia, writes the history of renal disease treatment in B.C. from the time Dr. Russell Palmer had a machine built in 1951 to the design of the Dutch pioneer Dr. W.J. Koff's machine.

The training of patients for home hemodialysis was started in B.C. in 1967.

Approval of the construction of the Victoria Cancer Clinic was announced by Health Minister Jim Nielson.

February, 1985 *Journal* article: "Premenstrual Syndrome—A Review" by T.C. Rowe MB, BS, MRCOG, FRCSC and Shaila Misri MB, BS, FRCPC.

March, 1985 A message to the doctors of British Columbia about a psychiatrist, Dr. Fanny Pollarolo, being held in Chile was described by Annette Horton MB, BS, FRCPC and Janine O'Kane MB, FRCPC.

In reply to Dr. W.A. Dodd's editorial in the *BCMJ* of 1984, 26:784 making a plea for information as to why women physicians need their own medical organization, there were several replies to his comments. Dr. Vera Frinton wrote, "No Superwoman, I," and states: "It is because of such groups as the Federation of Medical Women of Canada that we Canadian women physicians have comparatively minor concerns compared to women physicians in other countries, who have no societies to demand and protect their rights." Dr. M. Elizabeth Patriarche of Victoria wrote, "I would suggest that the reason is mainly biological. It is not as yet possible for male physicians to become pregnant and bear children. The women's group provides a support network for sharing part-time post-graduate and part-time practice." Dr. Carol Herbert wrote, "Gentlemen, No Guilt, Please," and Dr. Shelley Ross and Dr. Susan Laubenstein of B.C. Branch FMWC executive, wrote, "The Federation of Medical Women of Canada Meets Unique Needs."

It was noted that the Medical Women's International Association held its Congress in Vancouver in August, 1984, and 600 women doctors from 43 countries attended. It was a great success, thanks to the local committee of the B.C. Branch FMWC.

April, 1985 In the *Journal* Dr. Patricia Rebbeck writes about "Thieving Patients" who do not keep up with their MSP premiums.

In the Annual Reports of the BCMA, Dr. Hedy Fry reported on the CMA Council on Health Care, and also reported on the Convention Sub-Committee. Dr. Susan Laubenstein reported for the B.C. Branch

FMWC. Women doctors on BCMA Committees include Dr. Bluma Tischler, the Mental Retardation Committee; Dr. Shirley Rushton and Dr. Anne Gagne, the Athletic and Recreation Committee; Dr. Carol Herbert, the Child Care Committee; Dr. Hedy Fry, the Nutrition Committee; and Dr. Susan West, the Prison Care Committee.

May, 1985 *Journal* article: "Changing Concepts in Early Childhood Autism" by Helena Ho, MD, CM, FRCPC. Dr. Ho is Assistant Professor, Department of Pediatrics UBC, and Co-ordinator, Child Development Program, B.C. Children's Hospital.

Dr. Doris Kavanagh-Gray was made a Prince of Good Fellows at the VMA Osler Dinner. Dr. Sheldon Naiman was the Osler Lecturer.

Justice Allan McEachern struck down the limitation of billing numbers proposal and enshrined in judicial precedent doctors' rights to freely move within the province to set up practice.

June, 1985 Dr. Gerry Karr assumed the duties as President of BCMA for 1985–1986.

Dr. Angela Penny has retired from the Victoria office of the Workers' Compensation Board.

July, 1985 Dr. Dorothy Goresky wrote an article: "Take Steps to Disarmament."

BCMA 16 member Body Mechanics Team won the YMCA Sunlife Corporate Cup for the third year in a row, outdoing 98 teams. Members of the team include Dr. Cheryl Mason, Dr. April Sanders, Dr. Shirley Schwab, Dr. Connie Lebrun, and Dr. Jennifer McCormick.

Two literary submissions tied for first place in the VMA first literary contest, and awards were given to Drs. Ronald Calderisi and Kirsten Emmott.

Medical offices in British Columbia are advised to use computers for their MSP billing.

The Canadian and Australian Royal Colleges of Physician and Surgeons will meet in Vancouver September 8–12, the biggest meeting of its kind. It is expected to draw more than 2,500 specialists, interns, and residents from North America, Australia, and other parts of the world.

Dr. B. Lynn Beattie, a Fellow of the Royal College of Physicians and Surgeons of Canada, took office as President of the American Geriatric Society at the 42nd Annual Meeting in New York, July 12, 1985. Dr. Beattie was born in Nelson, B.C., and graduated from UBC in 1965. In 1983 she became Associate Professor and Head, Division of Geriatric Medicine UBC. She also holds the posts of Clinical Director, Geriatric Medicine, Health Sciences Centre Hospital and Head, Department of Geriatrics and Continuing Care, Shaughnessy Hospital.

The in-vitro fertilization program has moved from the UBC campus to Shaughnessy Hospital. Heading the team is Dr. Victor Gomel, head of the Department of Gynecology at both UBC and Shaughnessy Hospitals.

Dr. Hedy Fry wrote for the *Journal* an article: "Be Aware of Eating Disorders as one in 100 to 200 Adolescent Females Are Affected."

August, 1985 *Journal* article by Carol Herbert, MD, CCFP: "Examination of the Sexually Assaulted Person."

Dr. Carol Herbert of Vancouver was one of six outstanding women honored by the YWCA for 1985. She was selected for her contributions in the area of health science and social services. Dr. Herbert is a family physician who has been involved in studies concerning sexual abuse, family violence, and stress management, and also has contributed significantly to the health care of immigrant families. She is Director of the Family Practice Behavioural Division of the Department of Family Practice, Faculty of Medicine, University of British Columbia.

An article by Millie Cumming MD, CCFP of Wrinch Memorial Hospital, Hazelton, B.C.: "No Smoking is feasible." She states that smoking has been banned in her hospital since 1972.

The approval of construction of the Victoria Cancer Clinic was announced by Health Minister Jim Nielson.

Dr. Hedy Fry has been elected Chairman of the Canadian Medical Association Council on Health Care.

September, 1985 *Journal* article: "Hepatitis B Prophylaxis." The authors are Linda Rebeneck MD, FRCPC and Noel Buskard MD, FRCPC, FACP.

Dr. Rebeneck is a Clinical Assistant Professor UBC and a member of the active staff in the Department of Medicine, St. Paul's Hospital.

October, 1985 The *Journal* has as a special topic: "Women in Medicine" with an article by M. Elizabeth Patriarche MD, "Vive La Difference!" With female enrolments in medical schools increasing from nine percent to 50% in the past 15 years, the author insists "that the role of women in medicine is no different than any other aspect of culture that prospers by the participation of both sexes." This topic "Vive La Difference" was the Listerian Oration by Dr. Patriarche for the Victoria Medical Society in 1982.

November, 1985 The Canada West Medical Congress is planned for June 29–July 5, 1986.

The Canadian Medical Association is opposed to home deliveries either by midwives or physicians (except where hospital-based care is not available).

There are 5,594 members of the British Columbia Medical Association. Of interest, there are 135 earning spousal members (women doctors).

At a special meeting on October 19, 1985 there was a proposal made to relocate the BCMA offices to 1665 West Broadway.

December, 1985 "Doctor, Doctor," BCMA's weekly half-hour TV show, has been on the air for 10 weeks of its 26-week run. Dr. Art Hister and Barbara Constantine chair the program, and three Vancouver physicians appear as weekly columnists: Dr. Paul Kent on sports medicine, Dr. Hedy Fry on medical issues relating to women, and Dr. Peter Grantham on diet and nutrition.

January, 1986 Article: "Conservative Breast Surgery." The twelve authors include Dr. Ann Worth, Pathologist with the B.C. Cancer Agency; Dr. Vivien Basco, radiation oncologist at the B.C. Cancer Agency; and Dr. Patricia Rebbeck, surgeon at St.Vincent's Hospital and Health Sciences Centre UBC.

February, 1986 Several articles in the February *BCMJ* by women doctors, reflecting the great increase of women in medicine.

An article: "Food and Fluids During Labour" by M. Joanne Douglas MD, FRCP(C) and Graham McMorland MD, FRCP(C).

"Epidural Analgesia During Labour; Alternative Methods of Labour Analgesia," an article by Margaret Bylsma-Howell MD, FRCPC; Renata G. Matthias MD, FRCPC; and Joanne Douglas MD, FRCPC.

Article: "Guidelines of Caesarean Section" by Gillian Moll MB, ChB, FRCP(C) and Susan Leacock MD, FRCP(C), both of Victoria, B.C.

"Are Your Labour and Delivery Rooms Safe?" by Peggy Ross MD, BSc (Meds), FRCP(C), and Jean Swenerton MD, FRCPC.

Article "Drugs and Sports: What Doctors Should Know" by Ann Gagne MD, Chairman, Athletics and Recreation Committee.

Vancouver General Hospital Lithotropter Unit opened in November, 1986.

Department of Pediatrics is now centralized at Children's Hospital. There were 8,000 patients admitted with 80,000 patient days; 8,000 operations, 70% as Day-Care surgery; 80,000 OPD patients, and 20,000 through Emergency. The Department of Pediatrics includes 33 geographic full-time hospital doctors and 67 clinical faculty. Ten of the latter are hospital-based, reflecting an increasing requirement in tertiary care institutions for full-time hospital doctors in addition to geographic full-time university faculty.

March, 1986 The VMA Osler Lecturer for 1986 is Dr. Patricia Rebbeck.

There are 6,069 practising doctors in British Columbia.

The manufacturer of the Dalkin Shield is advising that patients injured by use of the Dalkin Shield may file a claim.

Dr. Ruth Issacsen died in February, 1986.

April, 1986 Stephen Rogers is the Health Minister, replacing Jim Nielsen who was the longest serving Health Minister in Canada, who now becomes the Minister of Human Resources.

An article re Bill 41, by Dr. Pat Rebbeck: "The Profession Needs the Young." She thinks the Government should be encouraging older doctors to retire to make way for the young.

May, 1986 *Journal* article: "Aids: Introduction and Management Approach for Primary Physicians." Authors: W. Allistair McLeod MD, FRCPC; Hilary Wass MD, FRCPC; Linda Rebenek MD, FRCPC. Of the 400 Canadians diagnosed with Aids, 100 are in British Columbia.

Dr. Margaret Mullinger received the Primus Inter Pares (First Among Equals) award, an honour given her at the Osler Dinner, along with Drs. Phil Ashmore and Jack Whitelaw. The award was formerly known as the Prince of Good Fellows. Dr. Patricia Rebbeck was the Osler Lecturer. Her topic was "Communications: Things Osler Never Taught Me."

The British Columbia Medical Association relocates to 1665 West Broadway, Vancouver.

Dr. Pat Rebbeck is now a member of Council of the College of Physicians and Surgeons.

Dr. Eve Gulliford of Salmon Arm, B.C. writes in the Personal View column of the *Journal* that she is against the decision that BCMA does not endorse PSR (Physicians for Social Responsibility). She states, "The PSR membership is increasing. We happen to be part of the Nobel Prize winner group and that should make the BCMA proud of us, if you were not so biased. Perhaps you should raise your sights."

Dr. Gerry Karr is the President of BCMA.

Several women doctors are on BCMA Committees as noted in the reports of the BCMA Annual Meeting: Dr. Lynn Beattie of the Geriatrics Committee; Dr. Bluma Tischler and Dr. Kathleen Carter (Chairman) of the Mental Retardation Committee; Dr. Hedy Fry and Dr. Kathy Caidenhead of the Nutrition Committee; Dr. Evelyn Shukin and Dr. Mary Burgess of the Constitution and By-laws Committee; and Dr. Beverley Tamboline is on the Committee of Salaried Physicians. Dr. Dorothy Wishart reported on the B.C. Branch Federation of Medical Women of Canada; Dr. Ann Worth and Dr. Linda Warren are members of the Accreditation for Clinical Labs Committee; Dr. Alice Suiker, Committee of Public Affairs; and Dr. Hedy Fry, Communications Committee. The Athletics and Recreation Committee members include the following women: Dr. Ann Gagne, Dr. Paula Gordon, Dr. Shirley Rushton, and Dr. Anne Vogel. Dr. Carol Herbert is a member of the Child Care Committee, and Dr. Doris Kavanagh-Gray is continuing on the sub-committee on Cardiac Care which is part of the Pro-

fessional Advisory Committee to the Minister of Health. Of the Sections of BCMA, Dr. Annette Lam is Secretary-Treasurer of the Section of Dermatology; Dr. Marion Tipple is Vice-President of the Section of Pediatrics.

The incoming President of BCMA is Dr. John O'Brien-Bell for 1986–87. Dr. Hedy Fry is a District #3 delegate to BCMA.

June, 1986 The *Journal* articles were on: "Sleep and its Disorders."

July, 1986 Dr. Annette Horton writes that a group of concerned professionals, including several Vancouver psychiatrists, is interested in forming a treatment centre for people who have been tortured. It will depend on proving there is a need.

The Canada West Medical Congress was a huge success, the largest ever hosted by the BCMA. More than 1,200 doctors were registered. Sir Roger Bannister was one of the five renowned guest speakers.

WCB gave $270,000 for research into Occupational Diseases. Dr. Moira Yeung heads the UBC Research Unit responsible for the studies.

August, 1986 Dr. Archie Hardyment, who has been Editor of the *BCMA Journal* for the past eight years, retires as Editor.

The Council on Health Promotion: Dr. Marion Tipple writes: "Fecal Coliform Levels . . . What Do They Really Mean?" Dr. Tipple is Chairman, Sewage Disposal Sub-committee of the Environmental Health Committee. She recommends that the B.C. Ministry of Health review its water quality monitoring standards and consider changing from fecal coliforms to Enterococci or E coli standards.

September, 1986 Dr. Dorothy Goresky writes an article on "Psychological Aspects of a Nuclear Arms Race." Dr. Goresky is Past President of Physicians for Social Responsibility (Canada) and a President of the B.C. Chapter.

October, 1986 Guest Editorial: "Pediatric Trauma: Physician's Role in Prevention" by Judith Vestrup MD, FRCS(C). Dr. Vestrup is Director of Trauma at Vancouver General Hospital and Assistant Professor, Department of Surgery, UBC.

November, 1986 *Journal* articles on Genetics. Dr. Judith Hall writes "The Impact of Genetics on Daily Medical Practice." Dr. Hall is Director UBC Clinical Genetic Services, Grace Hospital, Vancouver.

Dr. Dagmar Kalousek writes on "New Developments in Chromosome Studies as they Relate to Cancer." Dr. Kalousek is Associate Professor of Pathology, UBC, and program head Cytogenetics and Embryo Pathology, B.C. Children's Hospital.

Dr. Pat Rebbeck writes an article on "Rudeness of Doctors Compromises Care."

The new President of the Vancouver Medical Association is Dr. Roberta Ongley.

December, 1986 *Journal* articles: "Biopsychosocial Model" by Dr. Carol Herbert, CCFP, FCFP.

"Food Irradiation" by Dr. Hedy Fry who stressed limitation of irradiation.

A history note: Internship was made mandatory in 1935 by the Royal College of Physicians and Surgeons of Canada.

Peter Dueck is now the Health Minister.

Dr. Gail Harvey has joined the Workers' Compensation Board in the Claims Unit 1.

Dr. Margaret Norman has written an "Update on Newborn Screening: Biotinidase Deficiency." Dr. Norman is Director of C.H. Wills Newborn Screening Laboratory.

January, 1987 In the Personal View column of the *Journal*, Dr. Marlene Hunter, who has been very much involved with the practice of Hypnosis and Hypnotherapy for the past 14 years, has written that she is very concerned over the Hypnotherapy advertising. The *BCMJ* is an ideal forum for the presentation of such concern about lay Hypnotherapists.

In the January *Journal* there are eight pages of advertisements for Rogaine topical solution for baldness.

Interesting statistics about the changing population of B.C. noted in the article on "Cancer in British Columbia." In 1983 in B.C. there were 1,402,000 males and 1,421,000 females. B.C. population increased by 29% since 1971. Of this increase only 15% were Canadian. British Columbia consistently had the oldest population in Canada, median age being 32.1 years in 1983. The proportion of British origin population declined from 58% in 1971 to 51% in 1981. About 78% of the population of B.C. is urban. Women's share of the labour force increased from 39% in 1971 to 52% in 1981.

February, 1987 Shirley Baker-Thomas MD, FRCPC writes on: "Court Order Creates Crisis." This court order demands clinical records of patients from doctors and if a doctor is not compliant, a court order with costs is sent.

It is disturbing to many doctors to watch the word "client" becoming more popular, replacing the word "patient."

Dr. Frank Turnbull writes an interesting article: "Starting a Medical School in British Columbia."

From the Victoria File in the *Journal*: The proposed five-year phase-out of Riverview Hospital caused so much reaction that the Minister of Health, Peter Dueck, felt compelled to make a ministerial statement to explain the draft plan of the Mental Health Consultation Report, which was the result of two years of study. Mr. Dueck assured the House that "We will not release people (Riverview patients) into the community and not have a place for them to go."

Journal article: "Medical Genetic Services in B.C." by Patricia Baird MD, CM, FRCPC, FCCPC, FCCMG. Dr. Baird is Professor and Head of the Departments of Medical Genetics at the Grace Hospital and at University of British Columbia.

"Fragile X Mental Retardation," an article by Barbara McGillivray MD, BSc. Dr. McGillivray is Assistant Professor and Co-Director of the Prenatal Diagnosis Program in the Departments of Medical Genetics, Grace Hospital, and University of British Columbia.

Mammography screening has the potential to reduce deaths from breast cancer by 1,000 a year in Canada.

In Memorium: Dr. Marguerite B. Shea Carrol and Dr. Valentina Marken.

March, 1987 *Journal* article: "Osteoporosis and the Menopause." Authors Dr. Eugene Cameron, Dr. Roger Sutton, and Dr. Jerilynn Prior are members of the Faculty of Medicine UBC.

Another article: "Psychological Issues Associated with the Menopause" by Shaila Misri MD, FRCPC. Dr. Misri is a practising psychiatrist and Clinical Assistant Professor, Department of Psychiatry and of Obstetrics and Gynecology, Faculty of Medicine, UBC.

April, 1987 Editorials discussed early retirement and Bill 41 (restriction of billing numbers).

Dr. Gordon Fahrni is 100 years old, and is interviewed for the *Journal* by Dr. C.E. McDonnell.

Article on "Ritalin for Attention Deficit Disorder with Hyperactivity" by Dr. Tanya Wulff, *et al.*

May, 1987 *Journal* article "Differential Leukocyte Counting" by Deborah J. Griswold MD, FRCP(C), who is a pathologist at Royal Columbian Hospital.

It was announced by the Minister of Health, Jake Epp, that Dr. Patricia Baird, Professor and Head, Department of Medical Genetics at UBC, has been appointed to the Medical Research Council of Canada for three years.

Dr. David Boyes retires as Director of the Cancer Control Agency.

In the Personal View column, Doctors V.H.A. Black, K. Jokhani, D.P.Y. Loh, Estelle Stevens, and Tanya Wulff discuss treatment with Ritalin (methylphenidate) for ADDH (Attention Deficit Disorder with Hyperactivity).

Vancouver Medical Association recognized the contribution of three outstanding members with Primus Inter Pares (first among equals) degrees on March 19, 1987: Dr. C.E. McDonnell, Dr. Beverley Tamboline, and Dr. William Thomas. The occasion was the Osler Dinner. Dr. W.A. Dodd gave the Osler Oration. The VMA President is Dr. Roberta Ongley.

June, 1987 Judith L. Issac-Renton MD, DPH, wrote on "Giardiasis: A Review." She is an Assistant Professor of Microbiology at UBC.

Dr. Ann Gagne of the Council on Health Promotion wrote on "Cyclists and Helmet Use."

July, 1987 Dr. Katherine Carter MB, ChB, of the Mental Retardation Committee of the Council of Health Promotion, writes on the contentious issue "Selective Abortion: Now is the time for reflection," and ends with,

"After all, who among us can claim that we are the 'perfect' child our parents expected when we were in the womb."

August, 1987 Opposition to Bill 41, which restricts billing numbers, was stated in letters to the *Journal*.

October, 1987 Editorial "From Bad to Worse" by Dr. Patricia Rebbeck criticizes Bill 34, which gives the Minister of Health or his agents the right to obtain confidential records such as those from doctors' offices.

November, 1987 Chairman of the General Assembly is Dr. Hedy Fry. The President of BCMA is Dr. David Jones. At the BCMA Annual General Meeting it was noted that Dr. Mary Donlevy of Burnaby was the only female member who spoke in the all-morning voting for counselling in malpractice lawsuits.

December, 1987 At the BCMA Annual Meeting in Victoria, B.C. in October, 1987 the Annual Reports were presented and later printed in the December *Journal*. In the lists of Annual reports the following women are on committees: Dr. Hedy Fry, CMA Council on Health Care; Dr. Carol Herbert, Child Care Committee; Dr. Bluma Tischler, Mental Retardation Committee; Dr. Hedy Fry, Nutrition; Dr. Karen Kruse, Occupational Health Committee; Dr. Barbara Allan and Dr. Jacqueline Fraser, Palliative Care; Dr. Joanne Blaxland, Dr. Ann Gagne, Dr. Paula Gordon, Dr. Connie Lebrun, and Dr. Shirley Rushton, Athletics and Recreation Committee; Dr. Mary Burgess and Dr. Evelyn Shukin, Constitution and By-Laws Committee; Dr. Roberta Ongley, Medical Services Commission Liaison; Dr. Hedy Fry, Allied Health; Dr. Patricia Rebbeck, *B.C. Medical Journal*; Dr. Linda Warren, Cancer; Dr. Virginia Kilby, Communications; Dr. Shirley Reimer, Insurance; Dr. Alice Suiker, Public Affairs; Dr. Barbara Baxter, B.C. Branch FMWC; Dr. Lynn Simpson, Chairman of the Section of Obstetrics and Gynecology; Dr. Lynn Beattie, Geriatrics Committee; Dr. Anne (Patty) Vogel, Chairman of the Annual Meeting Convention; Dr. Patricia Rebbeck, member of the Council, College of Physicians and Surgeons of British Columbia; Dr. Doris Kavanagh-Gray, consultant for cardiac care, a subcommittee of the Professional Advisory Committee to the

Ministry of Health; Dr. Marion Tipple, President of Section of Pediatrics; Dr. Debbie Griswold, Dr. Ann Skidmore, and Dr. Ann Worth on the sub-committee on Accreditation for Clinical Labs; Dr. Janet Kusler, on the Impaired Physicians Committee.

The 1987–1988 Executive members of the B.C. Branch Federation of Medical Women of Canada: President, Dr. Barbara Baxter; Past-President, Dr. Dorothy Wishart; Vice-President, Dr. Mary Donlevy; Secretary, Dr. Peggy Lundeville; Treasurer, Dr. Jean Swenerton; Members at Large, Drs. Gillian Arsenault, Lois Davies, Robin Gunn, Georgia Immega, Susan Laubenstein, Shirley Reimer, Patricia Warshawski, and Denise Werker.

January, 1988 Bill 34: It appeared that any research organization could get access to medical records, but the Bill made it clear that only the Cancer Control Agency of British Columbia could demand records for research.

Bill 41: Restriction of billing numbers is still being criticized as it has not helped the northern areas. Young doctors refuse to go north.

In the January *BCMJ* there are 10 articles on Oncology and the Cancer Institute.

Dr. Vivien Basco MB, ChB, FRCPC, FRCR, writes on "Plans and Prediction for CCABC" (Cancer Control Agency of British Columbia). Dr. Basco is chairman of the Breast Tumor Group, and a Radiation Oncologist at the Cancer Control Agency of British Columbia.

February, 1988 Editorial by Dr. Pat Rebbeck on "An MD's Workload" stressing the too-long hours on duty.

Journal article "Early Detection of Breast Cancer" by Dr. Linda Warren Burhenne MD, who is Clinical Associate Professor in the Department of Radiology at UBC.

Dr. Vivien Basco wrote the Guest Editorial on "Mammography." In 1985, 1,553 females were diagnosed as having invasive breast cancer; 461 died.

BCMA members are 64% General Practitioners and 36% Specialists. An Association for Specialists has been organized, and will be another Section in the BCMA.

March, 1988 *Journal* article by Stephen Wood PhD, James S. Popkin MD, and Barbara McGillivray MD on "Duchenne Muscular Dystrophy: Carrier Detection and Prenatal Diagnosis." Drs. Wood and McGillivray are with the Department of Medical Genetics at UBC and Dr. Popkin is with the Medical Genetics Service at Victoria General Hospital.

Letters from members of BCMA on the abortion issue appeared in the March *Journal* following the announcement of the B.C. Government that there is a lack of funding for abortion services, were critical of the weak stand of the BCMA and the President, Dr. David Jones. Dr. Frances Rosenberg and Dr. Mary Donlevy, President of the B.C. Branch FMWC, wrote letters asking why the BCMA has not spoken out against the recent action of the B.C. Government.

Margaret Norman MD, Director of C.H. Wills Newborn Screening Program, Children's Hospital announced, that, as of January, 1988, B.C. Children's Hospital started using a primary TSH screen with immuno-fluorescent assay to screen for congenital hypothyroidism. This takes fewer laboratory days for diagnosis than radio immunoassay.

Dr. Martha L. Donnelly has been appointed the Mount Pleasant Legion Professor of Community Geriatrics UBC, succeeding Dr. Richard Ham.

April, 1988 *Journal* articles: "Depression in the Elderly" by Martha Donnelly MD, CCFP, FRCPC, Director of the Short-term Assessment and Treatment Centre at the Vancouver General Hospital. "Confusion, Delerium, and Dementia" by B. Lynn Beattie, MD, FRCPC, who is Head of the Division of Geriatric Medicine, UBC, the Department of Geriatrics at Shaughnessy Hospital, and also Clinical Director of the Alzheimer's Clinic at UBC Health Centre.

The abortion issue dominated the Legislature under Premier Vander Zalm during the month of February.

In the Personal View column, Dr. Denise Werker writes her views on BCMA and Abortion.

Dr. Mary Donlevy urges BCMA adopt non-sexist language in its communications. The *BCMJ* of the BCMA as a whole supports the principle of non-sexist language in its communications.

An article "The Poorly Motivated in Acute Care" by Lyn MacBeath MD, FRCPC, who is Director of Psychiatry for the Elderly Program at the Greater Victoria Hospital Society.

May, 1988 Theresa K. Isomura MD, FRCPC and Michael Myers MD, FRCPC write on "Women Doctors and Their Relationships."

Dr. Carol Herbert writes on "Family Medicine Research: Alive and Well in B.C."

"Gene Therapy": Dr. Pat Baird, Chairman of the Medical Research Council's new committee on guidelines for human gene therapy, invites comments and input from physicians and others with a position or suggestions on gene therapy.

Judith Hall, MD, FRCP, Professor of Medical Genetics and Director of Clinical Genetics Services at UBC, is on a Sabbatical year at Oxford University, July, 1988 to June, 1989 studying genetic animal modules, to explain the homologies with humans using human congenital anomaly syndromes.

Linda Rebeneck MD, FRCPC, a gastroenterologist at St. Paul's Hospital in Vancouver and Clinical Assistant Professor at the University of British Columbia, has been awarded a Detweiler Travel Fellowship to enable her to do a two-year Sabbatical at Yale University School of Medicine in gastrointestinal research.

June, 1988 Dr. Pat Rebbeck announces, "Good News: The Government supports the Breast Screening Program." The Director of the Breast Tumor Group is Dr. Vivien Basco. Women over 40 years of age in Greater Vancouver are invited to participate in the first mammography screening pilot project in Canada.

Journal article on "Strep Tests" by Alison Clarke MD, FRCPC, Chairman, B.C. Chapter of the Canadian Association of Microbiologists, and Chairman, Microbiology Science Section B.C. Association of Laboratory Physicians.

The following was part of the BCMA brief to the Royal Commission on Education: "The Challenge of Living: Schooling for Health and Competency," and was the work of the BCMA School Ad Hoc Committee chaired by Dr. Hedy Fry, Chairman of the Council on Health Promotion. Committee members included Drs. Fred Bass, Andrew McNab, Bill Mackie, Kate Parfitt, and Susan West, each representing a committee or specialty concerned with education and /or child health.

There will be a mandatory health curriculum developed and implemented in all B.C. schools, for all students in the province.

Planning and fundraising is under way for the University of British Columbia Medical Student and Alumni Centre.

July, 1988 Article on "Seatbelt Injury" by authors Jean Hlady MD, FRCPC, D.F. Smith MD, FRCPC, and G.C. Fraser MB, ChB, FRCS(E). Dr. Fraser is a pediatric surgeon on staff at Children's Hospital where Drs. Hlady and Smith are staff physicians.

An article on Aids Update: "Gastrointestinal Manifestations of Aids" by Linda Rebeneck MD, FRCPC, Clinical Assistant Professor, Faculty of Medicine UBC, and M.L. Reckart MD, DTM&H, FRCPC, Director STD Control, B.C. Ministry of Health.

August, 1988 From the Victoria File, *BCMJ*: Although UBC graduates 120 doctors per year, according to the Minister of Health Mr. Peter Dueck, 228 permanent billing numbers were given out last year, with only 41 UBC graduates receiving permanent billing numbers.

VMA Osler Lecturer is Dr. Wallace Chung, whose topic is "Osler and Multiculturism."

September, 1988 *Journal* article "Rheumatology Referral: Is It Necessary?" The author is Alice Klinkhoff MD, FRCPC who is a consultant rheumatologist at St. Paul's Hospital, and is on staff at the Vancouver Arthritis Centre. She states that the family doctor is able to deal with many musculoskeletal problems without referral.

Article: "Shoulder Pain in Practice" by A. Caroline Patterson MB, FRCPC. Dr. Patterson is Associate Medical Director of the Arthritis Society of British Columbia and Yukon Division and a rheumatologist at Vancouver General Hospital.

Article: "Rheumatology Disease: A View from General Practice" by Gwen Warren MD, CCFP, who is a family physician in White Rock, B.C.

Aids Update: "Blood Donor Screening and the Lookback Program" by

Penny Ballem MD, FRCPC, Deputy Director Canadian Red Cross Society Blood Transfusion Service, Vancouver, and Clinical Associate Professor, Faculty of Medicine UBC.

M.L. Reckart MD, Nasir Jetha MD (co-chairman of Lower Mainland Campaign), and Roberta Ongley MD urge doctors to donate to United Way.

Re: Bill 41: B.C. Court of Appeal decided that the Government's rules restricting the issue of Medicare billing numbers were "so procedurally flawed, manifestly unfair in substance that they violated doctors' constitutional rights." The primary moving forces behind the legal challenge have been PARI and the BCMA. PARI was represented by the named parties Dr. Peter Wilson and Dr. Christyanne Maxson, and BCMA by Dr. Jo Ann Arnason, Dr. Graham Conway, Dr. David Lee Williams, and Dr. Raymond Sui Hong Kwan.

From 1963 to 1987 there were 15 cases of leukemia occurring in patients with hypopituitarism treated with Growth Hormone. In Canada 1,047 children have received human or biosynthetic Growth Hormone in the past 22 years.

Dr. Carol Herbert has been appointed Royal Canadian Legion Professor and Head of the Department of Family Practice, UBC as of July, 1988. Born in Vancouver, B.C., she obtained a BSc from UBC in honours biochemistry concurrently with her first year of Medical School, graduating with an MD in 1969. She interned at St. Paul's Hospital and did a six-month pediatric Residency at Vancouver General Hospital. She practised as a family physician at the Reach Centre from 1971–1982. In 1982 she became a full-time faculty member of UBC.

October, 1988 Article by Dr. Cindi Clark and Dr. Pam Doig "Ski Injuries at Whistler."

A winning article of Health Care Research Foundation Competition was "Outcome Study of Brief Hospitalization of Psychiatrically Disordered Children" by Drs. Susan Penfold, Lynn Doyle, and R.S. Manley.

November, 1988 In the Personal View column of the *Journal* Dr. Mary Trott of Williams Lake, B.C. writes a letter about the lack of locums in rural areas. Dr. Trott is a radiologist covering a large area surrounding Williams Lake.

BCMA Annual Meeting was held in October. The new BCMA President is Dr. David Blair. The Chair of the General Assembly is Dr. Hedy Fry. New BCMA Board members are delegates Barbara Kane MD, FRCP and David Gray MD.

December, 1988 Article "Self-Help Groups" by Carol Herbert MD, CCFP, FDFP and Barbara Grantham BA (Hons), MA (PAdm).

BCMA Annual Reports include: Dr. Kathleen Carter reports for the Committee on Gender Issues; Dr. Hedy Fry reports on the CMA Council on Health Care and the report of the Council on Health Promotion; Dr. Mary Donlevy reports on the B.C. Branch FMWC; and Dr. Lynn Simpson, Chair for the Section of Obstetrics and Gynecology, reports for the Section.

January, 1989 Dr. T.F. Handley assumes the post of Registrar for the College of Physicians and Surgeons of British Columbia January 1, 1989.

Dr. Hedy Fry, Chair of the Council on Health Promotion, announces a conference on "Preparing for a Healthier Tomorrow" to take place January 27th, 1989.

A poem "Manikin," by Dr. Kirsten Emmott of Vancouver is printed in the *Journal* from her chapbook: *Are We There Yet*, published by $Dollar Poems$, Brandon, Manitoba.

February, 1989 An article by Verity Livingstone MB, CCFP, IBCLC, Director of Vancouver Breastfeeding Centre, and Kathleen Caidenhead MD, CCFP, Chair of the Nutrition Committee of BCMA.

March, 1989 *Journal* articles are mainly on Anorexia and Bulemia.

Ophthalmologists Drs. Perry Maerov and Jean Carruthers of Vancouver object to the insertion of an announcement by the B.C. Optometric Association in the December issue of an invitation to physicians to a seminar on eye disease given by an optometrist.

April, 1989 *Journal* article by Penny Ballem MD, FRCPC, "Platelet Disorders and Transfusion Therapy." Dr. Ballem is Deputy Medical Director, Canadian Red Cross Society Blood Transfusion Service, and Clinical Assistant Professor Department of Medicine, Division of Hematology UBC.

Another article by Enid Edwards MD, FRCPC: "Autologous Blood Transfusions." Dr. Edwards is a pathologist at St. Vincent's Hospital and former member of Canadian Red Cross Sub-committee Transfusion Services.

Dr. Shirley Baker Thomas notes that there were many errors in the first few months of Computerized Billing.

Shaughnessy Hospital joined UBC Health Sciences Centre in 1988 and is now called University Hospital, Shaughnessy Site.

Dr. C.E. Robinson MD, FRCPC writes in the *Journal*: "The History of Shaughnessy Hospital 1918–1974." The Federal Government, Department of Veterans Affairs was in charge of the hospital until 1974 when it was transferred to British Columbia as a Community Hospital.

May, 1989 Dr. Joan Ford, a family practitioner in Burnaby, writes an interesting account of "A Day in Nepal" where she has worked as a locum at Kundi, Nepal on five different occasions.

Dr. Kathleen Caidenhead writes on "Diet and Cancer."

The President of Vancouver Medical Association is now Dr. Hedy Fry.

At the VMA Osler Dinner, Dr. Roberta Ongley and Dr. Clement Beckett were the recipients of Primus Inter Pares awards. The Dean of Medicine, Dr. William Webber, was the Osler Lecturer, and his topic was "Osler and Present Day Health Care."

Dr. Tom Perry won a seat as NDP MLA in the Legislature and was sworn in April 14, 1989.

June, 1989 Dr. Pat Rebbeck calls her protest "Out of Joint" after hearing that the University of Victoria is opening a Faculty of Chiropractic.

July, 1989 Lynn Doyle MD, FRCSC, writes on "The Diagnosis of DVT" (deep vein thrombosis).

September, 1989 Guest Editorial and article for the *Journal*: "Psychiatry and Obstetrics Clinical Interface" by Shaila Misri MD, FRCPC, Associate Clinical Professor of Obstetrics and Gynecology, University Hospital, Shaughnesy Site, Director Psychosomatic Obstetrics and Gynecology Clinic, Grace Hospital; and she also writes another article "Psychiatric Disorders in Pregnancy."

Journal article: "Postpartum Disorders" by Kristin Sivertz MD, FRCPC, Clinical Associate Professor, Department of Psychiatry UBC, and Consultant at Grace Hospital.

October, 1989 Dr. William Webber, after 13 years as Dean of Medicine, UBC steps down.

In the *Journal* an interview with the new President of BCMA, John Anderson MD, by Editorial Board member Dr. C.E. McDonnell and Managing Editor Polly Thompson.

November, 1989 *Journal* article "Laser-assisted Balloon Angioplasty" by Peter Fry MB, FRCSC, FRCS(I), Lynn Doyle MD, FRCSC, and York N. Hsiang MB, FRCSC. Dr. Peter Fry is Clinical Associate Professor of Surgery and Head of the Division of Vascular Surgery, University Hospital, Vancouver. Drs. Doyle and Hsiang are Clinical Assistant Professors in the same Division.

FMWC B.C. Branch President wants BCMA to address Child Care for the profession as well as for the public.

Clinical Research: Aids: The multicentre Canadian AZT (azidothymidine) Trial is investigating the nature, dose, and natural course of the drug zidovudine (previously known as AZT) in 72 subjects in earlier stages of HIV infection. The study is nationally based in Montreal, Toronto, and Vancouver. (Dr. Karen Gelmon is one of the researchers.)

In Clinical Research, Dr. Penny Ballem is currently studying the pathophysiology of the thrombocytopenia syndrome often seen in HIV infected patients. Recently, this study has been expanded to look at the mechanism of action of zidovudine in those subjects

December, 1989 BCMA Section and Committee reports included Dr.

Roberta Ongley's report for the Section of Dermatology; Dr. Barbara Kane's report for the Section of Psychiatry; and Dr. Hedy Fry gave her report for the Council on Health Care. B.C. Branch FMWC report was given by Dr. Jean Swenerton. Committee reports were as follows: Dr. Kathleen Carter's report for the Developmental Handicapped Committee, and Dr. Kathleen Caidenhead's report for the Nutrition Committee. As in 1988 there were many women doctors who were members of BCMA committees, some for several years.

Dr. Hedy Fry is Chair of the General Assembly.

In the reorganization of the Health Ministry's Community and Family Health Services Division, the most notable change is the addition of a Health Promotion Office under Dr. Patricia Wolczuk, who reports to the Deputy Minister of Health Mr. Stan Dubas.

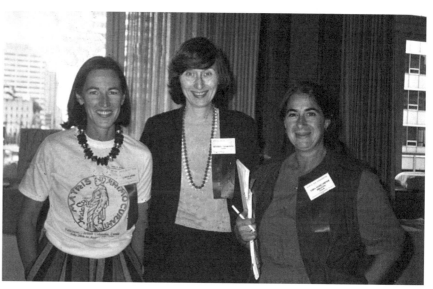

Dr. Lori Kanke, Dr. Beverley Tamboline (1963), Dr. Vera Frinton (1969) at the MWIA Congress in 1984

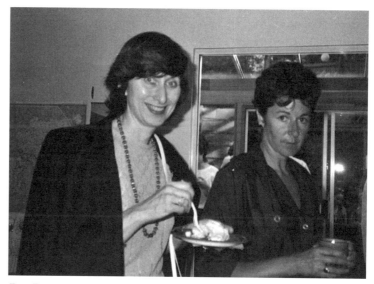

Dr. Beverley Tamboline (1963) and Dr. Mary Burgess at MWIA reception, 1984

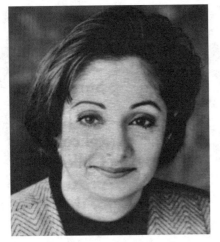

Dr. Rozmin Kamani, 1980

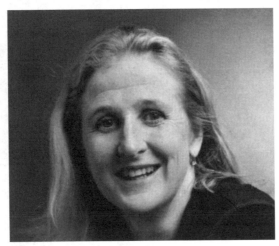

Dr. Chris Loock, 1981

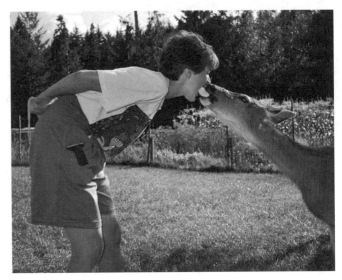

Dr. Doreen Tetz, 1983

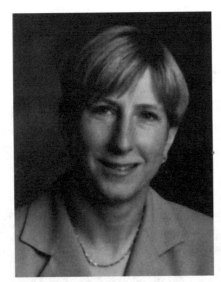

Dr. Heidi Oetter, 1985

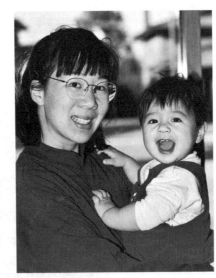

Dr. Alice Huang, 1988

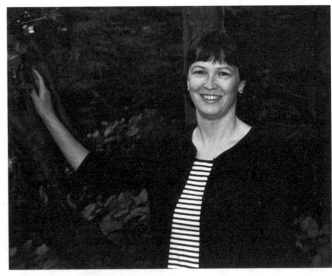

Dr. Davinia Kazanowski, 1989

Stories from **1990 – 1993**

This 100-uear history ends with 1993.

1990
Dr. Carmen Jadick
Dr. Davina Kazanowski
Dr. Frieda Justina Reddekop
1991
Dr. Pauline Alakija
Dr. Jane Hailey
Dr. Marian Catherine Cushing Reed
1992
Dr. Maria Daszkiewicz
Dr. Susan Finch
Dr. Marie Hay
Dr. Aileen McConnell
Dr. Heidi Martins
Dr. Ruth Joy Simkin
Dr. Sallie Jean Teasdale-Scott
Dr. Liz Zubek
1993
Dr. Deborah Bircham
Dr. Janice Mason
Dr. Stacey Leigh McDonald
Dr. Mary Wall
Dr. Marianne Willis

DR. CARMEN JADICK

In high school I was interested in sciences, but none of my friends were; it wasn't really a popular thing to do. I graduated with a specialty in both arts and science. I was not the most dedicated student. I hardly ever did homework because I had to walk to school and avoided bringing my books home as they were heavy to carry. My friend and I used to design dress patterns in biology instead of looking for things under the microscope. I was adjusting the bunsen burner in Chemistry and it fell apart, causing a gas fire in the lab that went right up to the gas outlet. Our teacher was a short Japanese man who used to work in a research lab and was not used to teaching high school; he got so excited he jumped up on the lab bench. I generally found high school boring and usually read a novel a day during class. I remember taking an aptitude test and it said I would have a good career as a rancher. I couldn't really relate to that as I had grown up in Vancouver. Counsellors said if you liked sciences you should go into nursing; you have to be really smart to go into medicine. So I entered nursing at St. Joseph's School of Nursing in Victoria. I worked in CCU, then ended up in ER, which I liked, but I came to the realization that I could keep up with these so-called geniuses I was working with. It quickly got frustrating for me to watch interns struggle to figure things out so they could order me to do things I thought should be done. It was even worse when they did not get it, like when they couldn't realize by looking at the patient or hearing the history that this person was sick and needed things done urgently. I watched a man walk in with severe low back pain, really high blood pressure, looking shocky and ill, rupture his abdominal aortic aneursym in front of me, because I couldn't get the ER doctor to attend him.

So I started taking science courses at college to make up for the things I missed in high school, still working in ER. That summer I got married and my husband was apparently all in favour of my plans to go into medicine. When we moved to Vancouver, I had planned to go to the University of British Columbia full-time, but my husband was starting a business,

worked long hours, made little money, and I went back to working as a nurse in St. Paul's Hospital Emergency Department to pay the bills. I got pregnant that year, and that seemed to give me the motivation I needed to pursue my dreams of becoming a doctor. I quit work and went to school part-time the year my daughter was born. I was the only one pregnant that year in my class. I remember in a class of 300 in chemistry, Rick Hansen and I had to sit in the back row as we were the only ones who could not fit into the regular desks.

I took organic chemistry in summer school the summer before my daughter was born, trying to avoid the more toxic substances. She was born in October and I did miserably in my Christmas exams, especially inorganic chemistry. My husband was going to look after her, but never seemed to make it home in time to babysit so I could get to class. After Christmas I got a babysitter on campus, the wife of a foreign student who was doing a PhD in forestry. She had her MSc in biochemistry from Brazil. Maria had two children, but she had wanted one more and my daughter was the the baby she wanted. I took my classes in the morning, went to get Lisa at lunchtime, and usually brought her home unless I had a lab in the afternoon.

My husband and I separated that summer and I carried on with my studies as a part-time student. I also went to spring and summer sessions, then went full-time the next year because the Dean of Medicine told me that any courses I took when I was part-time would not be considered in my GPA as I had an unfair advantage. He told me that lots of undergraduate students had part-time jobs. I was very angry with him: it seemed to me that being the mother of an infant was more time-consuming than working at a part-time job after school. Nevertheless, he made the rules and I went full-time in my third year at UBC when my daughter was two.

The next year I started medicine at UBC. I found that year to be very hard as the hours at school were very long and I did not have much time for studying. I moved into student housing on campus to save time commuting; Lisa's first animal word was cockroach. I then transferred to the University of Calgary Medical School, as the schedule was more geared to mature students. We lived in student family housing. I quite enjoyed my undergraduate studies there. I interned at Victoria General and Royal Jubilee Hospitals in Victoria. I had been planning to do family practice, but I fell in love with surgery after spending time with one of the surgeons there. He was a true mentor for me, as I could see that he had a family life, and interests in windsurfing, etc. He had a good sense of humour and a sort of 'with it' personality that I could relate to—unlike the navy blazer, grey flannel-pants mentality in surgery at the teaching hospitals. I assisted him in surgery as much as I could, even after my surgery rotation, to the detriment of missing the family practice sessions I was supposed to be attending, making up excuses to my mentor.

I had already made plans to do the second year of family practice training back in Calgary, but I hated every minute of it and quit as soon as I got into a surgery residency. I had difficulty being seen as a credible candidate, as most of my surgery interviews focussed on how I planned to organize child care. I was even told by one person who interviewed me that women do not do well in their program; that I would probably quit after the first year; that if I even thought I could do it, it showed how little I knew about the program. I got sort of mad at him and told him he did not know me if he thought I would quit, that I would never quit, and practically walked out.

I did eventually get a surgery residency back east, (and then Calgary even offered me a spot!). It was difficult, the hours were long, and we spent a lot of time doing scutwork and on call. I think we normally worked a hundred hours a week. The staff was not supportive of residents, and one of our program directors tried his best to eliminate the women in the program. I remember I had my exit interview with him and he told me he would 'let' me write my fellowship exam, but I had to promise him I would never practise east of the Great Lakes! I was happy after I got ninety percent in the CAGS two years in a row, not because it was a good mark, but because it was an outside method of evaluation and made it really hard for them to keep me from writing my fellowship exam.

Since then I have been practising in a remote and rural small town in south-eastern British Columbia. It is a beautiful town that I chose, not only because of the mountains, skiing, the lake, and beautiful summers, but because of the laid-back lifestyle, and because my daughter's best friend lives here. She has been happy to spend her teenage years here, has done well at the local high school, and had a season's pass at the ski hill and a job at the local store.

Living in a small caring community like this has advantages for raising children, especially for parents who work. I had a full report from several sources on my daughter's boyfriend before she even told me about him. I have been busy doing a real surgical practice and have patients who come a long way over the mountain passes in the winter and take the ferry over the lake to see me. I like my practice, as the patients are down to earth and very appreciative of the work I do. I have a personal relationship with my patients, as I do all the pre- and post-operative care as well as the surgery itself. They often bring me gifts from their gardens and sometimes fish from the lake.

DR. DAVINA KAZANOWSKI

My name is Dr. Davina Kazanowski (nee: Gilbert), a General Practitioner who is happily married with three beautiful children. I was born in North Vancouver, British Columbia, in 1963, following which I lived in Richmond for a couple of years. When my parents divorced when I was three, I moved to Kelowna with my mother and three older siblings. As I was growing up in Kelowna, I enjoyed the warm summers, spending a lot of time at the beautiful beaches cycling, playing tennis, jogging, and doing some waterskiing. In the winter months I skied at Big White mountain, where I also worked part-time on weekends as a teenager so that I would get free season passes.

Growing up with a single parent and three siblings was not always easy financially. In Grade 7, I really wanted to have a brand new 10-speed and realized that the only way I could get one was to pay for it myself. I then went out and got a newspaper route for the entire summer and saved up enough money to buy my bicycle, which I was very proud of, and actually rode for at least the next seven years. The bicycle cost me $100 and I sold it eight years later for about the same price. I then went on to have summer jobs every summer, and by Grade 10 I realized I had to start saving if I wanted to attend university. I was very active in many sports, including field hockey, basketball, soccer, and could be seen all over town riding my bike to various places. My summer jobs included picking cherries and peaches as well as tying grape vines, and I worked at a local bakery for many years, including the summers during university.

Sometimes I felt a little envious of my friends who did not have to work to save money for university; I can remember having to leave my after school field hockey practises a bit early in order to get to my part-time evening job. However, I learned how to balance fun with hard work and was able to save up enough money to attend the University of Victoria following graduation from Kelowna Senior Secondary School. I also won some bursaries which helped enormously. My mother was very good at teaching me how to save money and not to waste things. All of these childhood experiences provided the solid foundation for my aspiration of becoming a physician. I felt a strong desire to make a career where I could take care of myself and my own future children financially in case I was ever in the same predicament as my mother. While growing up I was very stubborn and determined to do things my way, which propelled me to search for a career that would allow me the flexibility and freedom to control my job situation. Such desire remained strong throughout my next eight years of university education.

We were the first class to have more women than men, and we often joked that we were the "experimental year," for we also had more racial minorities in our class.

Another important factor was that I had an aunt who was a physician. It never entered my mind that I could not become a doctor just because I am a woman. She was a brilliant pathologist and a great inspiration.

During the first year at the University of Victoria I was enrolled in the Bachelor of Science program, majoring in Human Performance, a program within the Physician Education Department. I thoroughly enjoyed the physical activity courses, especially the Anatomy and Physiology, which got me to start thinking seriously about medicine as a career. During my first year I had a lot of fun and revelled in the freedom of not living at home. By the second year I decided to concentrate more on my studies and see if I could get the grades required for admission to medical school. I found that when I applied myself, I could obtain the grades that were required, and I studied for very long hours.

I lived on campus for the first two years and off-campus in an apartment with various roommates for the next two years. I did not have enough money to buy a car, thus I often rode my bike to classes, which took about twenty minutes. There were moments I will never forget, such as riding home after the library closed at 11 o'clock at night in the dark, in the pouring rain. Throughout my four years at the University of Victoria, I was physically very active and had a great time playing on the Varsity Soccer Team. Again I found myself balancing studying with athletics, which proved to be a very good foundation for what was ahead of me with my career.

I can still remember the exact feeling and moment when I opened my admission letter to the medical school of the University of British Columbia. I was home in Kelowna for the summer and was alone when the letter arrived. I cried in disbelief when I opened it. I bought my brother-in-law's old Toyata Celica for less than $1,000, and off I went to Vancouver, again in disbelief that this was happening to me. I was fortunate that my aunt and uncle had neighbours who would rent me their basement suite for about $125 a month. They were a wonderful, older couple, and I could not have found a more suitable place. My father and his wife also lived in Vancouver and that was a comfort as well.

During the first year in medical school my most vivid memories are of the anatomy lab. I found dissecting a cadaver on one hand to be a bit shocking, but on the other, to be absolutely fascinating. It was mind-boggling to memorize all the names of body parts, nerves, muscles, and blood vessels. But it was truly fascinating to follow a nerve from its origin to its site of function. All of the muscles that I had learned in my original anatomy courses back at the University of Victoria were starting to come back to me as I now could actually see them being dissected and how they worked. This was September 1985 and I was twenty-two years old. I met a lot of great friends through medical school, and the camaraderie within our class of 120 students was wonderful. We were the first class to have more women than men, and we often joked that we were the "experimental year," for we also had more racial minorities in our class. During the first year of medical school I was on the women's varsity soccer team, but I had to give it up by the second year as it was just too time consuming. We did have an annual soccer tournament and this was always great fun. I also participated in the annual UBC event called Storm the Wall which was very exhilarating.

Throughout the four years of medical school, I studied a lot, but I also had a close-knit group of friends who spent much time supporting and encouraging each other when times were tough. We also managed to fit in the occasional tennis game or jog, which was very good for stress relief. Internship began in our fourth year, and we received $175 a month. I remember the shock of a classmate when she found out that I was actually able to pay my rent and food on that monthly salary. I was glad to have those great money-management skills that my mother had taught me.

The day of graduation in 1989 was a very proud day for me. I felt like "The Little Train that Could" as I walked across the stage, received my diploma, and saw my family in the audience.

I then went on to do my internship in Victoria from June 1989 to June 1990. I had always loved the city of Victoria for its beauty and charm, and it was during my internship that I met my husband, Greg. Again, this was a very challenging year as there were many time pressures on interns. We had a lot of thirty-four-hour shifts with little sleep, and Greg used to take me up to Nanaimo to visit his family on the occasional weekend; they teased him that I was not a very exciting person as I would usually fall asleep in exhaustion on their couch for most of the weekend.

During this year, the Association of Interns and Residents came up with a new rule that if an intern or resident had worked twenty-four hours straight with less than two hours of sleep, they were to be relieved of their duties at the hospital. Of course, most of the consulting physicians that we were training under were older gentlemen who were absolutely appalled at this ruling, and if you mentioned it, you could tell by the look in their eyes that they thought you were a very lazy person because they had worked twice as many hours and we were getting off easy. I remember feeling very frustrated that most of us would continue working about thirty hours because of that pressure. Greg was a great support to me during that time. Following the internship, I did locums in the Victoria area for about six months, and it was during this time that I received an offer to join a clinic in Nanaimo, as they had heard that I was thinking of moving there.

Greg had started to sell real estate and we felt that moving to his home-town of Nanaimo was a smart move with regards to his career. Since that time, we have bought a house on seven acres and are thoroughly enjoying the wooded area on our property and the privacy. We now have three beautiful children born in 1994, 1996, and 1998.

Prior to having children, I was delivering about 100 babies a year and was very busy. There was one occasion early in my pregnancy when I had to leave a Caesarean section because I was starting to faint, and of course the obstetrician knew right away that I was pregnant. I also recall leaving part-way through several deliveries for a quick trip to the washroom to vomit. During the pregnancy with my second son, I remember being about seven-months along and feeling very tired, having been up all night for a delivery with some complications. I was physically exhausted and had some back discomfort, and at that time there were only two on-call rooms for us to sleep in. The little bit of sleep that I tried to get in between checking on my patient was in the second on-call room which was basically a hospital room with a lazy-boy chair in it. I remember feeling quite resentful at the time of the older male obstetrician sleeping on a comfortable bed in the other on-call room while I was feeling extremely uncomfortable trying to get a little bit of sleep in this lazy-boy chair, being pregnant and having back pain and nausea. I felt a little sorry for myself at that moment, but I also thoroughly enjoyed delivering babies and, in fact, found myself in tears on many occasions at the beautiful moment of the birth and seeing the mother holding the baby in her arms. However, I stopped delivering babies after the birth of my second son, as I realized that I could not possibly be available on a moment's notice with two children at home unless I had a live-in nanny, which was not the type of lifestyle that I chose to have.

I have always marvelled at the miracle of birth; it helped me to deal with the death of some of my patients. During the days when I was delivering a lot of babies, I often found that when one of my elderly patients died, I would have a birth within twenty-four hours, and this was comforting. I always shared this with the grieving families; I hoped they could also see the cycle of life carrying on.

During my third pregnancy, I had to deal with gestational diabetes, which fortunately was mild and diet-controlled. However, again this was just another thing to juggle into my busy life. It was difficult to find time to exercise to bring my sugar down and frequently monitor my sugar. Despite all these challenges, the birth of my daughter was probably the greatest moment of my life, and I have enjoyed every second with her since. Being a crazy, hardworking, self-employed person, I worked until two days before I delivered each of my children. During one of my pregnancies, a male partner watched me "waddle" down the hallway at our office in my eighth month and commented that I should be at home. This was not a financial reality. I breastfed all three of my children until they were about thirteen months, which was a feat in itself, given that I went back to work after five months with each of them. I would carry an ice-cream bucket into the office in the mornings with all of my pumping equipment in it. A colleague came into my office one day and saw the ice-cream bucket and assumed it was full of some sort of cookies or goodies. He opened it up and was very shocked to see which was inside; red-faced, he quickly left the room. I felt like a bit of a cow double pumping in my small office every lunch hour for twenty minutes, but it helped ease the guilt of being at work and not home with my children. Since that time, I have always tried to put my children first. However, I am constantly torn between the needs and the challenges of my patients and my family.

Some days at work I wonder if I am being appreciated for the long hours that I put in and the extra time I take for my patients with phone calls, etc. But it is amazing how patients' compliments get me through some of the rougher moments of the day. It is wonderful that the occasional card of thanks from a patient remains in my mind for years.

When my eldest son was four years old, I was explaining that a father of his friend was a doctor, and much to my pleasant surprise his comment was, "Oh . . . I didn't know boys could be doctors too!" I enjoy my work, but on a busy, stressful day I always look forward to my "bright light" waiting for me at home—my family. I usually work three days a week from 8:30 a.m. until 6:30 p.m. without any breaks and then do paperwork for an hour or two at home after the kids are asleep. Then I work an evening shift for four to five hours each week. These shifts allow me to spend two days with my kids and to join in on the occasional school field trip or birthday party. My husband and I do a log of "tag teaming" with our jobs, which allows us to spend more time with our children. Fortunately, we have met a wonderful person who cares for our children two days per week. She is now like a member of our family and we feel very lucky to have her.

I am somewhat of a perfectionist, and unfortunately, that makes it hard for me, because I am constantly battling between my feelings of wanting to give 100% to my career as well as 100% to my family. I am extremely busy, but when I reflect back on my life, I see that I have always been extremely busy because I have always worked very hard at whatever stage I was at. I do not think that this will ever change, yet at this time I have probably reached the right balance. My husband is very supportive and for that I am grateful. I think that I have come a long way from the little girl riding her bike everywhere in the sunny Okanagan, yet at heart, I am still the same person.

DR. FRIEDA JUSTINA REDDEKOP

I moved to Penticton in the summer of 1989. I had lived in Vancouver during my 1969–1970 internship at St. Paul's Hospital, but had never enjoyed being in B.C. In 1989, however, I brought my heart with me—my husband wanted to live here when he retired.

Horndean, Manitoba, was my birthplace, and I spent my childhood between Manitoba and Ontario. In 1956, my family moved from Morden to Hamilton, Ontario, where my father obtained employment in an effort to improve the fortunes of his family.

So I started high school at the age of twelve years, spending three years at Delta Secondary School and Grade 12 at Hillpark Secondary School. My first summer job was at Cudney's fruit packing company, then I worked for the librarian at Delta Secondary School, and finally the Bell Telephone company as an information operator. I even had a short term job as a clown at the Eaton's Store in Hamilton. All positions were great opportunities for learning and growing.

After completing high school, I worked as a stenographer at a law firm. When my boss, John S. Millar, left to establish his own law firm, I was invited to join his new firm. The practice eventually became Millar, Alexander & Tokiwa. I worked for Mr. Millar, but occasionally took dictation from Mr. Lincoln Alexander (later Lieutenant-Governor of Ontario) and

Mr. Paul Tokiwa (a gentleman who put himself out to provide work for me when I later left for university). I was privileged to have worked for these fine men!

I worked for two years as a legal stenographer, but I had decided that medicine was what I wanted to do. So, during my first year of work, I taught myself Grades 9 and 10 mathematics. During my second year of work, I attended night school from Monday to Thursday, taking Grades 11 and 12 mathematics and Grades 11 and 12 German. Then I returned to Hillpark Secondary School to complete Grade 13. The guidance counsellor told me that my marks were better than many of my male classmates who were trying to enter medicine. I think that good references from my high school teachers helped my acceptance at the University of Toronto where I finally completed my MD degree.

Supporting myself financially was challenging. From 1965 to 1966, my weekly food budget was $5. Without my mother's homemade vegetable beef soup I would not have survived. My luxury in those days was the Saturday edition of the *Toronto Star*. How I looked forward to that paper. My oldest brother, Abe, came to visit occasionally and brought a brown paper bag filled with various snacks.

I was blessed to be exposed to good teachers during my time at university. The intravenous team at the Toronto General Hospital taught me how to take blood and start IVs. One evening, I was needed to start an IV on a patient who was a physician. Of course, I did not conquer that vein with my first stab, but the doctor-patient reached over, felt the tip of the catheter under his skin, and said to me, "Try deeper." I did, and it worked. Thank you, sir.

During my last year in medical school, I worked at Wellesley Hospital in the evenings, nights, and weekends. The job entailed drawing blood, starting IVs, and covering hematology and urinalysis services as well as cross matching blood in the blood bank.

During my internship at St. Paul's Hospital, anesthesiologists inspired me with their enthusiasm and knowledge, and I became interested in what was to become my specialty. My first love had been Obstetrics & Gynecology, but several events transpired to change my aspiration. A summer job doing gynecological study fell through at the last minute because of a lack of funding, and my application to U. of T. for an obstetrical residency was turned down. Both events were tragedies in my life at the time. Later, I thanked God that I had opted for anesthesia.

My anesthetic practice started in Brampton, Ontario, at Peel Memorial Hospital. Again, I was privileged to work with and learn from men who had developed skills which I needed to acquire. I learned much from my first chief, Dr. Brian Nixon, who seemed to have a knack for looking at situations in totality, and who had a deep understanding of human behaviour.

In late 1980, I met a man who was a widower with five children and several grandchildren. When we became engaged two or three months later, I was astonished at my own impulsiveness. When I informed my family that I was getting married, they laughed, thinking that I was joking as they had long ago given up on the idea of me getting married. In July 1981, Fred and I exchanged wedding vows. He came to the marriage with twenty-three-and-a-half years of marriage experience, and I came with none! As they say, it was the beginning of an interesting journey. No matter how old you are, you approach marriage with the same starry-eyed expectations that an eighteen-year-old has.

I struggled to balance work and looking after a husband, two teenaged children, and one dog named Fury. There were days when the dog was my best friend. I was working hard to establish relationships with the two children at home, as well as the three girls who had started their own families. As usual, the nurses at work were a wonderful source of information, support, and advice. How I treasured those people.

My husband, of course, had a lifetime of experience which became a gold mine for me. One day he turned to his son, Peter, and announced: "Peter, you are the biggest challenge Frieda has ever had." Little did I know how accurate that statement was. Today, Peter is the owner-operator of his own printing business. I am so proud of that young man.

Humour got us through many family challenges. At the dinner table one night, we smelled an odour which was competing with the dinner I had prepared. Everyone denied being the source of the problem. My husband suggested that we each remove our socks and pass them to the person on our right. Immediately there were howls of protest from Peter's sister who sat on his right side.

The children left home eventually: Louise in 1986, and Peter 1987. My husband and I became newlyweds on our own for the first time. Shortly thereafter, he started planning his retirement, and we relocated to Penticton, B.C., in the summer of 1989.

At Penticton Regional Hospital, I met another interesting group of people: Gordon Aitken, David McCurry, and Rick Wickett who made up the Department of Anesthesia. I became the vacation relief, golf relief, fatigue relief—my name became the "golden goose." TGIF stood for "Thank God it's Frieda" for some. Those were interesting days!

When Dr. Aitken and Dr. McCurry retired, I resumed full-time practice. Everything old is new again.

These days I collect medical supplies, old linen and equipment, and anything else that hospitals discard, and with the help of others arrange to send these supplies to clinics and hospitals in developing countries.

In spite of the frustrations of practising medicine today and the unrealistic expectations of some patients, it is still very rewarding to hear the patient say, "Thank you, I feel human again."

1991

DR. PAULINE ALAKIJA

Curriculum Vitae

Born: February 2, 1965.
Citizenship: Canadian.
Present Positions: Assistant Chief Medical Examiner, Office of the Chief Medical Examiner, Southern Region, Province of Alberta (since July 1, 1998); Clinical Assistant Professor, Department of Pathology and Laboratory Medicine, Faculty of Medicine, University of Calgary.
Other Experience: Forensic pathologist on Canadian Forensic Team investigating war crimes in Kosovo, Sept-Nov 99.
Education: Fellowship in Forensic Pathology, University of New Mexico, Albuquerque, New Mexico, U.S.A., 1997–98; Anatomical Pathology Residency Program, University of Calgary, Foothills Hospital, Calgary, Alberta, 1993–97; Rotating Internship, University of Toronto, St. Michael's Hospital, Toronto, Ontario, 1990–91; Medical Doctorate Program, Faculty of Medicine, University of British Columbia, Vancouver, B.C., 1986–90; Honours Physiology Program, Faculty of Science, University of British Columbia, Vancouver, B.C., 1983–86; Penticton Secondary School, Penticton, B.C., 1981–83.
Degrees and Certificates: Fellow of the Royal College of Physicians of Canada, 1999; Diplomate of the American Board of Pathology in Forensic Pathology, 1998; Diplomate of the American Board of Pathology in Anatomic Pathology, 1996; National Board of Medical Examiner's Certification, 1991; Licentiate of the Medical Council of Canada, 1990; Medical Doctorate, University of British Columbia, 1990.
Current Medical Licences: The College of Physicians and Surgeons of Alberta, 1997; The College of Physicians and Surgeons of British Columbia, 1991.
Past Positions: General Practitioner, Kelowna General Hospital, Kelowna, B.C., 1991–94; Rural Doctor Program, student doctor, Penticton Regional Hospital, Penticton, B.C., summer 1988; Phlebotomy Technician, Metropolitan Laboratories Ltd., Vancouver, B.C., summer, 1987; Research Assistant for Dr Hugh McLennan, Department of Physiology, University of British Columbia, Vancouver, B.C., performing binding assay studies for glutamate in rat hippocampus, summer 1986; Research Assistant for Dr. Donald Brooks, Department of Pathology, University of British Columbia, Vancouver, B.C., funded by the Natural Sciences and Engineering Council of Canada (NSERC grant). Studied monoclonal antibody and fibrinogen binding to red blood cells, summer, 1985.
Awards: Gold Star Letter for Outstanding Teaching in Lectures presented by the Class of 2001, Faculty of Medicine, University of Calgary, 1999; First Prize for Best Resident paper in Pathology/Biology at the American Academy of Forensic Sciences

Annual Meeting in New York, 1997; First Prize at University of Calgary, Department of Histopathology, Resident Research Day, 1996; Lange Medical Publications Award for Outstanding Achievement in Medical School, 1990; Nadel Medical Award for Top Medical Student on Hematology/Oncology, 1990; Florence E. Heighway Summer Research Award, 1988; Penticton Women's Club Scholarship, 1987; Medical Services Association Medical School Entrance Award, 1987; The Chris Spencer Foundation Special Scholarship, 1983/7; The Chemical Institute of Canada Award for top first year chemistry student, 1984; Norman MacKenzie Alumni Scholarship, 1983; H.D. Prichard Award for top overall graduating student, 1983.

Publications:

Nolte K.B., Alakija P., Oty G., Shaw M.W., *et al.* "Influenza A Virus Infection Complicated by Fatal Myocarditis." *Journal of Forensic Medicine and Pathology.* Accepted

Palmer R.B., Alakija P., Cde Baca J.E., Nolte K.B. "Fatal Brodifacoum Rodenticide Poisoning: Autopsy and Toxicologic Findings." *Journal of Forensic Sciences, 1999; -44 (4): -851-855*

Alakija P., Dowling G.P., Gunn B. "Stellate clothing defects with different firearms, projectiles, ranges, and fabrics." *Journal of Forensic Sciences.* 1998;-43(6):-1148-1152

Auer R.N., Alakija P., Sutherland G.R. "Asymptomatic large pituitary adenomas discovered at autopsy." *Surgical Neurology,* 1996; -46: 28-31

Garces P., Romano C.C., Vellet A.D., Alakija P., Schachar N.S. "Adamantinoma of the tibia: plain film, computed tomography and magnetic resonance imaging appearance." *Canadian Association of Radiologists Journal,* 1994; -45 (4): 314-317

Presentations/Posters:

"Child Abuse and SIDS." Office of the Chief Medical Examiner's Symposium, March 1999.

"Fatal Brodifacoum Rodenticide Poisoning: Autopsy and Toxicologic Findings." Poster at the American Academy of Forensic Sciences Annual Meeting in Orlando, 1999.

"Influenza A Virus Infection Complicated by Fatal Myocarditis." Poster at the National Association of Medical Examiners Annual Meeting in Albuquerque, 1998.

"Stellate Clothing Defects in Firearms Injuries." Podium presentation at University of Calgary Department of Pathology Resident Research Day and the American Academy of Forensic Sciences Annual Meeting for February 1997.

"Breast Carcinoma Synopsis." Presented at Princess Margaret Hospital, Roseau, Dominica in March 1996.

"Intracranial Neoplasms in Childhood." Presented at Princess Margaret Hospital, Roseau, Dominica in May 1996.

"Cytoplasmic Inclusions in Chondrosarcomas Arising in Enchondromas and Osteochondromas." Poster at the Canadian Association of Pathologists' Meeting on September 16, 1995; presentation at Foothills Hospital Residents' Research Day in October 1994.

"Asymptomatic Large Pituitary Adenomas Discovered at Autopsy." Podium presentation at Foothills Hospital Residents' Research Day October 1995.

Professional Affiliations: American Academy of Forensic Sciences, National Association of Medical Examiners, The Forensic Science Society, Canadian Society of Forensic Science, The Calgary Medical Legal Society, Calgary Association of Laboratory Pathologists, Alberta Society of Laboratory Physicians, Canadian Association of Pathologists, United States and Canadian Academy of Pathology, American Society of Clinical Pathology, College of American Pathologists, The Calgary Medical Society, Alberta Medical Association, Canadian Medical Association.

Teaching/Administration Experience: Instruct and examine residents in Anatomical Pathology, 1998–current; Teach University of Calgary Medical Students Cardiovascular Pathology Course, 1998–current; Chief Resident Foothills Hospital-Anatomical Pathology Program, July 96–Jan. 97; Instructor of gross pathology to medical students at Ross University in Dominica, Mar.–May 96; Preceptor for Principles of Medicine Course–Undergraduate Medicine, University of Calgary, 1995.

DR. JANE HAILEY

Jane Hailey, MA, MB, BChir, FRCPC is currently a pediatrician in private practice and a Clinical Associate Professor at the University of British Columbia. After qualifying as a physician in England, she returned to Canada to complete her pediatric residency in British Columbia's Children's Hospital, spending her final year as Chief Resident. For the last ten years she has worked in a group practice, working with children of all ages—from newborns to adolescents. She has also written and narrated a weekly medical column on CBC AM Radio, discussing a wide variety of topics in general medicine—from newborns to geriatrics!

Curriculum Vitae

Born: April 30, 1954, Toronto, Canada.
Education: Stanford University, California, BA Psychology (with Distinction), 1971–1975; University of California at Berkeley, California State Teaching Credenitial, 1975–1976; San Francisco University High School, English Instructor, 1976–1978; University of London, England, Advanced Level Certificate in Biology, Chemistry, and Physics, 1979–1981; University of Cambridge School of Medicine, Cambridge, England, MA, MB, BChir, 1981–1985; House Officer in Medicine and Surgery, University of Cambridge, 1986–1987; Pediatric Residency, B.C. Children's Hospital, 1987–1991; Chief Resident, FRCPC, 1990–1991; Clinical Assistant, Special Care Nursery, B.C. Children's Hospital, 1991–1992; Private Pediatrician and Clinical Associate Professor, Department of Pediatrics, B.C. Children's Hospital and B.C. Women's Hospital, 1992–present.

DR. MARIAN CATHERINE CUSHING REED

My father was a Protestant clergyman. My parents had many expectations of my two brothers and me. I am sure the psychological insecurities which I felt as a teenager and young adult especially helped determine my choice of psychiatry as a career. I have also had a life-long interest in spirituality and the role it plays in our lives and our decisions.

I should add that I have been in psychotherapy and psychoanalysis myself, in an attempt to understand my psychological difficulties and to deal with them in a more productive way. When I lived in Toronto, after my two years at the Gestalt Institute there, I went to live with a spiritual group in a communal house. This was quite an interesting experience, though I left the group when I moved to London, Ontario, in 1980.

I enjoyed my year in London, and that was where I met my husband, David Reed, a French professor at the University of Western Ontario. He also headed the French Immersion Summer School, which was located in Trois-Pistoles, Quebec. My French improved significantly because of him, and I learned that having a happy marriage could be very challenging. We were subsequently divorced after I moved to Penticton in November, 1996.

At present I am enjoying living in the Okanagan, and am not working as hard as I was in Vancouver—which is a relief. I am very interested in complementary or alternative medicine as it has greatly improved my health.

Curriculum Vitae

Born: Montreal, P.Q., Canada.
Marital Status: Divorced.
Education: BA McGill University, Montreal, 1960; MD, CM, McGill University, 1964; LMCC Licenciate, 1965; American Board exams, 1965; Passed exams for Certificate as Psychiatry Specialist, Royal College of Physicians and Surgeons Canada (CRCP(C)), 1970; Received Fellowship in Specialty of Psychiatry (FRCP(C)), 1974; Rotating Internship, Royal Victoria Hospital, Montreal, 1964–65; Junior Resident in Pediatrics, Hospital for Sick Children, Toronto, 1965–66; Resident in Adult Psychiatry, University of Cincinnati Medical College, 1966–68; Resident in Child Psychiatry, University of Cincinnati Medical College, 1968–70; Fellow in Child Psychiatry, University of Cincinnati Medical College, 1970–72; Trainee, Gestalt Institute of Toronto, two courses in Neurolinguistic programming, 1975–77.

Practice Experience: Private practice of Psychiatry, Hamilton, Ontario; Consultant to Student Health Services, Miami University, Oxford, Ohio, 1972–73; Private practice, Scarborough, Ontario, 1973–74; Private practice,Toronto, Ontario; Consultant, Sacred Heart Children's Village, Toronto, 1974–79; Consultant to Adolescent In-patient cottage, Thistledown Regional Hospital Downsview, Ontario, 1978–79; Staff Psychiatrist, Ontario Patient Clinic and Day Care Hospital, Thistledown, 1979–80; Private Practice, London, Ontario; Consultant, Salvation Army Children's Village, 1980–86; Private practice, Winnipeg, Manitoba, 1988–91; Psychiatric Consultant (half-time) to Child Guidance Clinic, Winnipeg, 1989–91; Private practice, primarily with adults, Vancouver, B.C. Part-time consultation sessions for: Delta Mental Health Centre, White Rock Mental Health Centre, and Surrey (Newton) Mental Health Centre, 1991–96; Private practice (adults), Penticton, B.C., 1997–present.

1992

DR. MARIA DASZKIEWICZ

My Life Through Various Cultural Windows
I was born in Poland, behind an Iron Curtain. When I say that, it sounds very dramatic, almost an attention-seeking statement. In fact, I was born behind the iron curtain, in the eastern part of Poland, which, after the Second World War, became a part of the Lithuanian Republic. Polish frontiers were discussed and further established at the Yalta Major World War II Conference by the allied leaders, President Roosevelt, Prime Minister Churchill, and Premier J. Stalin. That was why my mother decided to escape from the Soviet Union to Poland with her mother and me. This trip took place mostly on a bike; unfortunately, my mother was caught by Russian soldiers and placed in a prison. I was taken to a Russian orphanage. My mother, who was in her early twenties, went on a hunger strike to try to force the Russian soldiers to free her. She never said much about her time in the Russian prison, but she told me one story two or three times. She was taken for interrogation regarding her involvement in a conspiracy against the Soviet government. In fact, she was never involved in any organized conspiracy. One of the Russian guards commented, "You Polish people don't want to understand that Poland is just a playground for us to play out matches with Germany from time to time." All of them laughed quite vigorously at this comment.

When my mother eventually found me, I was living with an otherwise childless couple. They were quite wealthy, as he was an owner of the bank. They told my mother that they were quite used to having me and were very disappointed at losing the chance of having a baby. My mom recalled that I was able to say few simple words such as "Ma-Ma" (mother) and "Ta-Ta" (father). Apparently, however, according to my foster parents, I was quite cranky and cried a lot at the beginning of my stay with my new family. This occurred mostly when I would spill some milk or food on my clothing. They commented that probably I had received quite harsh feeding training at the orphanage so that the staff wouldn't have to change the clothes too often.

My parents married quite young. My father had just graduated from Cadet School and my mother had just completed private Catholic high school when the Second World War began. My father and his father were ordered into the Army right away. My father was only twenty-one when he was seen for the last time at the railway station among a big group of Polish officers greeting their family and friends from the train windows. The train was surrounded by Russian soldiers and taken into the Russian interior. Apparently, my father was not too careful in trying to locate his father, Erwin Daszkiewicz, and was caught on the street. He was quite optimistic, and had not imagined that he would not be able to return to his family. We've never learned what happened to him.

When I was a teenager, my mother tried to get some information through the Red Cross, which you would think would be easy. The information via the Red Cross was transmitted on western stations. We would listen to the news secretly, trying to muffle the noise by placing blankets on the doors and windows. I no longer recall which station produced lists of names, which were read alphabetically, including information regarding where soldiers were found or had died. One day we heard the name of Zbigniew Daszkiewicz, who was located working in a gold mine in Vladivostok in the Soviet Union. Could this have been my father? My mother wrote a letter to the Russian Embassy asking about him and received the answer that Zbigniew Daszkiewicz was not found in the Soviet Union. Obviously, we had to consider this statement as final because my mother would not dare to appeal. She never remarried because she did not know if she was a widow or still married. When I was thirteen or fourteen years of age, I had various fantasies about my father suddenly returning home from somewhere. The majority of my girlfriends had at least one man in their family—father, grandfather, or a brother. We had four women—my grandmother, my mother, my aunt, and me. I think that I was jealous and curious about how it would be to share the same roof with a man.

I never met my father's parents. My grandfather was a victim of the Katyn mass murder where Polish soldiers, mostly commissioned officers, were prisoners of the Red Army in September 1939. Thousands of these defenseless prisoners were shot at the edge of their open graves. My Grandpa's body was identified by his bankbook during the exhumation and a report was recorded in the International Medical Commission. As I grew up in this Communist-dominated country, there was a silence about the Katyn mass murder. My mother taught me a made-up family history. She warned me that I should never admit the truth about my father and grandfather. According to her story, my father and grandfather, who were Post Office employees, were probably killed by the Germans during the Second World War.

I was able to read the true history when I visited London in the late 1970s in the book titled *The Crime of Katyn—Facts and Documents*.

Despite the fact that we were forced to become refugees from Poland, when I look back at my childhood and teen years, I have mostly good and pleasant memories. First of all, I was very close to my grandma on my mother's side who was a lovely, caring, optimistic, and warm person. My mother was a gym teacher. She obtained a University Diploma after the Second World War, mostly through correspondence and summer courses. She was very busy and quite often, after school was finished for the day, my

mother would take me with her to various practices, to her gym class, or to study. I had many friends and, in fact, I missed out on nothing. My grandmother was a great protector. I remember that once when I was about ten years old, I was bothered by some older, local hooligans. My grandmother yelled at them through the window. She had a strong Russian accent due to the fact that the Russian border kept changing and we had to speak Russian more than Polish. The Polish boys started teasing her, laughing at her because of her accent. I felt hurt and extremely angry, so I jumped on one of the boys, pulling his ear and punching his face with my fists until his nose was bleeding and I felt relieved. I was somewhat of a tomboy as a young girl—I would get into fights with boys and I loved risky sports. To this day I have an old rib fracture which I sustained in a fight over a little crow which had fallen out of its nest. I tried to rescue the bird from a group of boys and one of them threw a stone at me while I was running away with the bird.

When I look back at my medical career, I think that my experience with my grandmother's suffering, and the contact with the hospital, made a profound impact on me. Grandma died at the age of fifty-four. Only a few years later, she was followed by my aunt, who was only forty-eight. She also died from cancer, which had metastasized to her lungs. She suffered a great deal and developed a huge ascites. My aunt firmly refused to be hospitalized. She was probably fully aware that she would share my grandmother's fate.

Choosing medicine was really simple—I felt that it was the only choice for me. However, I had significant opposition from my mother. I had spent a lot of time with her at summer camps, biking, camping on the riverbanks, and sleeping in haystacks. She was expecting me to follow in her footsteps. It was quite unusual, as most parents wanted their children to study medicine. "Why do you want to spend your life in hospitals, surrounded by sick and unhappy people?" she asked me. "Look at me, I am with young, healthy boys and girls and I enjoy doing what they like to do. You are not bad in sports." That was true, in fact, I did enjoy sports and the outdoors, and to this day, it is still one of my passions.

The challenge of getting into Medical School was great. After high school, I had to move to a big city. I spent all summer working hard, studying for exams. Even after passing the exams, it was very difficult to get onto the short list for admission. Fortunately, the Medical School needed students who had some achievements in sports. I had an additional point towards admission, as my name had been in local newspapers from time to time due to my sports achievements.

My years as a student at the Academy of Medicine in Warsaw were very busy. I tried to continue with my long jump—I was a member of the team representing our Medical School as well as a full-time student. The summer sessions and exams were happening at the same time as the sports competitions. My sports competitions required training every day, going to bed at a decent time, and being present at various places for competition. Although I tried my best, I realized during my third year of Medicine that I could not share my time between my studies and commitment to sports. I decided to give up sports and concentrate on my studies. Ten years of competing in sports had left me with a great deal of self-discipline. Now I had more time for studying, but I also discovered that the majority of my friends had a very rich social life. I started to work as a waitress at the Medical Club, mostly because I had no more scholarships since I was no longer a member of the sports club.

After receiving my diploma, I went directly to the Children's hospital. I started my Fellowship in Pediatrics. Although I did not have a specific preference at that time, I knew that I needed to follow my studies. There was a shortage of Pediatricians, therefore after obtaining my Fellowship, I was posted in an under-serviced area approximately 150 kilometres away from Warsaw. It was the busiest time of my life. I was never able to see all the patients every day. Leaving the office at the end of the day was a challenge because there were parents still waiting with their children—even outside of the building. I also had emergency visits at home quite often. As a young, newly-graduated pediatrician, I was overwhelmed at the prospect of facing this huge responsibility. My senior colleague was even busier, as he had to carry an administrative workload as well. Seeing acute meningitis, advanced rickets, or tuberculosis in patients was not uncommon, and I could only see each patient for a few minutes at a time.

I decided to go back to school as I felt that I needed to learn more about my patients—not only about their physical health, but also about their psyches. I applied for Child Psychiatry. The Child Psychiatry program was the longest—six years. It was a tough decision. At that time, I did not realize that it would not be the end of my studies—that in the future I would have to go back to Medical School again. As part of the Child Psychiatry program, I had to complete, in full, the Adult Psychiatry program along with two years of Child Psychiatry rotations, followed by two exams—one in Adult Psychiatry and one in Child Psychiatry. This time studying was very different. I realized that the subject I had chosen would follow me through my whole professional life.

After a few years of practising in the Zagore Neuropsychiatry Child and Adolescent Hospital Complex, I became the Head of the program for adolescent girls. It is hard to imagine now that for eleven years I was in charge of a twenty-five-bed inpatient ward for girls from the ages of thirteen to eighteen. This program, although very different, could be compared to the Maples Residential Treatment Centre in Burnaby. A large number of the patients—forty-seven percent—had a diagnosis of Adjustment Disorder, Anxiety, and Mood Disorders. Conduct Disorders accounted for thirty-four percent; Drug and Alcohol misuse or addiction for seven percent; and Psychotic Disorders for two percent. Many of the patients suffered from ADHD and learning Disabilities. The major therapeutic approach was based on Group Therapy and a Therapeutic Community that placed a maximum of responsibility for themselves and others on them.

I was never able to see all the patients every day. Leaving the office at the end of the day was a challenge because there were parents still waiting with their children—even outside of the building. I also had emergency visits at home quite often.

The mid-seventies brought a huge wave of drug addiction which developed very quickly and placed Poland on the list of one of the top countries for drug addiction in youth and adolescents in Europe. The most popular drug was alcohol, but many teens were also sniffling glue and other industrial toxins. And there was "homemade" opium, made from poppy plants. They would dry the poppy seed plants and then boil them whole, producing a dark concoction which was called "Kompot" (Kompot usually meant a dessert drink made from fruits). It could be taken orally or injected.

Gathering statistics or publishing a paper about drug addiction in youths was a challenge. Our government did not want to admit that this was a problem in our country. It was officially considered a problem of the west and capitalist countries. My colleague, Zbigniew Thille, who was the head of a similar treatment centre for boys with addiction problems, ran into serious difficulties after presenting a paper at the International Conference, which included statistics of the drug abuse problem in Poland. These difficulties lasted for quite some time. Zbigniew had told me that some of his meetings with "officials" who investigated his case were somewhat comical. For example, he was blamed for wearing jeans or carrying a black umbrella, as both were considered to be "imperialistic requisites." In fact, this time was so stressful for Zbigniew that he ended up suffering a Mycocardial Infarction, which he eventually died from. He was only in his mid-forties. His funeral was a big event for those who wanted to be acknowledged and helped. It was attended by hundreds of youths, many of whom had been his patients.

Africa

The late 1970s and early 1980s were difficult years because of the increasing political tension. There was a huge migration of people out of Poland. I did not hesitate, when the opportunity arose, to sign a contract with Nigerian officials as a consulting psychiatrist to a newly opened teaching hospital. It was initially located in Bauchi, but two years later moved to Sokoto, in northern Nigeria. I left Poland alone, leaving my husband, two sons, and my mother behind, because the situation of going to a new place was still an unknown, especially as my youngest son, Andrew, was only three years old. My older son, Rafal, who was fifteen at the time, remembers the Martial Law that came into effect after I left for Nigeria. He saw Russian tanks on the street in Warsaw and specifically remembers the curfew, the noise of sirens, and the official announcement of Martial Law on television. This was a very stressful time for all of us in Nigeria, as we had no contact with Poland and did not know what was happening. How blessed we are today in the age of the Internet!

The political situation has changed dramatically in the past few years, but in 1981, after great stress to us all, a third world war was considered to be very imminent and inevitable. I made the decision not to return to Poland after I was reunited with my family.

My professional life in Nigeria was a big surprise. Hospitals were suffering from a shortage of everything—staff, equipment, and medications. Basically, I used mostly Haloperidol, Chlorpromazine, and Benztropine to treat patients. Occasionally, there was also Chloral Hydrate, and a medication I was not familiar with, which contained numerous combinations of neuroleptics and anti-depressants. There were no mood stabilizers available. Despite all of these limitations, I think that my success in treating patients was probably better, or at least the same, as it was in Poland. This could be related to having quite an optimistic expectation of the patients, better compliance with the treatment and follow-up, and also the great involvement of the patients' families. I rarely saw a patient coming alone to my office. Most often these patients were accompanied by a large number of family members and friends. I learned the hierarchy and order in the African family structure. My patients were usually represented by their Uncles; the Uncle was the spokesperson for the family and not the parents. Why? Because in the extended family, there is a group responsibility for everyone. Parents are considered to be too biased toward their children, and therefore the Uncle is the one who is responsible for the patient's health, as he won't get overly involved.

Canada

My life and career in Canada is best related to Erickson's *The Life of Cycle Stages*. This is a simple as well as a very complex and deep theory of how our life consists of orderly, organized cycles which we have to go through.

I came to Canada in a stage of Generativity vs Stagnation, as a mature psychiatrist, who had practised psychiatry in Poland and Nigeria for about twelve years. According to Erickson, this stage goal is to create a new generation. This means to start summing up all of life's experiences and to pass them on through creativity to our children and patients. In my case, I had to go back to school to study for medical exams. My life train made a U-turn, and I found myself becoming a student again. It was not really a surprise after discussing my career with the immigration officer in Lagos. He opened the book, looking for employment opportunities for psychiatrists, and said that there was a shortage of psychiatrists across Canada, but not to forget that going through the exam would take a good five years or maybe even longer.

The first few years in Canada were very difficult. I still remember the smell of books in the library. I spent close to three years at the VGH library meeting many other foreign doctors. We were able to form small groups to help each other prepare for the exams, which made it much easier for me. I felt guilty about Andrew, my youngest son, because I couldn't spend enough time with him. I would leave home quite early, when he was still asleep, and would not return until very late. Andrew is the only one in our family who, after coming to Canada, felt Canadian right away. He is the only one who does not have an accent. He brought a maple leaf home from school one day and said, "Mom, don't ever step on this leaf. This is on the Canadian flag." Andrew was at the right age for immigration. Even in Nigeria, he was the bridge between our family and the Nigerian environment. Andrew learned Hausa very quickly and was our translator, specifically on market days, negotiating the prices. In Canada, Andrew was the first to visit Canadian homes and tried to introduce "burgers" into our cuisine, without much success as my husband is French and we enjoy our Polish-French cuisine. Andrew had a great passion for hockey, which he retains still.

Regarding my professional career, eventually I saw the light at the end of the tunnel. I was called for an interview as a short-listed candidate for the Psychiatry Program at the University of British Columbia. I specifically remember the interview with the Head of the Psychiatry Department, Dr. James Miles. He was a tall, gray-haired, pleasant man who made me feel very comfortable. In fact, I forgot the purpose of the interview. Initially we talked about my professional career. He was familiar with some of the names of my professors from Poland. Eventually, he asked me questions regarding my family background. I was impressed with the knowledge that he had about the history and geography of the places that I had come from. At the end of the interview, I asked him what he thought about me as a candidate for the Residency Program. "Well," he answered, "as a psychiatrist, you proved three times to be committed to psychiatry—you went up your professional ladder in Poland, Nigeria, and now again you want to go back to psy-

chiatry . . . but your family background was very traumatic." He summarized how my family went through major historical tragedies, and continued to comment that he wondered how those intergenerational experiences might have affected me as a person.

I felt cold chills go up and down my spine. I had not expected the interview to go that way. Was I going to lose my career because I had been born at the wrong time in the wrong place? I said to him, "As you know, out of the population of 23-25 million people, over six million people were killed during the Second World War in Poland. So there are no intact families in Poland. To this day, each family remembers those whom they lost. I don't think that I am exceptional for this part of the world."

I was accepted into the Psychiatry Program and had been through four years of residency. I don't think that I was repeating my training in psychiatry. Psychiatry is such a broad knowledge, having so many schools, trends, and theories. The core of psychiatry, however, is usually biological and similar across the world. Polish Psychiatry has strong roots in German and Austrian Psychiatry. We learned from translated German textbooks, specifically organic psychiatry and neurobiology. At the end of my post-graduate training, I was involved in Psychotherapeutic Post-Graduate education. I had already completed the second year of post-graduate training to become a Psychotherapist. That ended, though, when I left Poland.

In Canada, many of the rotations were really excellent. As a mature student, I could appreciate the excellent teaching I received in the consultation service at VGH. I also discovered a completely new area of psychiatry in the Gender Dysphoria Clinic at VGH. Initially, I was thinking about going back to child psychiatry, but as this would have involved longer studies, I decided that I would not do any more schooling because I was very anxious to go back to practising psychiatry again. I was surprised by the shortage of beds in child psychiatry in the Vancouver area. I compared the unit that I

I said to him, "As you know, out of the population of 23-25 million people, over six million people were killed during the Second World War in Poland. So there are no intact families in Poland."

had worked at in Poland to the Maples Residential Treatment Centre in Burnaby. Through the Residential Program, I also discovered an under-serviced part of British Columbia. I went with the UBC Outreach Program to places like Fort Nelson, Fort St. John, Watson Lake, Vernon, and 100 Mile House. These places were very different from the European provinces and rural places. In Europe, houses were built to last for generations. People know each other for generations. In Canada, I discovered that many of these towns were very transient, being temporarily established around some form of industry such as the oil industry. Obviously the gold rush had brought many people to those places in search of fortune and adventure. Buildings were constructed for today and not for tomorrow. During my time with the Outreach Program, I witnessed many young children ending up in foster homes and eventually living a transient life themselves.

I continue to discover British Columbia. I moved out of Vancouver to settle in Maple Ridge, a community with a rural flavor, which has dykes that I can easily reach by biking from my house. Even though Maple Ridge is an under-serviced region, it is very strong in some aspects. In the Psychiatry Department, we are lucky to have Dr. Britt Bright as the Head of the Department. She knows Maple Ridge very well, having lived there for many years. Not only is she an excellent psychiatrist, she also has administration and leadership skills, which many of us physicians shy away from.

My practice is a continuation of my experiences from residency. The Chronic Care rotation was mandatory at Riverview Hospital. During this rotation, I went through volumes of patients' histories, some of whom had been at Riverview for years. Many of these patients' names could be considered to be Eastern European origin. Generally, these thick histories gave very little information about the backgrounds of the patients. Some patients, who came to Canada in their twenties or thirties after the Second World War, had only a few sentences written regarding their life prior to coming to Riverview. Their cultural identity was often unknown. Some of these patients had lost their mother tongue because of their long hospitalization, partially because of their mental illness, and because they had no opportunities to speak their native language. It made me wonder if these contributed to their thought disorder, or if it was due to the alienation from living in a psychiatric institution.

When I was approached by my rotation supervisor to present the rounds on Chronic Care, my immediate thought was a topic about immigrants and refugees in a psychiatric institution. I had a plan to invite Dr. Morton Beiser to be my moderator and guest. I met him via Mosaic before I had entered the residency. He was the Head of the Social Psychiatry Department at the University of British Columbia. When I shared this idea with my rotation supervisor, he was not overly enthusiastic. He suggested that it would be more appropriate to look at the history of Riverview Hospital and review charts of patients who had had a lobotomy in the past. That was an experience! We were preparing the Grand Round with Mike Cook who was a senior resident. I was reviewing old charts in the Riverview archives. How well kept they were—I was amazed to see black and white pictures of patients who looked very well-groomed and well-prepared for photos. I found a number of charts of patients who were still hospitalized. It was very impressive that the comments of the doctors who were performing the lobotomies were quite standard, stating that patients were improved following their procedure and were then discharged from hospital.

Riverview Hospital is a true psychiatric monument in British Columbia. The first asylum for insane was opened in Sapperton, New Westminster, in 1878 and was renamed Woodlands School in the 1950s. The next step, in 1905, Colony Farm was established, quickly gaining the reputation of being the best farm in Canada, and winning all the championships. In the 1930s, the hospital's population numbered 2,550. Finally in 1965, this hospital was renamed Riverview Hospital. These buildings have seen a number of therapeutic approaches to psychiatric conditions: in 1907, hydrotherapy was introduced; in 1954, psychotropic medications became available and it was the beginning of Chlorpromazine treatment; in 1951, the total patient count was 3,479. Since that time, Riverview Hospital has turned a number of historical pages. Some, as in downsizing, could have been problematic as it required simultaneous development of community resources, and this still needs improvement. As of today, the number of patients is 808. The so-called downsizing has slowed down.

Beautiful trees, some planted over 100 years ago, still stand on the hospital grounds. The patients and staff, who were working together, looked after all of the gardens. This big space for the hospital grounds is a unique and beautiful land and plays an important role in the patients' therapy. For those patients who improved, we used to attribute their improvement to our treatment with medications and rehabilitation. I wonder, though, how much of the credit should go to the surrounding grounds, where patients can go for long, safe walks, which often help them to alleviate the side effects from the psychotropic medications—for example, akatisia.

In 1994, our Cross Cultural Psychiatry Program was established at Riverview Hospital. It is the only program of its kind in a tertiary care institution in North America. The objective is to deliver culturally sensitive care to minority patients, mostly immigrants or refugees.

My Final Thoughts

I like to think that we humans are like trees. I would not mind being a maple tree—feeling all of the changes each year according to the four seasons. It must be wonderful to have brand new leaves each spring, to welcome the birds in the summer, or to change colours in the fall. I wonder if falling asleep for the winter is like having a rest after being so busy. Or would I become fearful knowing that this might be my last time to wake up in the spring and now I might have to die?

Most important, although invisible, is the root system. Once it grows healthy and strong, the tree can be transplanted to another place, even far away, and it will continue to grow—much like our cultural identity.

Acknowledgements

To my Mother—for being both my mother and my father. Thanks to my patients for helping me to fulfill my life. To Judy Brereton, for her guidance with English and for typing the original story. To Dr. Eileen Cambon, for the great idea of putting this book together.

DR. SUSAN FINCH

I haven't always wanted to be a doctor. Actually, I fancied myself a research scientist. The idea of medicine was not seriously considered until Grade 12. At that time, my history teacher said I would never be a research scientist because I cared too much. I guess he was right. Of course, I didn't figure that out until I had almost gone the full distance in science. I did switch back and forth between the options of medical school and a PhD several times in third and fourth year university. The decision was clinched by a Commonwealth scholarship to do a PhD in biochemistry at Cambridge University in England.

I went off to mix with the history and great minds of science. The idea of research putting together the information and applying the results really did appeal to me. The problem was that I did not like the practicalities and isolation involved in actually carrying out the research. After a year, and a great deal of thought, I moved back to Canada to try my hand at medicine. I think I must be the only person ever whose parents were disappointed when their child went into medicine!

Montreal was my destination, as my partner had just got a job there. There was a year of waiting and working because (of course) I had missed all the application deadlines. In that year I got married, on Friday the 13th in the middle of Lent, but it couldn't have been that unlucky because we are still married. Judging from the attitude of one of my McGill medical school interviewers, I am surprised our marriage lasted a year. But then he also asked me who I thought was more intelligent, my husband or myself, and argued that war was good because it allowed medical trauma treatment to progress so far. This was in response to my involvement in nuclear disarmament groups (as indicated on my CV). Anyway, I got in (with an entrance scholarship at that) and attended McGill medical school from 1987 to 1991.

Our class was about one-third women and represented all the provinces, with plenty of French Canadians and a significant number of Americans. Both the class and the school felt male-dominated and macho in attitude. The women's medical society (formed by members of our class) was referred to as the "dyke society" by some of the men. Being married to an engineer was a challenge during this medical immersion, but also kept me sane. I am not sure how he survived it all (endless hours of studying in the first two years, and endless hours of clinical work in the several years following that).

However, McGill gave me a good solid medical background and provided challenging levels of responsibility. I remember in first year the surreal experience of the anatomy lab with its pungent smell which permeated my clothes, hair, and pores as though I was the cadaver; and the timed histology and anatomy exams where within thirty seconds we had to look at a fresh specimen and write down exactly what it was. We studied the head and pelvis for the same exam, and we all had trouble determining if the specimen was even from the head or pelvis! When I started medicine, biopsychosocial was a key word, but it was amazing how many of my classmates mocked it.

In first year, a pair of students were teamed with a chronic patient. I had the privilege of meeting a fellow who became quadriplegic following a severe neurologic illness. We learned of the emotional, physical, and spiritual adjustments he had had to make. Through those years I met so many other people, such as the Holocaust survivors with ID numbers tattooed on their arms who faced the end of their lives in the oncology unit at the Jewish General Hospital, the French families, who knew no English, from whom I would haltingly gather a history in the middle of the night, and the culture-shocked Inuit flown down as an emergency from the north. As physicians we are so fortunate to be allowed the opportunity to get to know and hopefully help so many people.

Both the class and the school felt male-dominated and macho in attitude. The women's medical society (formed by members of our class) was referred to as the "dyke society" by some of the men.

I became pregnant with my first child towards the end of my clerkship year. My pediatrics and obs/gyn rotations are a bit of a blur as a result. I seemed to float through them, constantly nauseated and occasionally vomiting; being woken up in the middle of the night to do newborn exams with a bag full of crackers on hand. I am sure if I went into the Montreal Children's Hospital now I would get a conditioned response of nausea!

There was a *lot* of scut work as we were required to take virtually all blood work, including blood cultures at 2 a.m. And we had to run our own EKGs which always meant untangling all the leads which looked like an octopus tied in knots. Each time the bulbs were squeezed for contact, old cold gel would ooze out. Walking the halls of the old buildings with paint peeling on the drab walls became commonplace. It was only when I trav-elled to various sites interviewing for internship positions that I realized how remarkable it was. So many of the hospitals in other provinces seemed shiny new with bright sunny rooms.

When I entered medical school, I had wanted to be a neurologist, but by the end it was between psychiatry, family medicine, and internal medicine. I matched to a rotating internship at St. Paul's Hospital in Vancouver where I had grown up. We left Quebec with enthusiasm as the political climate was tense and unfriendly to anglophones. At thirty-four weeks pregnant we drove a U-haul with a car in tow across Canada in four-and-a-half days.

The internship year was exhausting! I know there is no good time to have a baby when you are in medicine, but internship was *definitely* not a good time! I had my beautiful daughter two weeks after starting internship, going into labour following a full day at work. I went back to work after only six weeks so I would not have to prolong the internship year. Obstetrics was my first rotation back, so I was pushing along with my patients. All that year when I was alone in the call room I ached to cuddle my baby.

Until, of course, the pager went off yet again. I swear I still have a conditioned anxiety response to the sound of a pager. Some of the most challenging experiences I had during internship at St. Paul's in inner-city Vancouver were in the ER during a Welfare Wednesday night shift. The two trauma rooms were full all night. Also night shift New Year's Eve in the ER was a nightmare. The waiting room scattered with young people strapped into wheelchairs vomiting into basins in their laps—with the intoxicated obnoxiousness of the young and healthy.

Internship was planned to be the first year of a family practice residency. However, shortly after starting the second year, I decided to do psychiatry. I pulled out and spent the next year doing locums. A couple of short locums in Vancouver started out the year. Then I spent three months in Salmon Arm/Sicamous, commuting back each weekend to be with my husband and daughter. This work was diverse, challenging , and there was more responsibility than with a city family practice. It provided an opportunity to do ER work, surgical assists, and to admit and follow patients in hospital. It was my first introduction to small towns. Everyone knew about the new doctor in town and often feigned reasons to come and check me out. It was a fun experience.

I rounded out the year working at a walk-in clinic in Burnaby. This allowed me more time with my family and a more relaxed lifestyle. There was much more than colds and rashes that came through the door, and there was even an opportunity for follow-up. Rectal bleeding, spontaneous pneumothorax, depression, and chest pain were some of the presentations that I saw.

My psychiatry residency started in 1993 at the University of British Columbia. This was a time when I felt that a lot of things came together for me. Psychiatry seemed the right career choice (finally after a few side-tracks). I had a beautiful little girl and was soon to be blessed with another lovely daughter, and I found the Baha'i Faith which answered my spiritual search. It felt like a shift in my life from a time of searching to a time of immersion.

For the most part I enjoyed my residency very much. I met some amazing patients, and enjoyed my co-residents and a number of inspiring supervisors. I found discussions and reading about psychology and the working of the mind fascinating. Particularly intriguing to me was psychodynamic psychotherapy, and I did try to emphasize this during training. I have given priority to ensure it is incorporated into my practice despite later working in very much a community setting.

My second daughter was born in my the second year of residency. I found out I was pregnant during a call night when I was experiencing severe epigastric pain and thus ended up in ER along with the patient I had been called to see! In the last trimester, I did my consultation-liaison rotation at St. Paul's Hospital. I bustled around the whole hospital running the service and totally overcompensating, outraged that no one was taking these situations as seriously as me. I also remember the lack of boundaries, with strangers telling me how huge I was, asking if I was having twins, and touching my belly without permission!

Pregnancy had a very interesting effect on my psychotherapy patients and also on my fellow residents. I was surprised by the number of needling comments made, particularly by male residents, who suggested I was shirking my call duty because I had the nerve to be on maternity leave! Well, I survived, and managed a three-month maternity leave. I also did grand rounds on Pregnancy in Residency to facilitate discussion of these issues and other patterns noted in the literature.

Psychiatry does have a lighter call schedule and more sane hours than some of the other specialties. However, working in psychiatry is emotionally exhausting, as we work with some of the most challenging and at times most aggressive patients in medicine. I feel so privileged to have been allowed to have shared many amazing people's most intimate thoughts, feelings, and memories. I strive to remain respectful at all times toward all the people I am asked to be involved with.

Following the residency, my family and I decided to move to Duncan on Vancouver Island. We were attracted by the idea of a quieter, more rural lifestyle. Unfortunately, as a specialist in a small community, life is busier. There is more accountability because the anonymity is gone. And you often see patients outside the office, which does affect therapy. All aspects of psychiatry are covered by all of the psychiatrists, including inpatients, outpatients, consultation-liaison, emergency psychiatry, and a large variety of referrals of all sorts. There is more opportunity for program development, but less time to do it. As a female psychiatrist the majority of my patients are young women, and I see a lot of mood disorders, Axis 2 issues, and reproductive psychiatry. Much important work gets done, but there is limited opportunity for research, reading, and medical education, and it is easier to get professionally isolated.

In our community in the last three years, we have worked to fully integrate hospital and community services, and to expand the community services to provide more specialized groups and programs. We endeavour to work closely with family practitioners. Our challenges lie in developing more efficient systems and processes whereby patients see specific assigned practitioners with various training.

I found out I was pregnant during a call night when I was experiencing severe epigastric pain and thus ended up in ER along with the patient I had been called to see!

Throughout my training, my biggest challenge has been to balance my family (husband and children) with my career. They help me to set boundaries around the time I spend working. Decisions are made according to family interests and influence all aspects of practice including type, location, and areas of interest. Fitting time in for myself is always difficult. After three years of psychiatric practice, I feel I am just barely coming out of the exhaustion of having babies and raising young children during clerkship, internship, and residency. Now my children are school age and family life is more fun. There is more opportunity to expand my own interests. I have always been academically inclined, and hope to further pursue development of myself as a therapist. Soon it may be time for another change in direction.

DR. MARIE HAY

I was born April 8, 1953 in Shirebrook, Derbyshire, United Kingdom. My parents were Irish immigrants to Britain after the Second World War. My place in the family was the middle child of seven offspring. I was born and reared in a working-class mining village in Derbyshire with five brothers and a sister. Another boy also grew up with us. He was the youngest son of Mrs. Carney, a wonderful woman who reared us and basically was a significant mother figure for us all.

Our home life as children was not very happy. We were many in a small house, with not much money to go around. My father was a workaholic who spent little time with his children, and my mother was a sad woman. After my youngest brother died, my mother became addicted to drugs and alcohol and this limited her ability to care for us. There was quite a degree of physical abuse in our home, and as children we lived in fear of being whipped with bamboo canes, straps, and spoons. In this stressful environment, Mrs. Carney loved us through thick and thin, and I credit her steadfast love and constant good humour for keeping my spirit alive and kicking.

When I was four years old, my nine-year-old, most senior brother was sent away to Ireland to be educated in a boarding school there. Year after year, as each of my brothers reached the age of nine, they too were sent away to boarding school in Ireland. Then it was my turn to be shipped away to this foreign country, far away from all my family and loved ones. I was sent to a cloistered, contemplative, convent boarding school. I remember vividly its twelve-foot-high walls, even to this day. There, we were only allowed to speak for about three hours per day, in specially designated places and times, like when outside playing, or in the refectory. During the rest of the time we were supposed to stay silent, so as not to disturb the inner sanctum of the monastic atmosphere. At this school we were not allowed to have access to 'corrupting' outside influences, such as phones, radios, TVs, modern music, books, or magazines. Essentially, I endured this punitive educational environment until my graduation from high school at the age of seventeen.

At the age of twelve, I attended a slide show given to us in the school by a missionary nun who was a doctor working in Africa. It was fascinating to me, but then there wasn't much else in the convent school to capture my imagination at that time! There and then, I decided I was going to be a doctor, and I would go to work in Africa like this adventurous nun, and I wanted to be a neurosurgeon!

In order to achieve this dream, I had to survive many more years at the boarding school. I was always rebelling against what I saw as unjust situations. The nuns were constantly 'on my case,' punishing me unmercifully for this, that, or the other infraction. When I graduated, in their parting comments to me, they said I would not come to much good in my lifetime and I would likely end up on the wrong side of the criminal justice system!

At seventeen, there were two main obstacles standing in the way of my entering into medical school: my parents, who thought I shouldn't study medicine as it was too hard a life for a woman, and I should get married and have a family; and I had no money.

At that time in history, the British Government gave educational grants to students going into third level education. The government agreed to pay for me to take a course at a college, a little three-year science degree, but they absolutely refused to pay for me to do six years in an expensive medical school. In Ireland where I wanted to study, students usually go directly into medical school from high school. The usual length for a medical degree in Dublin is six years in university with a year of internship, in order to graduate as a fully qualified physician.

I knew in my bones I was being discriminated against when the government refused to pay for my medical courses simply because I was a teenage woman. I remember burning up with anger at this injustice. So I made an appointment to see the Regional Minister for Education in Derbyshire. I told this head guy I thought he was being discriminatory towards me on the basis of my sex. And guess what, that very day I walked out of his office with a grant in my back pocket to pay for six years of medical school! This was no small triumph for a teenager coming out of years locked in silence behind a twelve-foot-high enclosure. It felt so great to have fought injustice and finally come out on top. This had never happened to me before. So much 'manure' had been dumped on me by the powers that be in school that my feisty spirit had almost been extinguished.

From 1970 to 1976 I studied in the medical school of Trinity College, Dublin University, Ireland. It was really tough going, and I also felt I did not fit in with the majority of people in my class. In addition, there were relatively few women in my class–just twenty percent. The medical school hierarchy was overwhelmingly male and it was really sexist in many of its attitudes and behaviours. Feminism was not too prevalent in the Ireland of that era!

The war of attrition between Catholics and Protestants really erupted in 1989, my last year of school. After this year, life in Ireland was dominated by the 'Troubles' as it was called. There were indiscriminate bombings and shootings throughout North and Southern Ireland. It was a scarey time for all of us who lived in Ireland then. One weekend, I was up in Belfast playing intervarsity tennis against Queens University when all members of our teams were nearly killed by three exploding car bombs. One car bomb in particular blew me to the ground. After these close encounters, I suffered from a degree of post traumatic stress for about a year afterwards, although I didn't know what PTSD was until many years later.

To escape the regimentation and oppressive sexism of those six university years, I worked to earn money so that during the summer vacations I could travel far and wide, to see the world that had been denied me during all those years in the convent school. I spent an incredible three months one summer in Israel, working on a kibbutz near Lebanon. We used to rise at three in the morning to start work by four. Each day we went out to the orchards to pick fruit. There was a sort of war going on at that time, so we were always accompanied by armed soldiers whose job it was to protect us from snipers. After the kibbutz I went to work on an archaeological dig in the Negev desert, at a place called Tel Beersheva. I remember many romantic nights sleeping out under the stars on the beaches of Galilee and Eliat. Skinny-dipping was the thing in those days! One day a wild Australian friend and I swam a mile off shore into the Indian ocean to swim around Coral Island. We snorkled all day amongst the famous corals abounding in tropical fish of every shape and colour of the rainbow. Unfortunately we had forgotten to bring much water with us and it was forty degrees Celsius, so we nearly died of thirst trying to walk the ten kilometres to Eliat, as we had missed the last bus back. But we survived to tell the tale, after we managed to get our dehydrated tongues unstuck from the roofs of our mouths! During some other summers at University, I took trains or hitch-hiked around Europe to see the different countries, meeting all sorts of diverse peoples, cultures, and creeds. It was an enlivening education, far better than anything I was learning in medical school.

During my last summer of freedom, I took off for three months to Africa. We were allowed by our university to do 'elective study' periods anywhere in the world. I chose to go to the world-famous Red Cross War Memorial Hospital for Sick Children in Capetown, South Africa. The social situation between blacks and whites there was truly appalling to witness. The whites had so much wealth and affluence, while the blacks were so poor and disenfranchised. Discrimination against the black South Africans was rampant. For the first time in my life I felt ashamed of being a white person. After completing my elective studies in the hospital in Capetown, I jumped on a train and travelled to Botswana. From there I journeyed into the country of Rhodesia, known today as Zimbabwe. A bitter war of independence was going on there between whites and blacks, so when we travelled anywhere in the car, we always took a loaded gun with us. Africa was everything I ever dreamt it to be and much more. I fell utterly head over heels in love with this continent of unparalleled beauty. My heart bonded forever to its indigenous peoples.

As my six years passed inexorably by, my personal self-confidence grew. During five of those six years, I had the privilege of working regularly as a volunteer in a suicide centre. There, at a young age, I learned a little of the

There were two main obstacles standing in my way of entering into medical school: my parents, who thought I shouldn't study medicine as it was too hard a life for a woman, and I should get married and have a family; and I had no money.

art of really listening non-judgementally to people, and of being with them where they were, in the midst of their often lonely, troubled lives.

At the age of twenty-three, much to the surprise of the vast majority of my classmates and family, not only did I pass my final exams, but with just four others, I graduated top of my class, *magnum cum laude*. The success blew me away, as I had never been a student who stood out as a top flier.

After graduating from University as a physician, I then set about doing post-graduate work and study needed to prepare myself to work in Africa. By this stage in my career, I realized I did not want to be a neurosurgeon, as pediatrics had stolen my heart totally. Thus I completed a year of rotating internship at the International Missionary Training Hospital, Drogheda, Ireland. Following this, I did six months as a resident in general surgery, followed by six months as resident in obstetrics and gynaecology at Galway University in Ireland. Along the way I suceeded in passing the Diploma examination from the Royal College in Obstetrics and Gynaecology in London, England.

It was made perfectly clear to me that I was an 'English Woman' who was working in Ireland, and I was taking away the jobs earmarked for the 'home-grown Irish boys.'

However, career-wise things were not going well for me in Ireland. During many of my job interviews, it was made perfectly clear to me that I was an 'English Woman' who was working in Ireland, and I was taking away the jobs earmarked for the 'home-grown Irish boys.' It was such a sickening dose of reality. I also did not know anybody in a position of power and influence who could have pulled strings for me. Thus at this stage in my life, I decided to return to the land of my birth, England. There I was successful in completing four years of pediatric residency training in Manchester, Leeds, and Aberdeen, landing my first teaching job as a Clinical Tutor at the University of Aberdeeen. My years of residency can only be described as hell on earth. For four years I worked every second day, twenty-four hours on emergency call, living in dingy hospital residences, with equally dismal hospital food. Day in and day out, I endured the monotony and considerable stress involved in working thirty-two hours straight, followed by sixteen hours off duty. During my sixteen hours off, I had to fit in the academic book-work needed to sit the specialty pediatric examination, the MRCP(UK). There was no time left over for socialization or fun. It was an inhuman, awful experience which I would never wish upon anybody else. In many ways life in boarding school had been preparatory for the endurance needed for those years.

In 1982, I passed both the Diploma of Child Health and the MRCP (U.K.). Now I felt ready to go to work in black Africa as a fully qualified doctor, the place of my childhood dreams. To this end, I succeeded in getting a position as a Consultant Pediatrician, working with a great bunch of religious sisters, the Medical Missionaries of Mary, deep in the jungle area of eastern Nigeria, West Africa. 'Alone and Buried' for two years in the depths of a West African rainforest, I used to often wonder why I felt so completely and intensely alive there. Part of the answer is, I think, that by a subconscious osmotic process I absorbed some of the thrusting pulse of life so characteristic of the people I met there as they lived, prayed, and struggled together. Much as I want to share the immense richness of my experiences in Nigeria, words seem inadequate.

Passionate emotions were the very essence of human existence in Nigeria. When the dawn broke at six, I stretched out like a cat on a sheetless bed, relishing the coolness of the early morning. I knew this was but a temporary respite from the blistering rays of the African sun risen to full glory, beneath which one is cooked faster than a chicken on a spit. Throughout each new day, human dignity was reborn through the special and personal greetings exchanged with each person. Indeed, among all the people there was an almost palpable spirituality which constituted a living source of encouragement and support. I was constantly humbled to observe the cheerful manner in which the over-burdened women carried their multiple daily crosses.

As for the children, they filled my soul to bursting. I recall the pleasure and amusement at having my white skin stroked by fascinated little ones who had plucked up enough courage to venture close. I can still feel the calm peace of the heavy, humid tropical evenings, all stillness except for the gentle hum of the nocturnal wildlife.

But not all life in Nigeria was sweetness and light. I cannot describe to you what it feels like to be forever drenched with sweat in the terrific heat and humidity, nor can I tell you what it is like to be driven demented by unseen, treacherous, malarial-infested mosquitos buzzing in your ears all night long as they hover around waiting to pounce for a feast of blood. Too vivid is my memory of extreme weakness and vulnerability associated with recurrent bouts of malaria and dysentry. On my sick bed, acute feelings of isolation from loved ones far away became almost unbearable and I was moved to write poetry:

> "Away in the darkness of the night
> the echoes of my loneliness abide.
> Beyond the furthest star of night
> the Infinite has known I cried."

In utter shame and confusion, I remember the physical and mental revulsion I felt when I saw my first leper with no feet who, on home-made crutches, hobbled toward me proferring the stump of his arm for me to shake.

If it is possible to go beyond terror, this was how I felt one day when I awoke to find a green mamba snake sitting not two feet from my feet as I lay prostrated on the bed. Too numerous to mention were the times I was utterly speechless from rage and frustration at the widespread inhuman injustices caused by bribery and corruption on a massive scale. I can still feel the savage intensity of my desire to kill the fathers who refused to donate their blood when their own children were dying, lest doing so would lessen their sexual prowess, as was their belief! I shall never forget the mortal anguish I felt when children I carried in my arms to the ward died before ever reaching a pillow to rest their weary heads. I can still, at times, hear in my dreams the cries of bereaved mothers as their wails resounded throughout the hospital verandas.

One Christmas in Nigeria, I had the honour of joining the other hospital workers to go and greet prisoners in the local prison. I had never been 'inside' before, so I was shaken by what I witnessed. The men's cell blocks were grossly overcrowded. There were few windows, which were just open holes in the walls criss-crossed with iron bars. Each small square bulged at the seams with bare hands and feet, arms and legs, and intent faces with watchful eyes. The men struggled to obtain a breath of fresh air and catch a glimpse of their visitors. Beneath the fiery sun under unshaded tin roofs, the prisoners cooped up in such confined spaces were visibly suffering from the intensity of the heat. The stench of unwashed bodies and stagnant human excrement brought to my mind at the time vivid images of slave-ship galleys. On death row eighteen young men awaited the dawn of their execution.

The most poignant moment I experienced was in the female section of the prison, where women and children were incarcerated. As we huddled together, mothers, warders, children, and hospital staff, we regarded one another in stunned silence. Initially the mothers' faces were masklike and expressionless. Dark brown circles were deeply engrained around their deadened eyes. They resembled zombies, ghosts of humanity dead to the world, forgotten . . . until a solitary voice quavering with emotion began to sing a much loved Christmas carol. A few moments later a volcano of song erupted out of the hearts and lips of all present. When the carols died down, those ghostly eyes had become alive again and were swimming with tears of a vigorous humanity. It was then, in commom with many others, I wept without shame or reserve. Such emotions were elequently captured by Virgil two thousand years ago:

> "Ever here, virtue hath her rewards and mortality her tears;
> Even here, the woes of man touch the heart of man."

Africa and its peoples touched my heart forever.

On returning from Nigeria, back into the affluence of the western world, I experienced a lot of culture shock in reverse. I felt anchorless and restless. So I took a couple of extra years of further post-graduate studies, doing a fellowship year in Neonatology followed by a year of Dysmorphology and Behavioural Pediatrics.

During my year in Neonatology, I met an Iranian physician. He had been allowed out of Iran to do two weeks of extra study, but his main reason for being there was that he had smuggled his two sons out of Iran to get them away from being drafted at a very young age into the revolutionary armies of the Ayatollah. He asked if I would help him find somebody to look after his twin boys. I took pity on him and agreed to help. This is how at about thirty, I became the guardian of two young boys, Ali and Reza. They proved to be a joy and challenge to journey with, as they have grown and evolved into their own independent personhoods. My life has been truly blessed with their presence.

In 1987 I had the honour of being invited to Iran for a three-week vacation. This was a time of war between Iran and Iraq. There were scud missiles landing daily in Tehran where I was staying, which made the experience a bit hair-raising. But other than this my trip to Iran was a fantastic highlight in my life. I found the people to be lovely, and the land they inhabit is awesome in its grandeur and beauty. The arts and culture of antiquity I found there were overwhelming; their archaeology stretches back for thousands of years. It taught me a lesson, too, about the strength of negative American propaganda within our culture, which has tried to turn us against Iranians, especially during that time in history.

As time went by, I began to realize I had reached the glass ceiling of my career in Europe and I would never get one of the few pediatric consultancies available in England or Ireland. I also had increasing financial responsibilities towards my two wards. After much soul-searching and with lots of encouragement from three of my siblings who had already emigrated to Canada, I packed my bags and in 1988 came west to its shores. My first job in Canada was in Newfoundland, where I worked for two years as a remote, rural community pediatrician.

It is not always easy for physicians in remote areas to find spouses for themselves at the best of times. When an individual happens to be a lesbian physician, then this becomes exceedingly difficult.

Then I had the opportunity to visit British Columbia and I fell head over heels in love with its stunning beauty, especially the Rocky Mountains. I was attracted also by its diverse cultures from all over the world. I knew I had to come and live in B.C. When the offer of a Pediatric Consultant post came up in Prince George, I packed my bags and moved west again.

Many people do not realize that to come to Canada as a foreign medical graduate is really tough. I had to sit an examination for foreign graduates first, then do the LMCC examination (twelve years after leaving medical school in Dublin). Then I had to sit for the Canadian Pediatric Specialty exam, the FRCP(C), which I passed in 1991. All of this meant a lot more study, sweat, and stress, which compounded the added stresses of leaving one's homeland and trying to adjust to a new culture. When I had succeeded in passing all these exams, I was then free to pursue Canadian citizenship. On the first day of July, 1995, I celebrated the joy of becoming a Canadian citizen. It was one of the proudest days of my life. To this day, the passion I feel for my adopted homeland burns with intensity.

I continue to work in Prince George, B.C. and have been very active as a Community and hospital-based pediatrician. In the early '90s, I tried to persuade Prince George City Council to make Prince George into a 'Spanking free zone,' to set an example in educating parents not to hit their children, and to fund courses for teaching positive parenting skills. Such an idea was much too advanced for the City Councillors for the time, and I also got a lot of ridicule and flak from many people in the community over this issue. Thwarted in Prince George, I turned my attention to persuading the B.C. Pediatric Society to support the concept of abolishing 'Corporal Punishment of Children.' Incredibly, with great leadership and courage, they did so. They are the first and only pediatric society in Cananda to do this. My next challenge was to try and get the Canadian Pediatric Society to advise the Federal Government to abolish "Section 43 of the Criminal Code of Canada," which makes it perfectly legal for parents to hit their children. I wanted the CPS to be very clear and unambiguous in their stance against physical punishment of children and to fully support the United Nations Convention on the Rights of the Child. Unfortunately, to this date, the CPS has, in my opinion, been rather wishy-washy in this regard.

I was the first pediatrician to work in and become the medical director of the Prince George Child Development Centre. I continue working there part-time to this day. I also work at the Prince George Regional Hospital as a consulting pediatrician, in addition to having my own office-based private practice. I was a key organizer in establishing the first multi-disciplinary, community based child protection clinic, set up in a shopping mall, becoming its first director in 1993. In 2001 the clinic was transferred to the Northern Regional Health Board and has become one of the leading SCAN (Suspected Child Abuse and Neglect) clinics in B.C. In addition to this I have been active in raising professional and community awareness about the blight of fetal alcohol effects which has damaged so many of our young people in northern B.C., especially among the First Nations. I am recognized as an expert in Fetal Alcohol Syndrome and Effects and have co-authored a book called *Fetal Alcohol Syndrome/Effects: Developing a Community Response*, published by Fernwood Press.

Because of these activities, I have been asked to speak all over B.C., in Alberta, and in California about issues relating to corporal punishment of children, child abuse, and fetal alcohol effects. I have discovered I actually love to teach the new generation of health care professionals, social workers, early childhood educators, and law enforcement officers some of the insights and knowledge which has been gifted to me by my life experiences and training to date. Since 1997, I have been given the title of clinical assistant professor at the University of British Columbia. My main role in teaching pediatrics now is to family practice residents going through the new family practice training program in Prince George. One of the things which has pleased me a lot in my work as a child advocate in Prince George has been my contribution to the team of community professionals who were instrumental in creating the first Canadian Infant Food Bank. As a community we decided to try and improve the nutrition of children living in poverty. Mothers who had been feeding their babies canned evaporated milk were offered free baby formula through the milk bank. We based the milk bank in the community far away from the hospital, so as not to jeopardize the encouragement of breast feeding among new mothers, according to World Health Organization guidelines. Obtaining free milk and other infant food articles is linked to the mothers receiving twenty minutes of nutritional counselling for their infants of less than a year.

Finally it was in Prince George that, after the completion of all my studies, examinations, and becoming a Canadian, for the first time in my life I had time to settle down and no longer be a rolling stone. At this stage of my life, I was wonderfully blessed to meet the love of my life, a beautiful, warm, loving woman called Philomena Hughes. Philomena has now become my spouse and life partner. It is not always easy for physicians in remote areas to find spouses for themselves at the best of times. When an individual happens to be a lesbian physician, then this becomes exceedingly difficult.

This is especially true in a town like Prince George, not well-renowned for its tolerance towards minority persons of the GLBT (gay, lesbian, bisexual, transgendered) community. As a gay doctor in Prince George, I have been very impressed by the acceptance I have felt from my fellow physicians. They have been incredibly supportive in this regard, and I could not speak more highly of them.

When I first got to know Philomena she already had a son Zak, and she was in the process of adopting her daughter Hanna, from China. On the first of July, 2001, Canada Day, having lived together for three years or more, a compassionate Anglican priest blessed our union. Phil and I shared our commitment ceremony to each other with a community of 140 family and friends from all over the world, right here in our garden in Prince George. My life is now replete with joy and happiness, with my beloved partner and our two children, Zak and Hanna, topped off with a frisky lab-husky named Trixie.

As a human being first and then as a physician, I know I continue to experience new things each day I live. My hope is that I will continue to grow more deeply in compassionate understanding, so to be better able to share with my family and clients not just good scientific knowledge and skills, but some of the rich love and deep wisdom which has been freely gifted to me by the many beautiful peoples, places, and cultures I have encountered thus far on my life's journey, through the four continents of Europe, the Middle East, Africa, and North America.

DR. AILEEN McCONNELL

It seems that the business of looking after sick people and animals has always been part of my life. My father, a family practitioner in Belfast Ireland, had been a pharmacist with his own pharmacy before finishing medical studies. In those days doctors could do their own dispensing, so when he began to practise he did most of his own dispensing. Under his supervision—of course—I learned to 'make up the bottles' for him. I well remember once when he was away for a weekend, a young patient with asthma needed a refill. I phoned the doctor covering Dad's practice, and got permission to give out the required medicine (ephedrine was then the magic ingredient). During those years there were many weekend visits to uncles and aunts with family farms where something interesting was always happening. I recall once we gave a duck chloroform so that I could remove a sebaceous cyst from its head.

I was at Victoria College, a much-respected girls' school in Belfast where it was the custom for the headmistress to invite those girls in their final year to her office for a chat about their future plans. I well remember her pained expression as I told her, "I would like to be a vet." She looked at me and slowly said, "Oh, Aileen, no lady ever does that!" For many reasons, I did not leave home to study veterinary medicine, but entered the Faculty of Medicine at Queen's University, Belfast. The six years I spent there remain among some of the best years of my life. After graduation I became a houseman at the Royal Victoria Hospital, and began my first rotation on the neurosurgical unit with the outstanding neurosurgeon Cecil Calvert, followed by periods on medical and later surgical wards, and a rotation through surgical outpatient and emergency units. This was followed by a six-month period in pediatrics with some gynecology, and another six months at the Royal Maternity Hospital, after which I took the Diploma of the Royal College of Obstetricians and Gynecologists, and spent eight months as an SHO (senior resident) in Obstetrics in a country hospital. At that time my father needed to have some surgery, so I came home and took over the practice.

It was a lot of fun being in charge and looking after all those patients who had known me as a little girl and were gracious enough to trust me as their doctor!

It was a lot of fun being in charge and looking after all those patients who had known me as a little girl and were gracious enough to trust me as their doctor! When Dad was ready to resume his place, the big question was, 'Whither, what?' The year was 1958, and of the sixty or so graduates of my class of '55, more than thirty were by then across the Atlantic, ten in eastern Canada. And so I sailed to Montreal, and did my residency in Internal Medicine under the guidance of Dr. Douglas G. Cameron at the Montreal General Hospital. The transition to residency life was not easy. I had had many responsibilities in my various positions in Ulster, so dropping a couple of years' seniority was tedious for a while. But there were many good things. Montreal was an exciting city, and I was very grateful for all the emphasis put on French at Victoria College, as I could work and speak in French, and enjoyed the many exciting facets of the French scene in Montreal.

It was in Montreal that I met Fleming, recently arrived as a radiologist on staff, and we were married back in Ireland in 1960. We stayed at the Montreal General until 1965. I was a Hosmer teaching fellow for several years, and also looked after the staff health service. I had Internal Medicine qualifications from both the Quebec and the Canadian Colleges.

In September, 1965, we headed west—Fleming to the Chair of Radiology at the University of Alberta, Edmonton, and I was asked to work with adolescents, becoming Consultant Physician to the Alberta Institution for Girls, the province's maximum security facility. Those were interesting but trying times, when solitary confinement was just being phased out. Dr. Jean Nelson, my predecessor, had become Deputy Minister of Health and was able to get some long overdue reforms underway. I recall showing a short educational film about drug use to the girls and having the wrath of the administration descended upon me with strict instructions not to repeat any such nonsense!

At the University of Alberta, the R. S. McLaughlin Examination and Research Centre (part of the Canadian College of Physicians and Surgeons) was established, with Dr. D.R. Wilson as Director. I began to work there in 1968 as the Internal Medicine Test Committee Secretary, remaining for nineteen years. One of the first projects, started by Dr. Bryan Hudson and with which I was involved, was writing case history programs for computer assisted instruction. During that time there was much interest in having a common written examination for the United Kingdom Colleges, the Royal Australasian College, the American Board of Internal Medicine, and the Canadian College of Physicians and Surgeons. Examination material from all four groups was reviewed at length to find acceptable common ground, and it seemed possible that a consensus might indeed be achieved. However, various immigration policies changed, so that the previously free movement of physicians among those countries was no longer a given. Because of this restriction, a common examination became less important.

For several years during that time I was also responsible for the Medical Council of Canada's Medicine Test Committee, as the R.S. McLaughlin Centre began to manage examinations for the Medical Council.

These commitments allowed me to pursue some other interests, such as getting my first horse, which had been on my list since I was six years old. I was most fortunate to begin my equestrian career at a well-known stable, a training ground for members of Canada's National Team (Jumping) and the top Canadian Cutting Horse Competitors. This was inspiring company, and I went on over several years with different horses, trained my own horses, and competed in both English and Western events. In time I taught at that stable, and also finished the Grant MacEwan College Western Certificate Program.

When we moved to a farm near Wetaskiwin, some twenty-six miles south of Edmonton, I had my own stable with outdoor and indoor training facilities and an eleven-horse barn. For twelve years we had horses and riders in for training. Living in the Wetaskiwin area led to some local medical opportunities. I became the Medical Officer of Health for the Wetoka Health Unit and the Medical Director when the Wetaskiwin General Hospital opened the Care Unit, a fifteen-bed in-patient substance abuse treatment facility. This was probably the most interesting, challenging, and rewarding time of my life! The Care Unit was specially funded for a trial period, admitting patients by medical referral with the aim of returning them to their various occupations as soon as possible. Patients included a school principal, an operating room nurse from a major teaching hospital, a bank manager, a sixteen-year-old school girl, and a seventy-year-old grandmother, to name but a few. And this group of patients from the general population suggested that substance abuse knows no boundaries. I had always had an interest in this field, so to be given such a unique challenge was wonderful. The staff of the unit became a great closely-knit team, and I look back on that time with much gratitude. Seeing many of the patients return to their professional positions was our greatest reward. During my time as Director of the Care Unit, there was a full-time manager at the stable to keep everything working.

Eventually my husband retired and decided that he no longer wished to live in Alberta. This led to a move to Metchosin, British Columbia, and a small farm, where there is now a flock of North Country Cheviots with their resident Border Collies. I obtained my B.C. Licence, but for various reasons, did not return to active medical practice. Without my horses and stable I turned to the sheepdog world, and with a young keen Collie, began to compete at local sheep dog trials. Later, a young dog, which I trained for another shepherd, finally settled down to work, and went on to win a nursery class in California. We competed at the U.S. national nursery finals. I now have three dogs competing and another youngster waiting in the wings. Because of some very lovely large fields, magnificent views, and one of the largest commercial flocks of sheep in British Columbia, it was obvious to me and another shepherd that we just had to get a trial going. That was nine years ago. With these essential ingredients Metchosin has become home to one of the largest Trials in the northwest, and the Ninth Annual Trial was held here in July 2000. Handlers came from as far away as Ontario and Missouri, as well as California, Oregon, Washington, Alberta, and British Columbia. Setting the standard for this Trial, we had previous national and international judges coming to both judge and teach. Organising the event as well as looking after our own flock (twenty-three lambs this spring) and training my own and some other dogs and has made my life quite full! Presently I am Chair of the Metchosin Healthy Community Advisory Commission, where I manage to keep in touch with many interesting and challenging health-related projects afoot in our community.

Pearson College of the Pacific, one of eleven United World Colleges, is in Metchosin, and my husband and I have been closely involved there since 1992. We have become host parents to the students from Victoria's sister city, Suzhou, China, and have had some of their parents come to visit us at home. With these Chinese connections we were able to take Mandarin language study sessions at two universities in China, and during our visits there we met families of all the students who have come to Pearson College. Several of these students are in undergraduate and post-graduate programs in the U.S. and Canada, but still call Metchosin their North American home. I find that there is rarely a day when I do not use some part of my varied medical and non-medical training. I have been fortunate to be able to follow so many of my dreams!

DR. HEIDI MARTINS

My parents were living in Mozambique, in then Lourenco Marques, and since my mother's family and doctors were in South Africa, I was born in Johannesburg on January 18, 1953. Medical services were basic in Mozambique, and as a child I was ill with asthma, so my mother was told to take me back to Johannesburg for consistent care and for the climate. My mother left my father behind in 1959 and took me and my one-and-a-half-year-old brother Etienne to Johannesburg where we lived for the rest of our school years. We would go back to Maputo, Mozambique, for summer vacation. I spoke Portuguese as a first language and learned Afrikaans (my mother's language) at six years of age and then English at ten, when my father insisted we should change to an English school. My parents spoke to each other in English.

At school, biology and art were my favourite subjects, and I wanted to be an artist. However, I was advised I'd "starve in an attic," so was pressured to do something in biology. My first plan was marine biology, but again I was advised to study medicine so I would "always have a job." Being obedient at that time, I studied medicine at the University of Witwatersand from 1970 to 1976.

We went on one safari as a group in 1973 and did a little local hiking during my university years, and I kept up the tradition of summer vacations in Mozambique. My parents' marriage was failing.

In 1977 I did a house job or internship in the Johannesburg Hospital in surgery, then medicine, and in my second year pediatrics, more medicine, and oncology. Then I joined the Internal Medicine Residency Programme for the next four years, rotating through four Johannesburg Hospitals.

My boyfriend of the last year of medical school and first year of internship also joined the Residency Programme, but the stresses of work and my need to pursue my own career caused the relationship to end. He subsequently emigrated to Canada and works and lives in Sudbury, Ontario.

At the completion of my residency, I failed my examination and took off with my life savings to have a year away. I lived in London for eight months and enjoyed the cultural life. To assuage my guilt, I did the Diploma of Tropical Medicine at the London School of Tropical Medicine. It was fun

and I loved living in the cosmopolitan world of the International Student Home at Mecklenbergh Square. During that year I went to Portugal with my father, visiting relatives and friends from Mozambique. We travelled throughout Portugal for a month, then I spent a month in Peru with a group from South Africa and another month in North America. This was my introduction to Canada and I loved the west coast, having stayed in Vancouver and on Mayne Island.

After that year I returned to do an extra year of residency and passed my exam, then went to Capetown to do a Haematology fellowship. It was a program in decay, and I was determined to leave South Africa with its increasing violence and social disorder. So I came to Toronto to do the LMCC exam and visit friends. I passed the exam and was given six months grace to be in Canada and working. My friend in Sudbury arranged a job for me there, since this was an underserviced area and non-Canadians could be employed. However, it was later discovered that two other oncologists from South Africa were prepared to come to this area, so I was offered a training position in Ottawa to do the fellowship. My ex-boyfriend also accepted the training arrangement.

I arrived in Ottawa on New Year's Day, 1987. It was a culture shock for me to come from mid-summer Capetown to minus twenty-five degrees Celsius in Ottawa. I was miserable, alone, and stressed out during the two-year fellowship. My ex-boyfriend had his wife with him and fared better. I had to do my fellowship in Internal Medicine exam during this period and failed it the first time, so I stayed for an extra six months and passed the exam in May, 1989.

To remain in Canada I had to apply for permission to work in an underserviced area. I chose to go to St. John's Newfoundland as there was no oncologist there. I loved the beauty and ruggedness and isolation of Newfoundland. I stayed two and a half years, and enjoyed my job and time there. I lived in a beautiful apartment for a year with a 180 degree view of the harbour. I later moved to a fisherman's cottage on the harbour, travelled throughout Newfoundland with various friends, and did pottery at the Blue Moon Pottery overlooking the Narrows.

However, the department could not recruit anyone for the next two and a half years, and I felt I would not be able to sustain myself without colleagues in the same field. My then male friend, a geologist, could not find work in Newfoundland in the long term either. So I moved out west to Victoria in 1991 when the job was advertised.

I have lived in a lovely west-coast style home and gardened a lot since being here. It is a wonderful area for me for hiking, kayaking, and skiing in winter. My geologist friend has been an inducement to travel and explore the world.

My family is still in Africa and I visit them every three years. My hobby of pottery has been a joy for the last twenty-five years and I have fixed up a workshop in my basement. It does make me sad to think that I did not get married and have children. However, I am thankful for being able to live in a beautiful area of the world and that I am healthy. I would like to do regular travelling and some volunteer work as I become older.

DR. RUTH JOY SIMKIN

Medical school and feminism entered my life at the same time, which was somewhat ironic as they combined somewhat less smoothly than oil and water. Almost from the beginning of my first year I was constantly involved in some sort of embroilment with the staff and male students.

I was in the first class of the University of Calgary Medical school. There were 1,200 applications for thirty-two places and there were 100 professors ready and waiting to begin educating a new generation of physicians. The year prior to the opening class of medical school was fiercely competitive. At the University of Calgary, most people would not share any class information with others for fear that they might give something away and fall behind. This was most distasteful to myself and two others, and so Ron, Mickey, and I formed a trio of sharing—notes, information, and discussion. This helped immensely while waiting for the selections to be made.

The medical school had not yet been built. In fact, it officially opened on the day that we, the first class, graduated. We used the old pathology labs on the twelfth floor of Foothills Hospital for our "med school" and it was there we had our classes, saw patients, dissected cadavers, and anything else medical school related. Our study areas were divided into eight areas of four—each quarter had four desks in an open-sided rectangle. Within the

first month, the fellows in my group started putting up playboy pin-ups all over the walls and general area. I went to the professor in charge of the student study area. He shook his head at me: "This is what we expect of our medical students, Ruth. If you can't handle it, maybe you shouldn't be here." Oh, I could handle it. For Christmas holidays I went to visit a friend in New York where I made a very special purchase. Upon my return, I waited until a tour group was about to come through the medical school, I then hung up a large repulsive pin-up of a naked man, right over my desk. That same professor came running over to me: "Take that down at once!" he exclaimed. "But sir, I am only trying to fit in, as you advised." We made a deal. I would take down my pin-up and the fellows would take down theirs. The tour passed through a very sterile-looking, bland study area. From that day on, I had my work cut out for me.

I could not understand why the washrooms in the doctors' lounge were for men only, or why the doctors' changing room of the OR and obstetrics was for men only. By the time I finished my residency, we had female washrooms and change rooms.

Before I began my residency, I had established myself as a troublemaker, although from my perspective, I was simply working for equal rights for women. When the preceptors were to pick their practice residents, they held a lottery and the 'loser' got me. I was quite hurt when I found this out. I was always very dedicated and my marks were good. I loved working with patients and was very conscientious. But the more traditional male physicians were not willing or ready to have anyone challenge the status quo. And so I became the 'other,' the troublemaker.

I was told that women could not do an ICU (intensive care unit) rotation because the doctors in charge felt it was too difficult. I objected and protested and they finally relented. Of course, since I was the first woman to do this rotation, I was watched far more closely and had much less chance for imperfection than my male colleagues. We had to wear little white miniskirts and white jackets. The first time I had to lead a cardiac arrest and get up on a gurney to do cardiac compressions, I realized that miniskirts were not appropriate. Yet in medical school, I had been sent home for wearing slacks on a day we had classes only! I started wearing white slacks like the male residents, much to the chagrin of the staff physicians. Today it seems like a silly issue, but it was a big thing then—for a woman to come to work in slacks. I finished my ICU rotation wearing slacks, feeling somewhat triumphant as the ICU physicians now accepted that women residents were able to manage the work.

My surgery rotation was a disaster at first. My assigned surgeon did not believe that women belonged in the OR unless they were patients or compliant nurses. He had heard that I spoke Greek and wanted me to teach him some. I was delighted—I said I would and looked forward to his teaching me surgery. He smiled. After several weeks of doing nothing more than holding a retractor and receiving virtually no surgical teaching, I went to the head of the department. I was ready to leave, I felt so frustrated. I felt I should at least learn how to take out a hot appendix and other basic surgical skills. We finally found a surgeon who was willing to have me on his team, and I went on to have an excellent rotation.

The rounds used to start off with "Gentlemen." When I was a resident, I used to hold up my hand every week and say: "Excuse me, sir, but we are not all gentlemen here." Then for months after, the rounds would start with: "Gentlemen. And Ruth," and most people would snicker. Years later, the rounds start with: "Ladies and Gentlemen." No one snickers.

In my second year residency, I did an elective in Israel. Dr. Ben Fisher was a superb dermatologist and teacher. After teaching at the medical school for four years, he had gone to work in a hospital outside of Tel Aviv. He had asked if I would be interested in doing an elective there. *Would* I? It was a wonderful four months. I learned a lot about how medicine is practised in other countries. There were things I found shocking, other things amusing. And I learned a lot of dermatology. As part of my elective, I was to do a research paper. I wrote and subsequently published a paper on basal cell epithelioma of the vulva. As a result of my research, the treatment of this disease changed from radical vulvectomies, which left the women terribly scarred both physically and emotionally, to local excisions and follow up. I was very proud of this contribution.

Prior to my going to Israel I had made arrangements for the resident preceptor to register me for my CCFP (Certificant of the College of Family Physicians of Canada). I was told everything was in order. After I returned, I didn't really think about it until all my fellow residents started talking about the letters they received regarding the CCFP exams. I did not receive such a letter. I went to the preceptor:

"Did you not register me for the CCFP exams as we discussed?"

"Oh no, Ruth, did I forget to tell you? We decided you weren't ready to write the exams."

"Why is that?"

"We didn't want you to bring the marks down. This is the first year University of Calgary students are writing the exams."

"But my marks have always been good."

"Well, we felt you would bring the marks down. Maybe next year. It's too late for this year."

I left the office in tears of frustration which soon gave way to resolve. I contacted another physician who was going to Ottawa who agreed to argue my case. Since the deadline for registration had long passed, he was not sure if he would be able to do anything or not. However, luck was with me and I was able to write the exams with my colleagues. My marks were in the ninety-eighth percentile in the whole country. So much for bringing disgrace upon my alma mater!

There are many more memories of my medical school training: working two years with "unwed mothers" as they were called then, and using hypnosis with them during delivery. The hypnosis was taught us by the expert Dr. Dave Kovitz. Under his guidance, I became skilled in its use. One of my favourite memories was representing the Department of Pediatrics and successfully treating a baby orangutan at the zoo for gastroenteritis.

I now had an MD, a CCFP, and wanted to go into practice right away. It was 1975. I applied for hospital privileges. To my amazement, they were denied. I found out they would consider privileges if I would go into an already existing practice. This is not what I wanted to do at all. I remember crying bitterly that night. The next day I entered into a practice with two fellows. I got my privileges. I was the first person from the University of Calgary ever to go into private practice. Within six months, my practice was so full that I had to move to offices down the hall because I needed more room. Things were good. I was practising family medicine, and loving it.

In 1975 there were no organizations for women physicians in Calgary. Apparently, the Federation of Medical Women of Canada used to have a chapter there, but the few female physicians had no real information about this. So several of us started a chapter. In the beginning there were only a few members, but over the years, as more women graduated, we built up our numbers. I was president for several years, and very active in the organization until I left Calgary. One of the highlights of my involvement with the FMWC was my presenting a paper at the Medical Women's International Association Congress in Manila, Philippines, in 1982.

In 1976, we realized that there was not really any opportunity for women in the general public to learn more about their bodies and medicine in general. I was a founder of From Woman to Woman: You and Your Health, which started in the mid-seventies. Of course, I was also a presenter. This was the first of yearly events that have spread across the country. The female physicians are instrumental in organizing a seminar for women in the community. It has always been very well attended and successful, with wide-ranging topics. When I see these conferences still going strong in the 21st century, I do feel proud of my contribution in starting them.

In 1976 I had my new offices, and my practice was full. I was a lecturer (1975-79) in the Department of Family Practice, University of Calgary. In 1979, I became an Assistant Professor, until I left the department in 1986. As well, in 1977, for an extra challenge, I became Chief Medical Officer at Alberta Vocational College. Life was pretty good.

I would go to family practice rounds every week and be one of two female physicians there initially. The rounds used to start off with "Gentlemen." When I was a resident, I used to hold up my hand every week and say: "Excuse me, sir, but we are not all gentlemen here." Then for months after, the rounds would start with: "Gentlemen. And Ruth," and most people would snicker. Years later, the rounds start with: "Ladies and Gentlemen." No one snickers. And no one knows about the tears of humiliation I fought back every week. I feel proud about helping to normalize the existence and validity of female physicians.

As soon as I finished my residency and had a bit more free time, I joined many feminist organizations in the community. I was on the Board of Directors of the Calgary Birth Control Association, and the Board of Directors of the Alberta Status of Women Action Committee. As well, I helped plan several large conferences, such as the Women and Madness Conference in 1975 with Dr. Phyllis Chessier, and the Women and Violence Conference in 1980.

As busy as I was in my community, I was getting busier in my professional life as a family physician. My practice was full, I was doing some teaching at the medical school, and I was on the Foothills Hospital Abortion Committee from 1976 to 1981. When I first started on the committee, women requesting an abortion used to have to come before a tribunal of doctors and answer their questions. In the majority of cases, this was a humiliating experience. I was very pleased to see things changed over the years to allow these women more dignity.

I had been getting interested in alternative medicine and, in particular, acupuncture. I went to China in 1977 on a tour and had seen some Chinese medicine practised there. I had taken some courses offered locally, and then in 1982, I went back to China to attend the Shanghai College of Traditional Chinese Medicine, where I received a Diploma in Acupuncture in a WHO-sponsored course. My four months away were months of wonder. The biggest gift from my experience in Shanghai was being able to accomplish a paradigm shift in my thinking. I remember an elderly gentleman who came to our clinic complaining of insomnia. Easy, I thought, just give him a sleeping pill. "Oh no," said our teacher. "He has too much fire in the heart." It took a long time for me to be able to understand that concept and to work with that. I will always be grateful for the flexibility it taught me in my thinking.

I came back to my private practice and incorporated acupuncture. In fact, I was the first MD in Alberta to be licensed to practise acupuncture. But I still continued to have a fairly ordinary family practice.

In 1983, I sold my practice and moved over to the Alexandra Community Health Centre. This position was quite a challenge, one which I adored. When I had started working at the clinic, there was one half-time physician. By the time I left five years later, we were three physicians, several counsellors, a lab, and myriad programs for seniors and others in the community.

As well during that time, I worked part-time evenings with the Planned Parenthood Teen Clinic.

I had noticed that PMS was a major complaint of many of our patients, and set out to learn more about it. In 1984, I went to England to study with Dr. Katarina Dalton, the physician who first identified PMS. I came back and started Western Canada's first PMS clinic at the Alexandra Community Health Centre. Within a very short time we had a six-month waiting list. We had patients coming to us from the United States and all over Canada. And I do believe we were able to offer them some relief. I was starting to get a lot of referrals from some psychiatrists and other physicians as well. About this time, one of the physicians who had been a resident with me wrote a letter to all the members of the Department of Family Practice. In the letter he wrote that I was running a PMS clinic, and that I was a charlatan, taking unfair advantage of patients. He wrote that everyone knew there was no such thing as PMS, that I had fabricated it, and that I was just making money off innocent patients. He was not aware that I was salaried, so more patients just meant harder work for the same pay. He wanted my licence revoked immediately and to have me dropped from the Department. No one had spoken to me about any concerns prior to my seeing this letter. I contacted my lawyer and sued him for libel. He apologized publicly but unhappily.

I founded the Calgary Lesbian and Gay Political Action Group and, in 1993, I did a four-part series for CBC TV on lesbian health. Also in 1993, I was profiled on TV as a lesbian health care educator.

In 1986, I left the Department of Family Practice at Foothills Hospital. I had been working very long hours and had decided to take Fridays off. Just weeks after I made this decision, I received a call from the secretary of the Department telling me that I had to take my turn on the death audit committee which met every Friday morning. I replied that I didn't work on Friday and couldn't be on it, and when she said that I *had* to be on it, I replied: "Well then, I quit!" And the next day I had my letter of resignation on her desk. I have always felt good about this, because there are parts of bureaucratic medicine that don't make sense to me. I had finally started to take care of myself, and working forty to fifty hours in four days, I just refused to go into a non-vital meeting at 7:30 a.m. on my day off.

During my time in Calgary, I also ran a production company, producing many concerts over the years. I gave over two hundred public presentations, as well as appearing on both radio and TV shows. I became very active in the area of lesbian health, and founded the Calgary Lesbian and Gay Political Action Group. In 1993, I did a four-part series for CBC TV on lesbian health. Also in 1993, I was profiled on TV as a lesbian health care educator. I also was involved in the making of two films, one on PMS and one on suicide, and was a member of the Task Force on Suicide for the Canadian Mental Health Association.

I have been published many times, with over a dozen papers in medical journals, a chapter in a medical book for women, and over seventy-five articles, opinions, etc. in community and national magazines. In 1999 I published the book *Like an Orange on a Seder Plate*, which is a lesbian-feminist-oriented haggadah for Passover.

I have always been very involved in my community, but no more than in Calgary. During my twenty-two years there, I was on the Board of Directors and Executive of the Alberta Theatre Projects, involved in the building and completion of the Calgary Centre for Performing Arts. I was an organizer for Judy Chicago's "The Dinner Party," and brought the show to Glenbow Museum, one of the most successful exhibitions they have ever had. I organized and ran a political action workshop, was volunteer co-ordinator of the counselling team for the AIDS quilt display, and the production manager for the Women's Legal Education and Action Fund (LEAF) Canadian Travelling Road Show. These were just some of my many activities over the decades in Calgary.

Throughout the years I have won several awards. The two of which I am most proud are Woman of the Year Award in Health and Fitness, jointly awarded with Dr. Maria Eriksen in 1981, and Speak Sebastian Award of Distinction, presented for work in the lesbian and gay community, 1991.

I worked very hard those five years at the Alexandra Clinic, and then wanted to try working part-time. Within a year, I was working less and had started a hologram gallery in Calgary. I ran the gallery for several years and then decided to relocate to British Columbia. Part-time practice didn't work for me. Patients do not get sick on Tuesdays and Thursdays only, and I found I ended up either working all the time, or not seeing my patients appropriately. Neither of these was acceptable to me.

I bought some property on Saltspring Island and ran an organic vegetable farm there for five years. But I missed medicine. I had been reading about Palliative Care, and had a definite interest in that field. I called Dr. Carole Herbert, of the UBC Department of Family Practice to ask her advice about further training and became the first Palliative Care Fellow in British Columbia. I did a fellowship from 1997 to 1999, and later that year was hired as a hospice staff physician at Victoria Hospice Society, where I had done the majority of my training. I still practise there and feel very privileged to be able to do this work. I love my work at the hospice and feel really lucky when I can wake up smiling in the morning because I am on my way to work that day!

I think any story about me would be incomplete without including my two wolf dogs. Their mother was an arctic wolf, their father a Belgian Sheepdog. They go with me everywhere and are official registered pet therapy dogs! They love coming to work with me as much as I love working. I feel I have been truly fortunate to have these two animal companions in my life.

When I first started my practice, I did a lot of obstetrics. At that time, it was a true privilege to help people into this world. And now that I practise Palliative Care, I again feel it is a privilege to help people leave this world with dignity and peace. Even though I have done many different things during my life, I have always enjoyed my work. I feel blessed to be a physician and to be involved in the work I do.

Curriculum Vitae

Education: RHI program, Palliative Care, University of British Columbia, 1998–1999; Fellowship, Palliative Care, University of British Columbia, 1997–1999; BA *Cum Laude*, Trinity College, Washington, D.C., 1966–1969; Further education, University of Calgary, Alberta, 1969–1970; MD, University of Calgary, Alberta, 1970–1973; CCFP Residency, Family Medicine, University of Calgary, Alberta, 1973–1975; Elective, Dermatology, Tel Hashomer, Israel, 1975;

Acupuncture Diploma, Shanghai College of Traditional Chinese Medicine, Shanghai, People's Republic of China, 1982; Intensive training, Premenstrual Syndrome Treatment with Dr. Katarina Dalton, London, England, 1984; Courses ranging from women's studies to film-making, 1970–present.

Employment: Hospice physician, Victoria Hospice Society, Victoria, B.C, 1999–present; Associate hospice physician, Victoria Hospice Society, Victoria, B.C., 1997–1999; Contractor, B.C. Women's Hospital. Developed recommendations for admission to residential drug and alcohol treatment, Vancouver, B.C., 1995; Physician, private practice, Family Medicine, Calgary, Alberta, 1988–1991; Staff physician, Alexandra Community Health Centre, Calgary, Alberta, 1983–1987; Part-time physician, Planned Parenthood Teen Clinic, Calgary, Alberta, 1983–1986; Chief Medical Officer, Alberta Vocational Services, Calgary, Alberta, 1977; Physician, private practice, Family Medicine, Calgary, Alberta, 1975–1983; Owner and manager, organic farm operation, Saltspring Island, B.C., 1992–present; Owner and manager, Holomagic, Calgary, Alberta, 1988–1991; Owner and manager, Circle Productions, Calgary, Alberta, 1975–1996.

Awards: Speak Sebastian Award of Distinction, Calgary, Alberta, 1991; Woman of the Year (with Dr. Maria Eriksen), Calgary YWCA, 1981; Hillebrand Junior Award, Chemical Society of Washington, Washington, D.C., 1968.

Teaching Appointments: Lecturer, Department of Family Practice, University of Calgary, Alberta, 1975–1979; Assistant Professor, Department of Family Practice, University of Calgary, Alberta, 1979–1984.

Publications:

Like An Orange on a Seder Plate: Our Lesbian Haggadah. Published in Canada, February 1999

Quarterly column "Not Only For Lesbians," *Federation of Medical Women of Canada Newsletter*, 1997–1999

"Not all your patients are straight," *Can Med Assoc J*, Aug 25, 1998; 159 (4), pps. 370-375

"Women's Health: Time For A Redefinition," Editorial, *Can Med Assoc J*, Feb. 15, 1995, 152(4), pps. 477-479

"Introduction," in Regan McClure and Anne Vespry, eds., *Lesbian Health Guide*, Queer Press, Toronto, 1994

"Creating Openness and Receptiveness with your patients: overcoming heterosexual assumptions," *The Canadian Journal of Ob/Gyn & Women's Health Care*, 1993, 5(4), pps. 485-489

"Unique Health Care Concerns of Lesbians," *The Canadian Journal of Ob/Gyn & Women's Health Care*,1993, 5(5), pps. 516–522

"Health Issues," *Healthsharing*, 1992, 13(L), pps. 40-42

"Lesbians Face Unique Health Care Problems," *Can Med Assoc J*, 1991, 145(12), pps. 1620-1623

"Lesbian Health Care," in Carolyn DeMarco, *Take Charge of Your Body*, The Well Women Press, 1989

"Premenstrual Syndrome: Approaches to Diagnosis and Treatment," *Can Fam Physician*, October 1985, 31, pps. 1959-1967

"Alternative Birthing," *Can Fam Physician*, June 1981, 27, pps. 1007-1010.

"Basal Cell Epithelioma of the Vulva," *Obstetrics and Gynecology*, May 1977, 49(5), pps. 617-619

"Methanolysis of 2-nitrophenyl acetate," *Chemistry and Industry*, with Alicja Kirkien-Konasiewics and Robin Murphy, 1968, pps. 1842-1843

Approximately seventy-five articles, opinions, etc. in community and national newsletters and magazines, 1972 to present

Presentations:

"Delirium and Confusional States," University of Victoria Continuing Education, Victoria, B.C., 2000.

"Working Effectively with Lesbian Clients," Women's Health Clinic, Winnipeg, Manitoba, 1995.

"Lesbian Health." Four-half-hour segments for "What On Earth." CBC TV, 1993.

Profiled on TV show "Women's Wellness" as a lesbian health care educator, Vancouver, B.C., 1993.

"Lesbian Health Issues in Family Medicine," keynote address, Women's College Hospital, Toronto, Ontario, 1993.

"An autobiographical reading," Women in A Violent Society Conference, Banff, Alberta, 1991.

"Lesbian Lives: Community as Family," Women Helping Women Conference, Calgary, Alberta, 1990.

"Discrimination on basis of sexual orientation," Canadian Advisory Council on the Status of Women, Ottawa, Ontario, 1989.

"Public Forum on PMS," Calgary Jewish Centre, Calgary, Alberta, 1988.

"A Profile of PMS Patients at the Alexandra Community Health Centre, Calgary, Canada," with Maureen Osis, first international conference on the Premenstrual Syndrome, Anaheim, California, 1985.

"The Uniqueness of the Feminine Perspective on Healing: A Consideration of Eastern and Western Medical Approaches," Medical Women International Association, Manila, Philippines, 1982.

Content specialist for "Cause of Death," video, Task Force on Suicide, Canadian Mental Health Association and Faculty of Medicine, University of Calgary, Alberta, 1982.

"Psychological Advantages Inherent in a Traditional Doctor-Patient Relationship which Lead to Inferior Health Care," The College of Family Physicians of Canada, Ottawa, Ontario, 1979.

"The Inadequacy of Health Care of Women," Canadian Research Institute for the Advancement of Women, Quebec City, Quebec, 1978.

Over two hundred presentations in person, on radio, and on television, on topics of women's health care, civil rights, and feminist politics, 1972–present.

Professional Service: Over twelve peer manuscript reviews for *Canadian Family Physician* and *Canadian Medical Association Journal*, 1983–present; Over twenty published book reports for *Canadian Family Physician* and *Canadian Medical Association Journal*, 1977–present; Examiner, College of Family Physicians of Canada specialty exams, Calgary, Alberta, 1976.

Volunteer Activities: Entertainment Committee Member, Canadian Palliative Care Association 2001 Conference, Victoria, B.C., 2000; Board of Directors, Planned Parenthood (Saltspring), Saltspring Island, B.C., 1997; Production Manager, LEAF Canadian Travelling Road Show, Calgary, Alberta, 1989; Volunteer co-ordinator, counselling team, AIDS quilt display, Calgary, Alberta, 1989; Founder, chair, and director, Calgary

Lesbian and Gay Political Action Guild, Calgary, Alberta, 1988–1991; Founder, organizer, and presenter, "Political Action Workshop," Calgary, Alberta, 1989; Physician and office staff, Michigan Women's Music Festival, Michigan, U.S.A., 1988–1995; Organizer, "The Dinner Party," Judy Chicago, Glenbow Museum, Calgary, Alberta, 1983; Board of Directors and Fundraising Chair, Alberta Theatre Projects, Calgary, Alberta, 1981–1987; Organizer, "Women and Violence Conference," Calgary, Alberta, 1980; Member, Task Force on Suicide, Canadian Mental Health Association, Calgary, Alberta, 1980–1983; Board of Directors, Alberta Status of Women Action Committee, Alberta, 1976–1980; Delegate to Destiny Canada Destinee, York University, Toronto, Ontario, 1977; Board of Directors, Calgary Status of Women Action Committee, Calgary, Alberta, 1975–1980; Board of Directors, Calgary Birth Control Association, Calgary, Alberta, 1976–1981; Member, Abortion Committee, Foothills Hospital, Calgary, Alberta, 1976–1981; Founder and President, Calgary Branch, Canadian Federation of Medical Women, Calgary, Alberta, 1976–1981; Founder and presenter, "From Woman to Woman: You and Your Health," Calgary, Alberta, 1976; Organizer, "Women and Madness Conference," Calgary, Alberta, 1976.

DR. SALLIE JEAN TEASDALE-SCOTT

I was born the third child of four (three girls, one boy) during the Depression in 1931 to a fruit farmer in the Niagara Peninsula, Ontario, and his wife, a primary school teacher. We had absolutely no money, but we had everything a child could want—lots of contact with both parents, horses and ponies to ride, tennis court, skating rink, high bar, swing, seesaw, etc., and parents who believed that play and sports were important. My father died when I was thirteen and my mother, always dominant in the child-rearing department, took over. It was a given that we would seek some form of higher education, although to any outsider, it seemed financially unlikely.

I was so into sports that I decided on Physical and Health Education, and chose the University of Toronto because it was only a three-year course at that time. A variety of scholarships and a good summer job made it all possible. I played on every team that I could for the faculty, and played intercollegiate tennis and basketball for U of T. Basketball was the love of my life; I was a high scorer throughout and captain elect four years out of six. I had a great time athletically and was among the first dozen students to be elected to the University of Sports Hall of Fame when this institution became established many years later.

While at university, I lived in residence and came to know a small group of girls studying medicine. These girls not only became my friends, but also won my admiration because they seemed to be striving to do something worthwhile for other people. I began to realize that perhaps I could, too. As a high school student I had never dreamed that I could study medicine. It was far too lofty a goal for a farmer's daughter like me even though I had always done well (first and sometimes second) throughout all my schooling.

My acceptance into medicine at the University of Toronto was a wondrous thing to me, and until this day I consider myself among the most fortunate in the world. Since the death of my father I had suppressed an unrealistic, juvenile thought in the back of my head that I might contribute somehow to the defeat of cancer. I still chuckle when I recall an interview I had with a physician, a member of the admissions committee, who asked me the routine question, "Why do you want to be a doctor?" Sitting there nervously with my hands clasped I replied with all the misguided earnestness of youth, "I want to find a cure for cancer." He looked at me a while and with a grin said, "Why don't we just write down that you want to do general practice?" This experience was sort of my first brush with reality, one might say.

I was the first person to jump from physical education into medicine at the University of Toronto without having to do pre-med, although many have since followed this path. U of T had a policy of accepting a maximum of ten percent women of the 150 students in first year at this time (1953). Thank goodness we were subsidized by the government (i.e., taxpayers) and did not have to mortgage our future like the present would-be MDs do.

Our class was encouraged to form two all-girl clinic groups (a practice subsequently discontinued, to the benefit of all, I'm sure), but I never felt that I suffered any gender bias while I was a student. In fact being young and female might even have been an advantage during the clinic years when most of the practising clinicians were fatherly males.

After graduation, though, gender took on a special meaning. As a woman there were some specialties that we knew were not for us. No one actually announced "males only," but few women applied for surgery, and the few who did were strongly discouraged. I completed a junior internship at the Toronto General Hospital (1,400 beds at that time) and decided that I would apply to the specialty of obstetrics which seemed a natural choice for a female. During my interview with the Chief of Obstetrics, he informed me that if I undertook a career in obstetrics I was not to marry, and of course there would be no place for me on the Toronto General Hospital Staff—my target should be Women's College Hospital. I was accepted for training the following year without any legally binding promises of celibacy because I planned to do a year of general practice first for financial reasons.

A member of the admissions committee asked me, "Why do you want to be a doctor?" I replied with all the misguided earnestness of youth, "I want to find a cure for cancer." He looked at me a while and with a grin said, "Why don't we just write down that you want to do general practice?"

I joined an established practitioner in my hometown along with another young male graduate. Family practice was challenging and extremely satisfying and often fun. But I worried whether I could possibly maintain the 'state of the art' knowledge in all fields as time went on. I felt I had to zero in on a smaller field of practice to remain an 'expert' consultant. As the only female general practitioner in Niagara Falls (the only other female physician was a part-time pediatrician) I attracted a sizable obstetrical practice and it became very clear to me that the unpredictability of the practice of obstetrics could become a real obstacle to marriage, which I was contemplating at the time, a family, and a reasonable home life. As I was in practice with two male general practitioners, I could not help but notice also the relationship they enjoyed with the young pregnant mother who had an elevating effect on their self-image, while I, on the other hand, seemed to get my highs from my in-hospital practice dealing with very sick patients.

I think that some time spent doing general practice is invaluable to the young doctor trying to make a sensible choice for a lifetime career (and that the current practice of having to pick a specialty in third year is foolhardy).

After two years of family practice I considered internal medicine, but settled on anaesthesia as it would always place me where the in-hospital action was, (albeit often 'contrived' by the surgeon), and often among the first to be called to an emergency. It represented pharmacology in action, sort of an instant evidence of how drugs work. I thought it was the right choice for someone like myself who has a "just the facts, Ma'am" kind of brain and prefers short action stories to long philosophical epistles. I also entertained the naïve expectation that my hours would be more reasonable. The young colleague with whom I was working had a wife and family to support while I had my mother (the rest of my siblings had taken their turns at financial support, and it was my turn). My colleague and I decided to train in anaesthesia close to home, in this case Buffalo, and to continue our general practice in evenings and on weekends. This arrangement was supported by our loyal patients, and with our willingness to give anaesthetics for our short-staffed colleagues during night-time hours, we managed to pay our bills. At this time anaesthesia training in the U.S.A. required two years ("board eligible" after passing written exams with a set of orals to be passed after a year of practice to be fully qualified).

My young colleague succumbed to the allures of California, but I had become engaged to marry a Torontonian, so I applied and was accepted to continue my training in the four-year anaesthesia program in Toronto. This switch allowed me to combine a very practical, independence- and confidence-building U.S.A. kind of training with a very academically oriented Toronto training—giving me a broader base on which to build my own career. The confident American style with which I entered my third year of training (after all I was qualified to practise in the U.S.A!) inspired the chief to ask me to stay on staff at the Toronto General Hospital once my training was completed. I was flattered and accepted the offer. I married that year and during my Medicine rotation gave birth to a son. A junior staff man at Sunnybrook Hospital and I (as a resident) were setting up the hospital's first coronary care unit, and I recall running down corridors in the middle of the night when eight months pregnant in response to a cardiac arrest call and having to climb on a chair as my five-foot-eight-inch frame had lost the necessary flexibility required to perform chest compressions. It was exciting but tiring.

As a junior intern in 1957, I had the good fortune to be the sixth assistant holding a retractor in an operating theatre full of the local media when the first open heart operation with heart-lung bypass was performed at the Toronto General Hospital. (I believe it was the first such heart operation in Canada.) Cardiac surgery was in its infancy and everything was at the pioneer stage. The staff cardiac surgeons had all trained in some other specialty, such as orthopedics or general surgery, and they were learning on the job. The anaesthetists (nowadays anesthesiologists) were pioneering their craft right along with them. The anesthesiologist was a big part of the team and constantly relied upon for help and advice. Communication between the surgeon and the anesthesiologist was constant. The patients offered up for surgery in those early years were those whom the cardiologists could no longer help. Any success was a victory. Without question, this was where I wanted to be, where I started out as a junior staff, and where I remained until leaving Toronto twenty-seven years later.

The hours I worked in cardiac anaesthesia were punishing in the early years. One operation could easily take eight hours or more, and then there was the resuscitative care required in the post-operative period—usually primarily the responsibility of the anesthesiologist. As time went on and the world's expertise improved we became much better in all aspects of our practice—but my, those early years were exciting! Through those years, I had the privilege of sorting out, with my surgical colleagues, the clinical effects of hypothermia and bypass on heart rhythm, electrolyte balance, coagulation, blood pressure, drug metabolism, consciousness, etc. We progressed through surgery on cold hearts, warm hearts, beating hearts, arrested hearts, unperfused hearts, perfused hearts, and finally we transplanted hearts. We progressed from keeping patients sedated and ventilated post-operatively (sometimes for days) to patients awake and extubated in the OR at the end of the procedure. Of course, all the major centres in the world were making similar clinical discoveries in parallel with us as we all pushed forward the learning edge of cardiac surgery/anaesthesia—but the challenge was to prove something first and to show the best results. Now, of course, surgery for coronary heart disease has become so routine and so successful that it is more common than a D and C.

During my practice my husband and I had four children—I took two to three months off with each. Maternity leave was frowned upon in the 1960s in my hospital. There was a seldom expressed but strong feeling that if you were going to take a man's job then you should work a man's hours. If you had any leadership ambitions at all you could not work less than full-time in academia. One Toronto hospital consistently refused to hire female anesthesiologists for over a decade on the premise that pregnancy or a sick child made them unreliable on a day-to-day basis. Thank goodness this attitude has changed.

My fourth child likes to hear the story of her birth each year on her birthday—so I remember it well. It went like this: I anesthetized a patient for an open heart surgery with our senior surgeon in the morning, and then anesthetized a patient for a closed mitral split with our junior surgeon in the afternoon. Just when this finished, I was called to give a colleague an anesthetic for an esophagoscopy. As I was resting in the doctors' lounge, the junior staff surgeon phoned and asked if I could re-anesthetize our patient who was experiencing a post-op bleed. I replied that I would if he could not find another anesthetist, but that I thought I was going into labour, having started to feel a few contractions. He hurriedly said "never mind, never mind," and I proceeded up to the labour floor and two hours later had Catherine.

My career at the Toronto General Hospital (1965-1992) also involved teaching, clinical research, and some administration. Much of my clinical research involved studying the effects of new drugs on the cardiovascular system and then introducing them in appropriate dosages into our clinical practice. For example, I recall being one of Canada's earliest clinical investigators of the drug bretylium. I had the very satisfying experience of being

One Toronto hospital consistently refused to hire female anesthesiologists for over a decade on the premise that pregnancy or a sick child made them unreliable on a day-to-day basis.

able to resuscitate a patient with recurring ventricular fibrillation following aortic valve replacement, after which the surgical team had given up all hope of saving the patient, using this new wonder drug unknown to clinical practice at the time. We continued to receive Christmas cards from this well patient for many years. Also, our research team was the first ever to establish the use of ancrod, venom from a viper, to anticoagulate blood for bypass for patients allergic to heparin.

Although combining a career and family is pretty routine nowadays, it was not quite so common in the 1960s and 1970s. I loved my work, but often worried that I might be short-changing my children. We were fortunate to have a young English nanny for a consecutive thirteen years, which provided great consistency in care, while Montessori schools provided the children's early education. Fortunately, our children have all enjoyed a university education, are well-established in their respective careers and seem, to me at least, to be well-adjusted citizens. I gave up seeking reassurance from them by asking them directly about their youthful deprivations as it seemed to encourage them to exercise their sense of fun at my expense.

However, there is no doubt that my marriage suffered from the demands of double careers in the family, and my husband and I divorced after the children had grown. I am now married to a wonderful man—also a physician—and we moved to Victoria in 1991.

After coming to Victoria I worked at both Victoria General and Royal Jubilee Hospitals on a part-time basis, as I was just completing a sabbatical, then spent the last few years at the Victoria General only. As these are not teaching hospitals I was unable to continue the same academic pursuits as I had in Toronto, but I thoroughly enjoyed the friendly atmosphere and the excellent medicine that was practised here.

I retired in 1998, and with my husband, also retired, we are enjoying our eight children and eight grandchildren, with a little gardening for him and some wood carving for me and some boating thrown in for both of us.

Curriculum Vitae

Born: 25 December, 1931, Niagara Falls, Ontario.
Marital Status: Married, 4 children.

Education: BPHE, University of Toronto, 1953; MD, University of Toronto, 1957.

Awards and Honours: Margaret Eaton Scholarship, University of Toronto, 1951; Margaret Eaton Scholarship, University of Toronto, 1952; Joseph Azziz Scholarship, Faculty of Medicine, 1957; Inducted into the Sports Hall of Fame, University of Toronto, 1988.

Post-Graduate Training: Rotating Internship, Toronto General Hospital, 1957–58; General Practice, Niagara Falls, Ontario, 1958–61; Resident in Anesthesia, Buffalo Veterans' Hospital and Myer Memorial Hospital, University of Buffalo, New York, 1961–62; Resident in Anaesthesia, University of Toronto, 1962–64; Chief Resident, Toronto General Hospital, 1964–65.

Licensure and Certification: College of Physicians and Surgeons Licence, 1958; Royal College of Physicians of Canada FRCP(C), 1965; American Board of Anesthesiology, 1965.

Professional Memberships: Canadian and Ontario Medical Associations until 1992; Critical Care Society, Division of OMA until 1992; Canadian Cardiovascular Society, life member; American Heart Association until retired in 1999; Canadian Anaesthetist's Society until retired in 1999; International Anaesthesia Research Society until retired in 1999; American Society of Cardiovascular Anesthesiologists until retired in 1999; American Society of Anesthesiologists until retired in 1999.

Academic Appointments: Lecturer, University of Toronto, Faculty of Medicine, Department of Anaesthesia, 1964–65; Assistant Professor, University of Toronto, Faculty of Medicine, 1966–72; Associate Professor, University of Toronto, Faculty of Medicine, 1972–87; Professor, Faculty of Medicine, University of Toronto, 1987; Professor Emeritus, Faculty of Medicine, University of Toronto, 1994.

Hospital Appointments: Staff Anaesthetist, Toronto General Hospital, 1964–75; Chief of Cardiovascular Anaesthesia, Toronto General Hospital, 1975–92; Associate Director, Cardiovascular Intensive Care Unit, Toronto General Hospital, 1976–90; Deputy Anaesthetist-in-Chief, Toronto General Hospital, 1979–87; Director of Post-Operative Recovery Room, Toronto General Hospital,

1979–87; Acting Anaesthetist-in-Chief, Toronto General Hospital, 1987–89; Sabbatical, 1991–92; Staff Anaesthesiologist, Greater Victoria Hospital Society, 1992–98; Retired from active practice, retained Locum Privileges at GVHS, 1998.

Dr. Sallie Teasdale-Scott was a member of numerous committees at the University of Toronto, Department of Anaesthesia from 1979 to 1992 as well as on many committees of the Toronto General Hospital from 1970 to 1992. She gave over fifteen presentations for Continuing Medical Education, University of Toronto. Her national/international presentations numbered nineteen in Canada, the United States, Nassau, England, Japan, and Belgium, from 1969 to 1992. She was co-author of forty-eight Abstracts and thirty-four publications listed in her CV. This is in addition to teaching, doing research, and practising her specialty of anesthesia.

DR. LIZ ZUBEK

Medicine is a career that I dove into blindly, with the naïve pre-med ideal of "I just want to help people." I entered my studies without an awareness of the sheer mental, physical, and emotional exhaustion of 100-hour work weeks on the wards, or of the pain of watching a young patient die despite all possible interventions. Conversely, I did not realize what an honour it would be to share in the most intimate moments of families' lives, from their joyous births to their overcoming of tragedies. I did not anticipate that my career would span Canada from Newfoundland to the Northwest Territories and to British Columbia, or that I would learn some of my most valuable lessons in a far corner of Africa. All that I knew was that medicine was a fascinating subject. Along the way I learned that it is a true art.

I obtained my medical degree in Winnipeg at the University of Manitoba. In the second year of my studies I toyed with the possibility of a political career, running in the 1988 Federal Election. Since I was a candidate for the Rhinoceros Party, my medical vocation was not in any real jeopardy.

On graduating in 1991, I entered the UBC Community-Based Family Practice Residency. I loved the options of travelling throughout the province to train. With my extreme wanderlust I found myself making ten moves in the two-year program. I became quite adept at packing all my worldly possessions, including an enormous aquarium for my pet iguana, into a compact Toyota Tercel. Bogart the iguana is perhaps remembered more than I am from all my travels. He had a penchant for escape. In the Queen Charlotte Islands it took three doctors, a principal, and the hospital administrator to form a posse to corner him in the bushes. In Kitimat, he got lost in the heating ducts that led between the hospital residence and the doctors' exam rooms. I had to make an emergency late-night call to the hospital engineer to extract the little green guy before he burst in on some unsuspecting lady having a PAP exam.

My initial experience of small-town B.C. medicine was in Hazelton. On my very first real day on call as an MD, I was suddenly faced with two comatose patients from a huge accident. As I raced to do the ABC's on each man with my so-newly-acquired ATLS skills, there arrived not one but *three* of the local family practitioners who had heard the ambulance siren and had shown up to pitch in. The teamwork was amazing. This was what medicine was about.

I found a similar community spirit among the medical personnel in the Queen Charlotte Islands, which are traditionally known as Haida Gwaii. In such an isolated community, weekly staff meetings are the key to resolving community health issues. In this setting, I became aware of the widespread use of traditional Native medicine alongside our own medical interventions, and when deciding on a residency research project this seemed to be the ideal topic. I proposed to determine, via questionnaire, how prevalent the use of traditional Native medicines was, and whether the First Nations people wished to have more access to their medicines while hospitalized. I was, quite naïvely, surprised when a sizeable faction of the Haida population did not support my thesis idea. A traditional healer described it succinctly: "Our people have been studied many times. How does that benefit us? You must ask your own people first." Of course! Why would they be willing to impart their own views until they knew the underlying attitudes in the medical system? I thus changed my perspective, and sent a questionnaire to a random sample of family physicians across B.C. This survey was to ascertain their knowledge base about traditional Native medicine, and their willingness to allow its use in a variety of settings, from preventive health and minor illnesses to hospitalized care. The results of this research can be found in *Canadian Family Physician*, Nov. 1994; 40: pps. 1923-1931.

My eight months working as a medical resident in Haida Gwaii was fascinating, Through our isolation, a one-day ferry ride or a six-hour Med-evac away from specialist care, we as family physicians were forced to deal with even the most complicated subspecialty-type problems. Tremendous credit must be given to the Vancouver specialists who were willing to help us through a crisis with telephone advice! Whenever one of these specialists flew into town for a clinic, it was a crash-course in medical diagnosis. We saved up all of our most difficult cases and they worked late into the night doing consultations. As a resident, I eagerly sat in on these marathon clinics with notebook in hand.

In the second year of my studies I toyed with the possibility of a political career, running in the 1988 Federal Election, but since I was a candidate for the Rhinoceros Party, my medical vocation was not in any real jeopardy.

Living on Haida Gwaii was isolated and difficult for a young single woman. The only regular social life revolved around the local bar, where I felt my presence would be unprofessional. I rented many videos, and had few excuses to procrastinate on my studying for the CCFP exams. However, there was a flourishing artistic community on the Island. I learned from local artists about argillite carving, First Nations symbolic painting, silk tie-dying, and world-class batik tapestries. I attended a local potlatch as the special guest of one of my patients, and enjoyed the camaraderie around the gift-giving, dancing, and traditional foods served. I just couldn't, however, develop a taste for oolichan oil or fried roe on seaweed!

B.C. coastal delicacies were commonplace, and I often opened my door to receive a gift of freshly caught salmon. Strangely enough, the one thing we craved on Haida Gwaii was good old fast food! The local school chartered in an airplane filled with McDonald's hamburgers as a successful fund-raiser.

Life after CBP graduation began with a series of locum tenens. The most exciting was in Churchill, Manitoba, a remote community where my biggest fear on emerging for a 3 a.m. hospital call was not any human danger, but rather whether there were eyes in that snow bank I passed. Great white polar bears were known to roam through the town. The hospital nurses even had it formally written in their contract that they would not be docked pay if they were unable to begin their shift due to a polar bear blocking the hospital entrance!

Churchill was an interesting community, with a blend of Cree people and a large population of us 'transients'—medical and military personnel who seemed to enter and exit through a revolving door. Our medical centre was responsible for referrals and on-call advice to a number of Inuit communities staffed by very competent nursing personnel. Each of these outposts was visited by one of us once a month, and we held a filled-to-the-brim clinic of all the toughest cases the nurses saved up for our visit. I spent my free time after my clinics in Baker Lake visiting the homes of some of the most talented soapstone carvers, and managed to hitch an airplane ride on my weekends off to meet artists in Rankin Inlet and Sanikiluaq.

Practising medicine with the Inuit was different. They tended to talk at an extreme minimum, and I had to ask endless leading questions to get any history. I also learned to watch every nuance of facial expression. A scrunch of the eyes signified no, and a raise of the eyebrows indicated yes, in response to my questions.

I had visited Churchill and Baker Lake once before, as a medical student doing my Family Practice rotation. In that capacity I did a research project which was a chart review to determine the breastfeeding rates and correlation with subsequent hospitalizations in the population. I was surprised to find in my review, not only a three times higher hospitalization rate among those not breastfed, but also that large numbers of babies were not breastfed because they were being adopted out to other family members. In fact, a high percent of Inuit babies studied in my review were adopted! I found a personal face to this statistic on meeting an Inuit health worker who was pregnant for the first time. She was married and anxious to have children of her own, but she was determined to give up her child to her sister (who already had a handful of children) because it was such an honour that her sister had offered to raise her child for her. I realized then the magnitude of difference there could be in cultural beliefs.

My other extreme experience with cultural differences in medicine came in my medical school elective. I backpacked solo for seven weeks learning about Third World medicine in Mali, a French-speaking nation in northwest Africa. My sojourn was arranged via one of my professors. Through his contact with Mali's "personal physician to the president-for-life," he found me quite a high-ranking personage who had accompanied the President on trips to the Kremlin and the White House. The problem was this President was also deposed in a revolution that transpired during, to just after, my trip! I realize that I had questionable safety staying as his guest in assorted City Halls across the country.

My first weeks in Mali were spent in the tiny town of Dioila, where I arrived to find a long line-up of people who spoke only native Bambara. I quickly learned the essentials: "Do you have a fever? Diarrhea? Where's the pain?" Diagnosis with a language barrier was difficult enough, but the auxiliary lab tests were nonexistent. Most people had only enough money for either the appropriate test or the likely treatment, and physicians were quick to prescribe chloroquine for any fever rather than ask for a costly malarial blood smear. Sexually transmitted diseases were devastating, as many men had three or four wives, and they could only afford treatment for the one ill person and not the contacts. I saw fulminant tetanus, leprosy, schistosomiasis, and secondary syphilis in routine clinics. We spent one day screening the entire population of a neighbouring town for onchocerciasis, not with any elaborate tests, but rather by feeling each person's hips for subcutaneous worms. We must have found a hundred cases, and hoped that our documentation might lead to funding for medications so that this village could fight the treatable disease of river blindness.

I assisted in Dioila's surgical suite, surprised to find a large dog ambling through the operating room to no one's chagrin. In the corner was a little old man with a pail of water and a scrub brush—this was the sterilization of the instruments. The majority of surgical cases were for hydrocoele, a common condition in Mali due to parasitic infections. Most men did not come to surgery until their scrotum was the size of a watermelon. Though cost was a factor, I was also informed that men delayed treatment because the size of the scrotum was seen as a sign of virility, and they were quite happy to have enlargement to a grapefruit degree.

I went on to learn about the practice of medicine in secondary care centres in the larger towns of Mopti and San. The physicians were so knowledgeable, but so limited in resources. San had only enough electricity for one procedure at a time, so that the dentist had to time his drilling between the examinations of the ophthalmologist and the radiologist. The village dentist sent me home one night with a three-page synopsis of "how to be a dentist in the Third World." The next morning I was injecting anaesthetic and extracting teeth in his office. He rationalized that this was a skill I may someday need if in a remote setting, and in fact most of the dental problems were so extensively abscessed that extraction *was* the only option.

My last stop in Mali was the most remote, in the land of the Dogon people who live in clustered cliffside huts and practise animistic beliefs. There was no local doctor, and the very capable nurse of the community took me under his wing as we learned from each other. One night we were approached by a messenger about a very ill woman in a nearby village, and I agreed to accompany the nurse with medical supplies for a house call. We spent a harrowing hour driving on a moped in the dark along a winding gravelly cliff-top road before reaching our destination, or so I thought. Disembarking, I asked where the village was, and he pointed— straight down. Flashlights in hand, we spent the next hour descending a steep cliff in the darkness. Every fifth step I felt myself treading on a loose boulder, and if I shone my flashlight to the side it illuminated only an extreme depth of nothingness. Finally we arrived to set up an intravenous infusion of antibiotics to treat her pneumonia, then slept on mats under the starry night sky. I awoke with a rooster crowing in my ear and chickens hopping over my legs. I looked up, aghast to see above me the monumental cliff-face that I had descended that night. I muttered something incredulous to the nurse, and he responded, "I thought it was far too dangerous to do in the dark. I would never have done it, except you said you wanted to go."

The trek back in daylight was much easier, but we couldn't leave until we had made respectful visits to the homes of the main families in the village, all of whom had just finished brewing their traditional beer, and all of whom insisted we take a ceremonial taste of their batch. One sip was

I have pushed a double stroller to the hospital to do my rounds, breastfed through our medical staff meetings, and learned to do my charts with pen in one hand and breast pump in the other.

powerful. I soon had to fake drinking if I was to make it back up the cliffside.

As I write this, in the year 2000, I realize how many more exotic adventures could have led from my medical degree. However, the adventure I now find myself on, nine years from graduation, is combining motherhood and practice in suburban Maple Ridge B.C. I've found, through necessity, adaptations that work. My twenty-odd hours of practice per week are at unusual times, to balance my husband Stan's work schedule so that one of us is always with our children (Erika and Adam Zubek-Nizol, aged four and two respectively). I have pushed a double stroller to the hospital to do my rounds, breastfed through our medical staff meetings, and learned to do my charts with pen in one hand and breast pump in the other.

To challenge myself professionally I did one year of post-graduate training in Addictions Medicine with the UBC Department of Family Practice, and extra training in travel vaccination and immunization. I've found myself becoming increasingly more involved in evaluating the scientific merit behind herbal remedies, an interest that began with Mali and Haida Gwaii and which continues to be nurtured by patient inquiries and requests for me to peer-review manuscripts and publications on the subject. The parameters change, but medicine, and life, remain an adventure and a challenge.

1993

DR. DEBORAH BIRCHAM

My licence to practise was issued in 1993, but my story started a considerable time before that. As a little girl in the late fifties, I remember 'playing doctor' with all my dolls as my favorite pastime. I watched Marcus Welby, Dr. Kildare, and Ben Casey with awe as they saved lives and made great impacts on their patients' lives. They occasionally featured women physicians on these programs, but growing up in the sixties, the daughter of a truck driver and a waitress, I thought that as a female, I would have to be a brilliant student to aspire to become a doctor.

I was always a good student and did especially well in Science and Math, but I wasn't brilliant, and my parents had never even met a woman who had entered university, so they couldn't understand my aspirations. I met my future husband when I was fifteen years old and almost immeditely knew that I also had a dream to become his wife and the mother of his children. We married when I was eighteen and I gave birth to a wonderful son two years later and a beautiful daughter several years after that. My life felt complete.

On our tenth anniversary, over a very intimate dinner, my husband asked me if I had any regrets in my life. I honestly answered that I had no regrets at all about the path my life had followed. I loved him and our children deeply and I enjoyed my work as an office nurse. I had completed some upgrading and a nursing course after being a full-time mom for the first few years of my children's lives. We had a beautiful home overlooking Okanagan Lake that my husband had designed and built. I did, however, reveal that I had always secretly dreamed of becoming a doctor. My husband, without any hesitation, strongly encouraged me to pursue my goal. I was surprised and excited by his response and knew immediately that my dream could become a reality. I also knew I was a very lucky woman to have a husband who loved me very much.

I was concerned about the sacrifice required by my family for me to follow this new path. We would have to sell our beautiful home, my husband's successful business, and eventually move our children to a new community. Some of our extended family and friends thought we were crazy. We would be giving up so much without even knowing I would be accepted into Medicine. There was also the long-term commitment of such a demanding career to consider. I had worked in our local hospital, both as a unit clerk and a nurse in areas such as Emergency and Labour/Delivery, and had five years medical office experience. I felt this gave me a realistic idea of the demands of medicine and that I could, with my family's support, now follow my dream and still be a good wife and mother.

I also had support from my employer, who was a family doctor and excellent role model. He accommodated my new schedule of attending college to attain my prerequisite courses and part-time work in the office. I worked very hard and was surprised to find myself at the top of my class in courses such as Physics, Chemistry, and Biology. Calculus, however, was my nemesis. I thought I was good in Math, but this was something else! I was sure that the C grade would shatter all my dreams and keep me out of Med School. Maybe this wasn't meant to be and I really wasn't bright enough or wasn't capable of working hard enough to realize my goal.

I continued to study long hours and hoped that I could make up for that poor grade by scoring well on the MCAT, and hoped that I could convince my interviewers that I was a good candidate. Our local college in Okanagan presented me with a Diploma in Science "with distinction" and it was now time to bite the bullet and uproot my family to Vancouver. There was no guarantee that I would be accepted into Medicine, but I was accepted by the the Faculty of Science, where I planned to work hard to complete the rest of my required courses and hope for the best.

To add confusion to this important decision of moving, I was offered a position in the third year of the newly created degree program in Nursing at our local college the same week that I was informed that they had a suite reserved for us in the family housing at UBC. The nursing degree offered me a career opportunity without having to uproot my husband and children, but it meant giving up on my dream. My husband had sold his business and we had sold our home to afford the expense of University. Our first year resembled a prolonged camping trip in very small quarters in family housing, but by the next year we settled into lovely new residences on campus, and my husband had established himself in another successful business in Vancouver.

I didn't get accepted to Medicine on my first try. I had selected an elective without researching it well and found myself with another C on my record. I don't think the Faculty of Medicine was aware that C was the highest grade given by the professor, and that most of the class failed the course. Again I wondered if I was good enough. Was it the one low grade or was it the interviews? I changed my major to Dietetics during my second year at UBC and fortunately did very well and was offered a position for a Master's degree in the Dietetics Department.

I, however, persevered and again went through the interview process. In addition to the many ethical questions I expected, I was asked in two separate interviews about my parents' work and what made me think I would be successful in a career in Medicine. Again self-doubt raised its ugly head. On return from a holiday with my family, I found a letter under our door that I had expected weeks earlier that had been mistakenly delivered to neighbours. It was from the Faculty of Medicine. With great anticipation and anxiety, I opened the envelope. I had been accepted!

The next few years were filled with excitement, exhaustion, and more determination and hard work than I ever imagined. It was now impossible to be the straight A student I had grown to expect. All my classmates had been the best in their class and they were young, bright, energetic, motivated, and without responsibilities of a family. In our fourth year, we worked many twenty-four to thirty-six hour shifts, often to return to the hospital twelve to sixteen hours later and repeat the cycle. Fortunately, my husband and family were extremely supportive. We made a date once a week to ensure we kept in touch and they knew they were still a priority in my life. I managed to make it through the four years without someone tapping me on the shoulder to tell me they had made a mistake in choosing me for this valued position.

I have delivered well over a thousand babies and I still love the experience and the privilege of being a part of one of the most important events in my patients' lives. I also enjoy the rest of my practice, particularly the very old and the very young.

Next, it was time to apply for Residency, and I felt much more confident in these interviews. I was placed in my first choice residency position in Victoria, but this meant moving my family again. My son had graduated from high school the same year I graduated from medicine, and my daughter was very settled with her life in Grade 10 in Vancouver. We planned to stay in Victoria after the Residency, so this would be our last move. My husband commuted for the first year while the children and I settled in. Shortly, my husband finally sold yet another business to join us. I was told that the second year of Residency would not be offered at Victoria, and I would have to complete my final year in a rural setting or back in Vancouver. I couldn't possibly uproot my family again. I chose to leave the Residency program and was in the last group of physicians to be allowed to practise in British Columbia with just one year of post-graduate training.

I practised for two years as a locum tenens in family practices that had a lot of Obstetrical patients, and I loved the work. I established my own family practice late in 1994, which has evolved to include many Obstetric referrals as more and more physicians in our community have given up this part of their practice. I have delivered well over a thousand babies and I still love the experience and the privilege of being a part of one of the most important events in my patients' lives. I also enjoy the rest of my practice, particularly the very old and the very young. I teach Residents in the Family Practice program, and encourage them to continue with full service Family Practice, including Obstetrics, as it is so personally rewarding. I am Vice-Chief of Obstetrics in Family Practice at Victoria General Hospital and have recently accepted a position as delegate on the Board of the Society of General Practice of British Columbia. I admit that I often find it difficult to work all night delivering a baby and then all day seeing patients in the office. I try to find a balance in a very busy schedule by making dates for holidays with my husband and children as often as I can find a locum tenens to take care of my busy practice.

My husband and I celebrated our thirtieth anniversary this year. He didn't ask me if I had any regrets. I wonder why? I would have assured him that I have none.

DR. JANICE MASON

Spots of light decorate the distant darkness outside my window—mast lights of sailboats anchored in the harbour. Periodically the rumble of a generator on a freighter a mile off-island disturbs the tranquility. Barely discernible, yet what an annoyance in the stillness! Awakened to a siren's call, the adrenaline surge subsides as I locate the source—across the water on a neighbouring island. Surrounded by dense, damp fog—the stillness and quiet are reminiscent of snow-covered mountain mornings. This peace and darkness—welcome to Lotusland. In my early years on Saturna Island when I was fresh out of internship in Victoria a wistful specialist from the city occasionally ribbed me—in my mid-thirties I was setting up my medical practice in the land where people go to retire. Wasn't I getting this a lit-

tle backward? It is funny how the Gulf Islands, once unknown bumps of land along the long trek from Victoria to Grandma's place in Vancouver, have now become home.

Doctoring in the Gulf Islands with a baby in tow—our first experience was as a locum, and the volunteer receptionist crew still recalls (eight years later) my little girl in her car seat being so patient in the waiting room. Juggling the nursing needs of an infant, the medical needs of a community, and fitness needs of myself led to hikes up the local mountain, late night calls to a woman in labour, and the late night sleep in the van while mom attended (with frequent dashes out to check on babe snuggled sound asleep) the needs of an unconscious teenage cyclist (someone else's baby) before the helicopter whisked her away to the city on a blustery, dark, and rainy September evening—all this was part of our lives.

We soon moved to Saturna where I became the resident doctor. The pager became a necessity . . . initially a forgotten one. It once took me an hour to figure out what that strange beeping emanating from the hall closet was, reminding me of the time as a medical student when I couldn't figure out why the floor of the hospital kept vibrating. Luckily neither page was for anything serious, at least not as far as my medical training was concerned. On the islands, though, if the pager or cell phone can't reach you (because often they don't work), they know where to find you . . . like the early morning knocking on the door as the ambulance crew rushed off to a 'chest pain' situation, or the friend busting into the local community hall calling out for me (and the concert hadn't even begun!). Initially, it seemed that nothing major ever happened when I was on the island—I'd return from a week away to hear of the suicide, the house fire, the only car accident in four years, and while at home the pager and phone seemed idle for weeks. After a few returns to hear of unpleasant events I decided that I should a) never leave the island, or b) go, but never return!

Perhaps the most challenging has been dealing with expectations—mine and of the community. What was a single mom, a medical doctor, relatively young and intent on enjoying life on the islands, doing here anyway? Islanders are here because we love the way of life, the environment, the water (I still fantasize about making my living being on the water every day), and I certainly was not planning on spending my life working full-time, tied to a pager, especially with a young child. There are too many stories of burnout due to lack of backup, lack of privacy, lack of a chance to enjoy one's own backyard, always being on call. But it has been tough, as I am supposed to be a male, married with wife and kids at home, happily available twenty-four hours a day, seven days a week. Isn't the hospital supposed to be only five minutes away? I often wondered why people with such health fears would bother living on an island. And then there was the cardiologist I was trying to urgently refer a patient to—what kind of place was this that had no stretokinase available? He was definitely going to look elsewhere to have his heart attack while on vacation! Gee, we didn't even have a 12 lead ECG, or X-rays, or a lab or . . . but we had a great volunteer ambulance crew! In a land where one-half the population (or more) is retired and grew up in the city watching the Brady Bunch or in the world of Leave it to Beaver, single moms just aren't doctors, even to those 'progressive, independent' retired women. It has been a rather eye-opening experience.

The attempts at commuting between the islands to work using the ferry system can be a challenge—so close and yet so far. Many have suggested that I travel by private boat—the two-to three-hour trek by kayak in the summer could be fun, but maybe not in the winter wind, rain, and dark. I haven't yet traded my human-powered boats in for the high-speed power ones. So like most I rely on, and periodically complain about, B.C. Ferries. But I can also sit atop the Bluffs (with a gorgeous view stretched out in front of me) eating dinner, watching my ferry cruise through Active Pass, and I still have ample time to swallow those last few bites and head down the hill to the ferry terminal. It is twenty minutes by float plane, or three hours by ferry! A 'day at work on Galiano' once meant leaving home on Saturna at 6 a.m. and returning at 10 p.m. that evening. The crazy, bumpy ride and a pilot commenting "that's about the limit we could fly in!" still hasn't deterred me from the thrills of a small plane, though I was glad that he waited until we were safely back on the water to make that comment! My hands and forearms were rather sore from gripping the seat and he still had to go back up for the journey home, across the Strait. The frustration of the time my daughter and I stopped on our way from Saturna for dinner on Mayne Island, only to arrive back at the ferry dock to be told that the ferry to Galiano had been cancelled. With wind howling, rain pouring down, a

leaky sunroof, and the predictable power outage, we woke to a calm and peaceful ferry ride home.

Once upon a time I turned away from a career in medicine—I did not want to be making life and death decisions (my young mind liked simple black and white) for others. The confidence we place in others I found frightening, amazing, and sad. Somewhere along the way we found that it wasn't our responsibility, it was someone else's, and if we got hurt or didn't receive the proper treatment, then it was going to cost someone else financially. It didn't matter that we were driving too fast, careless in our attention, smoked, drank, didn't exercise, and partied all night long. The words "I can't do that" are heard all too often. Someone was supposed to fix us now that we were broken and if they made a mistake—watch out. But somehow we became responsible enough to walk alone to the local store, spend our first few dollars, take the ferry by ourselves, get a driver's licence, have children, borrow money from a bank, decide what we are going to eat for dinner. It is amazing how it all just evolves. Here I am, now forty-three years old, with all these things surrounding me, responsibilities to myself, my daughter, those who consider me their doctor, the bank, my friends, the earth. Coming to the islands has dramatically increased my awareness of the world, and how truly sheltered we can get here on the amazing west coast of Canada. I feel that I am moving back to the earth, while much of the world wants to move away. We pump thousands of dollars into medical care, when wouldn't it be a wiser investment if we put it into health and believing in ourselves?

So—we come to the islands for breaks in our busy lives, for a holiday, a getaway . . . and a few of us end up living it, myself included. I've been an islander for eight years—four on Saturna and four on Galiano; thirty-eight in total if one counts the thirty years spent on the big island of Vancouver Island before that. And really, why an island, a place filled with

Once upon a time I turned away from a career in medicine—I did not want to be making life and death decisions (my young mind liked simple black and white) for others. The confidence we place in others I found frightening, amazing, and sad.

challenges—no movie theatres, no fitness centre, no bank, no laundromat, no hospital, no twenty-four-hour gas station or grocery store or . . . no traffic lights, no highrises, and my TV doesn't even clue in to the CBC! The only way 'out' is by boat or plane. We get stalled by winter storms—power out, phones out, cell phones don't work, wells run dry. The earth is green and warm as I pad barefoot around my place. My daughter can run around the marina, or row out in the bay with her cat and I know that she is safe. We see the same people day in and day out. Some think our population of crazies is higher than elsewhere, but I feel we just know each other better! I can hug my patients and no one seems to be threatening lawsuits. Would I trade it back for the city? I don't think so. The constant challenge of our lives—to find peace, balancing one's needs of solitude and community: one minute I long for the conveniences of the city, but the next longer minute I retreat from the busy pace, the noise, the concrete, the artificial green, and relish the comforting surroundings of the naturally quiet green of my island home.

DR. STACEY LEIGH McDONALD

Dr. Stacey McDonald is a family physician practising in Merritt, British Columbia, a town serving a population of approximately 10,000, where she has resided for seven years. Her medical interests include geriatrics, psychiatry, diabetes, and women's health issues. She especially enjoys spending time with her family (two wonderful children); her interests include swimming, volleyball, and ballet.

Curriculum Vitae

Born: January 15, 1968.

Education: College of Family Physicians of Canada (member), 1993–2002; LMCC, 1992; Family Medicine Residency, CDHG, Calgary, Alberta, 1991–1993; Medical Degree, Faculty of Medicine, University of Calgary, Alberta, 1988-1991; Bachelor of Science (1990) Major: Biology, Simon Fraser University, Burnaby, British Columbia, 1985–1988; Shad Valley Enrichment Programme, Canadian Centre for Creative Technology, University of Waterloo, Waterloo, Ontario, 1985; Centennial Senior Secondary School, Coquitlam, British Columbia (graduated with Honours), 1983-1985.

Papers and Publications:

"Endometrial Biopsy: a skill for Family Practice Residents?" (Abstract), 1993

"The clinical relevance of Pseudomonas cepacia in patients with cystic fibrosis: a study of the intrinsic antibacterial activity of the beta lactamase inhibitor, sulbactam, through susceptibility testing of P.cepacia sputum isolates from CF patients," 1990.

Joint authorship with Dr. Hermann Ziltener: "Immunoassay for Interlukin-3 using Polyclonal Antipeptide Antibodies" (Abstract), 1988

Scholarships and Awards: Calgary Family Medicine Resident Research Project—First Place, 1993; Dr. Douglas Cadger Award (CDHG) for exceptional proficiency in Internal Medicine, 1992; Nat Christie Foundation Medical Award, 1988–1991; SFU Open Scholarship, 1987-1988; B.C. Provincial Government Scholarship; B.C. Hydro Scholarship; SFU Designated Undergraduate Award; SFU Honour Roll; SFU Open Scholarship, 1986–1987; B.C. Provincial Government Scholarship; SFU Honour Roll; SFU Entrance Scholarship, 1985–1986; Chris Spencer Foundation Scholarship; Crown Forest Industries Award; Cam MacKenzie Citizenship Award; Coquitlam United Soccer Club Award; Gold Award (Centennial) for academic excellence.

Employment History: The Medical Clinic (Associate), Merritt, B.C., Geriatric Outreach Physician (Merritt and Logan Lake, B.C.), Long Term Care Co-ordinator (Meritt, B.C.), 1995–2002; Locum tenens (Prince Rupert, B.C., Calgary, and Provost, Alberta), 1994; Locum tenens (Calgary and Red Deer, Alberta), 1993; Medical Group Missions volunteer: Erandique, Honduras; Family Practice Resident, CDHG, Alberta, 1991–1993; Calgary Medical Examiner's Office autopsy assist/security (IL-3 detection assays) Calgary, Alberta, 1989; Biomedical Research Centre, University of British Columbia, Vancouver, B.C., 1988; Biotechnology Research Institute (peptide synthesis) NRC, Montreal, Quebec, 1987.

Positions and Committees: Mental Health Team sessional physician, Adult Psychiatry, 1988–99; Diabetes Education Co-ordinator, Medical Director, Nicola Valley Health Society, continuing care medical director, Long Term Care; Medical Co-ordinator, Library; Chairman, Continuing Medical Education Committee; Chairman, Pharmacy and Therapeutics Committe; Member, 1995–1996; Diabetes Education Co-ordinator; Medical Director, Long Term Care; Medical Co-ordinator, Library/Computer Committee; Chairman, Continuing Medical Education Committee; Chairman, Facilitator for CCFP problem based small group learning, 1996–1997; Vice-President Medical Staff Nicola Valley General Hospital, Diabetes Education Program; Medical Co-ordinator, Geriatric Outreach Program; Physician Consultant, Long Term Care Committee; Chair, Continuing Medical Education Committee; Chair, Facilitator for CCFP problem-based small group learning program, 1997–1998; 1998–2002, Diabetes Education Program; Medical Co-ordinator, Geriatric Outreach Program; Physician Consultant, Long Term Care Co-ordinator, Continuing Medical Education Committee; Chair (until 2000); Community speaker; Breast Health Education for Healthy Living; Pharmacy and Infectious Disease Committee; Co-ordinator, Provost Municipal Health Care Centre, 1994; Pediatric curriculum review committee for University of Calgary Family Medicine Program, CDHG Resident's Retreat Co-co-ordinator and Treasurer, 1992; Student Affairs Committee, University of Calgary Medical School, 1989–1991; Christian Medical Dental Society member, 1988-1991.

Certificates: BLTS/ATLS (1993); NALS (1996); PaedALS (1995); BCLS/ACLS (1995 and 1996); Royal Lifesaving Bronze Cross and Medallion, Sr. Resuscitation (1984); CPR A and C (1995).

Continuing Medical Education: CCFP course requirements met (50+ education hours per year), 1993–2002; Fellowship in Geriatric Medicine (Vancouver, B.C.), May 1997; Fellowship in Women's Breast Health (B.C. Women's Hospital/B.C. Cancer Agency/VGH), Vancouver, B.C., April 1999.

Associations: Catholic Physicians' Guild; Christian Medical Dental Society; B.C. Schizophrenia Society; Association of Geriatric Physicians; Canadian Diabetes Society; British Columbia Medical Association.

DR. MARY WALL

I feel the most interesting part of my life has been getting into medical school. I was born and obtained my early education in Newfoundland. I entered Memorial University Medical School in September, 1986, at the age of thirty-three. That in itself was a feat. I had obtained my RN at the age of nineteen, and my BN at the age of twenty-four. And I worked mostly in rural areas all through my nursing career. After graduating from Memorial University in June of 1990, I did a rotating internship in St. John's, Newfoundland, and started private practice with my husband in June, 1991, in New Harbour, Trinity Bay, Newfoundland. On July 4, 1991, I had my first son, but managed to see twenty patients in my first two weeks post partum and continued on from there.

On April 1, 1993, I arrived in British Columbia with my twenty-month-old son after staying six weeks on my own in Newfoundland, wrapping up the practice since my husband had come out to B.C. in February. It was one point in my life I will never forget, as I worked fourteen to sixteen hours per day, seeing up to sixty patients a day. And on March 31, 1993 at 10:30 p.m. I dictated my last referral letter and left at 4 a.m. to drive to St. John's to catch the 6 a.m. flight. Of course I packed in-between. My husband picked me up at the Vancouver Airport on April 1.

On April 2, we went to the College of Physicians and Surgeons to pick up my licence and headed for the interior of British Columbia. Now that I am thinking back to ten years ago, a lot of things seem a blur. However, there are several instances that still remain vivid in my mind. I was totally exhausted arriving in British Columbia and did not actually start my practice at Rock Creek until April 1993. My husband was working hard and got himself established with the hospital in Grand Forks, which is forty-five minutes away; he was using our car. I was left with doing calls in Midway on my bicycle. I remember going out in the mornings on my bicycle with my son in the little trailer to see someone at the clinic and thinking, "My god, what am I in for?"

I survived that, and began a practice in Rock Creek, which was quite good to start as it was being subsidized up to $100,000 per year as long as the clinic stayed open five days a week, eight hours a day. Of course it was slow at first. But still one can get caught off guard. I was only out there a couple of days when the husband of the President of the Medical Society came in with chest pain, and I set up an IV that must have been at least ten years old. And I had to give him morphine that was five years outdated. However, it settled his pain, and we got him off the hospital, and he is still living today.

Of course there is at least one story for every day. However, being a new doctor, a young mother with no family around was quite distressing. It is the people you hire to work for you that can make or break you, and I was very lucky with my staff.

To keep having to leave the house to a minimum in the evenings and at night, I set up suture and surgeon trays, and stored drugs in the top cupboard of my kitchen. However, more than one night at two in the morning I would have to rouse the boys and say that "a little kid is sick," and they would walk in their sleep to the truck and jump in.

Within a year and a half, I was working at Rock Creek clinic in the mornings and Midway clinic in the afternoons, and working in the clinic at Grand Forks one day a week. I had my second son on September 19, 1994.

Working in a rural area and being female and a mother requires you to set principles and priorities if you want to succeed in each role. Of course, my priority was my sons. Things were fine at the beginning. I had a young woman who enjoyed looking after my three-year-old, and up until four months of age, my second son came to work with me wherever I went. I remember, when he was just two weeks old, at two in the morning I was at Boundary Hospital with a patient in labour. I called in another doctor and we were lucky enough to have an intern at the time. So the doctor I called in was sitting at the resuscitation unit. The intern was watching the perineum and I was standing beside her breast-feeding my baby while the mother was pushing. We always joke we should have taken a photograph and sent it to the family practice.

By the time Alistair was four months old, he was too rambunctious to keep in the office, so I left him with the babysitter and my three-year-old. On the first day I went out to Rock Creek in the morning to work, and at lunch time came back to start my afternoon clinic in Midway. My babysitter's home was next to the clinic in Midway, so I popped in to feed him. As I was coming through the door, I heard the baby screaming at the top of his lungs and saw the babysitter sitting at the table. When she noticed the look on my face, she casually said, "Oh, I'm trying to teach him that if he cries he won't get picked up, and if he stops he will." So I took him to the office with me, fed him, and had my secretary babysit while I saw the patients. The next day was my Grand Forks day, so my babysitter came up to the house as usual. And I had to ask her again what she was thinking. The only thing she could say to me, "Well, I never was very good with babies." And I thought, "Well, you had nine months to tell me about it," and I picked up the baby to take him to Grand Forks with me. I carried him out, placed him in my truck, started it up, and backed out of my garage right into my babysitter's car, costing $2,500 for the damage. I could not fire her, so I ended up hiring two babysitters, one for the three-year-old and one for the baby, because there was no one around at the time that was willing to care for two small children.

Our lives in this babysitting business got much better for me in August 1995, when a Japanese lady, well-known in the community, came to work for me. She is still with me today, and now the boys are eight and eleven.

Over the years I had to reinvent the ways things got done, and always tried to make sure I was there for my children and also for my patients. I had my office number routed to ring in my home. That was fine except, especially in the spring, the phone would ring at four in the morning when people just wanted to check office hours. Also, to keep having to leave the house to a minimum in the evenings and at night, I set up suture and surgeon trays, and stored drugs in the top cupboard of my kitchen. However, more than one night at two in the morning I would have to rouse the boys and say that "a little kid is sick," and they would walk in their sleep to the truck and jump in.

I think I am probably one of the few physicians who still carry the old black bag around with all the basic necessities in it. I also keep a travel emergency kit in my truck with IV, syringes, scopes, and drugs for highway accidents because the ambulance and police will call me when things are messy. And I am always very conscious about keeping up-to-date with my skills and techniques since I am a solo physician. I do this by providing complete service as much as I can for the patients at the clinic. I am what you call the dispensing physician, so I keep the first line of drugs such as antibiotics, anti-flammatories, and inhalers. It is only in the past year that we now have a small drugstore in our community, but it is only open three days a week, so I still keep my dispensing. I draw my patients' blood on Wednesday mornings; teach an antenatal patient program at the hospital in Grand Forks twice yearly, and teach the diabetic clinic at my clinic in Midway and Rock Creek when the diabetic nurses are doing their rounds there. I maintain privileges at the hospital even though it kills my schedule if I have to go daily just to keep contact with the other physicians, to do some emergency work, or assist in the OR. I make sure I do at least two continuing education programs per year. It seems that in assessing my skills and performance, they are at the extremes of life, with obstetric and palliative care. We have a very excellent home-care nurse in our area, and between the two of us we give our palliative care patients comforting service by allowing them to stay at home until the end. Sometimes it means two or three visits a day, but it is worth it for the family comfort.

Certainly after being here for ten years I am a lot smarter than I was when I first came. I still put in long hours at work and am on call seven days a week when I am here. But now that my children are older, I need to spend more time with them. The school requires a lot of attention with our present situation: I have started a community soccer league for the kids on Saturday morning, which I funded through my office. The boys have their sports—hockey, swimming, baseball—and they are both doing music. One of my other priorities now is to make sure I can go home to Newfoundland every year for at least two weeks with the boys; I consider myself a displaced Newfoundlander and would really like to be back there. But I am not unhappy here in B.C. The people are wonderful, the climate is excellent, and the lifestyle is what you make it. However, being brought up as an Irish Catholic Newfoundlander, there is always a sense of responsibility deep within me that makes me feel that I still have dues to pay for all that was given to me, especially when my hometown is presently without a doctor. So it is constantly on my mind. Of course, I have a husband and two little sons who think Midway is the centre of the universe, and cannot see themselves being anywhere else.

I certainly do not have any regrets about entering medicine and working rural medicine. This is what I enjoy, and I realize that my background as a nurse, especially in Newfoundland, has helped me to be a good rural physician. I have also learned to just take things as they come because Rock Creek and Midway are quite isolated, and one never knows what is going to walk through the door. You have to just assess the situation and do the best you can.

Being brought up as an Irish Catholic Newfoundlander, there is always a sense of responsibility deep within me that makes me feel that I still have dues to pay for all that was given to me, especially when my hometown is presently without a doctor.

I remember a time in the early days at Rock Creek when I had an older gentleman come in. He was in his eighties and had been in the woods Christmas-tree hunting, when he had a cardiac arrest. Some folks brought him in so the first thing I did was to intubate him, and had one of the people who brought him in doing the CPR. I had taught my secretary how to do resuscitation with the bag, so I got her there going "squeeze-two-three, squeeze-two-three" while I was setting up an IV on him. We actually got him resuscitated and into the ambulance on the way to the hospital only for him to arrest half an hour later. I am not sure if that was a success, and I never realized before that my secretary had never really been around somebody that critically ill or, basically, dead. When I think of it now, she probably had some elements of post-traumatic stress. However, she is still with me today, and has been my most fearless and loyal supporter for the past ten years.

I had two full-time secretaries, Bonnie and Nelly, and also a spare secretary. Over the ten years I have been here, I think I must have hired about twenty people on and off for house cleaning and various tasks, and those workers never lasted long. These days I am trying to organize my life better, as my children require more time to get on with their school, and because of all the cutbacks I have tried to organize my practice at Rock Creek to one full day a week rather than three mornings a week. I am still working the same number of hours and seeing the same number of patients, but with fewer expenses. And in Midway I work one full day on Mondays and Fridays, afternoons on Tuesdays and Thursday, and Tuesday and Thursday mornings at the hospital.

The most frustrating part for me is finding time; I really need to become more computer literate so that I can co-ordinate the two practices in order to make life a lot easier. But the thought of the process of reorganizing is daunting. When I first came out to B.C., I told myself that I would be here for five years at the most, and then move on to something else. It is hard to believe that I have been in one place for ten years. People have certainly come to depend on me now, and I feel that having an established medical practice here has certainly added to the community. Midway is actually quite a small community, supported by a sawmill, and the employment rate is about eighty to ninety percent, which is excellent. The surrounding communities of Rock Creek and West Bridge are farming areas, so it is quite a pleasant area to live in.

One of the most interesting features of my practice was that when I first came here, there were men who would stay away unless their finger was falling off or they had a large cut that needed suturing. But now they come to me for their physical and prostate exams, so it is not a problem anymore.

I see myself eventually moving into part-time teaching, and doing something with palliative care in a university setting, because I find it satisfying to help people in their dying process, something that a lot of people do not do very well. And I think coming from such a large extended family and being exposed to death as a part of life at a very young age, there is an acceptance there that it is important to grasp if one is going to live life to the fullest.

It is interesting that people tend to think that when they have a heart attack and have recovered from their MI, that their lives are not in jeopardy. However, when you tell someone they have cancer, it is very difficult for them to try to keep living everyday the same as if they had not had the diagnosis. It is quite a challenge, and once you can get people to understand that, even when they are at the palliative stages, it becomes a comforting and a rewarding experience.

I am very blessed in the fact that I have two healthy and bright children who are interested in everything in life. I have an extended family in Newfoundland that keeps me balanced and always makes me aware of where I come from and how much the experiences of childhood help you to be a good functioning adult. I feel I have lots of things left to be accomplished yet, both in medicine and in my personal life, even though I turned fifty this year. I do want to go on and do more continuing education, and once my children are on their own, I will start working for such things as Doctors Without Borders or the Red Cross doing relief work. I am not sure if my husband likes this plan or not.

I could go on and on, as I have a story for every day. Just yesterday a young lady was home for a visit. It was six years ago May that her mother had turned forty, and I got my little fellow, who was five years old at the time, up and we went at four o'clock in the morning and put forty pink flamingos on her lawn. She had breast cancer and died later that year. Her daughter was a teenager then, and has since moved to Prince Edward Island where she met her husband and got married. She came to me yesterday as a newlywed and had had no experience in sexual activity before. She had waited until she came back after three months of marriage to ask me the questions she needed answers for.

When I sit down to think about it, I cannot even begin to fathom the questions that people come in to me to ask about bodily and sexual functions or the personal stories they tell me. When I first started hearing them, I got very overwhelmed by all this information. They say with age comes wisdom, and that is true, because now I think I am just a safe sounding board, and people know what they say is going to go nowhere. All they want is to get their problems off their chest. I can tell you that I have been asked every possible question about Viagra, about sex and the positions—how and when and where—and some questions I have never even thought of myself.

One of the most interesting features of my practice was that when I first came here, there were men who would stay away unless their finger was falling off or they had a large cut that needed suturing. But now they come to me for their physical and prostate exams, so it is not a problem anymore. When I listen to the stories of a female physician who was here about twenty years ago and see the ability of my gender in my practice now, I do not know if it is I or the male patients who have come a long way, but now my practices are probably sixty percent female and forty percent male.

During the process of having our two sons, we had a foster daughter in 1999 for one year. She graduated from high school, and is now in her second year at university. This year we have taken on a seventeen-year-old fellow who also graduated this month, but he definitely has been more challenging, and I am not going to say that he is a success. But because I have practised so close to the high school, I know every student and they are quite comfortable coming in. I shudder at times at the questions they ask and the answers they want, and the young age of sexual activity. I have tried various scenarios to get them to think about their decisions and the consequences. But I also have to be upfront and open, and to protect them for whatever lifestyle they choose. Of course, as with all areas, drugs are quite free around here. Certainly, I have to deal with a lot of cocaine and marijuana use, which people see as quite normal. Because many parents consider marijuana use as normal, especially those who grew up in the 1960s when a lot of American citizens came up to this area to avoid the Vietnam War and to live communally, you still see the remnants of that today. We used to have a Spanish school for children in this area, which has now become a Buddhist colony. Being mixed up into all of these cultures has been quite an experience.

Of course, there are people who do not like pills, as they want all natural things. So they will go to a health food store and buy $300 worth of natural ingredients that have been through a chemical process, but they certainly do not want to take any medication for their blood pressure.

Before the women initiative studies, probably about five years ago, I had a young woman who had ovarian endometriosis and a hysterectomy when she was thirty-two years old, and she has been on hormone replacement therapy for about fifteen years. She came in one day and wanted something more natural. To her disappointment, I could only say to her, "I can't think of anything more natural than pregnant horse urine."

Your medical degree is only one little component that helps you get through the day sometimes. A lot of times you need to use your common sense when a problem arises. Being a good physician also means listening to patients and keeping your eyes open to see where things are going.

DR. MARIANNE WILLIS

I was born in Cape Town, South Africa in 1955, the youngest child in my family. My parents were not professionals, their college careers having not materialized because of the Second World War. However, from an early age they instilled in me and my two brothers the assumption that we would go on to some kind of university training after school. I spent a year after high school working as a nurse and then registered in the Medical Faculty at the University of Cape Town and duly completed the six years required to obtain my medical degree. It was a time of political upheaval, with blacks being excluded from the medical school by law. The university policy at the time was non-discriminatory, however. We spent a large amount of time working with black patients, and I attended a medical outreach program to the black townships where students volunteered time in the evening to supply medical services for no charge. There would always be a qualified doctor in attendance to help with challenging cases.

I qualified in 1980 and did my internship in Windhoek, Namibia, which at that time was still regarded as part of South Africa. I clearly recall my first night as a surgical intern or 'houseman' as I was thrown in at the *I clearly recall my first night as a surgical intern or 'houseman' as I was thrown in at the deep end and had to deal with two patients with stab wounds to the chest, one with a pneumothorax and the other a haemopneumothorax.*

deep end and had to deal with two patients with stab wounds to the chest, one with a pneumothorax and the other a haemopneumothorax. The expectation of one's seniors was that they were only to be called if there was something which was totally beyond my capabilities, so with some trepidation I prepared to put in a chest tube for the first time. Although I knew what to do and how to do it, I would have been happy to have someone standing by to give a hand had I needed it! Anyway, both patients survived my treatment and recovered uneventfully. And I inserted many more chest tubes, as knife wounds were extremely common.

Another memorable occasion that year was another night on call, this time in the internal medicine department. One was expected to stay on the premises and if there was any time for sleep, there was a room at the end of the large medical ward for the interns' use. I had fallen into an exhausted sleep for an hour or two when suddenly I was aware of a male patient next to my bed. I was instantly awake, and convinced that I was going to be raped by an aggressive patient, my heart hammering. I clutched the sheet around me as he explained in broken English that I needed to get up as the ward was flooded. Sure enough a pipe had burst and there was water ankle-deep in my room and in fact throughout the ward. After quickly donning some more respectable clothing, I splashed barefooted through the water and helped with moving patients elsewhere until things returned to some degree of normality.

After a complicated pregnancy I ended up with a C-section for breech at thirty-five weeks with preterm ruptured membranes. I took all of ten days off as I was not eligible for maternity benefits and my husband had no income at all, so there was not really any choice about it.

The following year I returned to Cape Town as my engineering husband, intrigued with my tales of medical life, decided to register for medicine himself. His reason, among others, was that he thought the hours would be better!

I spent a year doing a senior house officer position in Pediatrics and Obstetrics and Gynecology, based at the Red Cross Children's Hospital and the Groote Schuur Hospital. It was a busy lifestyle; I don't think I saw very much of my spouse at that time. We worked a one in three call, which was exhausting. Obstetrics included being part of the flying Squad Ambulance Service which would bring patients in from outlying Midwife Obstetric Units which were in an area consisting of about thirty kilometres around the hospital. These calls were sometimes done by the consultant and sometimes by the resident or senior house officer, depending on the assessed difficulty of the case. There are two that stand out in my memory, one where I was sole medical attendant and had to perform a difficult forceps delivery of a face-to-pubis present fetus. The MOU, as it was called, was thirty minutes from the hospital, a long way to travel with an already distressed fetus. The other one was to a home where an unqualified midwife was in atten-

dance and the large baby had impacted shoulders. I will never forget the expressions of despair on the faces of the family as we walked in (fortunately, on this occasion the consultant was with me and I was merely the helper). The labouring mother and the midwife were in a poorly-lit bedroom with newspaper spread over the bed and we were greeted with the sight of a very purple fetal head, which unfortunately had been in this position for about twenty minutes. The delivery was not too difficult subsequently, but the fetus was stillborn and weighed in at five kilograms. Since then, I have not been a supporter of home births.

Another memorable occasion in this rotation was my first breech delivery, this time at night in the hospital with more experienced doctors around to supervise me. The first part of the delivery went according to plans and the breech was hanging. I was about to start delivering the head when we were plunged into darkness. It was a mere thirty seconds or so till the auxiliary power came on, but by then the babe was born. A quick-thinking nurse had grabbed a flashlight and the delivery of the head fortunately went smoothly.

I decided after that rotation to find a specialty that had less demanding hours, and with the intention of going into ENT, I took a part-time position in the Anatomy Department in the Medical School in Cape Town. This involved helping students with dissections and taking tutorial groups, and gave me time to study for my surgical primary exam which I needed to get a position in the ENT Department. My husband was one of the students in that year's class, which was a bit tough on him! As if our life wasn't busy enough already, we chose that year to start a family, and after a complicated pregnancy I ended up with a C-section for breech at thirty-five weeks with preterm ruptured membranes. I took all of ten days off as I was not eligible for maternity benefits and my husband had no income at all, so there was not really any choice about it. I did go on and complete the surgical exam, with memories of breast-feeding while studying endlessly, or was it studying while breast-feeding endlessly?

Maternal instincts having kicked in, I couldn't face going back to full-time work and leaving my new baby for the long hours that residency demanded. So I stayed on for the next four years as a lecturer in the Anatomy Department. This allowed me Monday to Friday work and some flexibility in that some of my preparation time could be done at home.

Babysitters were not always reliable in that politically unsettled time and there were occasions when I took my young daughter with me. On one occasion when she was about two years old she was sitting on the floor in my office, busy with puzzles and toys, while I was preparing a hand dissection showing the course of the radial artery. I was startled when a little voice next to my shoulder said, "Oh, poor hand" . . . and I had to try to gently explain that I wasn't hurting the hand. My daughter plans to be a doctor herself, and fortunately doesn't appear to have any permanent psychological trauma from seeing that rather morbid sight!

When my husband Stuart finally qualified we left the city for a rural area in northern Kwazulu (just south of Mozambique) and spent the next two-and-a-half years there. By now we had two children, four and two years old. I worked part-time in primary health care, involved in training African RNs to work as nurse practitioners. Some of these women had already been working for years in these positions, but were not expected to get certification. One of them had even successfully delivered triplets at a remote health centre where she was the only medically trained attendant and the nearest hospital was four hours away by rough dirt road! I felt very inadequate in teaching these wonderful women, but they all passed their exams and went back to continue their work in their communities. I spent some time visiting these communities; each one would have a doctor visit about every second week, for a day. It gave me the opportunity to see what rural medicine really means and it was an education in its own right. I think I learned more in that time than I ever could have taught any of them.

In 1990, now with three children, we left South Africa and travelled for three months in Europe and England. In retrospect we must have been crazy, with the youngest, being all of seven months old when we set off. Then to Canada to Saskatchewan where Stuart had arranged a locum for three months in order to make some money to pay for the next leg of the journey, which was to New Zealand. We had left South Africa with only a few thousand rands to our names (about $500) and borrowed money from my father for air fares.

We had ten months in New Zealand and then came to British Columbia in July 1991, and have been in Vanderhoof ever since. Until about two years ago I was the only female physician between Prince George and Burns Lake—a distance of about 250 kilometres. I had the dubious distinction of having female patients come for Pap tests from as much as four hours away! Now I am happy to say there is another female physician here and one in the neighbouring community of Fraser Lake, so no longer do I need to do ten or twelve Pap tests a day!

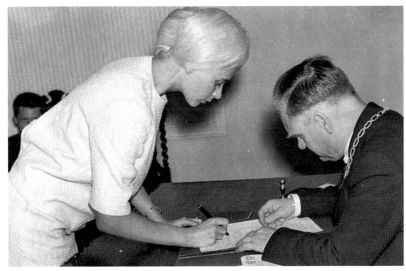

Dr. Maria Daszkiewicz (1992) graduating from medical school in Poland

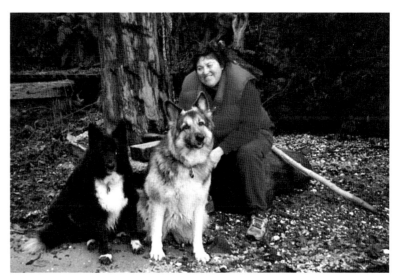

Dr. Ruth Simkin, 1993

Notes from BC MEDICAL JOURNAL 1990–1993

January, 1990 Several articles in the *Journal*, On Stroke: on carotid surgery, stroke rehabilitation, and socioeconomic impact of stroke.

Shirley Baker Thomas MD writes on "Who Grinds the Medicare Bill?" with figures that "belie the media representation that doctors' fees are bankrupting the medicare system."

The new Minister of Health is John Jansen.

The president of the BCMA is Dr. John Anderson.

Hospitals to receive block funding from the Ministry of Health for MRI.

Veterans Affairs Canada has entered into a national agreement with Blue Cross to process and pay for veterans' treatment accounts.

February, 1990 Dr. Christine Loock writes on "Developmental Handicaps." In this article she states that 15 of 30 babies born in one area of Vancouver in 1989 were born with preventable developmental handicaps, that is, prenatal exposure to alcohol causing Fetal Alcohol Syndrome.

After a long and valiant rearguard action in defence of the one-year rotating internship, the B.C. College of Physicians and Surgeons has recently endorsed a two-year pre-licensure requirement, in line with the rest of the Provincial Colleges of Physicians and Surgeons.

March, 1990 An article reviewing twin pregnancies at the Lions Gate Hospital: "Ultrasound Diagnosis of Twins" by Mary Graham MD, FRCP. Dr. Graham is Clinical Director of the Ultrasound Department at Lions Gate Hospital.

Dr. C.E. McDonnell of the Editorial Board wrote an "Irish Medical Odyssey," after a trip to Ireland to explore the hospitals of the Irish medical renaissance known as the Dublin School.

April, 1990: Dr. Marlene Hunter is interested in establishing a unit in Vancouver for the assessment and treatment of Multiple Personality Disorder as well as other similar problems. Dr. Hunter is the national co-chair of the Canadian Society for Studies in Multiple Personality Disorder and Dissociation.

May, 1990 The B.C. College of Physicians and Surgeons reports on physicians' illegible handwriting! The College of Pharmacy pleads: "Anything you could suggest which will raise the awareness of this problem with your members would be greatly appreciated."

The Federation of Medical Women opposes Bill C-43, Canada's new abortion legislation. Their statement: "FMWC objects to the Bill because it denies women the right to make choices about reproduction in consultation with their doctors and threatens the security of women as persons. . . . The Bill could lead to physicians withdrawing their services for fear of criminal charges."

Dr. David Williams, a recent visitor to Romania and as part of the Romanian Medical Relief, requests every kind of medical supplies to be collected for Romanian physicians.

The new University of British Columbia Medical Student and Alumni Centre had a grand opening in March. Since the first UBC medical class graduated in 1954, a total of 2,559 MD degrees have been granted. A very large number of UBC graduates remained, or have returned to practise in British Columbia.

June, 1990 At the BCMA Annual Meeting in the General Assembly reports were presented by Dr. Roberta Ongley as Chair of the Section of Dermatology, by Dr. Dorothy Wishart as Secretary-Treasurer of the Section of Anesthesia, by Dr. Lynne Simpson as Chair of the Section of Obstetrics and Gynecology, and by Dr. Pat Rebbeck as Chair of the Section of Surgery. The various committees presented reports: Dr. Hedy Fry as Chair of the Native Health Committee, and Dr. Kathleen Cadenhead as Chair of the Nutrition Committee. Dr. Barbara Kane and Dr. Evelyn Shukin are members of the Constitution and Bylaw Committee; Dr. Jean Hlady and Dr. Christine Loock are members of the Child Care Committee; Dr. Kathleen Carter and Dr. Bluma Tischler are members of the Committee of Developmental Handicaps; Dr. Caroline Terry and Dr. Susan Mann are members of the Environmental Committee; Dr. Martha Donnelly, Dr. B.

Lynn Beattie, and Dr. Janet Martin are members of the Geriatric Committee; Dr. Lysbeth McCrone is a member of the Native Health Committee; Dr. Barbara MacLeod is a member of the Nutrition Committee. The Joint Committee on Accreditation for Diagnostic Service has Dr. Ann Worth as Chair of the sub-committee Accreditation for Medical Imagining, and also on sub-committee Accreditation for Clinical Labs. The Cancer Committee has Dr. Linda Vickers and Dr. Linda Warren as members. Other women doctors on committees include Dr. Anne (Patty) Vogel on the Convention Committee; Insurance Committee has Dr. Shirley Reimer as a member; Patterns of Practice Committee has Dr. Denise Werker (FMWC) as a member.

Dr. Barbara Kane, Vancouver #3 District Delegate, and President Dr. Hedy Fry are the only two women on the BCMA Board.

Dr. Holly Stevens of the Section of Otolaryngology is the Canadian Otolaryngology Society representative for British Columbia.

Dr. Kwandwo O. Asante, a pediatrician in Terrace, B.C. writes about Fetal Alcohol Syndrome. From 15 years of experience in northwest of B.C. and the Yukon, he estimates 25 to 46 per 1,000 children are handicapped from the mother imbibing alcohol during pregnancy. The prevalence is estimated at two in 1,000 live births in British Columbia. More than $500,000 has this far been allocated over a three-year period to fund the Pregnancy Outcome Program (POP).

British Columbia's first mammography centre opened in 1988 and during the first nine months of operation discovered 29 cases of previously undetected cancer of the breast.

BCMA won an award chosen by the provincial Ministry of Environment in recognition of outstanding achievement in the protection and enhancement of the B.C. environment. President-elect Dr. Hedy Fry and Environmental Health Committee Chair Dr. Ian Gummeson recently accepted the award on behalf of the association at a special ceremony at Government House.

July, 1990 For the *Journal* Dr. Gordon Fahrni writes "Reflections on the Canadian Medical Association."

Dr. Hedy Fry is now the President of BCMA, the second woman to become President. The first was Dr. Ethlyn Trapp in 1946–47. In her first speech as President, Dr. Fry spoke of "the fruitless engagement in fee negotiation with the government."

The new Dean of Medicine, UBC is Dr. Martin Hollenberg, formerly associate Dean of Research in the Faculty of Medicine at the University of Toronto.

Council on Health Promotion: Dr. Kathleen Cadenhead, Chair Nutrition Committee, writes on low calorie liquid diets. She states, "There is no evidence these diets improve weight loss maintenance. Their use is not generally recommended."

August, 1990 Interview with President Dr. Hedy Fry, for the *Journal*.

A review of a widely read publication article with a bias against physicians: "Second Opinion" gets a critical analysis from Dr. Marcia Johnson. She is a resident in Community Medicine program at UBC.

Chris Lovelace is now Acting Deputy Minister of Health in British Columbia.

September, 1990: Several articles on Psychiatry. Dr. Shaila Misri, Dr. Diane Best, and Dr. Victoria Harris write on: "Referral Patterns in a Psychosomatic Obs/Gyn Clinic." Dr. Misri is clinical associate professor in the Department of Obstetrics and Gynecology, and in the Department of Psychiatry at UBC. Dr. Fast is clinical assistant professor in the Department of Psychiatry a UBC, and Dr. Harris is an intern.

Dr. Angus Rae was the Vancouver Medical Association Osler Lecturer for 1990. His topic: "Osler's Nightmare: The Rise and Fall of Bedside Medicine." Dr. Vivien Basco and Dr. Francis Ho were the Primus Inter Pares award winners at the 69th Annual Osler Dinner.

The number of Aids patients in British Columbia is 766 as of June, 1990. Of this number, 689 are homosexual.

October, 1990 In the Personal View Column Dr. Denise Werker writes an excellent letter in response to Dr. Gutowski's comments in the *Journal* of August, 1990, who admits that statements such as FMWC's on abortion always intrigue him.

Bill C-43 discussions about payment for abortions continue.

November, 1990 New President of the Federation of Medical Women of Canada is Dr. Mary Donlevy. She was President of the B.C. Branch FMWC in 1987–88. Dr. Donlevy, previously a Registered Nurse, currently is a family physician and mother of two small children.

Dr. Barbara Copping has attained the NDP nomination for her riding. She practises at the Student Health Services, BCIT.

December, 1990 There were six articles in the *Journal* on Congenital Craniofacial Deformities. Jean Carruthers writes on "Craniofacial Dyostosis," "Hyperteleorism," and "Strabismus." Dr. Carruthers is a Clinical Professor in the Department of Ophthalmology UBC and ophthalmology consultant to the craniofacial team at B.C. Children's Hospital.

Dr. Margo Fluker writes about "New Reproductive Techniques." Dr. Fluker is a Professor in the Department of Obstetrics and Gynecology UBC and presented this paper at the Annual Meeting of BCMA in June.

A Royal Commission on Health Care has been appointed in British Columbia. The five-member Commission is chaired by Mr. Justice C. Seaton. Members are Marguerite Ford, former alderwoman Vancouver City Council 1976–86; Dr. Robert Evans, a health research scientist UBC; Dr. Ken J. Fyke who has been previous President of the Greater Victoria Hospital Society; David Sinclair, a senior partner in accounting firm Coopers and Lybrand; Dr. William Weber, former Dean of Medicine, UBC.

President of BCMA Dr. Hedy Fry commenting on the Royal Commission on Health Care in B.C. states: "Why don't they ask the doctors?"

The B.C. Branch FMWC President Dr. Rozmin Kamani for 1990–1991; the Past President is Dr. Jean Swenerton; President-elect is Dr. Peggy Ross; Treasurer is Dr. Patricia Warshawski. Dr. Chris Hill, Ottawa, the first female urologist in Canada, was speaker at the FMWC B.C. Branch Annual Meeting. Dr. Elspeth McDougall is the first female urologist in western Canada, and Dr. Lynn Stothers is a urology resident.

January, 1991 Three articles on penicillin-resistent gonorrhea, an emerging epidemic.

In the Personal View column of the *Journal* Dr. Don Farquhar asks: "Where are the women on the BCMA Board of Directors?" There are only two female faces on the BCMA Board. The Editor Dr. W.A. Dodd replies: "The number of women on the Board is a direct reflection of women physicians' interest or lack of interest in Board membership."

One of the District #3 Delegates is Dr. Janet Martine.

UBC awarded a WCB research grant to Dr. Moira Yeung of the Respiratory Disease Research Unit of the UBC Department of Medicine. She receives the grant for four years to investigate the exposure to chlorine gas on workers in pulp mills, and to continue her investigation of red cedar dust as contributing to occupational asthma.

There are nearly 7,000 practising physicians in the province, compared to 3,500 in 1972.

February, 1991 The *Journal* has five articles on Sinusitis, including one by Dr. Holly Stevens on "Chronic Sinusitis." She is the Head of Otolaryngology at the University Hospital, Shaughnessy Site.

Dr. Elizabeth Whynot reviewed a book: *Trauma in Our Midst —A Study of Child Sexual Abuse in Surrey*, by Mr. Robert Kissner. Dr. Whynot is Assistant Professor in the Department of Family Practice UBC and co-director of the Sexual Assault Service, and also Medical Officer at the Vancouver Health Department, North Unit.

March, 1991 Since 1985 when it was found that some growth hormone is contaminated with Creutzfeldt-Jakob disease, there are now 10 such cases worldwide.

Dr. Christine Loock of the Child Care Committee, Council on Health Promotion writes, "Are We Disease Professionals, Not Health Professionals?"

A MRI Scanner has been approved for Children's Hospital.

April, 1991 Excellent articles for the *Journal*: "Stressful Issues for Physicians and Their Families" by Dr. Michael Myers, "Women Physicians and Their Families" by Dr. Carol Herbert, "The Foreign Medical Graduate" by Dr. Shaila Misri, and "Doctors and Psychiatric Illness" by Dr. Kristin Sivertz.

Dr. Hedy Fry states that "After 22 months of frustrating negotiations a barely acceptable compromise fee-for-service agreement was made."

With Bill Vander Zalm's departure as Premier of British Columbia, Rita Johnston is now Premier. Dr. John Jansen is Minister of Health.

May, 1991 An article by Dr. Jean Carruthers and Dr. Ross Kennedy on: "Botulisum Toxin in Treatment of Eye Disorders." Dr. Carruthers is Clinical Professor and Dr. Kennedy is Clinical Assistant Professor in the Department of Ophthalmology UBC.

Dr. Patricia Baird is the Vice President of the Canadian Institute of Advanced Research (CIAR). Dr. Baird is the 1991 VMA Osler Lecturer and has chosen the topic: "Changes in Society, Changes in Technology: A Duel Challenge."

Dr. Hedy Fry in the Comment column, *BCMJ* writes: "Time to take care of ourselves," and quotes from Dr. Kirsten Emmott's poem "The Naked Physician."

> We are as kind as we knew how.
> This was not enough. There was death
> now and then, and considerable pain
> for the patients. We tried to care about
> them. Nobody cared about us, not
> even ourselves.

June, 1991 There are six articles on "Sleep Disorders" in the June *Journal*.

Dr. Josephine Mallek is the President of the Vancouver Medical Association.

July, 1991 The Armorial Bearings of the British Columbia Medical Association, Quaerite-semper-veritatem, are on the cover of the July *Journal*.

Barbara Foxwell MB, BS, writes on "Percutaneous Discectomy." She is assistant director of the Rehabilitation Centre of WCB of British Columbia.

Canadian infant mortality is 7.3 per thousand, the fifth in the world.

Dr. Mary Donlevy of Vancouver is elected to the Council of the College of Physicians and Surgeons of British Columbia.

Dr. Patricia Rebbeck heads the sexual misconduct committee. B.C. is the third after Alberta and Ontario to undertake review of sexual misconduct by physicians.

The pamphlet in the BCMA April *Journal* advertising Elizabeth Bagshaw Women's Clinic providing abortion services upset some doctors.

New President of the Council of the College of Physicians and Surgeons of British Columbia is Dr. Patricia Rebbeck, who has been a member of the Council of the College since 1985. She graduated in Medicine from Edinburgh and obtained a FRCSC in 1967. She is Associate Professor in the Faculty of Medicine, UBC and is on the active staff of the University Hospital, UBC Site and St. Vincent's Hospital. She is Consultant in General Surgery to the B.C. Cancer Control Agency where her area is breast cancer, and is the first female General Surgeon in British Columbia.

Dr. Elizabeth Patriarche was presented with the BCMA Medal of Service by Dr. Hedy Fry. Dr. Carole Guzman of Ottawa is President-Elect of Canadian Medical Association 1991.

At the BCMA Annual Meeting in Kamloops, Dr. Gur Singh becomes the BCMA President.

Dr. Joan Ford was awarded the David Bachop Gold Medal at the Annual Meeting. (She was also named a member of the Order of Canada in 1991.)

In the Annual Reports new names on committees include: Dr. Janet Martini, the Geriatric Committee, also a member of the Board of BCMA; Dr. Janet Kusler a member of the Section of Psychiatry and the Committee of Physician Support Program; Dr. Frances Rosenburg a member of the division of Chemistry and the Section of Laboratory Medicine; Dr. Kirsten Emmott a member of the Section of General Practice.

Dr. Peggy Ross is the new President of the B.C. Branch FMWC.

Dr. Frances Rosenburg is the Editor of the *Newsletter* of the Federation of Medical Women of Canada.

August, 1991 Bruce Strachan is the new Health Minister of British Columbia.

The August *Journal* has several articles on Breast Cancer including one on "Screening Mammography Program" by Dr. Linda Warren Burhenne. She is the executive director of the Screening Mammography Program of B.C.

Another article "Management of in Situ Breast Cancer" by Dr. Ivo Olivotto, Dr. Robert Baird, Dr. Dorothy Harrison, and Dr. Ann Worth.

September, 1991 An article "Early Breast Cancer: Breast Conservation" by Dr. Vivien Basco, who is a Clinical Professor, Department of Surgery UBC, a radiation oncologist, and past chair of the Breast Tumor Group at BCCA.

Dr. Patricia Rebbeck and Dr. Graham Clay write on: "Surgical Approach to Early Breast Cancer."

Dr. Kathleen Cadenhead *et al* write: "Is meat Obsolete? Risks and Benefits of Vegetarian Diets."

The College Library moves to 8th and Hemlock.

October, 1991 Article "Osteoporosis and Arthritis" by A. Caroline Patterson MD, MRCP, FRCPC, FRCP Rheum. and John Wade MD, FRCPC, FPCP Rheum.

Dr. Carol Herbert writes: "70% of UBC Family Practice graduates who completed training in the Community Based Residency Training Project since 1982 are practising in small communities or are taking further training for rural practice."

First article on "Chronic Fatigue Syndrome" by H. Grant Stiver MD, FRCPC, and Jerry J.Vortel MD, FRCPC, noted in the *BCMJ*.

November, 1991 More medical articles appearing in the *Journal* of BCMA. In the November *Journal* there were nine, four by women physicians. "Recurrent Pregnancy Loss; Habitual Abortion: An Overview" by Mary D. Stephenson MD and Timothy Rowe MD; "Significance of Luteal Phase Defects" by Margo Fluker MD; "Detection and Management of Anti-Phospholipid Antibodies in Pregnancy" by Penny Ballem MD; "Psychological Response" by Shaila Misri MD.

At the Canadian Medical Association meeting the B.C. delegates were active participants with interesting exchanges during the meetings of the Council on Health Promotion, Aboriginal Land Claims, Special Funding for Native Students, and Funding for Drug and Alcohol Treatment Centres.

December, 1991 Obituaries of Dr. Robert Langston and Dr. Kathleen Langston. Dr. Kay Langston died 24 days before her husband.

January, 1992 The front cover of the *Journal* has a picture of the most senior member of BCMA, Dr. Gordon Fahrni, receiving a gift of a cedar talking stick from BCMA. The talking stick was carved by Kwakiutl artist Bill Wilson.

Elizabeth Cull is now the Minister of Health.

The Royal Commission on Health Care presented 650 recommendations, one of which is Regional Health Councils.

The *Journal* Editorial by Dr. A.J. McMahon commented on other recommendations which included a program to limit the number of physicians practising in British Columbia; also that contractural arrangements will be promoted as an option to fee-for-service.

Health Conference 1991 attracts 2,000.

February, 1992 Theme Issue: "Breast Feeding." Guest Editorial: "Managing Common Problems" by Dr. Verity H. Livingstone, Medical Director of Vancouver Breastfeeding Centre and Associate Professor UBC Department of Family Practice.

An article "Virus Transmission in Breast Milk: Practical Implications" by Dr. Anne Junker.

"Physician Sexual Misconduct" pamphlet written by Barbara Fisher, Legal Consultant, and Dr. Mary Donlevy, co-chair of the College of Physicians and Surgeons of B.C. Committee on Physician Sexual Misconduct. The pamphlet will be sent to all doctors in B.C. on request.

March, 1992 Dr. Shaila Misri and Dr. Kristin Sivertz wrote on "Postpartum Depression and Affective Disorder: Is there a Difference?"

An article: "The Impact on Patients of Diversion from Grace Hospital in May and June, 1989" by Dr. Elizabeth Vreede-Brown and Faith Gagnon BSc.

For the Council on Health Promotion, the chair of the Geriatrics Committee, Dr. Martha Donnelly, wrote on "Health Promotion with the Frail Elderly."

April, 1992 Theme of the April *Journal*: "The Management of the Multi-Problem Mentally Disordered Person." There were five articles on the subject for the *Journal*.

In the Personal View column: Dr. Mary Wonder of Nanaimo, B.C. wrote a letter "In Defence of Homeopathy."

May, 1992   In Vancouver the Federation of Medical Women of Canada had a special session May 9, 1992, hosted by the B.C. Branch and chaired by the FMWC President, Dr. May Cohen. There were five local presentations: "Visions for Women's Health in the '90s," by Dr. Penny Ballem, Medical Director of the University Hospital Women's Centre; "Coronary Heart Disease in Women," by Dr. Doris Kavanagh-Gray; "The Older Woman Patient—Issues in Geriatric Care," by Dr. Lynn Beattie; "What's New in Ultrasound, Breast Exam, Women and HIV, and Contraception?" by Drs. Paula Gordon, Elizabeth Whynot, and Dorothy Shaw; and "Newborn Screening and Early Discharge," by Dr. Margaret Norman, Director of Newborn Screening.

Drs. Shaila Misri, Victoria Harris, Diane Fast, Carolyn Ferris, and Marion Warrington RN write on: "Late Luteal Phase Dysphoric Disorder and Concurrent Psychiatric Illnesses," for the Council on Health Promotion: "The Medium is the Message: Changing Children at Risk into Children of Promise" by Dr. Joan Fraser and Dr. Zita Mary Rutkanus, members of the BCMA Child and Adolescent Committee.

June, 1992   Ophthalmology update: "Retinoblastoma" by Dr. J. Rootman and Dr. Jean Carruthers. (The incidence of Retinoblastoma has doubled in the last 50 years owing to an increase in gene pool and mutation rate.)

Council on Health Promotion: B.C. Autism Initiative: "Can functional assessment replace medical diagnostic evaluation?" by Dr. Helena Ho, of the Committee on Development Handicaps. Autism is relatively rare, 600–800 people in B.C., or 4 to 5 in 10,000 population.

Dr. Steve Hardwicke is BCMA President, 1992–1993.

July, 1992   Manitoba, Quebec, and New Brunswick have eliminated mandatory retirement in all occupations, but 65 years remains the retirement age for B.C., Saskatchewan, Ontario, Nova Scotia, and Prince Edward Island.

At the BCMA Annual Meeting June 4–6 at Whistler, Drs. Phil Ashmore, Robin Bell-Irving, Fred Ceresney, Joan Ford, John D. Hamilton, J. War-ren Irvine, and Raymond LeHuquet were awarded Senior Membership by the Canadian Medical Association. Dr. Carol Guzman, President of the Canadian Medical Association, presented the awards.

Dr. Diane Thompson received the David Bachop Silver Medal.

Dr. Janet Martini, as a District #3 (Vancouver) delegate is on the BCMA Board, the only woman other than Dr. Hedy Fry, the Past President.

August, 1992   Guest Editorial for the Theme Issue: "Management of Intersex," by Dr. Barbara McGillivray of the Department of Genetics.

Another article "Psychosexual Considerations" by Dr. George Szasz and Dr. Stacy Elliott. Four other articles discuss the problem.

Dr. Patricia Baird has been awarded the Order of British Columbia for her remarkable contribution to the field of Research.

September, 1992   An article on "Caesarean Section Rates in Primagravidas in British Columbia in 1988" by Mary Ellen Thompson, PhD, of the Research and Evaluation Branch of the B.C. Ministry of Health. The rate in 1988 was 22% of primagravidas.

In Memorium: Obituary of Dr. Betty Poland, was written by Dr. Fred Bryans.

October, 1992   There were seven articles for the *Journal* on Asthma. Dr. Moira Chan Yeung writes on "Increasing Morbidity and Mortality."

Dr. Judith Hall and Dr. Margot Van Allen, UBC Faculty of Medicine, are among the country's first group of 12 medical geneticists certified by the Royal College of Canada. Dr. Judith Hall is head of the Department of Pediatrics and Dr. Margot Van Allen is Clinical Associate Professor in the Department of Medical Genetics at UBC.

November, 1992   The article on Caesarean Section Rates in B.C. in the September *Journal* resulted in criticism from some doctors. Dr. Kirsten Emmott writes that in her own survey with Dr. K.F. King, the rate at Grace Hospital was 78% primipara, and 30% had no labour trial.

December, 1992   *Journal* Articles on Migraine, Hepatitis, and Chronic Leukemia.

Physicians Sexual Misconduct Report is now available.

December *Journal* had the first advertisement of Proscar for prostatic hyperplasia.

Dr. Anne Priestman is the head of the Professional Association of Residents and Interns of British Columbia (PARI-B.C.) Education Committee.

Dr. Peter Jepson-Young bursary has been donated for the Dr. Peter AIDS Foundation.

Dr. Frances Wong has been appointed head, Department of Radiation Oncology, BCCA Surrey Clinic, when the clinic opens in the spring of 1995.

January, 1993 A *Journal* Article "Tamoxifen: New Indications for an Old Drug?" by Cicely Bryce MD, FRCPC, Urve Kuusk MD, FRCSC, FACS, and Ivo A. Olivotto MD, FRCPC. Dr. Bryce is a medical oncologist at the BCCA, Vancouver Clinic. She is a Clinical Instructor in the Department of Medicine UBC. Dr. Kuusk is a general surgeon, University Hospital, Shaughnessy Site, Clinical Assistant Professor in the Department of Surgery UBC, and the principal investigator of the Breast Cancer Prevention Trial in B.C. Dr. Olivotto is a radiation oncologist, chairman of the Breast Tumor Group at BCCA, Vancouver Clinic, and Clinical Associate Professor in the Department of Surgery UBC.

Another article: "Hemochromatosis" by Stephanie G. Ensworth MD, FRCPC, et al. Dr. Ensworth is a clinical assistant Professor, Division of Internal Medicine and Pharmacology, Department of Medicine UBC.

Dr. Patricia Rebbeck wrote an editorial on "The Pleasures of Practice."

February, 1993 *Journal* article "Inflammatory Bowel Disease: Epidemiology" by Hanna Binder MD, FRCPC and Frank Anderson MD, FRCPC. Dr. Binder is a Fellow in gastroenterology UBC. Dr. Anderson is Associate Professor Department of Medicine UBC and Head Division of Gastroenterology, Vancouver General Hospital.

From the B.C. Centre for Disease Control, Marcia Johnson MD, MHSc, and Alison Bell MD, CM, MHSc, FRCPC wrote on "British Columbia's Hepatitis B Immunization Program." Dr. Johnson is the Federal Field Epidemiologist with the B.C. Centre. Dr. Bell is the Centre's Acting Director.

B.C. College of Family Physicians has as President, Dr. John Edworthy; Honourary Secretary, Dr. Joanna Bates; and member at large Dr. Darlene Hammell of Victoria.

March, 1993 In the College Report: On July 1, 1993, a two-year post-graduate training requirement to obtain a licence to practise medicine in British Columbia will begin.

April, 1993 Dr. Margaret McGregor wrote a letter on "Depression Concerns."

Dr. Debbie Carlow wrote a letter on "Sports Medicine not a luxury medicine or elitist."

Shaughnessy Hospital is to be closed in September, 1993, with many opposed to this move by the government. The announcement has taken professional perceptions of the current government to a new low.

May, 1993 *Journal* article "Management of Ectopic Pregnancy" by Timothy Rowe MB, FRCPC, and Sara Fisher MD. Dr. Rowe is Associate Professor, Division of Infertility and Reproductive Endocrinology, Department of Obstetrics and Gynecology UBC. Dr. Fisher is a Resident in the Department of Obstetrics and Gynecology UBC.

At the Vancouver Medical Association 72nd Annual Osler Dinner, Dr. W. Allan Dodd and Dr. Josephine Mallek were chosen for Primus Inter Pares awards.

Dr. Graham Fraser was the Osler Lecturer. His topic, "Osler and the Ward."

June, 1993 Article: "Child Sexual Abuse," by Jean Hlady MD, FRCPC, and E. Hunter MSW. Dr. Hlady is Director of the Child Protection Service Unit at Children's Hospital. E. Hunter is a Social Worker at Children's Hospital.

In the Council on Health Promotion report Dr. Hedy Fry writes: "NDP Ideology Ignores Practicality."

Walk-In Clinics begin in Vancouver.

July, 1993 Theme Issue: Cystic Fibrosis. Seven articles on this topic including "Lung Transplantation in Cystic Fibrosis," by Edina M. Nakielna MB, ChB, MRCP(UK), FRCPC and Dr. Guy Fradet MD, FRCSC. Dr. Nakielna is Clinical Associate Professor, Department of Medicine UBC, and Director of Adult Cystic Fibrosis Clinic, University Hospital, Shaughnessy Site. Dr. Fradet is Assistant Professor in the Division of Cardiovascular and Thoracic Surgery UBC and Vancouver General Hospital.

Article: "Multidisciplinary Care of the Cystic Fibrosis Patient" by Janine O'Kane MB, BS, FRCPC, et al. Dr. O'Kane is Clinical Associate Professor, Department of Psychiatry UBC.

Across Canada, a two-year post-graduate clinical requirement for licensing is in place, with a two-stage LMCC exam.

The College of Physicians and Surgeons of B.C. has decided to publish its own quarterly bulletin and will no longer have a College page in the *BCMJ*.

A British Columbia medical couple is honoured. Drs. Don and Sharon Blacklock who practise family medicine together in Comox have been chosen by the College of Family Physicians of Canada as the winners of the annual Family Physician of the Year Award. This is the first time two people have been selected.

Unionization issue of doctors was the popular debate at the 1993 BCMA Annual Meeting in June at Harrison Hot Springs Hotel.

New President of BCMA is Dr. Arun Garg.

Dr. Hedy Fry was given a sculpture by the members of the Council on Health Promotion in recognition of her years of dedication to the Council.

The David Bachop Silver Medal was presented to Dr. Arja Elisabet Moreau at the BCMA Annual Meeting.

August, 1993 Article on "Home Mechanical Ventilation in Adults" by Kathleen Ferguson MD, FRCPC and Pearce Wilcox MD, FRCPC. Dr. Ferguson is a Canadian Lung Association research Fellow at University Hospital UBC. Dr. Wilcox is an Associate Professor of Medicine UBC and a respirologist at University Hospital UBC.

Dr. Patricia Rebbeck was honoured as a Woman of Distinction by the YWCA.

Dr. Vivien Basco was chosen to be the BCMA Terry Fox Lecturer at the College of Physicians and Surgeons AGM on September 13, 1993.

Dr. April Sanders is a delegate to BCMA for District #3.

September, 1993 Theme Issue: Menopause. *Journal* articles numbered six. Margo Fluker MD, FRCSC wrote on: "Perimenopausal Attitudes: A Self-fulfilling Prophecy." Dr. Fluker is an Assistant Professor in the Division of Reproductive Endocrinology, Department of Obstetrics and Gynecology, UBC.

Jerilynn Prior MD, FRCPC, and John D. Wark MB, BS, PhD, FRACP, wrote on: "Osteoporosis After Menopause: An Update." Dr. Prior is Associate Professor of Endocrinology and Metabolism UBC and Vancouver General Hospital. Dr. Wark is Associate Professor of Endocrinology and Metabolism at the University of Melbourne and the Royal Melbourne Hospital, Melbourne, Australia. Dr. Wark was Visiting Professor at UBC in 1992.

In the Personal View column, Dr. Mary Winder of Nanaimo, B.C. wrote "Right to Practise." She is studying homeopathic medicine and wishes to use homeopathy in her practice.

BCMA petitions the Government to prohibit handguns.

October, 1993 In the *Journal* there were three articles on: "Post-traumatic Stress Disorder in Victims of Motor Vehicle Accidents."

Dr. Wendy White, et al, wrote on "Sporadic Typhus in British Columbia." Dr. White is with the Canadian Forces Hospital in Esquimalt, B.C.

Dr. Hedy Fry is the Liberal candidate for Vancouver Centre.

November, 1993 Theme Issue: Organ Transplantation. There were seven articles on this subject including: "Heart Transplantation" by Virginia Gudas MD, FRCSC, Donald Ricci MD, FRCPC, and Guy Fradet MD, FRCSC; "Lung Transplantation" by Virginia Gudas MD, FRCSC, Bill Nelems MD, FRCSC, David N. Ostrow MD, FRCPC, Guy Fradet MD, FRCSC, and Sue Howard RN.

Council on Health Promotion article "Beating Occupational Stress" by Janet H. Schechter MD, FRCPC, Chair of the Occupational Health Committee.

In the Personal View column Drs. Henry and Julia Van Norden write "Evanescent Extras."

Dr. W. Allan Dodd is retiring from the *BCMJ* editorship. The new editor is Dr. J.A. Wilson.

Dr. Vivien Basco, chosen to be the BCMA's Terry Fox lecturer, had as her topic for the lecture "Somewhere the Hurting Must Stop," a sentence written by Terry Fox. Dr. Basco presented her lecture at the Annual General Meeting of the B.C. College of Physicians and Surgeons, September 13, 1993.

December, 1993   Article on "New Reproductive Technologies in British Columbia" by Margo Fluker MD, FRCSC and Basil Ho Yuen MB, ChB, FRCSC. Dr. Fluker is Assistant Professor in the Division of Reproductive Endocrinology in the Department of Obstetrics and Gynecology UBC. Dr. Ho Yuen is Professor in the Division of Reproductive Endocrinology, Department of Obstetrics and Gynecology UBC.

Dr. Shirley M. Baker Thomas has retired as a Neurologist and is now enrolled in the Law Faculty at University of British Columbia.

Shaughnessy Hospital is now closed.

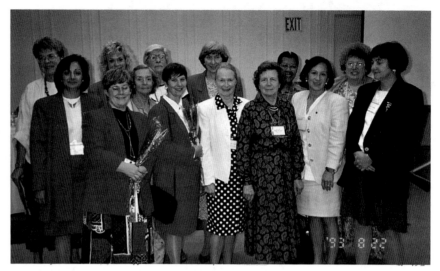

The B.C. members of the FMWC at the annual meeting of FMWC in Calgary in 1993. Front row: Dr. Rozmin Kamani, Dr. Shelley Ross, Dr. Magda Laszlo, Dr. Jean Swenerton, Dr. Eileen Cambon, Dr. Frances Forrest-Richards, Dr. Lorna Sent, Dr. Dorothy Woodhouse. Back row: unidentified, Dr. April Sanders, Dr. Lois Mckenzie-Sawers, Dr. Beverley Tamboline, Dr. Mary Trott, Marion Hutt

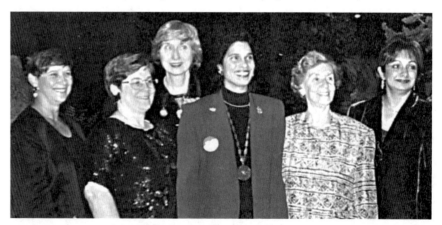

Canadian contingent at AMWA Conference in Chicago. Left to right: Dr. Jean Swenerton, Dr. Shelley Ross, Dr. Beverley Tamboline, Dr. Mano Murty, Dr. Magdalene Laszlo, and Dr. Rozmin Kamani, all from B.C. except Mano Murty, president of FMWC 1997–1998

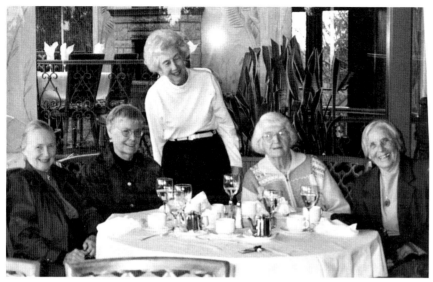

Dr. Eileen Cambon, Dr. Mavis Teasdale, Dr. Joan Ford, Dr. Agnes Weston, Dr. Laine Loo

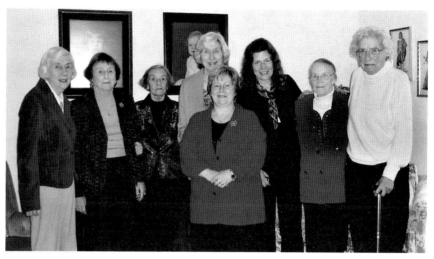

Dr. Joan Ford, Dr. Mary Hallowell, Dr. Magda Laszlo, Dr. Beverley Tamboline, Dr. Pat Warshawski, Dr. Eileen Cambon, Dr. Lois Mackenzie-Sawers. Front: Dr. Shelley Ross

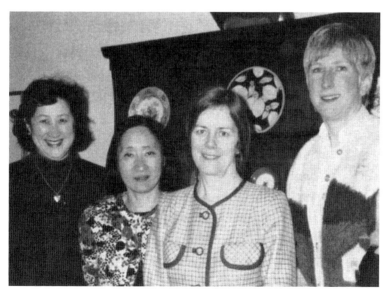

Dr. Charmaine Kim-Sing and Dr. Hiroko Watanabe, speakers, and Dr. Lynn Doyle (past-president, Vancouver Branch) and Dr. Heidi Oetter (both on BCMA executive)

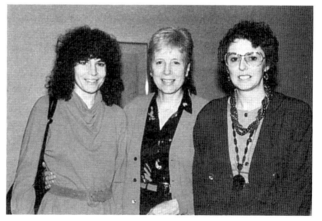

Dr. Patricia Warshawski (1980), FMWC secretary, Dr. Mary Donlevy, FMWC president, and Dr. Peggy Ross (1958), Vancouver Area Branch president, in 1991

APPENDIX 1:
WOMEN GRADUATES IN MEDICINE IN CANADA

1883 – 1895

	Medical College Kingston	Medical College Toronto	Other
1883	1	1 Toronto	
1884	3		
1885	2		
1886	2		
1887	3	2 Trinity	
1888	5	3 Trinity	
1889	1	2 Trinity	
		1 Toronto	
1890	6	4 Trinity	
		1 Toronto	
1891	3	4 Trinity	1 Bishop, England
1892	6	4 Trinity	1 Manitoba
		1 Toronto	
		1 Victoria	
		1 Ohio	
1893	2	4 Trinity	
1894		5 Trinity	1 Bishop
			1 Dalhousie
1895	1	9 Trinity	3 Bishop
		1 Toronto	1 Dalhousie

1896–1905

	Ontario Medical College For Women	Other
1896	3 Trinity	1 Bishop
	2 Toronto	1 Dalhousie
1897	4 Trinity	2 Bishop
	2 Toronto	1 Dalhousie
	1 Queen	
1898	6 Trinity	2 Bishop
	1 Toronto	1 Manitoba
	1 Western	
1899	8 Trinity	1 Dalhousie
1900	7 Trinity	2 Bishop
	2 Toronto	2 Dalhousie
1901	5 Trinity	1 Dalhousie
1902	6 Trinity	1 Dalhousie
1903	4 Trinity	2 Dalhousie
	1 Toronto	
1904	3 Trinity	4 Dalhousie
	1 Queen	
1905	2 Trinity	1 Dalhousie
	8 Toronto	

	Ontario Medical College For Women	Other
1906	9 Toronto	1 Dalhousie
1907	4 Toronto	
1908	5 Toronto	
1909	4 Toronto	
1910	3 Toronto	1 Dalhousie
1911	5 Toronto	2 Dalhousie
1912	2 Toronto	
1913	1 Toronto	1 Dalhousie
	1 Manitoba	
1914	3 Toronto	
1915	3 Toronto	1 Dalhousie
	2 Manitoba	
1916	4 Toronto	1 Dalhousie
	1 Queen	
1917	4 Toronto	
1918	5 Toronto	
1919	8 Toronto	1 Dalhousie
	1 Manitoba	
1920	4 Toronto	2 Dalhousie
	2 Manitoba	
1921	10 Toronto	1 Dalhousie
	1 Manitoba	
1922	14 Toronto	5 Dalhousie
	5 McGill	2 Manitoba
1923	13 Toronto	2 Dalhousie
	4 McGill	2 Manitoba

University	1924 to 1928	1929 to 1933	1934 to 1938	1939 to 1943	1944 to 1948	1949 to 1953	1954 to 1958	1959 to 1963	1964 to 1968	1969 to 1973	Total
Alberta	5	5	8	15	14	18	16	10	33	69	193
British Columbia							20	25	24	40	109
Calgary										3	3
Dalhousie		10	4	1	3	10	14	15	25	36	118
Laval				4	11	10	20	30	31	87	193
Manitoba	18	16	21	21	21	28	20	13	24	30	212
McGill	11	15	8	31	35	37	29	42	52	74	334
McMaster										7	7
Montreal					12	24	36	37	79	101	289
Newfoundland										4	4
Ottawa						4	10	25	36	50	125
Queen					2	16	18	20	30	52	138
Saskatchewan							9	13	22	20	64
Sherbrooke										33	33
Toronto	46	56	41	55	61	84	68	79	95	172	757
Western Ontario	2	13	11	13	14	18	18	20	31	56	196

(From the book *The Indomitable Lady Doctors*, by Carlotta Hacker, with permission from the publisher, Clarke, Irwin & Company Limited; pgs. 242–249.)

Registration Year	Total Number of Women Medical graduates registered in B.C.	Women Graduates of UBC Medical School registered in B.C.
1960	8	0
1961	19	3
1962	21	6
1963	12	3
1964	14	2
1965	11	2
1966	20	8
1967	27	5
1968	15	1
1969	27	1
1970	30	6
1971	31	2
1972	43	7
1973	42	6
1974	57	15
1975	44	10
1976	48	12
1977	62	10
1978	56	6
1979	53	12
1980	95	17
1981	69	15
1982	104	21
1983	113	28
1984	62	21
1985	107	37
1986	84	31
1987	96	35
1988	127	44
1989	118	32

The British Columbia Medical Act came into effect in 1886. Those physicians who registered before 1886 under the provisions of the Medical Ordinance of 1867 were now registered under the Act of 1886.

The registration fee was $10. The examinations were written and oral in eleven subjects:

Obstetrics
Diseases of Women and Children
Theory and Practice of Medicine
Pathology
Physiology
Chemistry
Materea Medica
Surgery
Clinical Medicine
Clinical Surgery
Medical Jurisprudence

By the year of 1887, 58 physicians were on the B.C. Register, and by 1893 when the first woman physician was registered, there were 116 registered in total.

From the yearly Medical Registers of British Columbia at the Library of the B.C. College of Physicians and Surgeons, the names of women physicians registered in B.C. are shown following each decade of biographical listings.

APPENDIX 4:
GLOSSARY

A

ACLS	Advanced Cardiac Life Support
ACTH	Adreno Corticotropic Hormone
ADDH	Attention Deficit Disorder with Hyperactivity
AGM	Annual General Meeting
ALS	Advanced Life Support, or Amyotrophic Lateral Sclerosis
APP	Associated Press of Palestine / Alenes Pharmaceutical Products
APSAC	American Professional Society on the Abuse of Children
ARP	American Registry of Pathology / Associate Reformed Presbyterian
ATLS	Advanced Trauma Life Support

B

BCCI	B.C. Cancer Institute
BCCH	B.C. Children's Hospital
BCG	Bacillus Calmette Guerin
BCIT	B.C. Institute of Technology
BCLC	B.C. Liquor Control Board / B.C. Lottery Corp.
BCLS	Basic Cardiac Life Support
BCLTS	Basic Life Trauma Support
BLTS / ACLS	Basic Life Trauma Support / Advanced Cardiac Life Support
BS	Bachelor of Science

C

CACC	Centre for Advanced Computing Communication
CAGS	Canadian Association of General Surgeons
CANTAB	University of Cambridge
CASC	Continuing Advisory Sub-Committee
CBC	Canadian Broadcasting Agency
CCA	Cancer Control Agency
CCABC	Cancer Control Agency of B.C.
CCFP	Canadian College of Family Practice
CCSA	Canadian Centre on Substance Abuse
CCU	Cardiac Care Unit

ChB	Bachelor of Surgery
CIAR	Clinical Institute of Advanced Research
CLEO	Consideration for Law, Ethics, and Organization of Health Care
CMAJ	Canadian Medical Association Journal
CPR	Cardio Pulmonary Resuscitation
CPS	College of Physicians and Surgeons
CRCPC	Certification by the Royal College of Physicians of Canada
CSGM	Canadian Society of Geriatric Medicine
CUP	Cambridge University Press

D

DCH	Diploma in Child Health
DMRT (London)	Dept. of Medical and Research Technology
DPH	Diploma in Public Health
DPM	Diploma in Psychological Medicine
DRCOG	Diploma of the Royal College of Obstetrics and Gynecology
DTM&H	Diploma in Tropical Medicine and Hygiene

E

ECT	Electroconvulsive Shock Therapy
EMAS	European Menopause and Andropause Society
ENT	Ear, Nose, and Throat

F

FAAP	Fellow of American Association of Pediatrics
FACC	Fellow of American College of Cardiology
FACP	Fellow of American College of Physicians
FAS	Fetal Alcohol Syndrome
FCCMG	Fellow of Canadian College of Medical Geneticists
FFA	Fellow of Faculty of Anesthesia
FMWC	Federation of Medical Women of Canada
FPCR	Foundation for Promotion of Cancer Research
FRCR	Fellow of the Royal College of Radiologists
FRCOG	Fellow of the Royal College of Obstetrics and Gynecology

FRCP	Fellow of the Royal College of Physicians
FRCPC	Fellow of the Royal College of Physicians of Canada
FRCSC	Fellow of the Royal College of Surgeons of Canada

G

GPA	Grade Point Average

I

IBCLC	International Board Certified Lactation Consultant
ICU	Intensive Care Unit
IND	International Nomenclature of Diseases (WHO)

L

LM	Licenced Midwife
LMCC	Licentiate of the Medical Council of Canada
LMRCP	Licentiate in Midwifery of the Royal College of Physicians
LRCP(L)	Licentiate of the Royal College of Physicians of London
LRCPS(I)	Licentiate of the Royal College of Physicians and Surgeons of Ireland
LRCS(Edin.)	Licentiate of the Royal College of Surgeons of Edinburgh

M

MA	Master of Arts
MAMBCh (MA, MB, ChB)	Bachelor of Medicine / Bachelor of Surgery (Edinburgh)
MASH	Mobile Army Surgical Hospital
MB & MB, BS	Bachelor of Medicine (other than Oxford) / Bachelor of Surgery
MDBS	Medical Doctor and Bachelor of Surgery
MDMS	Medical Doctor and Master of Surgery
MHSC	Master of Health Sciences
MRCGP	Member of Royal College of General Practitioners
MRCOG	Member of Royal College of Obstetrics and Gynecology (London)
MRCP	Member of the Royal College of Physicians of England
MRCS	Member of the Royal College of Surgeons of England
MRI	Magnetic Resonance Imaging
MWIA	Medical Women's International Association

N

NALS	Neonatal Advanced Life Support
NCIC	National Cancer Institute of Canada
NRC	National Research Council
NRP	Neonatal Resuscitation Program
NSAB	National Security Advisory Board (India)

P

PPD	Postpartum Depression
PSP	Physician Support Program

R

RCAF	Royal Canadian Air Force
RCP & SC	Royal College of Physicians and Surgeons of Canada

S

SIDS	Sudden Infant Death Syndrome
SMP of B.C.	Standard Medical Practice / Screening Mammography Program of B.C.

U

UIC	Unemployment Insurance Commission

V

VAD	Vascular Access Device
VSD	Ventricular-Septal Defect

BIBLIOGRAPHY

Barman, Jean, *The West Beyond the West: A History of British Columbia*, University of Toronto Press, 1991.

Bernazzani, Odette, Gold, Judith H., Lalinec-Michaud, Martine, *Pioneers All: Women Psychiatrists in Canada: A History*. Ottawa: Canadian Psychiatric Association, 1995.

Burrows, Bob, *Healing in the Wilderness: A History of the United Church Mission Hospitals*. Madeira Park, B.C: Harbour Publishing, 2004.

Converse, Cathy, *Mainstays: Women Who Shaped* BC. Victoria, B.C: Horsdal & Schubart, 1998.

Duffin, Jacalyn Mary, *History of Medicine: A Scandalously Short Introduction*. Toronto: University of Toronto Press, 1999; reprinted University of Toronto Press and Macmillan, 2000, 2001.

Ehrenreich, Barbara and English, Deirdre, *Witches, Midwives and Nurses—A History of Women Healers*. New York: The Feminist Press, 1973.

Hellstedt, Leona McGregor, *Women Physicians of the World: Autobiographies of Medical Pioneers*. Washington / London: Hemisphere Publishing Corporation, 1978.

Hill, Robert, *Paediatrics in B.C: A History, with Particular Emphasis on the UBC Academic Department*. Vancouver: Paediatric Department, UBC, 1997.

Hacker, Carlotta, *The Indomitable Lady Doctors*. Toronto: Clarke, Irwin, 1974

Jack, Donald, *Rogues, Rebels and Geniuses—the Story of Canadian Medicine*. Toronto: Doubleday Canada Limited, 1981.

Jensen, Vickie, *Saltwater Women at Work*. Vancouver: Douglas & McIntyre Ltd., 1995.

Lee, Eldon, *Scalpels and Buggywhips: Medical Pioneers of Central BC*. Surrey: Heritage House Publishing Company Ltd., 1997.

Leon, Vicki, *Uppity Women of Medieval Times*. New York: MJF Books Fine Communications, 1997.

MacDermot, H.E., *One Hundred Years of Medicine in Canada, 1867-1967*. Toronto: McClelland and Stewart, 1967.

MacEwan, Grant, *. . . and Mighty Women Too: Stories of Notable Western Canadian Women*. Saskatoon: Western Producer Prairie Books, 1975.

MacLeod, Enid Johnson, *Petticoat Doctors: The First Forty Years of Women in Medicine at Dalhousie University*. Nova Scotia: Pottersfield Press, 1990.

Murray, Florence J., *At the Foot of Dragon Hill*. New York: E. P. Dutton & Company, Inc. 1975.

Negodaeff-Tomsik, Margaret, *Honour Due—the Story of Lenora Howard King*. Ottawa: The Canadian Medical Association, 1999.

Waugh, Douglas, *Maudie of McGill : Dr. Maude Abbott and the Foundations of Heart Surgery*. Toronto: Hannah Institute & Dundum Press, 1992.

Acton, Janice et al., *Women at Work 1850-1930*. Toronto: The Women's Press, 1974.

Journals
British Columbia Medical Journals
Canadian Medical Association Journals
Medical Alumni News (Quarterly)

LIST OF PHOTOS

INDEX OF DOCTORS